A Lange Medical Book

W9-CEH-308

EMERGENCY MEDICINE ON CALL

Edited by

Samuel M. Keim, MD
Associate Professor and Residency Director
Department of Emergency Medicine
The University of Arizona College of Medicine
Tucson, Arizona

Series Editor
Leonard G. Gomella, MD, FACS
The Bernard W. Godwin, Jr., Professor
Chairman, Department of Urology
Jefferson Medical College
Thomas Jefferson University
Philadelphia, Pennsylvania

Lange Medical Books/McGraw-Hill
Medical Publishing Division

New York   Chicago   San Francisco   Lisbon   London
Madrid   Mexico City   Milan   New Delhi   San Juan
Seoul   Singapore   Sydney   Toronto

Emergency Medicine On Call

567890 DOC/DOC 09876
ISBN: 0-07-138879-6
ISSN: 1554-628X

Notice

Medicine is an ever-changing science. As new research and clinical experience broaden our knowledge, changes in treatment and drug therapy are required. The authors and the publisher of this work have checked with sources believed to be reliable in their efforts to provide information that is complete and generally in accord with the standards accepted at the time of publication. However, in view of the possibility of human error or changes in medical sciences, neither the authors nor the publisher nor any other party who has been involved in the preparation or publication of this work warrants that the information contained herein is in every respect accurate or complete, and they disclaim all responsibility for any errors or omissions or for the results obtained from use of the information contained in this work. Readers are encouraged to confirm the information contained herein with other sources. For example and in particular, readers are advised to check the product information sheet included in the package of each drug they plan to administer to be certain that the information contained in this work is accurate and that changes have not been made in the recommended dose or in the contraindications for administration. This recommendation is of particular importance in connection with the new or infrequently used drugs.

The book was set in Helvetica by Circle Graphics.
The editors were Janet Foltin, Janene Matragrano Oransky, and Regina Y. Brown.
The production supervisor was Philip Galea.
The index was prepared by Herr's Indexing Service.
The art manager was Charissa Baker.

RR Donnelley was printer and binder.

This book was printed on acid-free paper.

INTERNATIONAL EDITION ISBN 0-07-121972-2
Exclusive rights by The McGraw-Hill Companies, Inc., for manufacture and export. This book cannot be re-exported from the country to which it is consigned by McGraw-Hill. The International Edition is not available in North America.

Contents

Contributors

J. David Barry, MD
Professor
Department of Emergency Medicine
Division of Clinical Toxicology
University of California, San Diego
San Diego, California

Kathlene Bassett, MD
Assistant Professor
Department of Pediatrics
University of Utah School of Medicine
Salt Lake City, Utah

Mike Beeson, MD
Program Director
Department of Emergency Medicine
Summa Health System
Professor of Clinical Emergency Medicine
Northeastern Ohio University College of Medicine
Akron, Ohio

Burton Bentley, III, MD
Attending Physician
Department of Emergency Medicine
Northwest Medical Center
Tucson, Arizona

Howard A. Bessen, MD
Program Director, Residency Training Program
Department of Emergency Medicine
Harbor-UCLA Medical Center
Torrance, California

Louis Binder, MD
Associate Program Director and Director of Education
Department of Emergency Medicine
MetroHealth Medical Center Professor of Emergency Medicine
Case Western Reserve
Cleveland, Ohio

Diane M. Birnbaumer, MD, FACEP
Associate Program Director, Residency Training Program
Professor of Medicine
Department of Emergency Medicine
Harbor-UCLA Medical Center
Torrance, California

Paul A. Blackburn, DO
Director, Emergency Medicine Residency
Department of Emergency Medicine
Maricopa Medical Center
Phoenix, Arizona

Andra L. Blomkalns, MD
Assistant Professor and Associate Residency Director
Department of Emergency Medicine
University of Cincinnati
Cincinnati, Ohio

Ioliene B. Boenau, MD
Professor of Emergency Medicine
Department of Emergency Medicine
Eastern Virginia Medical School
Norfolk, Virginia

Michael Bohrn, MD
Associate Program Director, Emergency Medicine Residency
Clinical Assistant Professor
York Hospital/Penn State University
York, Pennsylvania

Robert Bolte, MD
Professor of Pediatrics
University of Utah School of Medicine
Division of Pediatric Emergency Medicine
Primary Children's Medical Center
Salt Lake City, Utah

Kristine L. Bott, MD
Chief Resident
Department of Emergency Medicine
Truman Medical Center
University of Missouri–Kansas City School of Medicine
Kansas City, Missouri

William J. Brady, MD, FACEP, FAAEM
Associate Professor of Emergency Medicine
Vice Chair and Residency Program Director
Department of Emergency Medicine
Clinical Associate Professor
Department of Internal Medicine
University of Virginia Health System
Charlottesville, Virginia

Kenny Bramwell, MD
Assistant Professor of Clinical Emergency Medicine
Department of Emergency Medicine
University of Arizona College of Medicine
Tucson, Arizona

Douglas Brunette, MD
Senior Associate Physician and Program Director
Hennepin County Medical Center
Department of Emergency Medicine
Associate Professor
University of Minnesota School of Medicine
Minneapolis, Minnesota

Jonathan L. Burstein, MD, FACEP
Medical Director
Emergency Preparedness and Response
Massachusetts Department of Public Health
Assistant Professor of Emergency Medicine
Harvard Medical School
Assistant Professor
Harvard School of Public Health
Boston, Massachusetts

Katherine Cassidy, MD
Clinical Assistant Professor of Emergency Medicine
Department of Emergency Medicine
Michigan State Kalamazoo Center for Medical Studies
Kalamazoo, Michigan

Lisa Chan, MD
Associate Professor of Clinical Emergency Medicine
Associate Residency Director
Department of Emergency Medicine
University of Arizona College of Medicine
Tucson, Arizona

Andrew Chang, MD
Assistant Clinical Professor
Department of Emergency Medicine
University of California, Irvine
Irvine, California

Michael Chansky, MD
Chairman, Department of Emergency Medicine
Cooper Hospital/University Medical Center
Camden, New Jersey

Jason Cillo, MD
Physician
Department of Emergency Medicine
Chippenham & Johnston-Willis Medical Center
Chippenham Campus
Richmond, Virginia

Richard Clark, MD
Professor, Department of Emergency Medicine
Medical Director, San Diego Division of the California Poison
Control System
Director, Division of Medical Toxicology
Director, Fellowship Program in Toxicology
San Diego, California

Samuel Coleman, MD
Resident, Internal Medicine Program
University of Pittsburgh Medical Center
Pittsburgh, Pennsylvania

Sarah Coleman, MD
Attending Physician
Department of Emergency Medicine
Sacred Heart Medical Center
Eugene, Oregon

Howard Corneli, MD, FAAP, FACEP
Professor of Pediatrics
University of Utah College of Medicine
Division of Emergency Medicine
Primary Children's Medical Center
Salt Lake City, Utah

Francis L. Counselman, MD, FACEP
Chairman and Program Director
Distinguished Professor of Emergency Medicine
Department of Emergency Medicine
Eastern Virginia Medical School
Emergency Physicians of Tidewater
Norfolk, Virginia

Tim Coury, MD
Attending Physician
Department of Emergency Medicine
Central Maine Medical Center
Lewiston, Maine

Brian Cullison, MD
Resident, Department of Emergency Medicine
Case Western Reserve University
MetroHealth Medical Center
Cleveland Clinic Foundation Emergency Medicine Residency
Cleveland, Ohio

Virgil Davis, MD
Attending Physician
Mad River Community Hospital
Arcata, California

Christopher Davison, MD
Resident
Department of Emergency Medicine
University of Pittsburgh School of Medicine
Pittsburgh, Pennsylvania

Peter DeBlieux, MD
Professor of Clinical Medicine
LSUHSC School of Medicine
Staff Physician, Pulmonary/Critical Care
Program Director, LSUHSC Emergency Medicine Residency
Director, LSUHSC Medical Student Skills Lab
New Orleans, Louisiana

Wyatt V. Decker, MD
Chair
Department of Emergency Medicine
Mayo Clinic and Mayo Medical School
Program Director, Emergency Medicine Residency
Mayo Graduate School of Medicine
Rochester, Minnesota

Ameet Deshmukh, MD
Attending Physician
Department of Emergency Medicine
St. Mary's Hospital
Blue Springs, Missouri

Travis Deuson, MD
Attending Physician
EMANON PA
Southwest Texas Methodist Medical Center
San Antonio, Texas

Jno Disch, MD
Resident
Department of Emergency Medicine
Case Western Reserve University
MetroHealth Medical Center
Cleveland Clinic Foundation Emergency Medicine Residency
Cleveland, Ohio

Ian Doten, MD
Staff Physician
Department of Emergency Medicine
Valley General Hospital
Monroe, Washington

Nanette C. Dudley, MD
Associate Professor of Pediatrics
University of Utah School of Medicine
Pediatric Emergency Medicine
Primary Children's Medical Center
Salt Lake City, Utah

Matthew Evenhouse, MD
Resident
Department of Emergency Medicine
MetroHealth Medical Center
Professor of Emergency Medicine
Case Western Reserve University
Cleveland, Ohio

Carol S. Federiuk, MD, PhD
Fellow, Sports Medicine
Jefferson Medical School
Thomas Jefferson University
Philadelphia, Pennsylvania

Trevor Fisher, MD, FACEP
Physician, Emergency Medicine
Legacy Meridian Park Hospital
Portland, Oregon

Kelly Anne Foley, MD, FACEP
Assistant Professor
Department of Emergency Medicine
Eastern Virginia Medical School
Norfolk, Virginia

Fun H. Fong, MD, FACEP
Assistant Professor
Emory–Adventis Medical Center
Director, Radiation Medicine
Oak Ridge Associated Universities
Medical Sciences Division
Smyrna, Georgia

Kim Friedman, MD
Resident
Department of Emergency Medicine
Cooper Hospital/University Medical Center
Camden, New Jersey

Ronald Furnival, MD
Associate Professor of Pediatrics
University of Utah School of Medicine
Pediatric Emergency Medicine
Primary Children's Medical Center
Salt Lake City, Utah

Gus M. Garmel, MD, FACEP, FAAEM
Stanford/Kaiser EM Residency Program
Medical Student Clerkship Director
Stanford University School of Medicine
Senior Emergency Physician
TPMG, Kaiser
Santa Clara, California

W. Brian Gibler, MD
Richard C. Levy Professor and Chairman
Department of Emergency Medicine
University of Cincinnati
Cincinnati, Ohio

Judd L. Glasser, MD
Resident
Department of Emergency Medicine UCSD Medical Center
San Diego, California

W. Shaun Gogarty, MD, FACEP
President
Southern Colorado Emergency Medical Associates
Pueblo, Colorado

Constance S. Greene, MD
Program Director
University of Chicago Emergency Medicine Residency
Associate Professor
Department of Emergency Medicine
Rush Medical College Cook County Medical Center
Chicago, Illinois

Carrie Gregory, MD
Emergency Medicine Physician
United States Airforce
Colorado Springs, Colorado

John Guisto, MD, FACEP
Associate Professor of Clinical Emergency Medicine
Medical Director, Emergency Services
Department of Emergency Medicine
University of Arizona College of Medicine
Tucson, Arizona

David Guss, MD, FACP, FACEP
Director
Department of Emergency Medicine
Professor of Medicine
Department of Emergency Medicine
UCSD Medical Center
San Diego, California

Greg Haugen, MD
Staff Physician
Department of Emergency Medicine
MeritCare Hospital
Fargo, North Dakota

Stephen R. Hayden, MD
Program Director, Emergency Medicine Residency
Associate Professor of Medicine
Department of Emergency Medicine
UCSD Medical Center
San Diego, California

Nathan Heaps, MD
Resident
Department of Emergency Medicine
Affiliated Residency in Emergency Medicine
University of Pittsburgh
Pittsburgh, Pennsylvania

Bruce Herman, MD
Associate Professor of Pediatrics
University of Utah School of Medicine
Primary Children's Medical Center
Salt Lake City, Utah

Robert Hockberger, MD
Chairman
Department of Emergency Medicine
Harbor-UCLA Medical Center
Torrance, California

Christopher Holstege, MD, FACEP
Director, Division of Medical Toxicology
Assistant Professor
Department of Emergency Medicine
University of Virginia School of Medicine
Charlottesville, Virginia

Debra Houry, MD, MPH
Assistant Professor of Emergency Medicine
Department of Emergency Medicine
Emory University School of Medicine
Associate Director
Center for Injury Control
Atlanta, Georgia

J. Stephen Huff, MD
Associate Professor of Emergency Medicine and Neurology
Department of Emergency Medicine
University of Virginia
Charlottesville, Virginia

Kenneth V. Iserson, MD, MBA
Professor of Emergency Medicine
Department of Emergency Medicine
Director, Arizona Bioethics Program
University of Arizona College of Medicine
Tucson, Arizona

Ken Jackimczyk, MD
Associate Chairman of Emergency Medicine
Department of Emergency Medicine
Maricopa Medical Center
Phoenix, Arizona

Geoffrey A. Jackman, MD
Assistant Professor of Pediatrics
University of Utah School of Medicine
Division of Pediatric Emergency Medicine
Primary Children's Medical Center
Salt Lake City, Utah

Gary Johnson, MD, FACEP
Associate Professor of Emergency Medicine
Vice Chairman for Clinical Operations
Department of Emergency Medicine
SUNY–Syracuse
Syracuse, New York

Melissa Johnson, MD
Resident
Department of Emergency Medicine
University of Arizona College of Medicine
Tucson, Arizona

Nicholas Jouriles, MD
Program Director
Emergency Medicine Residency
MetroHealth Medical Center
Cleveland Clinic Foundation
Associate Professor
Case Western Reserve University
Cleveland, Ohio

Howard Kadish, MD
Associate Professor of Pediatrics
University of Utah School of Medicine
Pediatric Emergency Medicine
Primary Children's Medical Center
Salt Lake City, Utah

William Kanich, MD, JD
Staff Physician
Department of Emergency Medicine
Charleston Emergency Services
Charleston, South Carolina
University of Virginia Health Sciences System
Charlottesville, Virginia

Paul S. Keim, PhD
Professor and Cowden Endowed Chair in Microbiology
Department of Biological Sciences
Northern Arizona University
Flagstaff, Arizona

Samuel M. Keim, MD
Associate Professor and Residency Director
Department of Emergency Medicine
University of Arizona College of Medicine
Tucson, Arizona

James Kempema, MD, FAAEM
Attending Physician, Brackenridge Hospital Emergency Center
Austin, Texas
Associate Medical Director, Critical Air Medicine
San Diego, California

Steven W. Kohler, MD
Physician, Emergency Medicine
Kaiser Foundation Hospital
San Diego, California

David Kramer, MD, FACEP
Program Director
Clinical Associate Professor
York Hospital/Penn State University
Clinical Associate Professor
Department of Emergency Medicine
Penn State University
York, Pennsylvania

Joseph LaMantia, MD
Program Director, Emergency Medicine
North Shore University Hospital
Manhasset, New York
Assistant Professor of Clinical Emergency Medicine
New York University School of Medicine
New York, New York

Shawna Langstaff, MD
Physician, Emergency Medicine
Penrose St. Francis Hospital
Colorado Springs, Colorado

Joseph Lauro, MD
Resident
Department of Emergency Medicine
Denver Health Medical Center
Denver, Colorado

David C. Lee, MD
Director of Research
Department of Emergency Medicine
North Shore University Hospital
Manhasset, New York

Evan Leibner, MD
Associate Program Director
Department of Emergency Medicine
Maricopa Medical Center
Phoenix, Arizona

Sion A. Levy, MD
Department of Emergency Medicine
LSUHSC School of Medicine
New Orleans, Louisiana

Ari M. Lipsky, MD
Resident
Department of Emergency Medicine
Harbor-UCLA Medical Center
Torrance, California

William B. Lober, MD
Acting Instructor, Division of Biomedical and Health Informatics
Department of Medical Education
Fellow, Department of Biological Structure
University of Washington School of Medicine
Seattle, Washington

Thomas Love, MD
Resident
Department of Emergency Medicine
Cooper Hospital/University Medical Center
Camden, New Jersey

Frank LoVeccio, DO
Medical Director
Department of Medical Toxicology
Good Samaritan Regional Medical Center
Attending Physician, Emergency Medicine
Maricopa Medical Center and Emergency Department Residency
Phoenix, Arizona

Boris Vladimir Lubavin, MD
Resident
Division of Emergency Medicine
University of California, Irvine
Irvine, California

Binh Ly, MD
Assistant Program Director, Emergency Medicine Residency
Division of Medical Toxicology
Assistant Clinical Professor
Department of Emergency Medicine
UCSD Medical Center
San Diego, California

Lori Lynch, MD
Chief Resident
Department of Emergency Medicine
Case Western Reserve University
MetroHealth Medical Center
Cleveland Clinic Foundation Emergency Medicine Residency
Cleveland, Ohio

K. Alexander Malone, MD
Resident
Department of Emergency Medicine
University of Arizona College of Medicine
Tucson, Arizona

Vince Markovchick, MD, FAAEM
Director, Emergency Medical Services
Professor of Surgery
Division of Emergency Medicine
Department of Surgery
Denver Health
University of Colorado
Denver, Colorado

Michael Martino, MD
Attending Physician
Department of Emergency Medicine
Saint Clair Memorial Hospital
Instructor of Emergency Medicine
Department of Emergency Medicine
University of Pittsburgh Medical Center
Pittsburgh, Pennsylvania

Harvey Meislin, MD, FACEP
Professor of Emergency Medicine
Head, Department of Emergency Medicine
Director, Arizona Emergency Medicine Research Center
University of Arizona Health Sciences Center
Tucson, Arizona

Gabrielle J. Melin, MD, PhD
Senior Associate Consultant and Instructor
Mayo Clinic
Rochester, Minnesota

Evan Minard, MD
Resident
Department of Emergency Medicine
Michigan State Kalamazoo Center for Medical Studies
Kalamazoo, Michigan

Scott Miner, MD
Division of Emergency Medicine
Department of Surgery
Denver Health
University of Colorado
Denver, Colorado

Eric Van Moorlehem, MD
Emergency Physician
Scottsdale Emergency Associates Ltd.
Scottsdale, Arizona

Jerry Moser, MD
Attending Physician
Department of Emergency Medicine
Northwest Tucson Emergency Physicians
Tucson, Arizona

Jay Mullen, MD
Attending Physician
Department of Emergency Medicine
Central Maine Medical Center
Medical Director, Four Winds Adventure Company
Lewiston, Maine

Doug Nelson, MD
Associate Professor of Pediatrics
University of Utah School of Medicine
Primary Children's Medical Center
Salt Lake City, Utah

Steve Offerman, MD
Professor of Emergency Medicine
Division of Clinical Toxicology
Department of Emergency Medicine
San Diego, California

David Overton, MD, FACEP
Director, Residency in Emergency Medicine
Professor
Department of Emergency Medicine
Michigan State Kalamazoo Center for Medical Studies
Kalamazoo, Michigan

Ryan Padgett, MD
Resident
Department of Emergency Medicine
University of Arizona College of Medicine
Tucson, Arizona

Kenneth Palm, MD
Resident
Department of Emergency Medicine
Mayo Clinic
Rochester, Minnesota

David Pawsat, DO
Attending Physician
Department of Emergency Medicine
Ingham Regional Medical Center
Michigan State University—Emergency Medicine Residency
Lansing, Michigan

Debra G. Perina, MD
Associate Professor
Department of Emergency Medicine
University of Virginia Health Sciences Systems
Charlottesville, Virginia

Jesse Pines, MD, MBA
Resident
Department of Emergency Medicine
University of Virginia School of Medicine
Charlottesville, Virginia

Paul Rega, MD, FACEP
Senior Medical Officer
Program Manager, Public Health/Medical Community
Center for Terrorism Preparedness
University of Findlay
Findlay, Ohio

Kevin Reilly, MD
Associate Professor of Clinical Emergency Medicine
Department of Emergency Medicine
Director, Medical Student Education
University of Arizona College of Medicine
Tucson, Arizona

Earl Reisdorff, MD
Attending Physician
Department of Emergency Medicine
Ingham Regional Medical Center
Michigan State University—Emergency Medicine Residency
Lansing, Michigan

Jared L. Richardson, MD
Department of Emergency Medicine
Program Director, Residency in Emergency Medicine
Truman Medical Centers
University of Missouri—Kansas City School of Medicine
Kansas City, Missouri

Lynn P. Roppolo, MD
Instructor of Emergency Medicine
University of Texas Southwestern Medical School
Division of Emergency Medicine
Dallas, Texas

Peter Rosen, MD
Associate Professor, Harvard University
Boston, Massachusetts
Visiting Professor, University of Arizona
Tucson, Arizona
Professor Emeritus, University of California San Diego
San Diego, California
Attending Emergency Physician, Beth Israel/Deaconess
Medical Center
Teaching Attending Physician, Massachusetts General Hospital
Boston, Massachusetts
Attending Emergency Physician, St. John's Hospital
Jackson Hole, Wyoming

Mike Rush, MD
Associate Professor
Department of Emergency Medicine
Assistant Program Director, Residency in Emergency Medicine
Truman Medical Centers
University of Missouri—Kansas City School of Medicine
Kansas City, Missouri

John Sakles, MD, FACEP, FAAEM
Assistant Professor of Clinical Emergency Medicine
Medical Director, AEMRC Paramedic Training Program
Medical Director, The Airway Site
Department of Emergency Medicine
University of Arizona College of Medicine
Tucson, Arizona

Joseph A. Salomone, III, MD, FAAEM
Associate Professor
Department of Emergency Medicine
Program Director, Residency in Emergency Medicine
Truman Medical Centers
University of Missouri—Kansas City School of Medicine
Kansas City, Missouri

Arthur B. Sanders, MD, MS
Professor of Emergency Medicine
Department of Emergency Medicine
University of Arizona College of Medicine
Tucson, Arizona

Raphael Santiago, MD
Fellow in Pediatric Emergency Medicine
University of Utah School of Medicine
Primary Children's Medical Center
Salt Lake City, Utah

James Sauto, MD
Resident
Department of Emergency Medicine
Case Western Reserve University
MetroHealth Medical Center
Cleveland Clinic Foundation Emergency Medicine Residency
Cleveland, Ohio

Aaron Schneir, MD
Assistant Clinical Professor
Department of Emergency Medicine
Division of Medical Toxicology
San Diego Division
California Poison Control System
San Diego, California

Jeffrey Schunk, MD
Director, Pediatric Emergency Medicine Fellowship
Professor of Pediatrics
University of Utah School of Medicine
Primary Children's Medical Center
Salt Lake City, Utah

Howard J. Shaps, MD
Attending Physician, Emergency Department
Jewish Hospital Health System
Louisville, Kentucky

Anuj A. Shah, MD
Department of Emergency Medicine
Summa Health System
Professor of Clinical Emergency Medicine
Northeastern Ohio University College of Medicine
Akron, Ohio

Scott C. Sherman, MD
Attending Physician
Department of Emergency Medicine
Cook County Hospital
Chicago, Illinois

Bryan Shiflett, MD
Resident
Department of Emergency Medicine
University of Arizona College of Medicine
Tucson, Arizona

Lee Shockley, MD, FACEP
Director, Emergency Medicine Residency
The Denver Health Medical Center Residency
in Emergency Medicine
Associate Professor, Division of Emergency Medicine
The University of Colorado School of Medicine
Denver Health Medical Center
Denver, Colorado

Paul R. Sierzenski, MD, RDMS, FAAEM
Chair, SAEM Ultrasound Interest Group
Director, Emergency Ultrasound Fellowship
Director, Emergency Medicine Ultrasound
Christiana Care Health System
Newark, Delaware

Adam Sigal, MD
Chief Resident
Department of Emergency Medicine
Cooper Hospital/University Medical Center
Camden, New Jersey

Elizabeth Guenther Skokan, MD, MPH
Assistant Professor of Pediatrics
Pediatric Emergency Medicine
University of Utah School of Medicine
Primary Children's Medical Center
Salt Lake City, Utah

Peter E. Sokolove, MD, FACEP
Associate Professor of Clinical Medicine
Residency Program Director
Division of Emergency Medicine
UC Davis Health System
Davis, California

Joyce Soprano, MD
Assistant Professor of Pediatrics
University of Utah School of Medicine
Primary Children's Medical Center
Salt Lake City, Utah

Sarah Stahmer, MD
Director, Residency Program in Emergency Medicine
Associate Professor of Emergency Medicine
Department of Emergency Medicine
Cooper Hospital/University Medical Center
Camden, New Jersey

Mari Stoddard
Associate Librarian
Head of Educational Services
Arizona Health Sciences Library
Tucson, Arizona

Jeffrey R. Suchard, MD, FACEP, FAAEM, DABMT
Assistant Clinical Professor
Director of Medical Toxicology
Department of Emergency Medicine
University of California Irvine Medical Center
Orange, California

Chad A. Surratt, MD
Department of Emergency Medicine
Truman Medical Centers
University of Missouri—Kansas City School of Medicine
Kansas City, Missouri

Noah Tolby, MD
Resident
Department of Emergency Medicine
University of Arizona College of Medicine
Tucson, Arizona

Terence Valenzuela, MD, MPH
Professor of Emergency Medicine
Department of Emergency Medicine
University of Arizona College of Medicine
Tucson, Arizona

Benjamin Vanlandingham, MD
Physician
Department of Emergency Medicine
University of Arizona College of Medicine
Tucson, Arizona

David Wachter, MD
Clinical Instructor
Department of Medicine
University of California at San Francisco
San Francisco, California

Richard Wagner, MD, PhD
Section Chair
Department of Emergency Medicine
El Dorado Hospital
Tucson, Arizona

Frank G. Walter, MD, FACEP, FACMT, FAACT
Chief, Division of Toxicology
Director, Medical Toxicology Fellowship
Associate Professor of Emergency Medicine
Department of Emergency Medicine
University of Arizona College of Medicine
Tucson, Arizona

C. Paige Waslewski, MD, FACEP
Staff Physician, Scottsdale Emergency Associates, Ltd.
Scottsdale, Arizona

John Ryan Whiteford, MD
Resident
Department of Emergency Medicine
Affiliated Residency in Emergency Medicine
University of Pittsburgh
Pittsburgh, Pennsylvania

Adrian M. Whorton, MD
Attending Physician
Department of Emergency Medicine
Evergreen Hospital Medical Center
Kirkland, Washington

Garry J. Wilkes, MBBS, FACEM
Director, Emergency Medicine
South West Health Service
Medical Director
St. John Ambulance Service
Clinical Senior Lecturer
Department of Medicine
University of Queensland
Western Australia

Allan B. Wolfson, MD, FACEP, FACP
Professor
Department of Emergency Medicine
Program Director, Affiliated Residency in Internal Medicine
University of Pittsburgh
Pittsburgh, Pennsylvania

Preface

I am honored to edit this first edition of *Emergency Medicine On Call*. The "on call" problem concept was first introduced in *Neonatology: Management, Procedures, On-Call Problems, Diseases, and Drugs*, edited by Tricia Gomella, MD, in 1988, and has been used as the model for the *On Call* series. The preceding books in the series, *Surgery On Call*, *Internal Medicine On Call*, *Obstetrics & Gynecology On Call*, and *Critical Care On Call*, have all served house officers extremely well in their times of greatest need: when a specific problem arises in a patient under their direct care. This complaint, or problem-based, approach is especially applicable to emergency medicine. Focusing on specific issues in the emergency department is crucial to the successful practice of emergency medicine. My hope is that this book will provide the house officer and student with a valuable tool to initiate effective evaluation and care of the emergency patient.

In general, the problems reflect issues that arise commonly in the emergency department. This initial guide to the evaluation and care should be augmented by more detailed standard textbooks when time permits. In addition to common adult emergencies, this book includes special sections devoted to Pediatric Emergencies, Geriatric Emergencies, Trauma Emergencies, Toxicology, Terrorism, Laboratory tests, Fluids and Electrolytes, Blood Component Therapy, Ventilator Management, Commonly Used Medications and Emergency Procedures. The Appendices Include many helpful tables for the busy emergency physician.

The chapters in this book each begin with a sample problem case, which illustrates one manner in which a patient might present with the topic problem. The immediate questions, differential, database, and plan sections are to assist with all relevant patients, not just the sample patient case. The diagnosis of the sample problem case is given near the end of each chapter. Each chapter lists some of the most common ICD-9 diagnoses that might be associated with the specific topic. This is meant to *assist* you in selecting the best diagnosis for your patient. Most topics end with a Teaching Pearls Question and Answer. For the teacher of emergency medicine, this is a suggested "pimp" question. For the student, this is a question with which you may be pimped! A limited number of pertinent references are included for most chapters for continued detailed reading. The reader is encouraged to use standard textbooks for further study whenever time permits.

I would like to acknowledge the tremendous efforts made by the contributors to this book. This group includes many of the best and brightest teachers in the emergency medicine community. The framework provided by the consulting editors of the other books in the *On Call* series is appreciated. I would also like to thank Janet Foltin at McGraw-Hill for her trust and guidance and Paulette Pierce for her outstanding administrative assistance. Please contact me with any suggestions you may have about how this book could be improved to assist you in providing emergency care of the highest quality in a cost- and time-efficient manner.

Samuel M. Keim, MD
Tucson, AZ
August 2003

Common Abbreviations and Acronyms

The following are common abbreviations used in medical records and in this edition.

/: per

÷: divided dose

≅: approximately equal to

±: with or without

<: less than, younger than

>: more than, older than

↓: decrease(d), reduce, downward

μm: micrometer

×: times for multiplication sign

↑: increase(d), upward (as in titrate upward)

+: with

A/G: albumin/globulin ratio

A-a gradient: alveolar-to-arterial gradient

AAA: abdominal aortic aneurysm

AaDO$_2$: A-a gradient

AAS: acute abdominal series

Abd: abdomen

ABG: arterial blood gas

AC: before eating (*ante cibum*), assist controlled, air conduction, alternating current

ac: before meals

ACE: angiotensin-converting enzyme

Ach-ase: acetylcholinesterase

ACLS: advanced cardiac life support

ACS: acute coronary syndrome

ACTH: adrenocorticotropic hormone

ad lib: as much as needed (*ad libitum*)

ADH: antidiuretic hormone

ADHD: attention-deficit hyperactivity disorder

ADL: activities of daily living

AED: automated external defibrillator

AEIOU TIPS: mnemonic for *A*lcohol, *E*ncephalopathy, *I*nsulin, *U*piates, *U*remia, *T*rauma, *I*nfection, *P*sychiatric, *S*yncope (diagnosis of coma)

AF: afebrile, aortofemoral, atrial fibrillation

AFB: acid-fast bacilli

AFP: alpha-fetoprotein

AHA: American Heart Association

AI: aortic insufficiency

AICD: automatic implantable cardioverter-defibrillator

AIDS: acquired immunodeficiency syndrome

AKA: above-the-knee amputation

aka: also known as

ALAT: alanine aminotransferase

ALL: acute lymphocytic leukemia

ALS: amyotrophic lateral sclerosis

ALT: alanine aminotransferase

ALTE: acute life-threatening event

AM: morning

amb: ambulate

AMI: acute myocardial infarction

AML: acute myelocytic leukemia, acute myelogenous leukemia

AMP: adenosine monophosphate

amp: ampule
AMS: altered mental status
ANA: antinuclear antibody
ANC: absolute neutrophil count
ANCA: antineutrophil cytoplasmic antibody
ANS: autonomic nervous system
AODM: adult-onset diabetes mellitus
AP: anteroposterior
APAP: acetaminophen
aPPT: activated partial thromboplastin time
APRV: airway pressure release ventilation
APSAC: anisoylated plasminogen streptokinase activator complex
ARDS: adult respiratory distress syndrome
ARF: acute renal failure
AS: aortic stenosis
ASAP: as soon as possible
ASAT: aspartate aminotransferase
ASCVD: atherosclerotic cardiovascular disease
ASD: atrial septal defect
ASHD: atherosclerotic heart disease
ASO: antistreptolysin O
AST: aspartate aminotransferase
ATLS: advanced trauma life support
ATN: acute tubular necrosis
ATP: adenosine triphosphate
A–V: arteriovenous
AV: atrioventricular
A–Vo₂: arteriovenous oxygen
AVPU: alert, voice response, pain response, unresponsive
β-HCG: beta human chorionic gonadotropin
B. burgdorferi: Borrelia burgdorferi
BAS: body surface area
BBB: bundle branch block
BC: bone conduction
BCAA: branched-chain amino acid

BCG: bacille Calmette–Guérin
BE: barium enema
bid: twice/day
bili: bilirubin
BiPAP: bilevel positive airway pressure
BKA: below-the-knee amputation
BLS: basic life support
BM: bowel movement
BMP: basic metabolic panel
BMR: basal metabolic rate
BMT: bone marrow transplantation
BOM: bilateral otitis media
BP: blood pressure
BPH: benign prostatic hypertrophy
BPM: beats per minute
BPPV: benign paroxysmal positional vertigo
BR: bed rest
BRBPR: bright red blood per rectum
BS&O: bilateral salpingo-oophorectomy
bs, BS: bowel sounds, breath sounds
BSA: body surface area
BUN: blood urea nitrogen
BVM: bag, valve, mask
BW: body weight
Bx: biopsy
C&S: culture and sensitivity
C. difficile: Clostridium difficile
C/O: complaining of
c: with (*cum*)
Cco₂: capillary oxygen content
Ca: calcium
CA: cancer
Cao₂: arterial oxygen content
CABG: coronary artery bypass graft
CAD: coronary artery disease
CAM: confusion assessment method
cAMP: cyclic adenosine monophosphate
C-ANCA: cytoplasmic-staining antineutrophil cytoplasmic antibodies

caps: capsule(s)
CAT: computed axial tomography
CBC: complete blood count
CBG: capillary blood gas
CC: chief complaint
CCB: calcium channel blocker
CCO: continuous cardiac output
CCU: clean-catch urine, cardiac care unit
CCV: critical closing volume
CD: continuous dose
CDC: Centers for Disease Control and Prevention
CEA: carcinoembryonic antigen
CF: cystic fibrosis
CFU: colony-forming unit(s)
CHD: coronary heart disease
CHF: congestive heart failure
CHO: carbohydrate
CI: cardiac index
CIS: carcinoma in situ
CK–MB: isoenzyme of creatine kinase with muscle and brain subunits
CK: creatine kinase
Cl: chlorine
CLL: chronic lymphocytic leukemia
cm: centimeter
CML: chronic myelogenous leukemia
CMV: cytomegalovirus
CN: cranial nerve
CNS: central nervous system
CO: cardiac output
COLD: chronic obstructive lung disease
conc: concentrate
cont inf: continuous infusion
COPD: chronic obstructive pulmonary disease
COX-2: cyclooxygenase-2
CP: chest pain, cerebral palsy
CPAP: continuous positive airway pressure
CPK: creatinine phosphokinase
CPR: cardiopulmonary resuscitation

CR: controlled release
Cr: creatinine
CrCl: creatinine clearance
CREST: calcinosis cutis, Raynaud's disease, esophageal dysmotility, syndactyly, telangiectasia
CRF: chronic renal failure
CRH: corticotropin-releasing hormone
CRP: C-reactive protein
CSF: cerebrospinal fluid, colony-stimulating factor
C-spine: cervical spine
CT: computed tomography
CTL: cervical, thoracic, and lumbar
cTnI: troponin I
cTnT: troponin T
Cvo_2: oxygen content of mixed venous blood
CVA: cerebrovascular accident, costovertebral angle
CVAT: costovertebral angle tenderness
CVP: central venous pressure
CXR: chest x-ray
D&C: dilation and curettage
d: day
D_5LR: 5% dextrose in lactated Ringer's solution
D_5W: 5% dextrose in water
DC: discontinue, discharge, direct current
DDx: differential diagnosis
DEA: United States Drug Enforcement Administration
DES: diethylstilbestrol
DFA: direct immunofluorescence
DHEA: dehydroepiandrosterone
DI: diabetes insipidus
DIC: disseminated intravascular coagulation
Diff: differential
DIP: distal interphalangeal joint
DJD: degenerative joint disease
DKA: diabetic ketoacidosis

dL: deciliter
DM: diabetes mellitus
DMSA: dimercaptosuccinic acid
DNA: deoxyribonucleic acid
DNR: do not resuscitate
DOA: dead on arrival
DOE: dyspnea on exertion
DP: dorsalis pedis
2,3-DPG: 2,3-diphosphoglycerate
DPL: diagnostic peritoneal lavage
DPT: diphtheria, pertussis, tetanus
DR: delayed release
DRG: diagnosis-related group
DRSP: drug-resistant *Streptococcus pneumoniae*
DS: double strength
DSA: digital subtraction angiography
DT: delirium tremens
DTR: deep tendon reflex
DVT: deep venous thrombosis
Dx: diagnosis
E. coli: Escherichia coli
EBL: estimated blood loss
EBV: Epstein–Barr virus
EC: enteric-coated
ECG: electrocardiogram
ECT: electroconvulsive therapy
ECVD: extracellular volume of distribution
ED: emergency department
EDC: estimated date of confinement
EDH: epidural hemorrhage
EDTA: ethylenediamine tetraacetic acid
EGD: esophagogastroduodenoscopy
ELISA: enzyme-linked immunosorbent assay
EMD: electromechanical dissociation
EMG: electromyelogram
EMS: emergency medical system,
EMV: eyes, motor, verbal response (Glasgow Coma Scale)
ENA: extractable nuclear antigen

ENT: ear, nose, and throat
EOM: extraocular muscle
EPO: erythropoietin
ER: endoplasmic reticulum, Emergency Room
ERCP: endoscopic retrograde cholangiopancreatography
ERV: expiratory reserve volume
ESR: erythrocyte sedimentation rate
ESRD: end-stage renal disease
ET: endotracheal
ETOH: ethanol
ETT: endotracheal tube
EUA: examination under anesthesia
Fab: antigen-binding fragment
FANA: fluorescent antinuclear antibody
FAST: focused abdominal ultrasound for trauma
FBS: fasting blood sugar
Fe: iron
FEV_1: forced expiratory volume in 1 s
FFP: fresh frozen plasma
FH: family history
FHR: fetal heart rate
Fio_2: fraction of inspired oxygen
FRC: functional residual capacity
FSH: follicle-stimulating hormone
FSP: fibrin split product
ft: foot
FTA-ABS: fluorescent treponemal antibody-absorbed
FTT: failure to thrive
FU: follow-up
5-FU: fluorouracil
FUO: fever of unknown origin
FVC: forced vital capacity
Fx: fracture
G: gauge
g: gram
G: gravida
G6PD: glucose-6-phosphate dehydrogenase
GABA: γ-aminobutyric acid

GBL: γ-butyrolactone
GC: gonorrhea (gonococcus)
GCS: Glasgow Coma Scale
G-CSF: granulocyte colony-stimulating factor
GERD: gastroesophageal reflux disease
GETT: general by endotracheal tube (anesthesia)
GFR: glomerular filtration rate
GGT: gamma-glutamyltransferase
GGTP: gamma-glutamyl transpeptidase
GH: growth hormone
GHB: γ-hydroxybutyrate
GHIH: growth hormone-inhibiting hormone
GI: gastrointestinal
GNID: gram-negative intracellular diplococci
gr: grain
GSW: gunshot wound
gt, gtt: drop, drops (*gutta*)
GTT: glucose tolerance test
GU: genitourinary
GVHD: graft-versus-host disease
GXT: graded exercise tolerance (cardiac stress test)
H&P: history and physical examination
H. influenzae: Haemophilus influenzae
H. pylori: Helicobacter pylori
H/H: hemoglobin/hematocrit
HA: headache
HAA: hepatitis B surface antigen (hepatitis-associated antigen)
HAV: hepatitis A virus
HBcAg: hepatitis B core antigen
HBeAg: hepatitis B e antigen
Hbg: hemoglobin
HBP: high blood pressure
HBsAg: hepatitis B surface antigen
HBV: hepatitis B virus
HCG: human chorionic gonadotropin

HCM: hypertrophic cardiomyopathy
Hct: hematocrit
HCTZ: hydrochlorothiazide
HD: hemodialysis
HDL: high-density lipoprotein
HEENT: head, eyes, ears, nose, and throat
HELLP: hemolysis, elevated liver enzymes, and low platelet count
HFV: high-frequency ventilation
Hgb: hemoglobin
[Hgb]: hemoglobin concentration
HIV: human immunodeficiency virus
HJR: hepatojugular reflex
HO: history of
HOB: head of bed
hpf: high-power field
HPI: history of the present illness
HPLC: high-pressure liquid chromatography
HPV: human papilloma virus
HR: heart rate
hs: at bedtime (*hora somni*)
HSM: hepatosplenomegaly
HSV: herpes simplex virus
5-HT$_3$: 5-hydroxytryptamine
HTLV-III: human T-lymphotropic virus, type III (AIDS agent, HIV)
HTN: hypertension
HUS: hemolytic uremic syndrome
Hx: history
HZO: herpes zoster oticus
I&D: incision and drainage
I&O: intake and output
IBW: ideal body weight
IC: inspiratory capacity
ICC: intercostal catheter
ICH: intracerebral hemorrhage
ICP: intracranial pressure
ICS: intercostal space
ICU: intensive care unit
ID: identification, infectious disease

IDDM: insulin-dependent diabetes mellitus
Ig: immunoglobulin
IHSS: idiopathic hypertrophic subaortic stenosis
IL: interleukin
IM: intramuscular
IMV: intermittent mandatory ventilation
in.: inch
INH: isoniazid
inhal: inhalation
inj: injection
INR: international normalized ratio
IPPB: intermittent positive pressure breathing
IRBBB: incomplete right bundle branch block
IRDM: insulin-resistant diabetes mellitus
IRV: inspiratory reserve volume
IT: intrathecal
ITP: idiopathic thrombocytopenic purpura
IUP: intrauterine pregnancy
IV: intravenous
IVC: intravenous cholangiogram
IVP: intravenous pyelogram
JODM: juvenile-onset diabetes mellitus
JRA: juvenile rheumatoid arthritis
JVD: jugular venous distention
K: potassium
katal: unit of enzyme activity
KB: Kleihauer–Betke test
kg: kilogram
KOR: keep open rate
17-KSG: 17-ketogenic steroids
KUB: kidneys, ureters, bladder
KVO: keep vein open
L: liter
LAD: left axis deviation, left anterior descending
LAE: left atrial enlargement
LAHB: left anterior hemiblock
LAP: left atrial pressure, leukocyte alkaline phosphatase

LBBB: left bundle branch block
LDH: lactate dehydrogenase
LDL: low-density lipoprotein
LE: lupus erythematosus
LFTs: liver function tests
LGV: lymphogranuloma venereum
LH: luteinizing hormone
LHRH: luteinizing hormone releasing hormone
LIH: left inguinal hernia
liq: liquid
LLL: left lower lobe
LLSB: left lower sternal border
LMP: last menstrual period
LMW: low molecular weight
LNMP: last normal menstrual period
LOC: loss of consciousness, level of consciousness
LP: lumbar puncture
lpf: low-power field
LPN: licensed practical nurse
LSB: left sternal border
LSD: lysergic acid diethylamide
LUL: left upper lobe
LUQ: left upper quadrant
LV: left ventricle
LVD: left ventricular dysfunction
LVEDP: left ventricular end-diastolic pressure
LVH: left ventricular hypertrophy
Lytes: electrolytes
M. pneumoniae: Mycoplasma pneumoniae
m: meter
MAC: *Mycobacterium avium* complex
MAO: monoamine oxidase
MAOI: monoamine oxidase inhibitor
MAP: mean arterial pressure
MAST: military/medical antishock trousers
MAT: multifocal atrial tachycardia
max: maximum
MBC: minimum bactericidal concentration

MBT: maternal blood type
MCC: motor cycle crash
MCDT: mixed connective tissue disease
MCH: mean cell hemoglobin
MCHC: mean cell hemoglobin concentration
MCT: medium-chain triglycerides
MCTD: mixed connective tissue disease
MCV: mean cell volume
MDI: metered-dose inhaler
MDMA: methylenedioxymethamphetamine
meds: medications
MEN: multiple endocrine neoplasia
mEq: milliequivalent
met-dose: metered-dose
Mg: magnesium
mg: milligram
MHA-TP: microhemagglutination–*Treponema pallidum*
MHC: major histocompatibility complex
MI: myocardial infarction, mitral insufficiency
MIC: minimum inhibitory concentration
min: minimum, minute
mL: milliliter
MLE: midline episiotomy
mm Hg: millimeters of mercury
mm: millimeter
MMEF: maximal midexpiratory flow
mmol: millimole
MMR: measles, mumps, rubella
MMSE: Mini Mental Status Exam
mol: mole
mon: month
MPGN: membrane-proliferative glomerulonephritis
MPTP: analog of meperidine (used by drug addicts)
MR: mitral regurgitation
MRI: magnetic resonance imaging

mRNA: messenger ribonucleic acid
MRS: magnetic resonance spectroscopy
MRSA: methicillin-resistant *Staphylococcus aureus*
MS: mitral stenosis, morphine sulfate, multiple sclerosis
MSG: monosodium glutamate
MSH: melanocyte-stimulating hormone
MTX: methotrexate
MUGA: multigated (image) acquisition (analysis)
MVA: motor vehicle accident
MVI: multivitamin injection
MVP: mitral valve prolapse
MVV: maximum voluntary ventilation
MyG: myasthenia gravis
N. gonorrhoeae: Neisseria gonorrhoeae
N. meningitidis: Neisseria meningitidis
N/V: nausea and vomiting
Na: sodium
Na⁺/K⁺-ATPase: sodium/potassium adenosine triphosphate
NAC: *N*-acetylcysteine
NAD: no active disease
NAPA: *N*-acetylated procainamide
NAVEL: mnemonic for *N*erve, *A*rtery, *V*ein, *E*mpty space, *L*ymphatic
NCV: nerve conduction velocity
NE: norepinephrine
neb: nebulization
NEC: not elsewhere classified
NED: no evidence of recurrent disease
ng: nanogram
NG: nasogastric
NIDDM: non–insulin-dependent diabetes mellitus
NKA: no known allergies
NKDA: no known drug allergy
nmol: nanomole
NMR: nuclear magnetic resonance

NNRTI: nonnucleoside reverse transcriptase inhibitor
NOS: not otherwise specified
NPO: nothing by mouth (*nil per os*)
NRTI: nucleoside reverse transcriptase inhibitor
NS: normal saline
NSAID: nonsteroidal antiinflammatory drug
NSR: normal sinus rhythm
NT: nasotracheal
NTG: nitroglycerin
OB: obstetrics
OCD: obsessive–compulsive disorder
OCG: oral cholecystogram
OD: overdose
OG: orogastric
oint: ointment
OM: otitis media
ophth: ophthalmic
OPV: oral polio vaccine
OR: operating room
ORS: oral rehydration solution
Osm: osmole
OTC: over-the-counter (medications)
P&PD: percussion and postural drainage
P. aeruginosa: Pseudomonas aeruginosa
P. mirabilis: Proteus mirabilis
p: para
P: phosphorus
PA: posteroanterior, pulmonary artery
PAO_2: alveolar oxygen
PaO_2: peripheral arterial oxygen content
PAC: premature atrial contraction
PAF: paroxysmal atrial fibrillation
PALS: pediatric advanced life support
PAN: polyarteritis nodosa
P-ANCA: perinuclear-staining antineutrophil cytoplasmic antibodies

PAOP: pulmonary artery occlusion pressure
PAP: pulmonary artery pressure
PAS: systolic pulmonary artery pressure
PASG: pneumatic antishock garment
PAT: paroxysmal atrial tachycardia
pc: after eating (*post cibum*)
PCA: patient-controlled analgesia
PCI: percutaneous coronary intervention
PCKD: polycystic kidney disease
PCN: penicillin
PCP: *Pneumocystis carinii* pneumonia
PCR: polymerase chain reaction
PCWP: pulmonary capillary wedge pressure
PD: peritoneal dialysis
PDA: patent ductus arteriosus
PDR: Physicians' Desk Reference
PE: pulmonary embolus, physical examination, pleural effusion
PEA: pulseless electrical activity
PEEP: positive end-expiratory pressure
PEG: percutaneous endoscopic gastrostomy
PEG-ES: polyethylene glycol electrolyte solution
PERRLA: pupils equal, round, reactive to light and accommodation
PET: positron emission tomography
PFT: pulmonary function test
pg: picogram
PGE_1: prostaglandin E_1
PICC: peripherally inserted central catheter
PICU: pediatric intensive care unit
PID: pelvic inflammatory disease
PIH: prolactin-inhibiting hormone
PKU: phenylketonuria
PMH: past medical history

PMI: point of maximal impulse
PMN: polymorphonuclear neutrophil
PND: paroxysmal nocturnal dyspnea
PNS: peripheral nervous system
PO: by mouth (*per os*)
POC: products of conception
POD: postoperative day
pod: postoperative day
postop: postoperative, after surgery
PP: pulsus paradoxus, postprandial
PPD: purified protein derivative
PPV: positive pressure ventilation
PQRST: palliation, provocation, quality, radiation, severity, timing
PR: by rectum
PRBC: packed red blood cells
preop: preoperative, before surgery
PRG: pregnancy
PRN: as often as needed (*pro re nata*)
PS: pulmonic stenosis, partial saturation
PSA: prostate-specific antigen
PSH: past surgical history
PSLAX: parasternal long axis
PSSAX: parasternal short axis
PSV: pressure support ventilation
PSVT: paroxysmal supraventricular tachycardia
Pt: patient
PT: prothrombin time, physical therapy, posterior tibial
PTCA: percutaneous transluminal coronary angioplasty
PTH: parathyroid hormone
PTHrP: parathyroid hormone-related protein
PTT: partial thromboplastin time
PTU: propylthiouracil
PUD: peptic ulcer disease
PVC: premature ventricular contraction

PVD: peripheral vascular disease
PVR: peripheral vascular resistance
PWP: pulmonary wedge pressure
Q: mathematical symbol for flow
q12h: every 12 hours
q4h: every 4 hours
q6h: every 6 hours
q8h: every 8 hours
qd: every day
qid: 4 times/day
QNS: quantity not sufficient
qod: every other day
Q_s/Q_t: shunt fraction
Qs: volume of blood (portion of cardiac output) shunted past nonventilated alveoli
Q_t: total cardiac output
R/O: rule out
R: right
RA: rheumatoid arthritis, right atrium
RAD: right axis deviation
RAE: right atrial enlargement
RAP: right atrial pressure
RBBB: right bundle branch block
RBC: red blood cell (erythrocyte)
RDA: recommended dietary allowance
RDS: respiratory distress syndrome (of newborn)
RDW: red cell distribution width
REAC: radiologic emergency assistance center
REF: right ventricular ejection fraction
REM: rapid eye movement
RhIG: Rh immune globulin
RIA: radioimmunoassay
RIND: reversible ischemic neurologic deficit
RL: Ringer's lactate
RLL: right lower lobe
RLQ: right lower quadrant
RML: right middle lobe
RMSF: Rocky Mountain spotted fever
RN: registered nurse

RNA: ribonucleic acid
ROM: range of motion
ROS: review of systems
RPR: rapid plasma reagent
RR: respiration rate
RRR: regular rate and rhythm
RSI: rapid sequence induction
RSV: respiratory syncytial virus
RT: rubella titer, respiratory therapy, radiation therapy, reverse transcriptase
RTA: renal tubular acidosis
RTC: return to clinic
RT-PCR: reverse transcriptase polymerase chain reaction
RU: resin uptake
RUG: retrograde urethrogram
RUL: right upper lobe
RUQ: right upper quadrant
RV: residual volume
RVEDVI: right ventricular end-diastolic volume index
RVH: right ventricular hypertrophy
Rx: treatment
S. aureus: Staphylococcus aureus
S. pyogenes: Streptococcus pyogenes
s: second
SA: sinoatrial
SAH: subarachnoid hemorrhage
SaO$_2$: arterial oxygen saturation
SBE: subacute bacterial endocarditis
SBS: short bowel syndrome
SCr: serum creatinine
SDH: subdural hemorrhage
segs: segmented cells
SEM: systolic ejection murmur
SG: Swan–Ganz
SGA: small for gestational age
SGGT: serum gamma-glutamyl transpeptidase
SGOT: serum glutamic-oxaloacetic transaminase
SGPT: serum glutamic-pyruvic transaminase
SH: surgical history
SI: Système International

SIADH: syndrome of inappropriate antidiuretic hormone
SIDS: sudden infant death syndrome
sig: write on label (*signa*)
SIMV: synchronous intermittent mandatory ventilation
SIRS: systemic inflammatory response syndrome
SL: sublingual
SLE: systemic lupus erythematosus
SLUDGE: *s*alivation, *l*acrimation, *u*rination, *d*efecation, *g*astrointestinal distress, and *e*mesis
SMX: sulfamethoxazole
SOAP: mnemonic for *S*ubjective, *O*bjective, *A*ssessment, *P*lan
SOB: shortness of breath
soln: solution
SQ: subcutaneous
SR, ER: sustained release, extended release
SRS-A: slow-reacting substance of anaphylaxis
SSKI: saturated solution of potassium iodide
SSRI: selective serotonin reuptake inhibitor
stat: immediately (*statim*)
STD: sexually transmitted disease
supp: suppository
susp: suspension
SvO$_2$: mixed venous blood oxygen saturation
SVC: superior vena cava
SVD: spontaneous vaginal delivery
SVR: systemic vascular resistance
SVT: supraventricular tachycardia
Sx: symptoms
T&C: type and cross-match
T&H: type and hold
T&S: type and screen
T: one
T$_3$ RU: triiodothyronine resin uptake

T_3: triiodothyronine
T_4: thyroxine
tabs: tablet(s)
TAH: total abdominal hysterectomy
TB: tuberculosis
TBG: thyroxine-binding globulin, total blood gas
TBLC: term birth, living child
TCA: tricyclic antidepressants
TCP: transcutaneous pacer
Td: tetanus–diphtheria toxoid
TD: transdermal
TEE: transesophageal echocardiogram
TFT: thyroid function test
TIA: transient ischemic attack
TIBC: total iron-binding capacity
tid: 3 times/day
TIG: tetanus immune globulin
TKO: to keep open
TLC: total lung capacity
TM: tympanic membrane
TMJ: temporal mandibular joint
TMP: trimethoprim
TMP-SMX: trimethoprim–sulfamethoxazole
TNFα: tumor necrosis factor alpha
TNKase: tenecteplase
TNTC: too numerous to count
TOPV: trivalent oral polio vaccine
TORCH: toxoplasma, rubella, cytomegalovirus, herpes virus (*O* = other [syphilis])
TPA: tissue plasminogen activator
TPN: total peripheral resistance, total parenteral nutrition
TRH: thyrotropin-releasing hormone
TSH: thyroid-stimulating hormone
TSS: toxic shock syndrome
TT: thrombin time
TTE: transthoracic echocardiogram
TTP: thrombotic thrombocytopenic purpura
TU: tuberculin units
TUR: transurethral resection

TURP: TUR prostate
TV: tidal volume
TVH: total vaginal hysterectomy
Tx: treatment, transplant, transfer
type 2 DM: noninsulin-dependent diabetes mellitus, type 2 diabetes mellitus
UA: urinalysis
UDS: ultra-Doppler sonography
UF: unfractionated
UGI: upper gastrointestinal
UGIB: upper gastrointestinal bleeding
URI: upper respiratory tract infection
US: ultrasonography
USP: *United States Pharmacopeia*
UTI: urinary tract infection
V/Q: ventilation–perfusion
V: volt
VC: vital capacity
VCUG: voiding cystourethrogram
VDRL: Venereal Disease Research Laboratory
VF: ventricular fibrillation
VHF: viral hemorrhagic fever
VIPoma: vasoactive intestinal polypeptide tumor
VLDL: very low density lipoprotein
VO: voice order
VSS: vital signs stable
VT: ventricular tachycardia
W: watt
WB: whole blood
WBC: white blood cell, white blood cell count
WBI: whole bowel irrigation
WD: well developed
WF: white female
wk: week
WM: white male
WMD: weapons of mass destruction
WPW: Wolff–Parkinson–White (syndrome)
XRT: x-ray therapy
y: year

Dedication

To Andrew, Colleen and Jude,
whom I love immeasurably

I. Adult Emergency On-Call Problems

1. ABDOMINAL PAIN

I. Problem. A 67-year-old male presents with generalized abdominal pain of gradual onset.

II. Immediate Questions

A. ABCs/Patient Stabilization

1. **Is the airway intact?** Manage appropriately. (See Section VIII, 15. Rapid Sequence Endotracheal Intubation, p 470.)
2. **What are the vital signs?** Does the patient look acutely ill or toxic? Quick assessment of mental status. Is the patient obtunded? Assess peripheral pulses. Initiate IV (two large bore if signs of hemodynamic compromise are present) and administer fluid bolus if appropriate; cardiac monitor, pulse oximeter, supplemental oxygen.

B. What was the timing of onset of symptoms? Sudden vs gradual, preceded by anorexia, N/V, constipation, diarrhea, fever, waxing and waning, or steady. (See 18. Constipation, p 60; 25. Diarrhea, p 82.)

C. Where does it hurt? *Generalized pain:* Peritonitis, ischemic bowel. Epigastric: gastritis, duodenal/gastric ulcer, pancreatitis, aortic pathology, early appendicitis, inferior MI, liver, or biliary tract disease. *RUQ:* Liver, or biliary tract disease, inferior pneumonia or MI, occasionally renal. *LUQ:* Spleen (especially if trauma), sometimes renal. *LLQ:* Diverticular disease, colitis, gynecologic, or genitourinary. *RLQ:* Appendicitis, gynecologic source, or genitourinary. *Radiation from back/flank:* Renal source. *Radiation from abdomen to back:* Pancreatitis, aortic aneurysm.

D. Are there genitourinary complaints? Dysuria, hematuria, back pain, penile discharge/bleeding. Sexual history, sexual practices, history of sexually transmitted diseases.

E. What is the quality of the pain? Burning/epigastric, consider gastritis or peptic ulcer. Penetrating or boring, consider pancreatitis. Pain out of proportion to physical findings, consider ischemic bowel. Patient can't find comfortable position or writhing on gurney, think colic (renal or intestinal). Patient avoiding movement, consider peritoneal irritation.

F. Are there GI complaints? N/V, diarrhea, hematochezia, hematemesis, prior history of same symptoms, any relation to food.

G. Respiratory Complaints. Cough, SOB, pleuritic pain.

H. Any history of trauma or prior surgeries?

I. Other Past Medical History. AAA, abdominal cancer, bowel obstructions, CAD, diabetes inflammatory bowel disease, peptic ulcer, pancreatitis, renal calculi, pyelonephritis, history of recurrent nonspecific abdominal pain.

    J. Additional Social History. Foreign travel, recent questionable food sources, diet history, ETOH or drug abuse, possibility of accidental poison/medicine ingestions.

III. Differential Diagnosis
  A. Gender-/Age-Neutral
    1. **Appendicitis.** Pain preceded by nausea, anorexia, fever; pain often vague initially, then localized to RLQ.
    2. **Biliary tract disorders.** Cholelithiasis/cholecystitis, hepatitis. (See 50, Jaundice, p 148.)
    3. **Peptic ulcer/GERD.** Think viscus perforation or hemorrhage if acutely ill.
    4. **Gastritis.** Food- or medication-related; viral.
    5. **Pancreatitis.** ETOH/diabetes history; rule out gallstones.
    6. **Bowel obstructions.** Distinguish from ileus.
    7. **Genitourinary and renal disorders.** Calculi, pyelonephritis, infections of the urethra, bladder, and reproductive organs. (See 70. Urinary Tract Problems, p 208)
    8. **Thoracic diseases.** Inferior pneumonias, pulmonary embolism, atypical cardiac angina/MI. (See 15. Chest Pain, p 51.)
    9. **Diverticulitis.** Severe, cramping LLQ pain associated with bloody diarrhea.
    10. **Inflammatory bowel disease.** Crohn's disease, ulcerative colitis (cramping, episodic, recurrent pain associated with diarrhea, sometimes bloody).
    11. **Sickle cell crisis.**
    12. **Diabetic ketoacidosis.** (See 23. Diabetic Problems, p 75.)
    13. **Irritable bowel syndrome.** Strictly a diagnosis of exclusion. Symptoms often only briefly present; a variety of symptoms, often crampy pain with intermittent diarrhea and constipation.
    14. **Mesenteric adenitis, gastroenteritis, constipation.** Diagnoses of exclusion.
  B. Adult Males
    1. Epididymitis. (See 59. Scrotal Problems, p 176.)
    2. Hernia. (See 41. Hernia, p 126.)
    3. Testicular torsion, torsion of appendix testis. (sudden onset, often presents with low abdominal pain).
  C. Females of Childbearing Age. (See 56. Pregnancy Problems, p 168.)
    1. Ectopic pregnancy
    2. Ovarian cysts/torsion
    3. Pelvic inflammatory disease
    4. Endometriosis
    5. Mittelschmerz
    6. Uterine/ovarian masses (fibroids, cancer)
    7. Pregnancy related (eg, placental abruption)
  D. Geriatric (See Section IV. Geriatric Emergency Problems, p 296.)
    1. AAA/aortic dissection
    2. Coronary disease (easy to overlook). (See Section IV, 2. Acute Myocardial Infarction in the Older Patient, p 298)

    3. Mesenteric ischemia/infarction (remember pain out of proportion to physical findings)

    4. Urinary retention (prostate disease, bladder stones, cancer)
      Note: Many elderly patients will have atypical presentations of abdominal catastrophes, such as only alteration in consciousness or nonspecific pain. Be suspicious and aggressive in management—this is a *very high-risk* population.

  E. Pediatric. (See Section II. 2. Abdominal Pain in Children, p 221.)

    1. Intestinal colic (usually in first 3 months of life, benign)

    2. Intestinal obstruction (midgut volvulus, pyloric stenosis, intussusception, incarcerated hernias, Hirschsprung's disease)

    3. Lead poisoning

IV. Database

  A. Physical Exam Key Points. Will vary with age/gender. (See Table I–1, p 3)

    1. General appearance. Mental status, signs of toxicity or hemodynamic compromise; is the patient acutely ill?

    2. Vital signs. Repeat frequently if patient acutely ill or with changes in condition.

    3. Thoracic. Crackles, rales, murmurs, wheezes; inspection of chest for signs of inferior chest trauma.

    4. Abdomen. Inspection (surgical scars, ecchymosis, caput medusae, petechiae), location of tenderness (see previous Immediate Questions section), rigidity, rebound tenderness, distension, peritoneal signs (toe tap, gurney shake), masses (liver/spleen

---

TABLE I–1. PHYSICAL FINDINGS WITH VARIOUS CAUSES OF ACUTE ABDOMEN.

Condition	Signs
Perforated viscus	Scaphoid, tense abdomen; diminished bowel sounds (late); loss of liver dullness; guarding or rigidity
Peritonitis	Motionless, absent bowel sounds (late); cough and rebound tenderness; guarding or rigidity
Inflamed mass or abscess	Tender mass (abdominal, rectal, or pelvic); punch tenderness; special signs (Murphy's, psoas, or obturator)
Intestinal obstruction	Distension; visible peristalsis (late); hyperperistalsis (early) or quiet abdomen (late); diffuse pain without rebound tenderness; hernia or rectal mass (some)
Paralytic ileus	Distension; minimal bowel sounds; no localized tenderness
Ischemic or strangulated bowel	Not distended (until late); bowel sounds variable; severe pain but little tenderness; rectal bleeding (some)
Bleeding	Pallor, shock; distension; pulsatile (aneurysm) or tender (eg, ectopic pregnancy) mass; rectal bleeding (some)

Reproduced, with permission, from Boey JH: Acute abdomen. In: Way LW, ed. *Current Surgical Diagnosis and Treatment,* 10th ed. Appleton & Lange, 1994.

edge, hernias), fluid shift/wave (ascites), auscultation for bowel sounds/bruits, presence of pulsatile mass.

5. Pelvic (females). Vaginal bleeding, discharge, cervical motion tenderness, masses or tenderness. Cervical os appearance. Look for RUQ pain in patients with pelvic findings to rule out Fitz-Hugh–Curtis syndrome (perihepatitis associated with PID).

6. GU exam (males). Testicular tenderness/ecchymosis, cremasteric reflex, penile discharge, hernias or masses, blue dot sign (torsion of appendix testis). Do NOT neglect the GU exam in males with low abdominal pain.

7. Rectal. Blood (occult or gross), reproduction of abdominal pain, masses, prostate tenderness/enlargement.

8. Back. Percussion tenderness, ecchymosis, costovertebral tenderness.

9. Extremities. Differential pulses (abdominal aortic aneurysm), psoas/obturator signs (appendicitis).

B. Laboratory Data. Tailored to history and physical findings.

   1. Urine pregnancy test in females of childbearing age to rule out pregnancy immediately. *Assume pregnancy* until proven otherwise.

   2. CBC with Diff, Lytes, BUN/creatinine, glucose.

   3. LFTs, amylase.

   4. UA (hematuria for renal calculi—think complete obstruction if absent; pyuria/bacteriuria).

   5. Cardiac enzymes in elderly.

   6. Type and cross for PRBCs if suspicious of significant blood loss.

C. Radiographic and Other Studies

   1. Acute abdominal series. To look for obstruction (dilated loops of bowel or air fluid levels), perforation (free air under diaphragm), or calculi (gall bladder, kidney), inferior pulmonary infiltrates, pleural effusions aortic calcification and diameter.

   2. CT scan. Often helpful when history/physical and labs are equivocal but suggestive of surgical pathology, especially in elderly and women of childbearing age with RLQ pain. Use in appendicitis and renal/ureteral calculi workup is increasing in prevalence.

D. Other Studies

   1. ECG in elderly

   2. Ultrasound. Abdominal (aortic diameter to rule out aneurysm; gall bladder, renal (stones/masses), obstetric/pelvic (ectopic pregnancy, adnexal or uterine pathology), testicular (torsion).

   3. Note on studies. NEVER let an unstable patient leave the emergency department unless going to OR, ICU, or other higher levels of care.

V. Plan

   A. Overall Plan. If there are signs of a "surgical abdomen," ie, obvious peritoneal signs, rigidity, or evidence of perforation or vascular catastrophe, immediate surgical or vascular surgical consultation is imperative (Table I–2, p 5. Delay in care may be fatal. As the patient's condition permits, other more time-consuming studies can be undertaken to address/manage other potential causes. Address pain early and adequately—abdominal exam may be more revealing after analgesics have been administered. Use of short-acting opioid analgesia is helpful (fentanyl), as well as antiemetics and glycopyrrolate.

- B. **Specific Plans**
    1. **Appendicitis, incarcerated hernias, bowel obstructions, perforated bowel from any cause.** Management on surgical service with admission, usually operative intervention. Initiate IV antibiotics to cover gram-negative bacteria and anaerobes early in ED stay if appropriate. Delay can be devastating.
    2. **Biliary tract disease.** Acute cholecystitis or ascending cholangitis mandates surgical consultation. If common duct stone suspected, consider GI consultation for ERCP. Remember antibiotics. If pain well controlled and no signs of infection, outpatient surgical consultation is appropriate.
    3. **Peptic ulcer disease/GERD/gastritis.** GI consultation if GI bleed present. Remember adequate resuscitation (fluids, blood, FFP). Screen for *H. pylori* and treat if appropriate, H_2 blockers

---

TABLE I–2. INDICATIONS FOR URGENT OPERATION IN PATIENTS WITH ACUTE ABDOMEN.

Physical findings
    Involuntary guarding or rigidity, especially if spreading
    Increasing or severe localized tenderness
    Tense or progressive distension
    Tender abdominal or rectal mass with high fever or hypotension
    Rectal bleeding with shock or acidosis
    Equivocal abdominal findings along with
        Septicemia (high fever, marked or rising leukocytosis, mental changes,
            or increasing glucose intolerance in a diabetic patient)
        Bleeding (unexplained shock or acidosis, falling hematocrit)
        Suspected ischemia (acidosis, fever, tachycardia)
        Deterioration on conservative treatment

Radiologic findings
    Pneumoperitoneum
    Gross or progressive bowel distension
    Free extravasation of contrast material
    Space-occupying lesion on CT scan with fever
    Mesenteric occlusion on angiography

Endoscopic findings
    Perforated or uncontrollably bleeding lesion

Paracentesis findings
    Blood, bile, pus, bowel contents, or urine

Reproduced, with permission, from Boey JH. Acute abdomen. In: Way LW, ed. *Current Surgical Diagnosis and Treatment,* 10th ed. Appleton & Lange, 1994.

and antacids as first-line treatment, proton pump inhibitors for treatment failures. Consider GI consultation for refractory cases.

4. **Pancreatitis.** Usually inpatient management unless very mild; complete bowel rest with IV fluids, NG tube suction, IV analgesia. Gallstone pancreatitis mandates surgical consult/admission (or GI consult for ERCP). Consider diabetes.

5. **Thoracic diseases.** Pneumonia, cardiac etiologies, PE. Manage accordingly.

6. **AAA/aortic dissection.** Get vascular surgery consult early, usually admission with operative management. High-risk patient for leaving ED for studies; use bedside ultrasound if available. (See Section VIII, 4. Bedside Ultrasound, p 424)

7. **Mesenteric ischemia, infarction.** Medical admission with surgical consult typical, depending on extent of disease; consider angiography.

8. **Diverticulitis.** If nonsurgical (no evidence of abscess or perforation), outpatient antibiotic management with pain control, or if pain intolerable, medical admission. Close follow-up to look for signs of developing abscess or perforation. If abscess or perforation present or suspected, IV antibiotics and surgical admission.

9. **Inflammatory bowel disease/irritable bowel.** Diagnosis rarely made in ED, usually falls under nonspecific abdominal pain unless diagnosis already established. Admit to hospital with GI consultation if patient has severe pain, unable to take fluids, or if diagnosis in question.

10. **Nonspecific abdominal pain.** A potential pitfall—if patient does not appear ill or toxic, and if exam not consistent with an acute process, consider discharge and reevaluation in 8–12 h in the ED. Beware of possible diagnoses being missed or patient's decompensating before follow-up. If there is any doubt, admit to medical or surgical service for observation and serial abdominal exams. An alternative to admission or discharge in worrisome patients is extended observation in either the ED or observation unit, if such resources are available. Be highly suspicious at extremes of age.

VI. **ICD-9 Diagnoses.** Abdominal pain (state which quadrant or location); Acute appendicitis—with rupture/abscess, acute cholecystitis, AAA, acute gastritis, ectopic pregnancy, mesenteric artery insufficiency, nephrolithiasis, acute pancreatitis, peptic acid disease, reflux esophagitis

VII. **Problem Case Diagnosis.** Acute appendicitis with perforation.

VIII. **Teaching Pearl Questions.** (1) What percentage of elderly patients (> 65 years) presenting with abdominal pain have an acute process requiring admission? (2) What percentage of elderly patients admitted through the ED with abdominal pain require an urgent or emergent operation?

IX. **Teaching Pearl Answers.** (1) > 50%, (2) > 33%.

REFERENCES

Graff LG, Robinson D. Abdominal pain and emergency department evaluation. *Emerg Med Clin North Am* 2001;19(1):123–136.

Kizer KW, Vassar MJ. Emergency department diagnosis of abdominal disorders in the elderly. *Am J Emerg Med* 1998;18(4):357–362.

Marco CA, Schoenfeld CN, Keyl PM, Menkes ED, Doehring MC. Abdominal pain in geriatric emergency patients: Variables associated with adverse outcomes. *Acad Emerg Med* 1998;5(12):1163–1168.

van Geloven AAW, Biesheuvel TH, Luitse JSK, Hoitsma HFW, Obertop H. Hospital admissions of patients aged Over 80 with acute abdominal complaints. *Eur J Surg* 2000;166(11):866–871.

2. ACID–BASE DISORDERS

I. **Problem.** A middle-aged alcoholic man with a seizure disorder presents to the ED with mild epigastric pain and vomiting for 12 h after his last beer. He has a 90-s grand mal seizure in triage and an ABG reveals a pH of 7.14.

II. **Immediate Questions**

    A. **Are the ABCs intact?** (Manage appropriately—See Section VIII, 15. Rapid Endotracheal Intubation, p 470)

    B. **What are the vital signs, level of consciousness and glucose?** A low serum glucose level can explain seizure activity, altered mental status.

    C. **Appear acutely ill?** Gasping respirations, cyanosis, altered mental status, and failure to respond appropriately to initial resuscitation effort all should suggest acid–base disturbance.

    D. **Recent trauma?** Head injury can lead to CNS pathology (subdural or epidural hematoma) that can cause mental status changes or seizures.

    E. **Has patient ingested ETOH or other substances?** (See Section V, 2. Alcohols, p 2)

    F. **Melena or hematemesis?**

    G. **Any family, friends, or witnesses that can provide additional information?**

III. **Differential Diagnosis of Acid–Base Disorder**

    A. **Is there an acid–base disorder? What type?**

TABLE I-A

		Respiratory	Metabolic
Acidosis	pH < 7.35	$Paco_2 > 45$	$HCO_3^- < 22$
Alkalosis	pH > 7.45	$Paco_2 < 35$	$HCO_3^- > 26$

B. Respiratory or metabolic? Mixed? Primary or secondary cause?
For every 10 mm Hg change of P_{CO_2}, pH should change 0.08 in the opposite direction. If measured pH does not equal calculated pH, a secondary acid–base problem exists. Respiratory acid–base disorders are caused by hypoventilation (acidosis) or hyperventilation (alkalosis). Metabolic acid–base problems are commonly attributed to the disorders of the kidneys but have many other causes. Mixed problems are common.

C. Specific Causes
    1. Anion gap metabolic acidosis
        A-lcoholic ketoacidosis
        M-ethanol
        U-remia
        D-iabetic ketoacidosis
        P-araldehyde
        I-soniazid, iron
        L-actic acidosis
        E-thylene glycol
        C-arbon monoxide
        A-spirin
        T-oluene
    2. Nonanion gap metabolic acidosis (check albumin level)
        F-istulas pancreatic or biliary
        P-yelonephritis
        U-reteral enteric fistulas/ureterosigmoidostomy
        S-aline, IV fluids
        E-ndocrine (hyperparathyroidism)
        D-iarrhea
        C-arbonic anhydrase inhibitors (acetazolamide), cholestyramine
        A-rginine HCl, hyperalimentation, ammonium Cl^- ingestion
        R-enal tubular acidosis
        S-pironolactone, sulfur
    3. Metabolic alkalosis (check albumin level)
        Saline responsive—urine $Cl^- < 10$
        Vomiting
        NG suctioning
        Postchronic hypercapnia
        Contraction alkalosis
        Diuretic therapy
        Saline resistant—urine $Cl^- > 20$
        Hypertensive
        Mineralocorticoid excess (hyperaldosteronism)
        Cushing's syndrome
        Renal artery stenosis
        Normotensive
        Hypokalemia
        Hypomagnesemia
        Bartter's syndrome

Licorice ingestion
Miscellaneous
HCO_3^- therapy
Acute alkali ingestion
Milk-alkali syndrome
Massive blood transfusion (citrate)
Cl⁻-wasting diarrhea
Hypoalbuminemia
4. **Respiratory acidosis**
Respiratory insufficiency or failure
Pulmonary edema
Laryngospasm
Myxedema
Foreign body aspiration
Mechanical ventilators; underventilation/leaks/human error
Obstructive sleep apnea
Chest wall trauma
Tension pneumothorax
Neuromuscular defects with chest wall or diaphragm involvement
Sedatives
General anesthetics
5. **Respiratory alkalosis**
Fever
Pain
Gram-negative sepsis
Thyrotoxicosis
Hypermetabolic states
Hepatic insufficiency
Hypoxemia
Early salicylate ingestion
Metabolic acidosis
Overventilation by mechanical ventilator
High altitudes

Appropriate Compensation

Metabolic acidosis $P_{CO_2} = [1.5 \times HCO_3] + 8 \pm 2$

Metabolic alkalosis $P_{CO_2} = [0.9 \times HCO_3] + 8 \pm 2$

Respiratory acidosis change in HCO_3

$= [0.1 \times \text{change in } P_{CO_3}] \times 4$

Respiratory alkalosis change in HCO_3

$= [0.1 \times \text{change in } P_{CO_2}] \times 2.5$

IV. **Database**
A. **Physical Examination Key Points**
1. **Mental status.** Mini mental status. (See Table A-4, p 658.)
2. **Vital signs.** Check carefully and monitor closely.

   3. Secondary survey examination. Observe for obvious abnormalities, evidence of track marks, trauma, infection.
   B. Laboratory Data. Chemistry panel and ABG should be drawn immediately, bedside glucose, CBC, LFTs, toxicology screen, UA. Consider testing for urine Lytes, serum osmolarity, and specific drug levels as indicated. Determine whether anion gap is present.
   C. Radiographic and Other Studies. CXR and 12-lead ECG are of limited value for assessing acid–base disturbances, but are readily available and can help identify related life-threatening problems.

V. Plan
   A. Overall Plan. Treat abnormalities identified on ABCs. If a specific precipitating cause is discovered for the acid–base disorder treat accordingly. Treat pH imbalance directly only if level approaches life–threatening numbers, such as pH < 7.10 or > 7.60. Don't rush to use $NaHCO_3$ because there are side effects, eg, hyperosmolarity.

VI. ICD-9 Diagnoses. Acidosis—metabolic or respiratory; Alkalosis—metabolic or respiratory; electrolyte imbalance; mixed acid–base disorder

VII. Problem Case Diagnosis. This patient has metabolic acidosis from an elevated anion gap caused by type A lactic acidosis from his seizure as well as alcoholic ketoacidosis from depletion of glycogen stores in a diseased liver. He may also have metabolic alkalosis from repetitive vomiting.

VIII. Teaching Pearl Questions
   1. How much time must elapse until the lactic acidosis of a grand mal seizure has cleared?
   2. What is the primary ketone produced in alcoholic (starvation) ketoacidosis?

IX. Teaching Pearl Answers
   1. 15–45 min for the lactic acid from a brief seizure.
   2. Beta-hydroxybutyrate. This is not usually measured in most hospital laboratories. The serum acetone and acetoacetate will actually increase as β-hydroxybutyrate is metabolized into these byproducts as the patient recovers. Alcoholic ketoacidosis treatment consists of administering IV fluids [D_5NS], thiamine, and food.

REFERENCES

Adrogue HJ, NE Madias. Management of life-threatening acid–base disorders. *N Engl J Med* 1998:338:26–34 and 107–111.
Gabow PA. Disorders associated with an altered anion gap. *Kidney Int* 1985,27:472–483.
Jourilles N. Acid–base disturbances. In: Silverstein S, Frommer D eds. *Management of Metabolic and Endocrine Disorders.* Aspen Press, 1988.
Rose BD. *Clinical Physiology of Acid–Base and Electrolyte Disorders,* 4th ed. McGraw-Hill 1994.

3. ALTERED MENTAL STATUS

I. **Problem.** 40-year-old male with bulging flanks, prominent veins on his abdomen and jaundice, is found by police wandering the streets at 4 AM disoriented and talking nonsense.

II. **Immediate Questions**
   A. **Is the airway intact?** Manage appropriately (see Section VIII, 15. Rapid Endotracheal Intubation, p 470.).
   B. **What is the oxygen saturation?** Begin oxygen.
   C. **What are the vitals and mental status?** Begin IV and monitoring.
   D. **What is the blood sugar?** Check bedside fingerstick (see Problem 23. Diabetic Problems, p 75).
   E. **Do you suspect alcoholism?** Give thiamine 100 mg IV.
   F. **Do you suspect opiate overdose?** Check for miosis and consider naloxone.
   G. **Get history** from friends, family, or EMS before they leave because patient is often unable to give adequate history. PMH, meds, drug abuse. Establish when patient was last at baseline mental status and quickness of change. Get details about the patient's baseline if elderly. History of trauma, drug exposure, environmental exposures.

III. **Differential Diagnosis**
   A. **Trauma.** (lateralizing signs) (See Section III. 3. Blunt Head Trauma, p 256)
      1. **Subarachnoid hemorrhage.** Sudden-onset headache (thunderclap) and retinal hemorrhages.
      2. **Epidural hematoma.** Trauma to the parietal-temporal area. Initial LOC, lucid interval, and progressive deterioration in mental status.
      3. **Subdural hematoma.** Have high index of suspicion in confused elderly or anyone on anticoagulation.
      4. **Concussion.**
   B. **Neurovascular**
      1. **Ischemic stroke.** Focal paralysis or paresis, dysarthria (See 65. Stroke/TIA, p 195.)
      2. **Hemorrhagic stroke.** (See 65. Stroke, TIA, p 195.)
      3. **Hypertensive encephalopathy.** (See 45. Hypertension, p 136.)
      4. **CNS vasculitis**
   C. **Cardiovascular**
      1. **AMI.** (See 15. Chest Pain/AMI/ACS, p 51.)
      2. **Dysrhythmia.** (See 11. Bradycardia, p 36, or 68. Tachycardia, p 202.) (See 67. Syncope, p 200.)
      3. **Hypotension.** (See 40. Hemorrhagic Shock, p 122, and 47. Hypotension, p 142.)
   D. **Neurologic**
      1. **Seizure or postictal state.** (See 60. Seizure, p 60.)
   E. **Infection**
      1. **CNS.** Meningitis or encephalitis. Fever, HA, mental status change.
      2. **Sepsis.** Fever and hypotension. (See 61. Sepsis, p 183.)

       3. Pneumonia

       4. UTI. Especially in the elderly.

  F. Major Organ Dysfunction

       1. Lung. Hypoxia or hypercarbia. (See Acid–Base Disorders) (Sec 58. Respiratory Distress, p 174.)

       2. Liver. Hepatic encephalopathy. Asterixis, fetor hepaticus, jaundice, ascites. (See 50. Jaundice, p 148)

       3. Kidney. Uremia. (See 24. Dialysis Patient Problems, p 79.)

  G. Metabolic (See Section IX. Fluids and Electrolytes. p 479)

       1. Hypernatremia or hyponatremia

       2. Dehydration

       3. Hyperglycemia or hypoglycemia (See 23. Diabetic Problems, p 75.)

       4. Hyperthyroid or hypothyroid

       5. Hyperthermia or hypothermia (see 46. Hyperthermia, p 139, or 48. Hypothermia, p 144.)

  H. Toxic. (See Section V. Common Toxicologic Emergency Problems, p 316.)

       1. Street drugs (narcotics, hallucinogens, etc)

       2. ETOH intoxication or withdrawal

       3. Carbon monoxide poisoning

       4. Anticholinergic poisoning. (See Section V, 4. Anticholinergic Poisoning, p 328, or 14. Organophosphate Poisoning, p 353.)

       5. Serotonin syndrome

       6. Other OTC/prescription OD

  I. Other

       1. Tumor or abscess. Papilledema and focal neurologic deficit.

       2. Dementia. Alzheimer's or cerebrovascular types. Get history from family on onset and duration of changes and patient's baseline. (See Section IV. 6. Functional Decline, p 310.)

       3. Neuroleptic malignant syndrome. Hyperthermia, rigidity, autonomic instability. (See 46. Hyperthermia, p 46.)

  J. Psychiatric. Seek other causes first. (See 57. Psychiatric Problems, p 57.)

       1. Depression

       2. Psychogenic coma

       3. Schizophrenia

IV. Database

  A. Physical Exam Key Points

       1. Vital signs. Pulse oximetry and blood sugar.

       2. General. Gross abnormalities. Signs of trauma.

       3. Mental status exam. GCS and/or Mini Mental Status Exam (See Table A-4, p 658.)

       4. Head and neck. Check for trauma (remember C-spine if appropriate) and nuchal rigidity. Bruits.

       5. Eyes. Miosis or lateralizing signs, scleral icterus, photophobia, papilledema or hemorrhages.

       6. Tongue. Laceration may be from seizure.

       7. CV. Rate, rhythm. S_3.

8. **Lungs.** Air exchange, crackles, rhonchi, wheezes. Focal abnormalities.
9. **Chest and abdomen.** Check for ascites, caput medusa, spider angiomata.
10. **Rectal.** Bleeding.
11. **Extremities.** Pitting edema.
12. **Skin.** Jaundice, rash, or needle marks.
13. **Neurologic.** Focal deficits or cerebellar deficits (ataxia). Asterixis.

B. **Laboratory Data.** History and physical should guide lab evaluation. In addition to blood glucose, ABG, CBC + Diff, BMP, LFTs, INR/aPTT, cardiac enzymes, urine tox screen, UA.
   1. **Hepatic encephalopathy.** Ammonia levels.
   2. **Thyroid disease.** TSH.
   3. **Seizure.** Antiseizure medicine levels if appropriate.
   4. **Toxicologic.** Salicylate and acetaminophen levels.
   5. **Febrile.** Blood, urine, and CSF analysis. (See Section VIII, 10. Lumbar Puncture, p 459.)
   6. **Neuroleptic malignant syndrome.** Calcium, CK, level

C. **Radiographic and Other Studies.** ECG, CXR, head CT, LP, EEG.

V. **Plan**

A. **Overall Plan.** Identify immediate life threats or any quickly reversible causes. Stabilize patient in preparation for admission. Follow ABCs. Almost all patients will be admitted unless cause is fully explained, reversible in ED, and patient is not at risk for increased morbidity or mortality upon discharge from the ED.

B. **Specific Plans in Addition to Admission**
   1. **Increased ICP, subarachnoid hemorrhage, epidural hematoma, or subdural hematoma.** Call early for neurosurgical consult. Consider ICP monitor, hyperventilation, mannitol, and elevating head of bed.
   2. **Cerebral hemorrhage of any type.** Lower blood pressure to premorbid levels. Call for neurosurgical consult.
   3. **Ischemic stroke.** Careful not to lower BP more than approximately 20% for fear of creating ischemic damage to parts of the brain from too rapid lowering of perfusion pressure. Follow hospital protocol for strokes.
   4. **HTN.** Assess for end-organ damage. Papilledema, mental status, pulmonary edema, kidney function, ECG, cardiac enzymes. Head CT. Careful not to lower BP more than approximately 20%. Assess for pregnancy-induced HTN. (See 45. Hypertension, p 136, and 56. Pregnancy Problems, p 168.)
   5. **Seizures.** If in status epilepticus, use lorazepam IV to abort. Consider loading dose of phenytoin 18 mg/kg IV with ECG and BP monitoring. (See 60. Seizure, p 180.)
   6. **AMI.** Aspirin, oxygen, nitroglycerin, morphine, metoprolol, heparin. Consider PTCA vs IV thrombolytics if patient meets criteria. Follow hospital protocol and call for cardiology consult. (See 15. Chest Pain, p 51.)

      7. Dysrhythmia. Stabilize if unstable. (See 11. Bradycardia, p 36, or 68. Tachycardia, p 202.)

      8. Infections. Begin appropriate antibiotics as soon as infection is identified or as soon as suspected if life-threatening.

      9. Toxic ingestion or exposure. (See Section V. Common Toxicologic Emergency Problems, p 316.)

   10. Metabolic. Treat accordingly.

   11. Neuroleptic malignant syndrome. Fluid resuscitation, manage BP, benzodiazepines, bromocriptine, and dantrolene.

   12. Psychiatric. Rule out other life threats first. Consider psychiatric explanations after other possibilities. For psychogenic coma, try dropping the patient's hand on the face to help with diagnosis. Psychiatry consult. Protective observation until disposition arranged.

C. Consider Discharge after appropriate treatment and observation if patient returns to baseline. Provide treatment instructions as well as criteria that require return to the ED. Make sure patient has way to follow up.

    1. Known epileptic with seizure. Load with antiseizure medicine and provide prescription. Patient not seizing during observation period.

    2. Minor concussion with return to baseline mental status.

    3. Carbon monoxide poisoning which is mild and returning to safe environment (eg, friend or family's home). Treated immediately with 100% oxygen for at least 4 h.

    4. Opioid or ETOH toxicity with clearing in the ED. Responsible adult accompanying the patient on discharge if uncertain mental status.

    5. Dementia mistaken for an acute change. Must confirm history. Best to have family present and discharge patient to family's care or to skilled nursing facility with family's consent. (See Appendix 5. Distinguishing Delirium, Dementia, Psychoses, p 659.)

VI. ICD-9 Diagnoses.

VII. Problem Diagnosis. Hepatic encephalopathy.

VIII. Teaching Pearls Question. With regard to carbon monoxide toxicity, what is the half-life of HbCO at room air, normobaric 100% oxygen, and hyperbaric 100% oxygen at 2.8 atm?

IX. Teaching Pearls Answer. 320 min at room air, 60 min at 100% normobaric oxygen, and 23 min hyperbaric oxygen.

REFERENCES

American College of Emergency Physicians. Clinical policy for the initial approach to patients presenting with altered mental status *Ann Emerg Med* 1999;33:251–281.

Ferrera PC, Chan LS. Initial management of the patient with altered mental status. *Am Fam Physician* 1997;55:1773–1780.

Lawrence CG, Nadel ES, Silvers SM, Brown DF. Acute change in mental status. *J Emerg Med* 2001;21(2):179–182.

O'Keefe KP, Sanson TG. Elderly patients with altered mental status. *Emerg Med Clin North Am* 1998;16(4),702–714.

4. ALTITUDE ILLNESS

I. **Problem.** A previously healthy 35-year-old male becomes increasingly lethargic and confused during a rest day at 4000 m above sea level while trekking in Nepal.

II. **Immediate Questions**
   A. **ABCs intact?**
   B. **Vital signs and mental status?** Pulse oximetry and full vitals (remember temperature and orthostatics); Mental status.
   C. **Trauma?**
   D. **Immediate Interventions.** O_2 to keep SaO_2 above 90 mm Hg on all patients.
   E. **Focused History.** Question observers/companions in addition to patient (often unresponsive or unreliable).
   F. **Altitude history?** Too rapid a rate of ascent? Focus on nightly sleep elevations (*Typical recommendation:* Average gain of 300–400 m/night, with additional no-gain night for every 1000–1200 m of ascent); Previous problems at altitude?
   G. **Onset/history of illness?** Early symptoms and rate of progression. Anything atypical of altitude illness?
   H. **Chronic illnesses?** Causative, complicating, or noncontributory to symptoms?
   I. **Meds/ETOH/recreational drugs?** What is used/abused chronically? What was taken/omitted leading up to illness?
   J. **Allergies?**
   K. **Immunization history?** Especially in developing world.

III. **Differential Diagnosis**
   A. **Nonaltitude/Hypoxia Illness.** Although altitude/hypoxia illness should be strongly considered given suggestive symptoms during ascent to high altitude (2000–2500+ m), still consider it a diagnosis of exclusion because any illness can present at altitude. Consider overexertion; dehydration; hypothermia; migraine; tension headache; URI; sinusitis; gastroenteritis; CVA; structural CNS pathology; CO toxicity (cooking in enclosed space); systemic illness with few localizing symptoms (eg, malaria, typhoid, meningitis, dengue fever, hepatitis, DKA, hypoglycemia, electrolyte imbalance, thyroid or adrenal disease); intoxication or withdrawal; psychiatric illness.
   B. **Altitude/Hypoxia Illness**
   C. **Acute Mountain Sickness (AMS).** Diagnostic criteria include headache, plus at least one of the following four symptom complexes: anorexia/nausea; fatigue/weakness; dizziness/lightheadedness; sleep disturbance. Some include changes in mood/mental status or dyspnea in diagnostic spectrum, but if significant, these suggest HACE or HAPE.
   D. **High-Altitude Cerebral Edema (HACE).** Diagnostic criteria include ataxia or mental status changes (confusion, delusions, hallucinations,

agitation, combativeness, stupor or coma) in patient with AMS or HAPE; headache, N/V and lethargy common; occasional blurred vision, diplopia, photophobia, meningismus. Signs include papilledema, retinal hemorrhage, ataxia, occasionally meningismus, extraocular muscle paresis, abnormal reflexes.

E. High-Altitude Pulmonary Edema (HAPE). Noncardiogenic, due to hypoxic pulmonary vasoconstriction and hydrostatic capillary endothelial damage with microvascular leak; dyspnea, cough (occasionally productive of white to pink frothy sputum), chest tightness, weakness, exercise intolerance are common. Orthopnea unusual. Signs include tachypnea, tachycardia, crackles, cyanosis, low-grade fever; Sao_2 generally below 75% (variable to normal range decreases with altitude, improves with acclimatization; comparisons with asymptomatic acclimatizers useful); desaturation with exercise may precede resting hypoxia.

F. High-Altitude Retinal Hemorrhage (HARH). May cause transient scotomata. Typically resolves with descent.

IV. Database

 A. Physical Exam Key Points. Careful exam for other causes.

 B. Mental Status. AMS/HACE spectrum from mild disinterest to frank psychosis and coma. Mini mental status exam for subtle abnormalities; do serial exams.

 C. Vital Signs. Hypoxia, mild temperature elevation, tachycardia, and tachypnea are typical of HAPE; BP often elevated, but in severe cases hypotension may occur. Orthostatics to evaluate hydration. Reevaluate frequently, as illness may progress rapidly, and treatment may alter vitals significantly.

 D. Funduscopic. Retinal hemorrhages (often incidental at altitude). Papilledema suggests HACE.

 E. Neck. Mild meningismus with HACE.

 F. Chest. Crackles, usually initially perihilar or basilar (often in right axilla or subscapular region), then generalized. Wheezes may indicate HAPE, but predominance of expiratory sounds more suggestive of bronchitis/pneumonia (may coexist with/predispose to HAPE).

 G. Cardiovascular. Dysrhythmia, loud/new murmurs, or S_3 gallop more suggestive of cardiac disease. Signs of RV strain (heave and accentuated pulmonary second sound) consistent with HAPE. Mild edema often incidentally present (legs, hands, face), but JVP generally normal.

 H. Skin. Central cyanosis in severe HAPE.

 I. Neurologic. Mental status changes and ataxia on tandem gait or sitting up (truncal ataxia) typical in HACE. Occasionally, extraocular muscle palsy, increased tendon jerks, and extensor plantar reflexes in HACE.

 J. Laboratory Data. Generally not available or necessary at altitude. Arterial blood gases usually reveal low Po_2 and Pco_2, elevated A-a gradient. WBC typically mildly elevated in HAPE. CSF typically normal aside from increased opening pressures in HACE. Glucose,

Lytes, cardiac injury markers, and drug levels may be useful to rule out other causes.
- **K. Radiographic and Other Studies.** CXR in HAPE reveals patchy infiltrates, generally perihilar, without cardiomegaly. X-ray findings may lag behind clinical exam. ECG may reveal right-heart strain pattern, but no evidence of acute primary cardiac pathology. Brain imaging in HACE or advanced AMS may show cerebral edema (MRI is most sensitive, with perivascular edema most typically in splenium of corpus callosum).

V. Plan
- **A. Overall Plan.** Immediate O_2 to reverse hypoxia; DESCENT critical in HAPE/HACE—although O_2 and hyperbaric treatment may actually reverse symptoms at a given altitude, all therapies should be considered temporizing measures, with descent being curative.
- **B. Specific Plans**
  1. **AMS.** Halt ascent if symptomatic. Extra rest day if symptoms mild, descend if symptoms intolerable or possible early HACE. General measures, eg, adequate hydration, rest, and analgesics/antiemetics may treat symptoms. Aspirin/ibuprofen proven effective for prophylaxis and treating altitude-related headache, respectively. Acetaminophen/paracetamol reasonable alternative. Avoid medications that depress respiratory drive. Acetazolamide (Diamox) 250 mg bid for treatment, or prophylaxis if unavoidable rapid ascent or prior acclimatization problems (125 mg bid empirically effective for prophylaxis and mild symptoms and better tolerated, but not studied). Acetazolamide also decreases nighttime periodic breathing and improves sleep, probably effective in doses as low as 125 mg qhs; Dexamethasone also effective AMS prophylaxis/treatment, but does not aid acclimatization, associated with rebound symptoms and more serious side effects—best reserved for treatment of severe symptoms and HACE (along with descent). Recent studies revealed therapeutic effect of Gingko biloba in doses of 80–120 mg bid
  2. **HACE.** Supplemental O_2. Dexamethasone 8 mg IM/PO initially, then 4 mg q6h. Hyperbaric treatment (portable altitude chamber or Gamov bag) also effective and does not require O_2 source. Drawbacks include difficulty with uncooperative patients (HACE/HAPE patients often claustrophobic or combative), and inability to access patient quickly to protect airway/ventilate in event of vomiting or respiratory arrest. DESCEND ASAP.
  3. **HAPE.** Supplemental O_2. Nifedipine 10–20 mg SR PO q8–12h has modest effect on oxygenation (SL route often recommended, but hypotensive complications may occur, particularly in severe cases). Inhaled beta agonists promising, but not well studied. Hyperbaric treatment as for HACE, and DESCENT. Avoid exertion, as exercise increases hypoxia and PAP, worsening clinical illness (nifedipine significantly protects against these effects).

      4. **HARH.** Usually spontaneous resolution within days or weeks following descent. No effective treatment except descent, which should be considered if visual acuity is significantly impaired.

VI. ICD-9 Diagnoses. High-altitude effect (same as "mountain sickness"), alkalosis (respiratory, metabolic), alteration of consciousness, dehydration, dizziness, electrolyte disorder, headache, hypoxia/hypoxemia, acute pulmonary edema, SOB.

VII. Problem Case Diagnosis. High-altitude cerebral edema.

VIII. Teaching Pearls Questions. What percentage of people presenting with HAPE also have AMS or HACE? What percentage with HACE have HAPE?

IX. Teaching Pearls Answers. Half of HAPE patients have AMS; 14% have HACE. Approximately one third of HACE patients have HAPE.

REFERENCES

Hackett P, Oelz O. The Lake Louise consensus on the definition and quantification of altitude illness. In *Hypoxia and Mountain Medicine.* Sutton J, Coates G, Houston C, eds. Queen City Printers, 1992:327–330.
Hackett PH, Roach RC. High-altitude illness. *N Engl J Med* 2001:345:107–114.
Hultgren HN. *High Altitude Medicine.* Hultgren Publications, 1997.

5. ANAPHYLAXIS

  I. Problem. Middle-aged female becomes short of breath after eating at a buffet.

  II. Immediate Questions
    A. Is the airway intact? Is oral swelling present? Apply oxygen, intubate if indicated (See Section VIII. 15. Rapid Sequence Endotracheal Intubation, p 470). Avoid paralysis if possible. Glottic opening may be narrow because of swelling. If intubation is unsuccessful, edema may prevent air entry via bagging.
    B. What are the vital signs? Apply monitors (ECG and pulse ox), start IV.
    C. Is urticaria present? Helps make diagnosis, but not always present.
    D. What was the precipitant? Medications (antibiotics. NSAIDs), Hymenoptera venom, food (seafood, nut, soy, or beer ingestion), contrast medium, latex gloves, vaccines.
    E. Any past medical history? History of allergic reactions or anaphylaxis? Did the patient use an epinephrine autoinjector?

  III. Differential Diagnosis
    A. Anaphylaxis. Allergic reaction including CV or respiratory compromise (or both). Includes both IgE and non-IgE-mediated (previously called anaphylactoid).

    B. Hereditary Angioedema. Angioedema of skin, upper airway, and gut, often simulating acute abdomen.

    C. ACE inhibitors. Causes angioedema of the tongue and palate.

    D. Scombroid. Poisoning from spoiled fish. N/V, headache, urticaria.

    E. Carcinoid Syndrome. Flushing, hypotension, GI disturbance. Precipitated by ETOH.

    F. Panic Disorder. Forced adduction of the vocal cords causes stridor.

IV. Database

A. Physical Exam Key Points

1. **Vital signs.** Repeat frequently. Look for tachypnea and tachycardia. Hypotension occurs from vasodilation and increased capillary permeability.
2. **HEENT.** Look for edema of the lips, eyes, uvula, tongue, and oropharynx. Conjunctivitis, rhinitis may be present.
3. **Respiratory.** Check for stridor or wheezing from bronchospasm.
4. **Skin.** Urticaria, angioedema.

B. Laboratory Data.
ABG, CBC, Lytes, bedside glucose, coagulation panel. Consider cardiac enzymes for myocardial ischemia from hypovolemia, hypoxia, and epinephrine. Blood cultures, thyroid and cortisol tests, tox screen, as indicated.

C. Radiographic and Other Studies.
ECG (look for sinus tachycardia, PACs, PVCs, AF, VT, ST-T wave changes), CXR.

V. Plan

A. Overall Plan.
Remove antigen if possible (stinger). Place patient in position of comfort. Oxygen, cardiac, and temperature monitoring. High-flow oxygen. Airway management. Fluid resuscitation with NS. (See following section.)

B. Specific Plans

1. **Airway management.** High-flow oxygen via mask immediately. Consider semielective intubation of patients with hoarseness or lingual or oropharyngeal swelling, who do not respond to initial treatment. Perform awake, sedated intubation without paralytics if possible. (see Section VIII, 15. Rapid Endotracheal Intubation, p 470.). If angioedema prevents intubation in a patient with impending respiratory failure, use alternative airway techniques such as fiberoptic tracheal intubation, digital tracheal intubation, needle cricothyroidotomy, or cricothyroidotomy.
2. **Administer epinephrine for all patients with airway swelling, respiratory distress, or clinical evidence of shock.** For swelling of lips, tongue, uvula, soft palate in the absence of shock: administer intramuscular or SQ epinephrine 0.3–0.5 mg (1:1000). Note that absorption of SQ epinephrine may be delayed with shock. For severe anaphylaxis as evidenced by profound hypotension or imminent airway obstruction: administer epinephrine 0.1–0.5 mg (1:10,000) diluted in 10 mL NS and given over 5 min. May also use

an epinephrine drip (1 mg/250 mL D₅W [4 μg/mL] at 1–4 μg/min). Consider high-dose epinephrine for patients in cardiac arrest.

3. **Second-line medications (mandatory).** *Antihistamine:* diphenhydramine 25–50 mg IV, IM, or PO. *Corticosteroids:* methylprednisolone 125 mg IV.

4. **H₂ blocker (recommended).** Cimetidine 300 mg IV, IV, or PO. Use famotidine 20 mg IV or ranitidine 50 mg IV if patient on β-blockers.

5. **Fluid resuscitation.** Rapid administration of 2–4 L of isotonic crystalloid as indicated (anaphylaxis may cause profound vasodilation)

6. **Vasopressors** may be indicated for blood pressure support. (*Final note on medications:* If patient is taking a β-blocker, epinephrine many have net α-adrenergic effect. Glucagon 1–2 mg IV every 5 min may be effective. Also may consider terbutaline 0.25 mg IV.)

7. **Observe all patients** closely for up to 24 h. Symptoms may recur despite an intervening asymptomatic period.

VI. **ICD-9 Diagnoses.** Anaphylaxis (same as anaphylactic shock/reaction). State whether due to food, specified drug, sting, allergic reaction. Angioedema—allergic or urticaria.

VII. **Problem Case Diagnosis.** Anaphylaxis triggered by peanuts ingested in eggroll.

VIII. **Teaching Pearl Question.** What percent of patients with serious anaphylactic reactions from insect stings will have systemic reactions on resting?

IX. **Teaching Pearl Answer.** Approximately 60%. (Reisman)

REFERENCES

American Heart Association. Anaphylaxis. Advanced challenges in resuscitation. *Resuscitation* 2000;46:285–288.

Cianferoni AC, Novembre E, Mugnaini L et al. Clinical features of acute anaphylaxis in patients admitted to a university hospital: An 11-year retrospective review (1985–1996). *Ann Allergy Asthma Immunol* 2001;87:27–32.

Reisman RE. Natural history of insect sting allergy: Relationship of severity of sting anaphylaxis to re-sting reactions. *J Allergy Clin Immunol* 1992;90:335–339.

6. ANEURYSMS

I. **Problem.** An elderly male has sudden chest and thoracic back pain that causes him to fall to his knees and become diaphoretic. Twenty minutes after onset, the pain suddenly disappears.

II. **Immediate Questions**

A. **Are there any deficits on primary survey exam?** Airway and breathing examinations should be performed as in all patients. Circulation exam may reveal an aortic murmur, distant heart sounds, and pulse deficits in the extremities. Stroke symptoms, including spinal cord stroke symptoms, may be present. Diffuse mental status changes may accompany a thoracic dissecting aneurysm.

B. What initial therapy is required? Large-bore IV access, supplemental oxygen, and cardiac monitoring is required. Abnormal blood pressures must be carefully monitored and treated.

C. What diagnostic studies are initially required? ECG and CXR must be promptly performed. Abdominal radiography may be helpful. Laboratory studies to prepare the patient for operation should be immediately performed (coagulation studies, Lytes, and hematocrit).

D. Additional History. Atherosclerotic risk factors and a history of connective tissue disease or valvular disease should be determined. Other pertinent history will vary as the manifestations of an aneurysm vary. CNS, intrathoracic, and intra-abdominal disorders will all be potential differential diagnoses.

III. Differential Diagnosis

A. Cardiovascular

1. **Aortic dissections** will most often begin in the thoracic aorta. Most will present abruptly and have severe pain in the chest or pain in the back between the scapulae. Neurologic symptoms occur commonly. Abdominal or flank pain may occur with dissection into the abdominal aorta. Patients often present with a dissection in progress and pain patterns may change with the changing anatomy of the dissection. Aortic insufficiency as well as pericardial effusion and tamponade may occur with proximal dissection.

2. **Thoracic aorta aneurysms** are commonly found by routine CXR but may be symptomatic if they compress adjacent structures.

3. **AAA** also commonly present on routine examination, however, they present with sudden abdominal or back pain. Syncope may occur with the abrupt injury of the aorta. Chronic contained ruptures can occur rarely.

4. **Other large arteries** (eg, splenic and ileac arteries) may also become aneurysmal and rupture.

5. **Other cardiovascular differential diagnoses** include valvular heart disease, CAD, and pericardial disease.

B. Noncardiovascular

1. **Mediastinal or pleural disease** may give pain that is similar to aortic dissection pain. Esophageal or tracheal disease may give symptoms that are similar to the compressive symptoms of a thoracic aorta aneurysm. Differential diagnoses for aortic aneurysms include all causes of abdominal pain, back pain, shock, and syncope. Because the aorta is retroperitoneal, other structures such as kidney and pancreas may give pain that is similar to aortic aneurysmal pain.

IV. Database

A. Physical Exam Key Points

1. **Vital signs.** A patient with hypotension may be in extremis soon.
2. **Cardiovascular exam is required.** Because aneurysms are a disease of the vessels, pulses must be documented in all four extremities. In addition, heart sounds with attention to pericardial and aortic valve findings need to be documented. Abdominal exam must include palpation for potential aneurysms of the aorta. Exam alone cannot rule out aneurysmal disease.
3. **Neurologic exam.** Check for evidence of CVA and spinal stroke signs.

B. Laboratory Data.
CBC, coagulation studies, electrolyte measurements, and cardiac enzymes should all be obtained.

C. Radiographic and Other Studies.
CXR will reveal nearly all thoracic aorta aneurysms and most dissecting aneurysms. However, dissections may give only a diffuse dilation of the mediastinal shadow and therefore the abnormality may be subtle. Plain films of the abdomen may reveal calcification of an abnormal aortic contour. CT scanning with a rapid IV bolus of contrast medium has a high sensitivity and specificity for thoracic aneurysms. Angiography is commonly considered a gold standard for aortic anatomy. In experienced hands, a TEE may be both sensitive and specific for thoracic aneurysm. Abdominal aneurysms may be reliably found with both CT scans and a technically adequate sonogram. (See Section VIII, 4. Bedside Ultrasound, p 424.)

V. Plan

A. Overall Plan.
Symptomatic patients with aneurysmal disease need prompt surgical evaluation. Some AAA patients may require emergent laparotomy without a radiographic study. BP must be carefully managed. Shock should be aggressively treated, however; if possible, excess IV fluids should be avoided. Surgical consultants should always be notified in patients with likely aneurysm rupture before radiologic studies obtained.

B. Specific Plans.
For patients with suspected dissection and HTN administer agents, eg, β-blockers or some calcium channel blockers, that can reliably decrease the shear force on the vessel. Vasodilators should not be utilized alone but may be used in conjunction with β-blockers.

VI. ICD-9 Diagnoses.
Aneurysm (state dissecting or ruptured if applicable and specific site); Abdominal aortic aneurysm; Aortic aneurysm (state ascending, descending, arch, thoracoabdominal); Dissecting aortic aneurysm; Syphilitic aneurysm; Thoracic aortic aneurysm.

VII. Problem Case Diagnosis.
Dissecting aneurysm of the ascending and descending thoracic aorta.

VIII. Teaching Pearls Question. Why did the patient in this problem case become pain-free?

IX. Teaching Pearls Answer. "Spontaneous cure" may occur with dissection back into the lumen of the native vessel through the intima. These patients are still at great risk of vessel rupture.

REFERENCES

Chen K, Varon J, Wenker OC et al. Acute thoracic aortic dissection: The basics. *J Emerg Med* 1997;15(6):859–867.

Cigarroa JE, Isselbacher EM, DeSanctis RW et al. Medical progress: Diagnostic imaging in the evaluation of suspected aortic dissection—old standards and new directions. *N Engl J Med* 1993;328:35–43.

7. ANXIETY

I. **Problem.** A 30-year-old female complains of a racing heart, SOB, light-headedness, sweating, numbness, paresthesias, and a sense of doom.

II. **Immediate Questions**
- A. **What are the vitals?** Apply monitors (ECG and pulse ox). Start IV, apply oxygen if vitals are abnormal.
- B. **What is the predominate symptom?** *Palpitations?* Dysrhythmia, drug, hyperthyroid. *Chest pain?* AMI or dissection. *Pleuritic CP?* PE, spontaneous PTX, pericarditis. *Dyspnea?* Asthma, PE, myocarditis. *Near syncope?* PE or dysrhythmia. *Panic, a sense of loss of control or going crazy?* Panic attack.
- C. **How did the symptoms begin?** *Sudden?* Consider PE, dysrhythmia panic attack. *With exertion?* CAD, valvular disorder, HOCM, or asthma. *At rest?* PE, dysrhythmia, panic attack? *After a meal or drug ingestion?* Food toxin or drug side effects. *After a stressful event?* AMI, panic attack. *History of drug abuse or withdrawal?* See section on Drug Intoxication and Withdrawal.
- D. **Risk factors for PE?** Previous PE, pregnancy, postpartum, smoking plus OCPs, lower extremity trauma, immobilization, family history of PE?
- E. **Risk factors for dysrhythmia?** Known cardiac disease, prolonged QT, or QT interval drugs (class IA, IC, antihistamines, phenothiazines, cyclic antidepressants), caffeine?
- F. **Risk factors for early CAD?** FH, high cholesterol, DM, HTN, smoker, Kawasaki's disease.
- G. **Risk factors for panic disorder?** Age < 40 (consider other diagnosis if patient > 40 years). Female (prevalence 2×). Separated or divorced. ETOH or drug abuse. Family history. Other psychiatric disorders.

III. Differential Diagnosis

A. Respiratory. Distress is *always* episodic with panic attacks.
  1. **Asthma.** Wheezing, poor air exchange, elevated peak flow.
  2. **Pulmonary embolism.** Causes SOB, hyperventilation, and anxiety. Consider with hypoxia or any risk factors. Can recur.

B. Cardiovascular
  1. **MI or angina pectoris.** Predominant symptom is chest pain or pressure, onset with exertion. Risk factor for early CAD.
  2. **Cardiac dysrhythmia.** If patient symptomatic in the ED most dysrhythmias will be evident on an ECG.
  3. **MVP.** Can be associated with panic disorder and is most often functional when it is. Anatomically significant with Marfan's syndrome.

C. Endocrine
  1. **Hypoglycemia.** History of DM? A normal glucose level with symptoms rules it out.
  2. **Hyperthyroidism.** Episodic anxiety that closely mimics panic attacks but also heat intolerance, hot skin, tachycardia, diarrhea, weight loss, proptosis.
  3. **Pheochromocytoma.** Half of patients with pheochromocytoma have anxiety attacks as well as headache, flushing, HTN, diarrhea, crushing back pain, and whole body sweats.

D. Neurologic
  1. **Seizure.** Some temporal lobe seizures present as anxiety, anger, or personality change. Fearfulness is the predominate symptom in up to 60% of partial complex seizures.
  2. **Combined systemic disease (posterolateral sclerosis).** Vitamin B_{12} deficiency can cause anxiety, panic, paresthesias, weakness, and hyperreflexia. Hyperventilation can occur with severe pernicious anemia.

E. Drug Intoxication and Withdrawal
  1. **Caffeine, cocaine, amphetamines, sympathomimetics, ma huang, yohimbine, amyl nitrate, cannabis, LSD, and khat in large amounts or chronic abuse can induce panic attacks.**
  2. **ETOH or sedative withdrawal.** ETOH withdrawal produces recurrent panic attacks in up to 80% of male alcoholics. Patients with anxiety or panic disorder have a higher rate of substance abuse. The intermediate acting sedatives cause the worst withdrawal symptoms.

F. Psychiatric
  1. **Panic attack.** This is *always* a *diagnosis of exclusion*. Strongly consider in patients with risk factors, normal exam and no other identifiable cause and fits the DSM IV-TR criteria (sudden onset, peaks within 10 min, 4–13 typical somatic or cognitive symptoms). Can occur unexpectedly or secondary to ingested substance, medical condition, or other psychiatric disorder.
  2. **Panic disorder.** *Recurrent (at least 2), unexpected* panic attacks followed by at least 1 month of apprehension over repeat attack

or significant behavioral change (panic disorder may occur with or without agoraphobia). Panic attacks are NOT due to a substance, medical condition or other psych dx.

3. **Mania** can present as dysphoria, irritability, anxiety, and panic attack in either manic or depressed state.
4. **Depression.** 20% of patients with major depression have panic attacks.
5. **Somatization disorder.** People with this disorder claim to have most symptoms they are questioned about.
6. **Generalized anxiety disorder.** Patients may have panic attacks but predominantly have uncontrollable worry about every day problems.
7. **Phobias and OCD** can be associated with panic attacks. In a phobic disorder, panic occurs only in relation to the specific phobia (in social phobias, panic is only connected with social situations).
8. **Posttraumatic stress disorder** can be associated with panic attacks. Panic attacks occur only when reexperiencing prior trauma. Later uncued panic attacks can occur.
9. **Schizophrenia-related** panic attacks are common especially early in the disease.

IV. Database
A. Physical Exam Key Points
General. Patients with PE may simply appear anxious.
1. **Vital signs.** SVT? HTN and tachycardia (sympathomimetic syndrome). Low-grade fever, hypoxia and/or tachycardia (PE).
2. **Conjunctiva and oral mucous membranes.** Pale (anemia) ETOH odor?
3. **Neck.** JVD? (large PE).
4. **Lungs.** Check for wheezing, retractions (asthma) or decreased breath sounds (PTX).
5. **Heart.** Hyperdynamic, (drugs, hyperthyroid, panic) accentuated pulmonic component of S_2 (PE), midsystolic click (MVP) pericardial rub (pericarditis)? S_4 (AMI).
6. **Neurologic.** Mydriasis and hyperreflexia (sympathomimetics), resting tremor (hyperthyroid, sedative-hypnotic and ETOH withdrawal panic attack).
7. **Psychologic.** Pacing, fidgety, posturing, red face, hallucinations.
8. **Skin.** Piloerection and diaphoresis (sympathomimetics, sedative-hypnotic and ETOH withdrawal), palmar sweating (panic attack), diaphoretic and hot (hyperthyroid).
9. **Extremities.** Calf tenderness, ankle edema, palpable cord (PE).

B. Laboratory Data.
If the patient has a history of panic disorder and presents with the same symptom constellation, minimal labs or none are required. If history or physical is suggestive, consider CBC and glucose or TSH.

C. Radiographic and Other Studies.
A normal ECG does not exclude all cardiac causes but can be reassuring to both patient and physi-

cian. Consider a CXR if prominent or pleuritic chest pain, abnormal O_2 saturation or lung exam. Consider spiral CT or VQ scan if risk factors or physical exam suggestive of PE. Very rarely does a patient require an echocardiogram or head CT.

V. Plan

A. Overall Plan. If PE or AMI cannot reasonably be excluded, based on history or studies in the ED, admission should be considered. Suicidality should be addressed, and the patient admitted if they are at risk. If the patient appears to have significant addiction or withdrawal symptoms a psychiatrist should be consulted or patient admitted to a detox facility. Patient should be instructed to avoid stimulants and ETOH.

B. Specific Plans

  1. **Isolated panic attacks.** One or two isolated panic attack does NOT suffice for the diagnosis of panic disorder and does not necessarily require medication.

  2. **New-onset panic disorder.** Short course of benzodiazepine (Lorazepam 0.25–1 mg PO bid). Alprazolam (Xanax) is shorter acting and more addicting but efficacious in a large trial. Give a test dose of 0.5–1.0 mg PO/IM in the ED. Low dose in elderly, dementia, traumatic brain injury, etc. Avoid if history of addiction. Benzodiazepines can cause disinhibition, respiratory depression, and ataxia.

     An SSRI at ½–⅓ the antidepressant dose (citalopram 10-mg, fluoxetine 5–10 mg, sertraline 25–50 mg, or paroxetine 10 mg/d) or a low-dose TCA (imipramine or clomipramine 10–25 mg/d) can be started in the ED but should be ordered in consultation with the follow-up physician. Anxious patients tend to experience more side effects and may C/O being "sensitive" medications. Start low and go slow.

     Referral to a psychiatrist or primary care physician is recommended. Psychotherapy, education, and reassurance for both the patient and family are important. Patients should be told that they have a well-defined, common syndrome that is treatable and that they are not going crazy.

  2. **Known diagnosis of panic disorder with similar symptoms.** Reassurance of diagnosis and referral back to patient's psychiatrist or primary care physician. Adjust medication in consultation with referral physician.

VI. ICD-9 Diagnoses.
Acute stress reaction; Anxiety; Drug-induced anxiety; Hyperthyroidism; Hyperventilation; Hypoxia; Mania; Panic attack; Pulmonary embolus.

VII. Problem Case Diagnosis.
Panic attack.

VIII. Teaching Pearls Question.
What percent of patients with panic disorder develop major depression?

IX. Teaching Pearls Answer.
50–65%.

REFERENCES

Bernstein CA. *On Call Psychiatry,* 2nd ed, 2001, WB Saunders Company.

Carlat, DJ: *The Psychiatric Interview, A Practical Guide.* Lippincott, Williams and Wilkins, 1999.

Kercher EE. Anxiety Disorders. In Marx: *Rosen's Emergency Medicine: Concepts and Clinical Practice,* 5th ed. Mosby, 2002.

Reus VI. Mental disorders. In: Braunwald E., Fauci AS, Kasper DL, et al, eds. Harrison's *Principles of Internal Medicine,* 15th ed. McGraw-Hill, 2001.

Strahl NR. *Clinical Study Guide for the Oral Boards in Psychiatry.* American Psychiatric Publishing, Inc, 2001.

Zun LS. Panic disorder: Diagnosis and treatment in emergency medicine. *Ann Emerg Med* 1997;30:92–96.

8. BACK PAIN

I. **Problem.** A 63-year-old, retired physician presents with back pain of 3 days duration that suddenly worsened this morning.

II. **Immediate Questions**
  A. **Are you dealing with a life-threatening emergency?** Is the patient conscious and alert with normal vital signs? If there is any question of mental status or vital sign abnormalities address the ABCs. If the patient is awake and alert then is it an imminent but pending disaster or simply a pain management and diagnostic case?
  B. **PPRST (Provocation Palliation Radiation Severity Timing).** What precipitated the event or worsened it? Did the situation begin during strenuous activity or was it sudden and unprovoked? Has anything eliminated the pain? Does the pain radiate down the buttocks, legs, or around to the testicles? On a scale of 1–10 how bad is the pain? Is the pain constant or does it wax and wane in intensity?
  C. **Neurologic and Vascular Considerations.** Has there been any numbness, weakness, or tingling in the legs? Have you had any trouble stopping, starting, or controlling bladder or bowel functions? Do your feet feel cold?
  D. **Infection Considerations.** Any fever? Any trouble with burning or frequency with urination?
  E. **Past History.** Is this an old, recurring problem? Have you ever had anything like this before? What surgeries have you had on the abdomen or back? Is there a history of HTN?

III. **Differential Diagnosis**
  A. **Musculoskeletal.** Muscle and/or ligament strain, disc herniation, osteoarthritis, spondylolisthesis.
  B. **Renal.** Stone.
  C. **Neoplasm.** Renal, spine, or metastatic (prostate).
  D. **Infectious.** Herpes zoster, pyelonephritis, epidural abscess.
  E. **Abdomen.** Aortic aneurysm, aortic dissection.

IV. Database
A. Physical Exam Key Points
1. **Vital signs.** Hypotension, tachycardia, or signs of shock.
2. **Abdomen.** Masses, tenderness, or bruits.
3. **Skin/Back.** Sores suggestive of varicella-zoster or discoloration suggesting bleeding. Pain at the costovertebral angle.
4. **Neurologic.** Strength and sensation in both lower extremities. Pay particular attention to whether it is normal and symmetric.
5. **Vascular.** Pulse strength in the dorsales pedis and posterior tibialis arteries. Pay particular attention to whether it is normal and symmetric.

B. Laboratory Data
1. **UA.** Look for evidence of blood, suggesting but not proving a kidney stone, or white cells, suggesting but not proving a UTI.
2. **Hemoglobin & hematocrit.** To determine if there is any evidence of blood loss necessitating more emergent management.

C. Radiographic and Other Studies
1. **Bedside U/S.** Although not diagnostic, radiography is capable of determining the degree of urgency of the patient's condition. Visualization of a large aorta in the setting of back pain should lead to more caution (ie, don't send patient to the CT scanner; call the OR and CT surgeon NOW). U/S can also pick up evidence of hydronephrosis, suggestive of ureteral obstruction.
2. **Abdominal CT scan.** Excellent for the stable patient. Very often diagnostic in AAA, ureteral stones, and even useful in disc herniation. However, the type of CT must be directed toward the most likely diagnosis. A plain abdominal CT could miss stones and won't even visualize the spine well.
3. **Lumbar spine plain films.** Only indicated if significant trauma, neurologic deficits, systemic symptoms, temperature > 100.4 °F, weight loss, drug or ETOH abuse, cancer, steroid use, or ankylosing spondylitis suspected.

V. Plan
A. Overall Plan.
The two immediate concerns with back pain are (1) hemodynamic stabilization if there is evidence of or potential for shock and (2) pain control. Pain control, once item 1 is addressed is an emergent need in many causes of back pain, especially renal colic.

B. Specific Plans
1. **Musculoskeletal.** For neurologic compromise (weakness, numbness, bowel or bladder control problems) an MRI and neurosurgical consultation should be obtained. Other pain should be managed with anti-inflammatories, narcotics, and/or muscle relaxants then appropriately referred.
2. **Renal.** Renal stones generally do not need emergency intervention other then pain control and appropriate urology referral—unless infected (urgent urology referral). In many hospitals a plain KUB and renal CT are the standard diagnostic approach.

3. **Neoplasm.** If plain films of the spine are ordered, then evidence of metastatic or primary neoplasm must be ruled out on the film.
4. **Infectious.** Pyelonephritis can be managed with antibiotics and pain medication on an outpatient basis if the patient appears/feels well, taking POs, and is not otherwise debilitated or pregnant. Varicella-zoster, if detected early should be treated with an antiviral and pain medication. Any question of infection/abscess in the lumbar spine (IV drug use, recent procedures, fever, immunocompromise) necessitates CT or MRI evaluation.
5. **Abdomen.** In the elderly a complaint of back pain necessitates a clear diagnosis or at least a complete rule out of life-threatening causes such as ruptured AAA (see 1. Abdominal Pain, p 1, and 6. Aneurysms, p 20.). Immediate resuscitation and simultaneous planning with surgeon and the OR are mandatory.

VI. **ICD-9 Diagnoses.** Abdominal aortic aneurysm; Acute pyelonephritis; Aortic dissection; Arthritis of spine; Epidural abscess; Intervertebral disc hernia; Low back strain; Nephrolithiasis; Spinal stenosis; Spondylolisthesis.

VII. **Problem Case Diagnosis.** Ruptured AAA.

VIII. **Teaching Pearls Question.** What is and causes the cauda equina syndrome?

IX. **Teaching Pearls Answer.** Central disc herniation compressing nerve roots that strand from the bottom of the spinal cord (horses tail = cauda equina) can cause difficult urination, incontinence, or impotence.

REFERENCES

Kuhn M, Bonnin RLL, Davey MJ. Emergency department ultrasound scanning for abdominal aortic aneurysm: Accessible, accurate, and advantageous. *Ann Emerg Med* 2000;36(32):19–223.

Stanford EK. Herniated lumbar disc. On-line *Textbook of Emergency Medicine* at http://www.medical-library.org/journals/secure/rheumorth/secure/herniated_lumbar.htm

9. BITES AND STINGS

I. **Problem.** A 17-year-old male complains of severe hand pain and swelling.

II. **Immediate Questions**

A. **What are the vital signs and mental status?** Is the airway intact? Is the patient stable and alert? If unstable or major trauma, apply monitors (ECG and pulse ox), start IV (contralateral extremity), apply oxygen. If airway compromise (or potential compromise), manage the airway. If signs/symptoms of anaphylaxis, begin appropriate treatment.

B. **What was the bite or sting from?** (See part III. Differential Diagnosis).

C. **How long ago did the bite or sting occur?** Was there prehospital care or intervention? Check for tourniquets, ice, and tight bandaging. These may NOT be appropriate.

    D. What are the reported injuries? Watch out for cranial (pediatrics), facial, vascular, or nerve injuries.

    E. Any past medical history? Prior history of similar bite or sting? Anaphylaxis? Street drug or ETOH use? Medications and allergies?

III. Differential Diagnosis

A. Bites

1. **Dog.** Most common bite. Provoked? Pet? Immunizations record available?
2. **Cat.** Treat deep scratches as bites. Consider retained teeth as foreign bodies. 80%+ become infected.
3. **Human.** Consider "fight bite" injuries to the metacarpophalangeal joints of the hands. High risk of infection.
4. **Rodent.** Seldom carry rabies.
5. **Bat.** Treat any exposure as a bite. Always consider rabies prophylaxis. (See Table A-2, p 654)
6. **Spider.** Black widow (*Latrodectus*) and brown recluse (*Loxosceles*) bites are occasionally clinically significant (pain and muscle rigidity; enlarging ulcer). Others usually not.
7. **Cone-nose bug.** (*Triatoma*) Painless bite at night, large area of erythema, pruritic. 5% of people bitten develop anaphylaxis. Seldom transmits Chagas disease in US. (See 5. Anaphylaxis, p 18)
8. **Gila monster (venomous lizard).** Seldom fatal. Extreme pain and local swelling. Found in the southwest US and Mexico.
9. **Crotalid bite (rattlesnake).** Localized pain, ecchymosis, edema, all may be progressive. Systemic signs/symptoms up to and including shock. Call regional poison center.
10. **Agkistrodon bite (cottonmouth and water moccasin).** Localized pain, ecchymosis, edema. Seldom fatal.
11. **Coral snake bite.** Neurotoxic, with minimal local effects.
12. **Exotic snakebite.** Often neurotoxic. Contact local poison center or zoo for identification.
13. **Nonvenomous snakebite.** Localized pain. No progression of swelling or ecchymosis from the bite site. No systemic signs or symptoms.

B. Stings

1. **Bee and wasp sting.** Localized pain and erythema. May cause anaphylactic reaction. (See 5. Anaphylaxis, p 18.)
2. **Scorpion sting.** Localized pain and paresthesias. Sting site often difficult to locate. Bark scorpion (*Centruroides*) causes extreme pain, agitation, and nystagmus in children < 3 years.
3. **Jellyfish and other Cnideria stings.** Pain and burning in areas of envenomation.

IV. Database

    A. Physical Exam Key Points. *Repeat exam frequently* in envenomated patients.

1. **Mental status.** Check if patient is awake and alert.
2. **Vital signs.** Check carefully and repeat during evaluation.
3. **HEENT and neck.** Check for lip and tongue swelling, oropharyngeal swelling, neck swelling, stridor, and change in voice.
4. **Lung sounds.** Check for wheezing (anaphylaxis or systemic toxicity), movement of air (neurotoxicity).
5. **Abdomen.** Check for muscle wall rigidity (*Latrodectus* envenomation)
6. **Neurologic.** Check for confusion (CNS toxicity), weakness (neurotoxicity).
7. **Extremities.** Check for deformity (fractures), compartment syndrome.
8. **Skin. Examine wounds carefully.** Check for progressive induration, erythema, ecchymosis, tenderness.

B. **Laboratory Data.** Often not needed, unless toxic appearing or history of snakebite. If suspected snakebite, CBC with platelets, Lytes, PT, PTT, fibrinogen, fibrin split products, *d*-dimer, UA. Wound cultures not indicated unless wound is old and infected.

C. **Radiographic and Other Studies.** Consider radiograph for retained foreign bodies (teeth). CT of head or radiograph for suspected skull fracture in children.

V. **Plan**

A. **Overall Plan.** Treat local wound as appropriate, diphtheria/tetanus prophylaxis, rabies prophylaxis, antibiotics if indicated, manage symptoms, consult a poison center if needed, disposition depending on specific clinical scenario.

B. **Specific Plans**

1. **Bites**

   a. **Dog.** Consider wound care, antibiotic (amoxicillin and clavulanate potassium (Augmentin) or other), rabies prophylaxis.

   b. **Cat.** Consider wound care, antibiotic (Augmentin or other), rabies prophylaxis.

   c. **Human.** Consider wound care, antibiotic (Augmentin or other).

   d. **Rodent.** Consider wound care, antibiotic (Augmentin or other).

   e. **Bat.** Treat any exposure as a bite. Always consider rabies prophylaxis.

   f. **Spider.** Black widow (*Latrodectus*) Antivenin available in parts of Arizona. Pain medication. Brown recluse (*Loxosceles*) localized wound care. Wide debridement is not effective in limiting progression of ulceration. Consider antibiotics.

   g. **Cone-nose bug (*Triatoma*).** Antihistamines. Treat anaphylaxis. Consider treatment for cellulitis if diagnosis is unclear.

   h. **Gila monster (venomous lizard).** IV pain medication, hydration if needed. Monitor blood pressure. Consider admission.

   i. **Venomous snakebite.** Antidotes (antivenin) are available for many venomous snakebites. Consult a poison center for more information. Manage the airway and BP IV pain medication, hydration, local wound care. No pressure dressings (except with elapid envenomation), no ice, no tourniquets, no incision/drainage. Mark progression of swelling/ecchymosis every 15 min.

   j. Nonvenomous snakebite. Local wound care, pain medication as needed. Consider antibiotics.

2. **Stings**

   a. Bee and wasp sting. Antihistamines, pain medication. Manage anaphylaxis.

   b. Scorpion sting. Pain medication in adults and older children. Consider a midazolam infusion with bark scorpion (*Centruroides*) envenomation in children < 3 years, with admission to a PICU. Consider antivenin.

   c. Jellyfish and other Cnideria stings. For most, apply vinegar to the envenomated areas for 30 min. For American sea nettle (*Chrysaora*), little mauve stinger jellyfish (*Pelagia*), or "lion's mane" jellyfish (*Cyanea*), apply baking soda instead of vinegar.

VI. ICD-9 Diagnoses. Insect, reptile, snake, or spider bite (use if venomous); Human and animal bites are coded as Wound, open (add location); Sting (animal, bee, fish, insect, jellyfish, wasp).

VII. Problem Case Diagnosis. Gila monster envenomation to the thumb.

VIII. Teaching Pearl Question. What organism(s) are most frequently isolated from both dog and cat bites?

IX. Teaching Pearl Answer. *Pasteurella* species. *Pasteurella canis* (50% of dog bite wounds) and *Pasteurella multocida* and *septica* (75% of cat bite wounds).

REFERENCES

Centers for Disease Control. Dog Bites. (Multiple other bite and envenomation-related publications). http://www.cdc.gov

Dart RC, McNally J. Efficacy, safety, and use of snake antivenoms in the United States. *Ann Emerg Med* 2001;37(2):181–188.

Olson KR, ed. *Poisoning and Drug Overdose,* 3rd ed. Appleton and Lange, 1999.

Talan DA, Citron DM, Abrahamian FM, Moran GJ, Goldstein EJ. Bacteriologic analysis of infected dog and cat bites. *N Engl J Med* 1999; 340(2):85–92.

Walter FG, Bilden EF, Gibly RL. Envenomations. *Crit Care Clin* 1999;15(2):353–386, ix.

10. BLEEDING PROBLEMS

   I. Problem. A young patient bumps his inguinal area and develops a large spreading hematoma.

   II. Immediate Questions

   A. What are the vital signs? Orthostatic? Is the patient alert? Obtain IV access. Apply oxygen and pulse ox and ECG monitors if vitals

markedly abnormal. Ensure airway is adequate, no bleeding into soft tissues in neck.
B. **History of bleeding disorders?** Problems with dental extractions? Easy bruisability, bleeding of gums. Prior need for transfusions, difficulties with prior injuries/operations? Problems with menses, labor and delivery, injections, nosebleeds? Spontaneous bleeding?
C. **Past medical history?** Liver failure, anticoagulant use, renal failure. lupus, DVT, PE, myeloproliferative disorder, malignancy, infection.
D. **Family history of bleeding disorder?** Any family members using anticoagulants? Negative family history does not rule out inherited coagulation disorder (30–40% hemophilia A patients have no family history).
E. **Medications?** ETOH, aspirin, NSAIDs, OTC drugs, herbals? *Thrombocytopenic drugs:* ranitidine, procainamide, carbamazepine, valproic acid, phenytoin, furosemide, thiazides, penicillins, sulfa drugs, chemo. *Coagulation factors inhibitors:* procainamide, phenothiazine, penicillin, aminoglycosides, isoniazid.
F. **Hematuria, hematemesis, melena, bleeding from other sites?** Hemoptysis only rarely associated with bleeding disorders.

III. **Differential Diagnosis**
A. **Coagulation Factor Deficiency.** Usually deep tissue bleeding. Hematomas, hemarthroses of joint, muscle, potential spaces (retroperitoneal). Presents with delayed bleeding after trauma.
   1. **Inherited coagulation factor deficiencies.** Hemophilia A (VIII), B (IX).
   2. **DIC, liver disease.**
B. **Thrombocytopenia/Functional Platelet Disorder.** Superficial surfaces, especially oral, nasal, GI, GU (menorrhagia, hematuria). Spontaneous bleeding or immediately after trauma. Major bleeding risk with platelets < 10,000.
   1. **Thrombocytopenia** from pooling, immunodestruction, ITP, DIC, dilution, TTP, HUS.
   2. **Dysfunction.** Von Willebrand's disease.
   3. **Iatrogenic.** Aspirin, platelet inhibitors.
C. **Pseudothrombocytopenia.** EDTA anticoagulant in blood tubes can cause platelet clumping.
D. **Hypercoagulable State.** Protein C, S, antithrombin deficiency.
E. **Vascular Disorders.** Similar to thrombocytopenia in presentation. Hemorrhagic telangiectasia, angiomas, TTP, hypoxemia, snake bite.
   1. **Aplastic anemia**
   2. **Anticoagulant overdose**

IV. **Database**
A. **Physical Exam Key Points**
   1. **Vitals and mental status.** Ensure patient is stable.
   2. **Neurologic.** Check for any deficits (CVA, spinal cord bleed).
   3. **Skin.** Petechiae, especially in areas of increased venous pressure (dependent areas, stockings), ecchymosis, purpura. IV sites

for bleeding, or bleeding from previously intact venipuncture sites (suggests DIC). Bleeding from superficial cuts and scratches. Signs of liver disease.
4. **HEENT.** Scleral icterus. Multiple small retinal hemorrhages common in patients with thrombocytopenia, other purpuric disorders. Mucosal bleeding (especially with vessel/platelet dysfunction).
5. **Abdomen.** Check size and shape of liver, spleen.
6. **Extremities.** Joint swelling, tenderness, hemarthroses, prior bleeding.
B. **Laboratory Data** (Table I–3, p 34.)
1. **CBC with platelet count.** Peripheral smear.
2. **PT.** Extrinsic pathway (factors VII, X, and V; prothrombin; fibrinogen). *Isolated PT prolongation:* Early liver disease, vitamin K deficiency, warfarin, early DIC.
3. **PTT.** Intrinsic pathway (prekallikrein, factors XII, XI, IX, VIII, X, and V; prothrombin; fibrinogen). *Isolated PTT prolongation:* Heparin, factors VIII, IX, XI, XII deficiency/inhibitor; lupus anticoagulant.
4. **Both PT, PTT prolonged.** High-dose heparin, prolonged warfarin (Coumadin), dilutional coagulopathy, vitamin K deficiency, moderate/severe liver disease, common pathway clotting factor deficiencies, DIC.
5. **Bleeding time.** Prolonged in thrombocytopenia, qualitative platelet abnormalities, defects in platelet-vessel wall interactions (von Willebrand's disease) and primary vascular disorders. Not increased in coagulation factor deficiencies.

TABLE I–3. COMMON CAUSES OF COAGULOPATHY DIFFERENTIATED BY ALTERATIONS IN PROTHROMBIN TIME, PARTIAL THROMBOPLASTIN TIME, AND PLATELET COUNT 1–3.

PT	PTT	Platelets	Most Common Causes
↑	—	—	Deficiency or inhibitor of factor VII (early liver disease, vitamin K deficiency, warfarin therapy, dysfibrinogenemia, some cases of DIC
—	↑	—	Deficiency or inhibitor of factors VIII, IX, or XI; vWD; heparin
↑	↑	↓	DIC, liver disease, heparin therapy associated with thrombocytopenia
—	—	↓	Increased platelet destruction, decreased platelet production, hypersplenism, hemodilution
—	—	↑	Myeloproliferative disorders
—	—	—	Mild vWD, acquired qualitative platelet disorders (eg, uremia)

DIC = disseminated intravascular coagulation; vWD = von Willebrand's disease.
Reproduced, with permission, from Haist SA, Robbins JB, Gomella LG, eds. *Internal Medicine On Call*, 3rd ed. McGraw-Hill, 2002.

6. **Consider inhibitor test.** If deficiency in one or more coagulation factors or an inhibitor (antibody) suspected, mix 1:1 patient and normal plasma. If complete deficient, this should correct the PT/PTT. If this fails, then inhibitor likely (ie, lupus anticoagulant, factor VIII antibody).

7. **Values > normal.** Virtually excludes any clinically significant systemic coagulopathy. *Exception:* Factor XIII deficiency (specific tests for it if suspected).

8. **Consider tests.** Fibrinogen, thrombin time, specific factor levels (if known deficiency to determine activity).

C. **Radiographic and Other Studies.** If pulmonary issues, consider CXR. Knee films for joint pain/hemarthroses. CT or U/S to assess retroperitoneal or deep tissue bleed.

V. **Plan**
   A. **Overall Plan.** Fluids for hemodynamic stability, order T&C. If pre-existing, check coagulation panel, factor levels as needed. *Severe bleeding/hypocoagulation:* Transfuse factor, FFP, or cryoprecipitate as needed. Admit newly diagnosed disorders, unknown cause disorders, also hemodynamically significant bleeding or inability to obtain hemostasis.

   B. **Specific Plans**
      1. **FFP.** Contains 100% of all clotting factors. Can always be used although may be consumed if DIC or inhibitor present.
      2. **Hemophilia A.** Transfuse with cryoprecipitate or factor VIII:C concentrate.
      3. **Hemophilia B.** Transfuse with factor IX or large doses FFP.
      4. **Von Willebrand's disease.** DDAVP, replace with factor VIII:C or cryoprecipitate (factors I, VIII, XIII, vWF).
      5. **DIC.** Diagnose, treat underlying cause. Replenish clotting factors with FFP, cryoprecipitate, blood.
      6. **Thrombocytopenia.** Transfuse with platelets to keep level > 50,000.

VI. **ICD-9 Diagnoses.** Bleeding disorder;
    Bleeding due to anticoagulants, Coagulopathy, Ecchymosis, Hematoma, Hemarthrosis; Hemophilia (A, B); Thrombocytopenia; von Willebrand's disease.

VII. **Problem Case Diagnosis.** Hemophilia A (factor 8 deficiency).

VIII. **Teaching Pearls Question.** What is the normal bleeding pattern for dental procedures?

IX. **Teaching Pearls Answer.** After a typical molar extraction, a normal person will have approximately 1 h of brisk bleeding and slight oozing for up to 2 days.

REFERENCES

Di Paola J, Nugent D, Young G. Current therapy for rare factor deficiencies. *Haemophilia* 2000;7 (Suppl 1):16–22.

Federman DG, Kirsner RS. An update on hypercoagulable disorders. *Arch Intern Med* 2001;161(8):1051–1056.

Mannucci PM, Tuddenham EGD. Medical progress: The hemophilias—from royal genes to gene therapy. *N Engl J Med* 2001;344(23):1773–1779.

Shapiro AD. Platelet function disorders. *Haemophilia* 2000;6 (Suppl 1):120–127.

Staudinger T, Locker GJ, Frass M. Management of acquired coagulation disorders in emergency and intensive care medicine. *Semin Thromb Hemost* 1996;22(1):93–104.

Triplet DA. Coagulation and bleeding disorders: Review and update. *Clin Chem* 2000; 46(8):1260–1269.

11. BRADYCARDIA

I. **Problem.** A 75-year-old woman has a syncopal episode in church. Her vital signs reveal a heart rate of 42.

II. **Immediate Questions**
   A. **Does the patient have an intact airway and is she spontaneously breathing?** If not, start basic life support measures and call for ALS.
   B. **What is her mental status and blood pressure?** Is there evidence of end-organ ischemia? (See 3. Altered Mental Status, p 11, 47. Hypotension, p 47, and 45. Hypertension, p 139).
   C. **What is her heart rhythm?** Sinus bradycardia, heart block, pacemaker failure, AF with high-degree AV block.
   D. **What medications is she taking?** Beta-blockers, calcium channel blockers, digoxin, type IA antiarrhythmics.
   E. **Does the patient have chest pain?** MI causing heart block or poor perfusion causing ischemia. (See 15. Chest Pain, p 51.)
   F. **Past medical history?** Pacemaker implantation, previous cardiac disease.

III. **Differential Diagnosis**
   A. **Medications.** See part D.
   B. **Ischemia.** Block at the AV node associated with inferior wall MI. (See 15. Chest Pain, p 51.)
   C. **Vagal Tone.** Presents with brief episode of bradycardia and hypotension, which resolves spontaneously. Often associated with pain, emotion, ocular manipulation, or Valsalva's maneuver.
   D. **Severe Hyperkalemia.** Dialysis patients. (See 24. Dialysis Patient Problems, p 79, and Section IX. Fluids and Electrolytes, p 479.)
   E. **Tachy-Brady Syndrome**
   F. **Infiltrative Process.** Amyloidosis, sarcoidosis, myocarditis, pericarditis, Chagas' disease.
   G. **Poisons.** Organophosphate (cholinergic), foxglove, monkshood, oleander. (See Section V, 14. Organophosphate Poisoning, p 353, and Section V, 8. Cardiac Glycoside Overdose, p 339.)

H. **Sinus Bradycardia.** Trained athlete or elderly with fibrosis of conduction system.

IV. **Database**
   A. **Physical Exam Key Points**
      1. **Vital signs.** Ongoing assessment is important. Hypotension or hypothermia.
      2. **Chest wall.** Pacemaker generator.
      3. **Cardiac exam.** Displaced PMI, murmur, gallop, diminished hear sounds. Signs of CHF (rales, JVD, pedal edema; See 16. CHF/Pulmonary Edema, p 54.).
      4. **Neurologic exam.** Altered level of consciousness, focal motor or sensory findings, slurred speech.
      5. **Skin.** Mottling, acrocyanosis, delayed capillary refill (signs of shock). Look for hemodialysis catheter or shunt.
   B. **Laboratory Data.** CBC, electrolytes, cardiac enzymes, and medication levels.
   C. **Radiographic and Other Studies**
      1. **ECG.** Look for MI, heart block, pacemaker capture.
      2. **CXR.** Look for pacemaker lead fracture.
      3. **Interrogate pacemaker.** Malfunction or low battery.
      4. **Urine output.** A good indicator of perfusion. Desired: 1 mL/kg/h.

V. **Plan**
   A. **Overall Plan.** Assess the effect of the bradycardia on end organs. Symptomatic bradycardia typically calls for an admission of observation in a telemetry unit at least.
   B. **Specific Plans**
      1. **Hypoperfusion**
         a. **Atropine** (0.5 mg IV, repeat until HR improves or total dose of 3 mg).
         b. **Transcutaneous pacemaker** to increase rate. Sedate as needed with transcutaneous pacer. Arrange for emergent transvenous pacemaker.
         c. **Isoproterenol** (1–10 µg/min titrate to effect).
      2. **Intact perfusion.** IV, continuous ECG monitor, observation, and address underlying problem.
      3. **Ischemia.** Treat MI, temporary transvenous pacemaker.
      4. **Heart block.** Permanent pacemaker.
      5. **Medications.** Support patient (pacemaker as required) and withdraw suspicious medications. (See Section V. Common Toxicologic Emergency Problems, p 316.)
         a. **Beta-blockers.** IV glucagon (See Section V. 6. Beta-blocker Overdoes, p 332.)
         b. **Calcium channel blockers.** IV calcium chloride. (See Section V. 7. Calcium Channel Blocker Overdose, p 334.)
         c. **Digoxin** (cardiac glycosides). Digibind. (See Section V. 8. Cardiac Glycoside Overdose, p 339.)

6. **Vagally mediated.** Self-limited. Place patient horizontal until episode resolves.
7. **Hyperkalemia.** (See Section IX. Fluids and Electrolytes, p 479.) IV calcium chloride (emergency drug of choice), insulin, glucose, sodium bicarbonate, sodium polystyrene sulfate (Kayexalate), dialysis.
8. **Tachy-brady syndrome.** Permanent pacemaker.
9. **Pacemaker failure.** Replace leads or generator.

VI. **ICD-9 Diagnoses.** Adverse effect medication; Heart block (specify type); Hyperkalemia; Hypothermia; Pacemaker-mechanical complication; Poisoning—specify drug; Sick sinus syndrome; Sinus bradycardia.

VII. **Problem Case Diagnosis.** MI with 3rd-degree heart block.

VIII. **Teaching Pearls Question.** List some common causes of sinus bradycardia.

IX. **Teaching Pearls Answer.** Inferior wall MI, vagal syncope, β-blockers, sinus node disease, athletic heart, hypothermia, hypothyroidism.

REFERENCES

Lampert R, Ezekowitz MD. Management of arrhythmias. *Clin Geriatr Med* 2000; 16(3):593–618.

Swart G, Brady WJ Jr, DeBehnke DJ, MA OJ, Aufderheide TP. Acute myocardial infarction complicated by hemodynamically unstable bradyarrhythmia: Prehospital and ED treatment with atropine. *Am J Emerg Med* 1999;17(7):647–652.

12. CANCER PROBLEMS

I. **Problem.** An elderly male with lung cancer is brought to the ED by his wife, reportedly "not acting like himself" and moaning incoherently.

II. **Immediate Questions**
   A. **Are the ABCs intact?** Manage appropriately (See Section VIII, 15. Rapid Endotracheal Intubation, p 470).
   B. **What are the vital signs?** Is the patient febrile? What is the mental status? Are the vitals stable? Apply monitors, obtain IV access, supplemental oxygen if needed. Confusion or fever may offer clues to specific oncologic emergencies.
   C. **What is the patient's underlying malignancy?** Specific cancers have known emergency complications.
   D. **What therapy has the patient received? When?** Radiotherapy and chemotherapy both have many side effects that may lead to an emergency complaint.

III. **Differential Diagnosis**
   A. **Cardiovascular**
      1. **Superior vena cava (SVC) syndrome.** Consider especially in patients with history of small cell cancer of the lung or lym-

phomas. May also be associated with long-term central venous catheters used for treatment of malignancy, hyperalimentation, or invasive hemodynamic monitoring.

2. **Malignant pericardial effusion with tamponade.** History of metastatic disease, especially lung and breast carcinomas.

B. Hematologic
1. **Neutropenia** (neutropenic fever). Particularly in patients who have bone marrow involvement or have recently received chemotherapy.
2. **Coagulation or bleeding diathesis.** Previous history of bruising or bleeding problems, metastatic lesions to liver or thrombocytopenia secondary to bone marrow involvement or chemotherapy.
3. **Anemia.** Especially in colon cancer, often presenting symptom of occult GI malignancy.
4. **Hyperviscosity syndrome.** Potential cause of acute ischemic injury to extremities, brain, myocardium.

C. Metabolic
1. **Hypercalcemia.** Usually has rapid onset; can cause confusion, stupor, vomiting, dehydration. Associated with advanced malignancy. Particularly associated with breast and lung carcinomas, multiple myeloma, lymphoma. (See Section IX. Fluids and Electrolytes, p 479.)
2. **Tumor lysis syndrome.** Seen after recent chemotherapy. Check potassium and uric acid levels.
3. **Infectious work-up.** Same as in nononcologic patients unless neutropenic, then work-up all potential sources and treat empirically. (See 32. Fever, page 32 and 61. Sepsis, page 183)

D. Neurologic. Consider compression of spinal cord or nerve root secondary to metastasis in any patient with back pain especially with motor or sensory losses or incontinence.

IV. Database
A. Physical Exam Key Points
1. **Mental status.** Mini mental status exam, orientation (sepsis/hypercalcemia).
2. **Vital signs.** Especially temperature, as fever can change management regardless of stability of other vital signs, clinical judgment of "sick" or "not sick." Hypotension may be sign of CV compromise secondary to critical effusion/tamponade.
3. **Head and neck.** Is there facial plethora or cyanosis (SVC), JVD (tamponade/SVC)? Are the mucosal surfaces dry (sepsis/hypercalcemia)?
4. **Cardiovascular.** Listen to the heart for rubs or distant heart sounds (effusion). Examine chest wall for engorged veins (SVC).
5. **Pulmonary.** Listen for rales (focal sign of infection). Is the patient dyspneic (SVC, tamponade, pneumonia)?
6. **Abdomen.** Examine for distension (hypercalcemia), tenderness (infectious source).

       7. **Neurologic.** Complete motor/sensory exam to delineate possible nerve/cord compression. Palpate spine for tenderness.

  B. Laboratory Data. Check CBC with Diff, basic metabolic panel with Ca, P, uric acid. Coagulation studies. UA and culture, blood and catheter tip cultures if febrile. CSF for analysis and culture if indicated. Assays for PTHrP (parathyroid hormone-related protein) can confirm hypercalcemia secondary to malignancy.

  C. Radiographic and Other Studies. CXR for mass lesion, obstructive lesion as cause of SVC syndrome. Look for cardiomegaly as sign of effusion. Look for focal infiltrate as source of infection. Contrast enhanced chest CT may be indicated to diagnose cause of SVC syndrome. ECG with low voltage or electrical alternans may indicate pericardial effusion. Echocardiography will demonstrate effusion or tamponade and can help guide pericardiocentesis. ECG with shortened QT interval may indicate hypercalcemia. Plain films of spine, and, if normal, consider CT/MRI/myelogram if suspect cord compression.

V. Plan

  A. Overall Plan. Quickly treat immediate life threats. If necessary, admit and begin therapy for other problems in consultation with patient's oncologist. Balance management of the medical problem with concern for patient's emotional and psychiatric needs, as these may be complex and significant. Adequate analgesia always and supportive care when indicated.

  B. Specific Plans

    1. **SVC syndrome.** Radiotherapy if in extremis. Otherwise admit for diagnostic evaluation (biopsy, thoracentesis, bronchoscopy, or mediastinoscopy), radiotherapy and/or chemotherapy. Surgical management and intravascular shunts less common.

    2. **Malignant effusion with tamponade.** Try IV fluid challenge with NS or LR. If no improvement, provide drainage via pericardial window (preferred) or pericardiocentesis (echo-guided preferred).

    3. **Neutropenia.** If febrile, pan culture, investigate for source and begin broad-spectrum antibiotics according to local resistance patterns.

    4. **Fever.** If neutropenic, admit and treat as in preceding item. Otherwise look for source and treat appropriately based on clinical judgment.

    5. **Hypercalcemia.** IV fluid rehydration with NS. IV pamidronate. Consider IV furosemide, calcitonin.

    6. **Spinal cord compression.** IV steroids, analgesics, emergent surgical decompression, or radiotherapy.

VI. ICD-9 Diagnoses. Anemia in neoplastic disease; Coagulopathy; Hypercalcemia; Hyperviscosity syndrome; Neoplastic pericarditis; Neutropenic fever; Pleural effusion of malignancy; Superior vena cava syndrome.

VII. Problem Case Diagnosis. Hypercalcemia.

VIII. Teaching Pearls question. What percentage of SVC syndrome cases requires emergent radiotherapy?

IX. Teaching Pearls Answer. 5% (Yellin).

REFERENCES

Bodey GB, Rolston KV. Management of fever in neutropenic patients. *J Infect Chemother* 2001;7(1):1–9.

Body JJ. Current and future directions of medical therapy of hypercalcemia: *Cancer* 2000;88(12 Suppl):3054–3058.

DeCamp MM, Mentzer SJ, Swanson SJ, Sugarbaker DJ. Malignant effusive disease of the pleura and pericardium. *Chest* 1997;112(4 Suppl):291S–295S

Grant R, Papadopolos SM, Sandler HM, Greenberg HS. Metastatic epidural spinal cord compression: Current concepts and treatment. *J Neurooncol* 1994;19(1):79–92.

Markman MA. Diagnosis and management of SVC syndrome. *Cleve Clin J Med* 1999; 66(1):59–61.

Nussbaum S, Younger J, VandePol CJ, et al. Single dose intravenous therapy with pamidronate for the treatment of hypercalcemia of malignancy: Comparison of 30-, 60-, and 90-mg doses. *Am J Med* 1993;95(3):297–304.

Schiff D, Batchelor T, Wen PY. Neurologic emergencies in cancer patients. *Neurol Clin* 1998;16(2):449–483.

Yellin A, Rosen A, Reichert N, Lieberman Y. Superior vena cava syndrome. The myth–the facts. *Am Rev Respir Dis* 1990;141(5 Pt 1):1114–1118.

13. CARDIAC ARREST

I. Problem. A middle-aged dialysis-dependent woman collapses in triage.

II. Immediate Questions

   A. Is the patient unresponsive? If no response to verbal and tactile stimulus, then call for defibrillator and check for signs of circulation (movement, breathing, pulse).

   B. Is the patient breathing? If so, roll patient into lateral decubitus recovery position. If not, open airway using head tilt-chin lift maneuver or jaw thrust (if trauma suspected). Assess for airway obstruction. Suction mouth and oropharynx. Consider placing oropharyngeal airway or two nasopharyngeal airways. Place a pulse-ox monitor. Apply 100% oxygen and provide positive pressure ventilations.

   C. Is there a pulse? Initiate chest compressions in an unmonitored patient only after taking 10 s to confirm the absence of breathing and a pulse. In contrast, a *monitored* patient who becomes unresponsive should receive immediate CPR if the rhythm is asystole or patient is in VF. Note that CPR is not effective if patient is on a soft mattress (use compression board). Consider a single precordial thump in a pulseless, apneic patient with *witnessed* arrest.

   D. Is the cardiac rhythm VF or pulseless VT? Attach defibrillator/ monitor after initiating CPR. If the rhythm is VF or pulseless VT, then defibrillate up to 3 × (200 J, 300 J, 360J). Check rhythm and pulse. Continue CPR if indicated and secure airway.

E. **Is the airway secure?** Secure airway with immediate tracheal intubation. If immediate intubation not possible, ventilate patient with bag-valve-mask ventilation. (See Section VIII, 15. Rapid Endotracheal Intubation, p 470.).

F. **Is there IV access?** Begin peripheral IV placement simultaneous to initiation of CPR, but do not delay resuscitation or defibrillation while placing IV. Lidocaine, epinephrine, atropine and naloxone can be given via ETT (pneumonic: "LEAN"). Obtain at least two peripheral IVs.

G. **What is the cardiac rhythm?** Identify rhythm and give appropriate IV agents and countershocks (see III. Differential Diagnosis).

H. **Is there a witness to the event or any known past medical history?** History of the event and PMH are less important in cardiac arrest. However, history may aid identification of reversible causes: renal failure (hyperkalemia); depression/suicidality (aspirin or tricyclic antidepressant overdose); diabetes (hypoglycemia); CAD or chest pain before event (acute MI, PE, aortic dissection); fever (septic shock); prescription medicines QT interval effects (IA, IC, antihistamines, phenothiazines, cyclic antidepressants).

I. **What is the temperature?** Use rectal thermometer. If hypothermic, then rewarm patient before terminating resuscitation.

III. **Differential Diagnosis**

A. **Ventricular Fibrillation.** Defibrillate × 3 (200 J, 300 J, 360 J). Check pulse and rhythm. If refractory, continue CPR, intubate trachea, obtain IV access. Epinephrine 1 mg IV push (repeat every 3–5 min) or vasopressin 40 U IV (single dose only). Defibrillate × 1 (360 J) between all drugs. For refractory VF, consider amiodarone 300 mg IV (repeat 150 mg × 1 in 3–5 min) or lidocaine 1.0–1.5 mg/kg IV (repeat 0.5–0.75 mg/kg × 2; max 3 mg/kg). Magnesium 1–2 gm IV if torsades de pointes or suspected hypomagnesemia (alcoholism, malnutrition). Consider procainamide infusion 50 mg/min (max 17 mg/kg) for intermittent or recurrent VF. Sodium bicarbonate only for hyperkalemia, aspirin overdose, or tricyclic overdose (Figure I–1).

B. **Pulseless Ventricular Tachycardia.** Treat as for VF (part A.).

C. **Asystole.** Confirm in more than one lead. Consider possible causes (see Specific Plans). Epinephrine 1 mg IV push every 3–5 min. Atropine 1 mg IV every 3–5 min (max. 0.04 mg/kg). Sodium bicarbonate 1 mg/kg IV (1 amp) if suspected hyperkalemia, tricyclic antidepressant overdose, or acidosis. Consider termination of efforts (Figure I–2).

D. **Pulseless Electrical Activity (PEA).** Consider possible causes (see Specific Plans). Epinephrine 1 mg push every 3–5 min. For pulseless bradycardia, Atropine 1 mg IV every 3–5 min (max 0.04 mg/kg). Fluid bolus for possible hypovolemia (most common cause of PEA). Consider sodium bicarbonate 1 mEq/kg IV (1 amp) for hyperkalemia, tricyclic antidepressant overdose, or acidosis. Calcium chloride for suspected hyperkalemia. Consider pericardiocentesis for tamponade. Consider needle decompression if pneumothorax (Figure I–3).

IV. Database

A. Physical Exam Key Points

1. **Primary survey for cardiac arrest.** Open airway. Provide positive-pressure ventilations. Chest compressions. Defibrillate VF and pulseless VT.

2. **Secondary survey.** Intubate trachea. Assess bilateral chest rise and ventilation. Gain IV access. Determine rhythm. Give appropriate agents. Search for reversible causes.

3. **Pulse.** Check carefully and repeat during evaluation for effective compressions and return of spontaneous circulation.

4. **Lungs.** Decreased air movement or chest rise suggests pneumothorax.

5. **Neurology.** Pupillary exam and reflexes, corneal reflexes and "doll's eyes" (only if not spine trauma expected) for signs of brainstem function.

6. **Mouth and neck.** Foreign body, inflammation (epiglottis, retropharyngeal abscess), trauma, or anaphylactic edema all suggest asphyxia.

7. **Cardiac.** Distended neck veins to suggest tamponade.

8. **Abdomen** Rigidity suggests abdominal catastrophe (ruptured aortic aneurysm, blunt trauma to spleen or liver) and hemorrhagic shock.

9. **Extremities.** Dialysis fistula (suggests hyperkalemia). Signs of illicit drug injection (suggests overdose).

B. Laboratory Data.
Bedside fingerstick glucose. ABG with Lytes, cardiac enzymes. No other labs indicated during resuscitation of cardiac arrest. CBC, Lytes, cardiac enzymes, and lactate will help management after successful resuscitation.

C. Radiographic and Other Studies.
Consider bedside Doppler to assess for arterial flow in PEA (prognosis is significantly different between flow and no-flow states). No other ancillary studies indicated during resuscitation of cardiac arrest.

V. Plan

A. Overall Plan.
Identify and treat reversible causes of cardiac arrest (see Specific Plans) while resuscitating. Obtain IV access and administer rhythm-appropriate medications and countershocks. Intubate trachea and provide positive pressure ventilation with 100% oxygen.

B. Specific Plans.
Consider the following causes for asystole and PEA.

1. **Hypovolemic shock.** Isotonic crystalloid fluid infusion. Blood products if suspected hemorrhagic shock.

2. **Septic shock.** Isotonic crystalloid fluid infusion. Vasopressors. Cultures and antibiotics.

3. **Tension pneumothorax.** Immediate needle decompression if suspected followed by chest tube thoracostomy.

Figure I–1. Algorithm for ventricular fibrillation and pulseless ventricular tachycardia (VF/VT). (Reproduced, with permission, from American Heart Association. Guidelines 2000 for cardio-pulmonary resuscitation and emergency cardiovascular care. *Circulation* 2000[August]:102.)

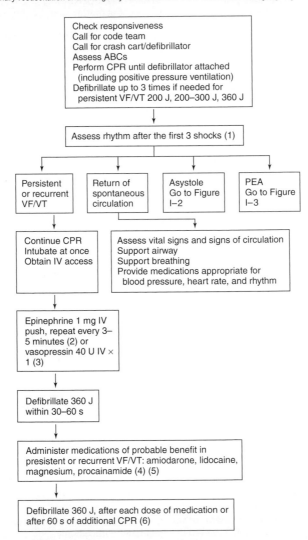

Footnotes to Figure I–1

(1) Hypothermic cardiac arrest is treated differently after this point. See Section I, Chapter 48, Hypothermia, p. 144

(2) The recommended dose of epinephrine is 1 mg IV push every 3–5 min. If this approach fails, consider high-dose epinephrine 0.2 mg/kg IV push, every 3–5 min; however, there is evidence this may be harmful.

(3) No evidence to support use of vasopressin for asystole or PEA or to support using more than one dose. If no response in 5–10 minutes after vasopressin, start or restart epinephrine administration,

(4) Amiodarone 300 mg IV push, consider additional dose of 150 mg IV. No more than 2.2 g should be given in a 24-hr period.
Lidocaine 1.0–1.5 mg/kg IV push. Consider repeat dose in 3–5 min to total loading dose of 3 mg/kg.
Magnesium sulfate 1–2 g IV (if hypomagnesemia present, or polymorphic VT [torsades de pointes])
Procainamide 30 mg/min in refractory VF (maximum total 17 mg/kg)

(5) Sodium bicarbonate (1 mEq/kg IV), for conditions known to provoke cardiac arrest:
If preexisting hyperkalemic,
If preexisting bicarbonate-responsive acidosis,
If overdose with tricyclic antidepressants,
To alkalinize the urine in drug overdoses (aspirin),
If intubated and continued long arrest interval,
Upon return of spontaneous circulation after long arrest interval.
Note: May be harmful in respiratory acidosis.

(6) Follow either CPR-drug-shock-repeat sequence or CPR-drug-shock-shock-repeat sequence.

4. **Cardiac tamponade.** Pericardiocentesis.
5. **PE.** After successful resuscitation, consider angiogram, thrombolytics, or surgical embolectomy.
6. **AMI.** 12-lead ECG. Consider pacing and emergent catheterization.
7. **Hypoxia.** Intubation, oxygenation, ventilation.
8. **Anaphylactic shock.** Rapid tracheal intubation. Isotonic crystalloid fluid infusion. Epinephrine.
9. **Hypothermia.** Passive and active rewarming (see 48. Hypothermia, page 144)
10. **Hyperkalemia.** Calcium chloride. Sodium bicarbonate. Insulin and glucose infusion.
11. **Hypoglycemia.** Glucose infusion.
12. **Hypokalemia.** IV potassium.
13. **Acidosis.** If patient has preexisting bicarbonate-responsive acidosis, then hyperventilate and administer sodium bicarbonate.
14. **Drugs.** See Section V. Common Toxicologic Emergency Problems, page 316. *Tricyclic Antidepressants:* Hyperventilate, administer sodium bicarbonate until pH 7.50–7.55, saline infusion 1 L/h, consider activated charcoal if gestation < 1–2 h, manage seizure and hypotension. *Digoxin:* ACLS for VF, give magnesium sulfate 2 mg IV plus 20 vials of Fab antibodies. *Calcium channel blockers:* Saline boluses, calcium chloride 5–10 mL IV (titrate to effect), dopamine 5–20 µg/kg/min IV, glucagon 1–5 mg IV, consider additional pressure agents and pacing as indicated. *Beta-blockers:* Saline boluses, glucagon 1–5 mg IV, Dopamine 5–20 µg/kg/min, norepinephrine infusion 0.5 µg/min IV *Opiates:* Naloxone 1–10 mg IV.

Figure I–2. Asystole treatment algorithm. (Reproduced, with permission, from American Heart Association. Guidelines 2000 for cardiopulmonary resuscitation and emergency cardiovascular care. *Circulation* 2000[August]:102.)

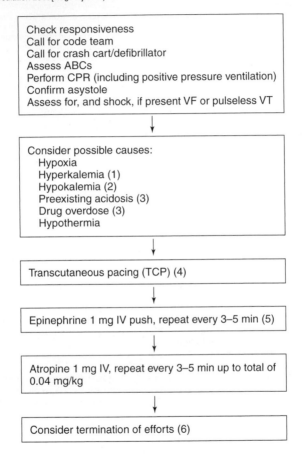

VI. **ICD-9 Diagnoses.** Asystole/Cardiac arrest; Cardiac tamponade (Unspecified diseases of pericardium); Hypovolemic shock; Myocardial infarction; Pneumothorax; Pulmonary embolism; Septic shock; Tension; Traumatic shock; Ventricular fibrillation; Ventricular tachycardia

VII. **Problem Case Diagnosis.** Ventricular fibrillation secondary to hyperkalemia.

Footnotes to Figure I–2

(1) Sodium bicarbonate 1 mEq/kg if patient has known preexisting hyperkalemia.

(2) KCl 40–60 mmol/hr IV, if >40 mmol/hr must be administered through a central line; for rates >15 mmol/hr cardiac monitoring is mandatory; be sure concomitant hypomagnesemia is not present.

(3) Sodium bicarbonate 1 mEq/kg:

If known preexisting bicarbonate-responsive acidosis,

If intubated and continued long arrest interval,

Upon return of spontaneous circulation after long arrest interval,

Hypoxic lactic acidosis,

If overdose with tricyclic antidepressants,

To alkalinize the urine in drug overdoses (aspirin),

Note: May be harmful in respiratory acidosis.

(4) Evidence does not support TCP for asystole.

(5) The recommended dose of epinephrine is 1 mg IV push every 3–5 min. If this approach fails, consider high-dose epinephrine 0.2 mg/kg IV push, every 3–5 min. Vasopressin is not recommended for asystole.

(6) Assess effectiveness of ABCs, IV access, and medications. If asystole has continued for >5–10 min despite resuscitation, then discontinue resuscitation efforts. If the cause is hypothermia, drowning, or reversible drug overdose, consider continuing for a longer period of time.

VIII. Teaching Pearls Question. Where do most cardiac arrests occur?

IX. Teaching Pearls Answer. At home. (Becker, et al)

REFERENCES

American Heart Association. Guidelines 2000 for cardiopulmonary resuscitation and emergency cardiovascular care. Part 6: Advanced cardiac life support. *Circulation* 2000;102(8 Suppl):186–189.

Becker L, Eisenberg M, Fahrenbruck C, Cobb L. Public locations of cardiac arrest: Implications for public access defibrillation. *Circulation* 1998;97:2106–2109.

14. CARDIAC TRANSPLANT PROBLEMS

I. **Problem.** A middle-aged female presents 3 weeks after heart transplantation with a fever and light-headedness.

II. **Immediate Questions**

A. **Hemodynamic Status.** Treat significant hypotension (dopamine), bradycardia (isoproterenol-denervated hearts don't respond to atropine), heart failure (dobutamine). Treat other arrhythmias according to ACLS protocols.

B. **What are the vital signs?** Low-grade fever can indicate rejection or opportunistic infection. Rejection and sepsis can both present with hypotension. Rejection can also present with hypoxemia from pulmonary edema.

C. **When was the transplant?** Acute rejection most common in first 6 weeks. Type of infection varies by time from transplant. (see under 6. Infections)

D. **What medications?** Cyclosporine and azathioprine have significant toxicity. Steroids are often tapered off after the first 6 months to 1-year posttransplant. High-dose steroid use significantly increases risk of infection. Consider adrenal insufficiency in patients on chronic steroids.

Figure I–3. Algorithm for pulseless electrical activity (PEA = rhythm on monitor without detectable pulse). (Reproduced, with permission, from American Heart Association. Guidelines 2000 for cardiopulmonary resuscitation and emergency cardiovascular care. *Circulation* 2000[August]:102.)

Check responsiveness
Call for code team
Call for crash cart/defibrillator
Assess ABCs
Perform CPR until defibrillator attached
 (including positive pressure ventilation)
Defibrillate up to 3 times if needed for persistent VF/VT 200 J,
 200–300 J, 360 J

↓

Continue CPR
Intubate at once
Obtain IV access
Identify rhythm
Administer appropriate drugs
Identify and treat underlying cause

↓

Consider possible causes (and immediate treatment):
 Hypovolemia (volume infusion)
 Hypoxia (ventilation)
 Cardiac tamponade (pericardiocentesis)
 Tension pneumothorax (needle decompression)
 Hypothermia (see Section I, Chapter 48,
  Hypothermia, p. 144)
 Massive pulmonary embolism (surgery, thrombolytics)
 Hyperkalemia (1) or Hypokalemia (2)
 Acidosis (3)
 Drug overdoses (tricyclics, digitalis, β-blockers, calcium
  channel blockers) (3)
 Massive acute myocardial infarction (thrombolytics,
  intra-aortic balloon pump, angiography with intervention)

↓

Epinephrine 1 mg IV push, repeat every 3–5 min (4)

↓

If bradycardia is absolute or relative, give atropine 1 mg IV.
Repeat every 3–5 min to a total of 0.04 mg/kg

Footnotes to Figure I–3

(1) Sodium bicarbonate 1 mEq/kg if patient has known preexisting hyperkalemia.
(2) KCl 40–60 mmol/hr IV, if >40 mmol/hr must be administered through a central line; for rates >15 mmol/hr cardiac monitoring is mandatory; be sure concomitant hypomagnesemia is not present.
(3) Sodium bicarbonate 1 mEq/kg:
   If known preexisting bicarbonate-responsive acidosis,
   If intubated and continued long arrest interval,
   Upon return of spontaneous circulation after long arrest interval,
   Hypoxic lactic acidosis,
   If overdose with tricyclic antidepressants,
   To alkalinize the urine in drug overdoses (aspirin),
   Note: May be harmful in respiratory acidosis.
(4) The recommended dose of epinephrine is 1 mg IV push every 3–5 min. If this approach fails, consider high-dose epinephrine 0.2 mg/kg IV push, every 3–5 min. Vasopressin is not recommended for asystole.

III. Differential Diagnosis

A. Acute Rejection. Occurs in first 6 weeks and presents with non-specific symptoms.

  1. Symptoms. Fatigue, dyspnea, low-grade fever, nausea, and vomiting.

  2. Signs of heart failure. Rales, hypoxia, S_3, murmur, edema.

  3. ECG, CXR. New atrial arrhythmias, tachycardia (most sensitive), decreased voltage, cardiomegaly (compare to priors–transplanted heart size varies), PE, effusions.

B. Allograft Vasculopathy. Chronic rejection that begins 3 months after rejection leading to coronary disease, CHF, AMI. May present acutely or insidiously.

  1. Insidious. Fatigue, cough, dyspnea.

  2. Acute. Heart failure, sudden death, infarction (note chest pain likely will not be associated with infarction as heart is denervated).

C. Infections. Recipients are at high risk for a variety of infections because of immunosuppressants.

  1. First month. Nosocomial bacterial infections, pneumonia, mediastinitis, UTI.

  2. First year. Opportunistic infections, community infections, CMV, HSV, *Legionella*, fungal, PCP.

  3. Steroids. If still on steroids, much higher risk of bacterial infections. Acute intra-abdominal processes and meningitis may have no signs on exam when on steroids.

D. Medication Toxicity

  1. Cyclosporine. Nephrotoxicity, hepatotoxicity, neurotoxicity (tremor, seizures).

  2. Azathioprine. Bone marrow suppression, leukopenia.

  3. Steroids. Osteoporosis, Cushing's disease.

E. Neoplasms. 3 × risk of general population from immunosuppression. Include skin and lip cancer, non-Hodgkins lymphoma, Kaposi's sarcoma, pelvic tumors.

IV. **Database**
   A. **Physical Exam.** Evaluate for signs of CHF (JVD, S_3, pedal edema, rales). Evaluate for source of fever, pulmonary rales, abdominal tenderness, meningeal signs.
   B. **Laboratory Data**
      1. Lytes, LFTs help evaluate medication toxicity.
      2. CBC, UA, and blood and urine cultures if febrile. Consider lumbar puncture for headache, seizures, altered mental status.
      3. ABG if patient is hypoxemic or has evidence of respiratory failure.
      4. Discuss with transplant service further tests, which could include cardiac enzymes, tests for CMV and HSV (titers or PCR, urine antigen, buffy coat), and cyclosporine trough level (random levels are not useful).
   C. **Radiographic and Other Studies.** Every patient should have an ECG and CXR (see Differential Diagnosis.). In conjunction with transplant service echocardiogram is often useful. Many patients will need cardiology consult for cardiac catheterization and myocardial biopsy.

V. **Plan**
   A. **Overall Plan.** Hemodynamically unstable patient should be stabilized. Differentiation should be made among rejection, infection, and medication toxicity. Transplant service should be involved early in patient's care. Patients with evidence of acute rejection, myocardial ischemia, dysrhythmias, moderate or severe CHF, fever, or suspected CMV or HSV should be admitted.
   B. **Specific Plan**
      1. **Acute rejection.** Requires stabilization (see Differential Diagnosis.). High-dose (1000 mg) methylprednisolone. Other antirejection medications per transplant team.
      2. **Infarction/allograft vasculopathy.** Aspirin, enoxaparin, angioplasty, retransplant.
      3. **Infection.** Discuss empiric antibiotics after cultures (especially if on steroids), consider ganciclovir for CMV (suspect with gastroenteritis, interstitial pneumonitis), acyclovir for HSV (suspected).
      4. **Medication toxicity.** Medication changes should be discussed with transplant service.

VI. **ICD-9 Diagnoses.** Complication of heart transplant (includes failure and rejection).

VII. **Problem Case Diagnosis.** This lady presents with acute rejection and pump failure causing her fever and light-headedness from hypotension. She requires dopamine for her blood pressure, high-dose steroids, and admission for her rejection. She also needs to be evaluated for possible infection with blood and urine cultures and CXR and is admitted to the transplant service in the ICU.

VIII. **Teaching Pearls Question.** What is the 5-year survival rate of cardiac transplantation?

IX. **Teaching Pearls Answer.** 69% (1-year survival is 85%).

REFERENCES

Chinnock R, Sherwin T, Robie S, et al. Emergency department presentation and management of pediatric heart transplant recipients. *Pediatr Emerg Care* 1995;11(5):355–360.

Johnson MR. Clinical follow-up of the heart transplant recipient. *Curr Opin Cardiol* 1995;10:180–192.

Mill MR, Grady MS. Cardiac transplantation. In: Tintinalli JE, Kelen GD, Stapczynski JS, eds. *Emergency Medicine: A Comprehensive Study Guide.* 5th ed. McGraw-Hill, 1999: 422–428.

Miniati DN, Robbins RC, Reitz BA. In: Braunwald E, ed. *Heart Disease: A Textbook of Cardiovascular Medicine.* 6th ed. WB Saunders, 2001:615–631.

15. CHEST PAIN

I. **Problem.** A 62-year-old female complains of chest pain and shortness of breath while climbing stairs to her bedroom.

II. **Immediate Questions**

A. **Is the airway stable?** How is the patient breathing? Is she talking and able to give a history? Manage airway as per Section VIII. 15. Rapid Sequence Endotracheal Intubation, page 470, if necessary.

B. **What are the vital signs?** Take vital signs including pulse oximetry. Is the blood pressure very low (SBP < 90 mm Hg) or high (SBP > 200 mm Hg)? Is the heart rate very low (< 60 bpm) or high (> 100 bpm)? Place patient on monitor, place IV, and administer oxygen (IV/O_2/monitor).

C. **What are the associated symptoms?** Are these symptoms associated with diaphoresis, nausea, vomiting, neck/jaw pain, shortness of breath, radiation of pain? Ask about radiation to back, abdominal pain, or pleuritic component of pain. Is the pain like a previous MI or bout of angina?

D. **What are the patient's medical problems (HTN, DM, hyperlipidemia)?** Any history of heart disease? Any history of recent surgery or immobility? What are the patient's present medications?

E. **Does the patient have any CAD risk factors (HTN, smoking, DM, hyperlipidemia, family history of CAD in first-degree relative < 50)?**

III. **Differential Diagnosis**

A. **Heart**
   1. **AMI**
   2. **ACS.** Includes unstable angina, non-Q wave MI, Q wave MI.
   3. **CHF**
   4. **Pericarditis/pericardial effusion**
   5. **Dysrhythmia**

B. **Aorta**
   1. **Dissection (type A and B)**
   2. **Aneurysm**

C. **Lungs**
   1. **PE**
   2. **Pneumonia**
   3. **Pneumothorax**
   4. **Pleurisy**

      5. **COPD/Asthma**
      6. **CHF**

IV. **Database**
  A. **Physical Exam Key Points**
     1. **Vital signs.** Monitor closely for hemodynamic instability. Check BP in both arms.
     2. **Neck.** JVD, carotid bruits.
     3. **Heart.** Rate, rhythm, rubs, murmurs, S_3 and S_4. Tachycardia suggests significant distress. With tachycardia and hypoxia, consider PE. New murmurs suggest papillary muscle dysfunction or aortic root pathology.
     4. **Lungs.** Assess breath sounds, respiratory effort, presence of crackles, wheezes, rubs.
     5. **Extremities.** Edema, pulses.
  B. **Laboratory Data.** Cardiac markers (myoglobin, CK-MB), cTnI, or cTnT). Serial determination of these may prove useful. Other recommended laboratory tests include CBC for tracking hematocrit and platelets, Lytes, ABG for PE suspicion.
  C. **Radiographic and Other Studies.** *ECG:* For acute changes such as ST segment elevation, ST depression, Q waves, reciprocal ST segment changes, dysrhythmias such as complete heart block. Old ECG can be very helpful regarding changes. *CXR:* Pneumonia, PE, mediastinal widening, pneumothorax, heart size, and silhouette. *V/Q scan or chest CT:* To look for PE, rest radionuclide imagine such as sestamibi to assess cardiac perfusion. *Echocardiogram:* To determine wall motion and ejection fraction.

V. **Plan**
  A. **Overall Plan**
     1. **Determine overall risk level for AMI/ACS.**
       a. **ST-segment elevation AMI.**
       b. **High risk for ACS.** Hx of CAD, PCI < 6 months, PE, rest pain, dynamic ST segment changes on ECG, positive cardiac markers.
       c. **Intermediate risk.** Appropriate Hx, 2–3 risk factors, nonspecific changes on ECG.
       d. **Low risk.** Atypical Hx, few to no risk factors, normal ECG.
     2. **Consideration of PE with those at risk**
       a. V/Q (ventilation/perfusion scan).
       b. Contrasted chest CT angiogram.
       c. Pulmonary angiogram (gold standard).
     3. **Thoracic aneurysm or dissection suspected by history and physical, papillary muscle rupture.**
       a. Immediate operative consultation if diagnosis suspected.
       b. Contrasted chest CT angiogram for diagnosis of aneurysm.
       c. Aortogram (gold standard).
  B. **Specific Plans**
     1. **Treatment of AMI/ACS/possible cardiac chest pain.**

       a. **AMI.** Need emergency therapy or intervention. All patients need aspirin, UF or LMW heparin. Beta-blockers should be used in patients that are not bradycardic or hypotensive. NTG and morphine used for pain relief with careful attention to blood pressure. Consider using glycoprotein IIb/IIIa inhibitors. For patients in cardiogenic shock, vasopressors such as dopamine or dobutamine may be required.

       b. **High risk for ACS.** Admission to monitored setting, anticoagulation with heparin, beta-blockade. Consider the use of IIb/IIIa inhibitor. NTG and morphine used for pain relief.

       c. **Intermediate risk.** Short stay admission or observation unit for serial markers, serial ECGs, rest, and provocative testing. All patients receive aspirin. Other therapies can be used as indicated.

       d. **Low risk.** ED evaluation consisting of thorough history, physical, ECG, and CXR.

  2. **Treatment of PE.**

       a. **Heparin (UF or LMW).** Consider this before definitive diagnosis if high suspicion.

       b. **Airway support.** Supplemental oxygen, mechanical ventilation as necessary.

       c. **ED thrombolytics.** Unstable patients with positive imaging test or clear evidence of RV dysfunction (ECG findings, bedside US, CVP).

  3. **Aortic aneurysm or dissection, papillary muscle rupture.**

       a. Immediate operative consultation.

       b. Tight blood pressure control (may need invasive hemodynamic monitoring, titratable IV antihypertensives such as esmolol, labetalol, or sodium nitroprusside). Aim for BP < 185/110 mm Hg.

VI. ICD-9 Diagnoses. AMI (state which wall involved); Acute pericarditis; Aortic aneurysm; Aortic dissection; Costochondritis; Dysrhythmia; Esophagitis; Pleurisy; Pneumonia; Pneumothorax; Pulmonary embolism.

VII. Problem Case Diagnosis. AMI.

VIII. Teaching Pearl Question. If a patient with chest pain presents with acute ECG changes in the inferior leads (II, III, and AVF) and becomes significantly hypotensive with administration of nitrates, what specific diagnosis must be considered?

IX. Teaching Pearl Answer. RV infarction! Get a right-sided ECG to look for elevation in V4R. Hypotension usually responds to fluids. Provide adequate preload in the form of fluids before considering vasopressors. Avoid nitrates in these patients.

REFERENCES

ACC/AHA Taskforce on Practice Guidelines (Committee on Management of Acute Myocardial Infarction). *J Am Coll Cardiol* 1996;28:1328–1428.

AHA 2000 Handbook of Emergency Cardiovascular Care for Healthcare Providers. AHA Publication, 2000.

ACC/AHA Guidelines for the Management of Patients with Unstable Angina and Non-ST-Segment Elevation Myocardial Infarction. *J Am Coll Cardiol* 2000;36(3):970–1062

16. CONGESTIVE HEART FAILURE/PULMONARY EDEMA

I. **Problem.** A 62-year-old white female presents with 2 days of progressive SOB, orthopnea, and PND. She has a respiratory rate of 38 and an SaO_2 of 72% on room air. She is in acute respiratory distress and is unable to answer questions secondary to dyspnea and decreased level of consciousness. Her husband informs you that she has had increased lower extremity edema and a cough productive of frothy white sputum.

II. **Immediate Questions**
   A. **Does the patient have a secure airway?** Immediately evaluate for respiratory rate, accessory muscle use, level of consciousness, ability to speak and swallow, and SaO_2. Secure airway if necessary before proceeding with the assessment and management. Consider BiPAP or immediate intubation and mechanical ventilation.
   B. **What are the vital signs?** BP very high or low, tachycardia or bradycardia, tachypnea or hypoventilation, fever.
   C. **What is the medical history?** Specifically, cardiac, renal, or pulmonary disease?
   D. **What medications is the patient taking?** Has the patient taken her usual medications today? Substance abuse?
   E. **What are the symptoms associated with the patient's complaint?** Symptoms of LV failure include dyspnea, PND, orthopnea, cough, pink or frothy sputum, wheezing. Right-heart failure symptoms include dependent edema, abdominal pain or increased abdominal girth, and nausea.
   F. **Acute or gradual onset?**
   G. **Associated chest pain?**
   H. **Exacerbating or alleviating factors?**

III. **Differential Diagnosis**
   A. **Cardiac.** AMI, subacute CHF, AF, AV block, BBB, VT, symptomatic bradycardia, valvular disease, ACS, pericarditis, myocarditis.
   B. **Pulmonary.** Asthma, COPD, PA, pneumonia, noncardiogenic PE, pneumothorax.
   C. **Other Causes.** Sepsis, anemia, anaphylaxis, acute renal failure, missed dialysis, opiate overdose, CVA, NSAID use, noncompliance with medication.

IV. **Database**
   A. **Physical Exam Key Points**
      1. **General.** Level of consciousness, extremely high or low BP, tachycardia or bradycardia, diaphoresis, agitation or lethargy.
      2. **Cardiac.** Murmurs, S_3 or S_4, JVD, hepatojugular reflux, peripheral edema.

3. **Pulmonary.** Respiratory effort, accessory muscle use, wheezing, rales, egophony, dullness to percussion (*Caution:* Rales may be obscured by concurrent respiratory disease).

B. **Laboratory Data**

C. **Radiographic and Other Studies.** *ECG:* The ECG in patients with PE is usually abnormal and may show conduction abnormalities, low voltage, inverted T waves, or evidence of chamber enlargement. The ECG should also be assessed for acute or old MI and for ongoing ischemia. ABG, CBC, Lytes, BUN, creatinine, and cardiac enzymes. Other labs such as urine drug screen as situation dictates. *CXR:* Frequently helpful in guiding initial management, particularly in the setting of concurrent respiratory disease. Will often show cardiomegaly, cephalization of pulmonary vasculature, and peribronchiolar cuffing. Bilateral, patchy, perihilar distribution of ground-glass-appearing lung density (batwing pattern) and Kerley B lines are also frequent findings. *Other tests to consider:* Echocardiogram, cardiac or pulmonary angiography, and radionucleotide studies. These tests are of limited utility in the ED but may be important in obtaining a definitive diagnosis and for ongoing management.

V. **Plan**

A. **Overall Plan.** Rapid recognition and treatment are necessary to prevent morbidity/mortality!

1. Place on cardiac monitor, obtain IV access, and administer oxygen to titrate to SaO_2 of $\geq 95\%$.

2. Consider BiPAP or rapid sequence intubation if the patient is obtunded, cannot maintain optimal SaO_2, or is fatigued. BiPAP has been shown effective in treating acute respiratory insufficiency/failure associated with PE and may reduce/eliminate the need for intubation.

B. **Specific Plans**

1. **Nitrates.** Start with sublingual NTG 0.4 mg and repeat every 3–5 min as needed. Some patients may require an IV NTG drip. The dose is 5–200 µg/kg/min, titrated to relief of dyspnea and striving to keep BP of ≥ 100 mm Hg systolic.

2. **ACE Inhibitors.** Give captopril 25 mg SL as a starter dose, in the absence of contraindications, oral ACE therapy should be started when patient is stable

3. **Diuretics.** Give furosemide 0.5–1 mg/kg IV, additional dose if no response in 15–30 min. If the patient is already on diuretics, give roughly twice the patient's usual PO dose IV.

4. **Morphine.** can be given in 1–2 mg IV boluses. (*Caution:* CNS and respiratory depression.)

5. **Inotropic agents.** when CHF/pulmonary edema is associated with hypotension/cardiogenic shock, Dopamine at 1–20 µg/kg/min IV and/or dobutamine at 0.5–20 µg/kg/min IV may be indicated.

6. **Digoxin.** The use of digoxin (digitalis) in acute PE is controversial. Studies have shown that a single IV dose of digoxin can improve LV stroke work index and decrease PWP. It may also be useful for rate control in AF.

7. **Nitroprusside.** Severe HTN that does not respond to NTG may be treated with nitroprusside at 0.3–10 µg/kg/min. Titrate to relief of dyspnea and approximately 25–33% reduction in BP.

8. **Beta-blockers.** In patients refractory to other therapies, short-acting beta-blocker such as esmolol may improve patients condition. All patients with mild to moderate CHF with no strict contraindications (lung disease, severe CHF, known AV block, or bradycardia) should be placed on beta-blocker therapy. Beta-blockers have been shown to improve LV function and long-term survival in CHF.

9. Treat known precipitating factors or suspected causes of pulmonary edema/CHF. Monitored bed generally required.

10. Patients may require invasive hemodynamic monitoring, positive airway pressure, or assisted circulation with an intra-aortic balloon pump and LV assist device.

VI. **ICD-9 Diagnoses.** Acute pulmonary edema; Congestive heart failure; High-output heart failure; Hypertensive heart failure with renal disease or renal failure; Pulmonary edema with left ventricular failure.

VII. **Problem Case Diagnosis.** The patient is showing signs of both right- and left-heart failure. This patient has a history of MI and CHF. She is also a smoker with COPD. The patient had recently been on vacation and had been neglecting her low-sodium diet. She also admits to forgetting to take her medicine "a few times" during her 1-week trip. This patient responded quickly to BiPAP, SL NTG, IV morphine, SL captopril, and IV furosemide. She was admitted to the ICU and was released 3 days later after an uneventful hospital course.

VIII. **Teaching Pearls Question.** What medication has been shown to increase both short- and long-term survival in patients with pulmonary edema/CHF?

IX. **Teaching Pearls Answer.** ACE inhibitors have been shown to decrease morbidity/mortality from pulmonary edema and also to halt the progression of heart failure and improve LV function in patients with CHF.

REFERENCES

Aronow WS, Ahn C, Kronzon I. Effect of beta blockers alone, of angiotensin-converting enzyme inhibitors alone, and of beta blockers plus angiotensin-converting enzyme inhibitors on new coronary events and on congestive heart failure in older persons with healed myocardial infarcts and asymptomatic left ventricular systolic dysfunction. *Am J Cardiol* 2001;88:1298–1300.

Garg R, Yusuf S. Overview of randomized trials of angiotensin-converting enzyme inhibitors on mortality and morbidity in patients with heart failure. *JAMA* 1995;235:1450–1456.

Hamilton RJ, Carter WA, Gallagher EJ. Rapid improvement of acute pulmonary edema with sublingual captopril. *Acad Emerg Med* 1996;3:192–193.

Sacchetti A, Ramoska E, Moakes ME, Moyer V. Effect of ED management on ICU use in acute pulmonary edema. *Am J Emerg Med* 1999;17:571–574.

Wigder HN, Hoffmann P, Mazzolini D, et al: Pressure support non-invasive positive airway pressure ventilation treatment of acute cardiogenic pulmonary edema. *Am J of Emerg Med* 2001;19:179–181.

17. CONSENT TO TREATMENT

I. **Problem.** A middle-aged male is brought to your ED by his wife who reports he "threw up a bunch of blood" 30 min prior to arrival. The triage nurse records a heart rate of 125 bpm but is unable to obtain a BP secondary to patient's agitation. The patient walks into an ED treatment room unassisted, but when the nurse approaches him, the patient refuses an IV and demands to be discharged saying he is "fine."

II. **Immediate Questions**
   A. **Is the airway intact?** Manage appropriately.
   B. **What are the vital signs and mental status?** Is the patient stable? If the patient will allow it, place on monitor, obtain vital signs, and assess for signs of hypovolemia and hypoperfusion, eg, tachycardia, hypotension. Is the patient confused? Does he answer questions appropriately? Oriented to place? Person?
   C. **Is the patient competent to refuse treatment in this situation?** Is the patient alert and oriented to person, place, and time? Does the patient appear to understand both the nature of his medical problem and the benefits and risks of treatment or nontreatment? Does his wife think he is at his baseline mental status? Does your initial evaluation suggest the patient may be under the influence of drugs or alcohol?

III. **Differential Diagnosis** (as pertains to patient's competency and ability to refuse treatment).
   A. **Patient is deemed competent.** If a patient is competent to make his own decisions he may do so even if the patient's decision appears irrational to you (see exceptions in IV. Database). An apparently irrational decision by a patient is not de facto evidence of incompetency; rather, it is the cognitive process that led to the ultimate decision that determines competency. It is incumbent upon the emergency physician to communicate the seriousness of the patient's condition to both the patient and family and to assure the patient acknowledges and fully understands the ramifications of treatment refusal. (See V. Plan for interventions in this regard.)
   B. **Patient is deemed incompetent to make decisions.** Patients incompetent to make decisions about medical care, whether incompetence is acute or chronic, must still provide consent to treatment. This is usually done through a surrogate such as a family member, a written power of attorney, or a court-appointed guardian. (See V. Plan for exceptions if surrogate methods of consent are unavailable.)

IV. **Database**
   A. **A Patient's Right to Refuse Treatment.** A patient's right to refuse treatment stems from several different aspects of the law.
      1. People are protected from **battery** (the unwanted touching by another) by state statutes.
      2. The United States Supreme Court has held that American citizens have a **right to privacy** emanating from the United States Constitution.

    3. The right to **self-determination** is woven into the fabric of American culture. People are allowed to make decisions that may not be in their own self-interest as long as they meet the following criteria:

        a. They are able to understand information about their condition, treatment options and benefits, and risks of nontreatment.

        b. They are shown to believe the information they are given.

        c. They are capable of weighing information and arriving at a conclusion.

B. Exceptions to the Right to Refuse. The right to refuse treatment is not absolute even in competent patients. Two exceptions exist (1) suicidal patients and (2) consent being denied for minor children, spouses, or other innocent parties who will suffer significant harm by refusal.

C. Pediatrics. In general, a minor needs consent of the legal guardian (most often a parent) for medical treatment. Exceptions to this rule are (1) emancipated minors (2) treatment for minors that are statutorily exempted from parental consent requirements (usually treatment for STDs, substance abuse, etc), (3) emergency treatment; however, every effort should be made to contact parents as soon as possible.

    1. Refusal of treatment for minors. Parents may also choose not to consent to treatment for their children because of religious, cultural, or other reasons. Courts have consistently sided with physicians who treat children to prevent death or disability despite the fact that the parents refused such care. It is important in such cases to include the hospital's ethics committee and risk management team.

V. Plan

    A. Overall Plan. Documentation is essential in all cases of refusal or competency issues. If you believe a patient is incompetent to judge his medical condition, state your opinion and why you believe the patient is incompetent. If a patient is competent but refusing treatment, the record should reflect

        1. the patient's condition,

        2. your efforts to educate the patient,

        3. involvement of family,

        4. why the patient refuses,

        5. your efforts to arrange follow-up.

        In pediatric cases the record should also reflect attempts to contact the parents (if they are not with the child).

    B. The Competent Patient Refusing Treatment. Reassess the patient with efforts to make the patient comfortable; discover and address the patient's fears.

        1. Sit with the patient; place yourself at or below the level of the patient; make eye contact; use the patient's name.

        2. Ask open-ended questions; what are the patient's concerns?

        3. Use a collaborative approach; involve patient's family members, social worker, clergy.

4. Reassure the patient that the final decision will be left up to the patient and you will answer all questions.
5. *A patient leaving AMA:* Document your discussions and efforts to convince him to stay. Give the patient discharge instructions, and reiterate to patient he may return to the ED at any time without prejudice in future medical care.
6. *The suicidal/homicidal patient:* For the patient's protection, he cannot be allowed to leave until evaluated by appropriate personnel. Involve social work and psychiatry, and have law enforcement personnel observe patient and restrain if necessary (see 3. The violent or uncooperative patient).

C. The Incompetent Patient Refusing Treatment

1. **Patient has life-threatening condition.** An emergency condition exists and implies consent to treatment. Treat as needed to ameliorate immediate medical threat; contact family, guardian, etc as soon as possible. In general, treatment should not continue beyond that necessary to correct the life-threatening situation unless further legal action is taken to declare the patient incompetent.
2. **Patient has medical condition requiring urgent attention.** Without treatment, the condition would become rapidly life- or limb-threatening. Attempt to contact a family member, guardian who holds power of attorney for this patient, or if none, involve a magistrate or judge to obtain an order for medical treatment. *Note:* Patients do not automatically fall under the emergency exception for consent simply because they are in an ED. A life-threatening condition or potential for such must exist. A magistrate or judge can declare the patient incompetent to make his own care decisions in two ways:
   a. **Temporarily incompetent.** Patient is not able to make decisions in the short term. This allows the caregiver to treat **only** the disease process or problem that is life- or limb-threatening. Once the crisis is over, the patient reassumes the right to self-determination.
   b. **Permanently incompetent.** Patient is judged to be chronically impaired and will never be able to self-determine care. This is much rarer and largely employed with patients who are demented or institutionalized.
3. **The violent or uncooperative patient.** You have a duty to protect the patient from himself and provide a safe environment for other patients and staff. If restraints are necessary, use least restrictive means first; frequently reassess patient.
4. **Patient tries to walk out.** If the patient has a life-threatening problem and is incompetent to make his own decisions and/or a danger to himself or others, you can have him held for evaluation. Each state has specific statues as to how emergency detention and evaluation will occur and who should evaluate the patient. This process will result in either commitment of the patient to a treatment facility and/or the patient being declared incom-

petent to make his own medical care decisions. In both of these cases the legal order usually has a time limit. Be familiar with the applicable state statues in your practice location.

VI. ICD-9 Diagnoses. None.

VII. Problem Case Diagnosis. This patient is likely not competent to make medical decisions because he has sustained enough blood loss to cause hypovolemia, hypoperfusion, leading to altered mental status. Further discussions with patient and family are necessary.

VIII. Teaching Pearl Question. Does an emergency treatment order allow you to provide any treatment you think necessary?

IX. Teaching Pearl Answer. No. You can only provide such treatment that is necessary to prevent death and disability.

REFERENCES

Adams J, Murray R. The general approach to the difficult patient, *Emerg Med Clin North Am* 1998;16:689–700.

Harrison DW, Vissers RJ. Approach to the difficult patient in the emergency department. In: Rosen P, Barkin R, Danzel DF, et al, eds. *Emergency Medicine: Concepts and Clinical Practice.* 4th Ed. Mosby Yearbook, 1997:2841–2852.

Hassan T, MacNamara AF, Bing A, et al: Managing patients with deliberate self harm who refuse treatment in the accident and emergency department. *Br Med J* 1999;319(7202): 107–109.

Lavoie FW. Consent, involuntary treatment, and the use of force in an urban emergency department. *Ann Emerg Med* 1992;21:25–32.

Lowery DA. Issues of Non-compliance in Mental Health. *J Adv Nurs* 1998;28(2):280–287.

Moskop JC. Informed consent in the emergency department. *EM Clin North Am* 1999;17:327–340.

O'Mara K. Communication and conflict resolution in emergency medicine. *EM Clin North Am* 1999;17(2):451–454.

Playne JF, Keeley P. Noncompliance and professional power. *J Adv Nurs* 1998;27(2): 304–311.

Sauvlescu J, Momeyer RW. Should informed consent be based on rational beliefs. *J Med Ethics* 1997;23(5):282–288.

Silverman H. The role of emotions in decisional competence, standards of competency and altruistic acts. *J Clin Ethics* 1999;8(2):171–175.

Simon JR, Dwyer J, Goldfrank LR. The difficult patient. *Emerg Med Clin North Am* 1999;17(2): 353–370.

Totten VY, Knopp R, Helpern K. Physician-patient communication in the emergency department: II. Communication strategies for specific situations. *Acad Emerg Med* 1996;3:1146–1153.

Workman S. Caring for difficult patients. *Hastings Cent Rep* 1998;28(4):4 Jul-Aug.

Zaubler TS, Viederman M, Fins JT. Ethical, legal, and psychiatric issues in capacity, competency, and informed consent, *Gen Hosp Psychiatry* 1996;18(3):155–172.

18. CONSTIPATION

I. Problem. A 60-year-old woman with a history of colon resection presents with constipation of 3 day's duration, worsening intermittent crampy abdominal pain, and vomiting of 1 day's duration.

II. Immediate Questions

A. How does the patient define constipation? Constipation is not a disease but a symptom interpreted subjectively by the patient. The simplest definition of constipation is a perceived change in bowel habits that results in more difficult or less frequent bowel movements.

B. Is the constipation a recent or chronic problem? Acute constipation such as described in this case is an intestinal obstruction until proven otherwise. Common but less serious causes of acute constipation include decreased fluid or fiber intake, changes in daily routine (ie, stress, immobility, travel), changes in defecation regimen (ie, failure to respond to the urge to defecate), and medication side effects.

C. What is the character of bowel movements? Reduced stool frequency compared with patient's normal bowel pattern, hard stools, excessive straining, intermittent diarrhea or incontinence of stool. Does the patient need to apply pressure on the perineum or posterior wall of vagina for evacuation (suspect rectocele)?

D. Are there any associated symptoms? Blood in the stool, painful defecation, abdominal distention or bloating, inability to pass flatus or excessive gas, abdominal pain, nausea and vomiting, anorexia, fatigue, fever, weight loss.

E. Does the patient have "alarm" symptoms concerning pathology?
1. **Intestinal obstruction.** May result in "obstipation" that is defined as the *inability* to have a bowel movement accompanied by nausea, vomiting, abdominal pain, and distention.
2. **Colorectal carcinoma.** Unexplained constipation of recent onset, persons older than 40 years of age, unexplained weight loss, rectal bleeding; may present with obstipation.

F. Does the patient have any medical conditions or surgeries that may cause constipation? See Differential Diagnosis. Constipation is common in pregnancy. Adhesions secondary to abdominal surgery are always a possible cause for an intestinal obstruction.

III. Differential Diagnosis

A. Anatomic or Mechanical
1. Neoplasm or other obstructive lesion (adhesions, diverticulum).
2. Rectal intussusception or prolapse.
3. Rectocele.
4. Perianal lesions (hemorrhoids, abscesses, fissures, fistulas, herpes).

B. Functional
1. Irritable bowel disease.

C. Pharmacologic
1. Anticholinergics.
2. Antidepressants.
3. Antiparkinsonian agents.
4. Antihypertensives (diuretics, calcium channel blockers, clonidine).
5. Sympathomimetics.
6. Cation-containing medications (aluminum, calcium, iron, bismuth).
7. $5-HT_3$ antagonists (ondansetron).
8. Phenytoin.

9. NSAIDs.
10. Laxative abuse.

D. Metabolic, Endocrine, Exocrine
1. Diabetes.
2. Hypercalcemia.
3. Hypokalemia.
4. Chronic renal failure.
5. Hypothyroidism.
6. Hypoadrenalism.
7. Cystic fibrosis.

E. Neurogenic
1. Aganglionosis (Hirschsprung's disease).
2. Intestinal pseudo-obstruction.
3. Multiple sclerosis.
4. Amyotrophic lateral sclerosis.
5. Dementia, stroke.
6. Parkinson's disease.
7. Spinal cord lesions.

F. Infectious
1. Chagas' disease

G. Psychogenic
1. Behavioral
2. Depression.
3. Psychosis.

H. Constipation of Unknown Cause
1. Slow colonic transit.
2. Pelvic floor dysfunction.

IV. Database
A. Physical Exam Key Points. Rule out organic causes of constipation.
1. **Abdomen/pelvis.** Distention, bowel sounds (high-pitched in bowel obstruction or absent with peritoneal irritation), areas of tenderness, hernias, abdominal or pelvic masses, ascites.
2. **Rectal and anoscopy.** Fecal impaction, hard stool, rectal mass, anal fissures, fistulas, hemorrhoids, perirectal abscess or prolapse of rectal mucosa; gross or occult blood; rectal tone. Evaluate for abnormal perineal descent (pelvic floor dysfunction) or formation of a rectocele with Valsalva's maneuver.

B. Laboratory Data. Fecal occult blood; hematocrit (especially if blood present in stool), metabolic profile (renal function, K^+ and Ca^{2+}), and thyroid function tests. Laboratory and radiographic data in general are not required in the evaluation of most cases of constipation. Order only as the clinical presentation mandates.

C. Radiographic and Other Studies
1. **Abdominal radiographs.** Document colonic loading; masses of stool have a speckled appearance and are easily visible on plain films. Rule out intestinal obstruction (dilated bowel loops, air fluid levels with upright film).

   2. **Abdominal and pelvic CT scan.** To evaluate for obstructive mass or lesion.
   3. **Barium enema radiography.** Evaluate for megarectum or megacolon.

V. Plan

  A. Overall Plan (empiric treatment). Steps 1 and 2 are the safest and most physiologic approach in the majority of patients.

   Step 1. Nonstrenuous exercise, adequate hydration (1.5 L/day in an adult), dedicated time for bowel movements, adequate fiber intake (10 g/day for an adult).

   Step 2. *Bulk-forming laxatives* (polycarbophil, psyllium, or methylcellulose); stool softeners with docusate sodium as needed (Table I–4).

   Step 3. *Osmotic laxatives* (magnesium citrate, magnesium hydroxide, sodium phosphates, lactulose, sorbitol); but avoid in patients with renal insufficiency or on sodium-restricted diets. Polyethylene glycol is the preferred osmotic laxative in selected patients due to fewer side effects (less bloating; does not affect salt and water absorption).

   Step 4. *Stimulant laxatives* (castor oil, bisacodyl, senna), to promote colonic secretion and motility. Only recommended if patient does not respond to initial measures.

  B. Specific Plans

   1. **Fecal impaction.** Must be manually disimpacted; mineral oil enema may assist in softening impaction.

TABLE I–4. LAXATIVES.

Type	Name	Dosage
Bulk—daily use	Effer-syllium	1 teaspoon (6–7 g) in fluid qd or bid
	Metamucil	1 teaspoon (6–7 g) in fluid qd or bid
Softeners/wetting agents—daily use	Docusate sodium (Colace)	50–200 mg qd or bid
		Available: Capsules 50–100 mg
		Solution 10 mg/mL
		Syrup 25 mg/mL
	Docusate calcium (Surfak)	240 mg qd or bid
	Lactulose (Chronuluc)	15–30 mL qd or bid
	Mineral oil	14–45 mL; one-time dose
Stimulants—prn	Bisacodyl (Dulcolax)	Oral 5–15 mg, 5-mg tablets
		Rectal 10 mg, 10-mg suppository
	Senna (Senokol)	1 tablet qd or bid
	Glycerine suppository	3 g; 1 PR
Osmotic—prn	Milk of Magnesia	15–30 mL qd or bid
	Magnesium citrate	200 mL; one-time dose
Enema—prn	Fleet enema	120 mL PR
	Oil retention enema	

Reproduced, with permission, from Haist SA, Robbins JB, Gomella LG, eds. *Internal Medicine On Call*, 3rd ed. McGraw-Hill, 2002.

     2. **Surgical evaluation.** For bowel obstruction and perirectal abscess.

     3. **Treat other underlying abnormalities and withhold causative medications.**

  C. **Referral to Specialist**

     1. **The patient should be referred to a specialist if the following criteria are met:**

       a. History and physical do not identify the cause of constipation *and*

       b. There is no relief by empiric therapy.

     2. **Evaluation may include:**

       a. Flexible sigmoidoscopy with barium enema or colonoscopy to identify lesions that narrow or occlude the bowel; colonoscopy preferable for older patients and in those with anemia or hemoccult-positive stools to identify polyps or other concerning lesions.

       b. Manometric and radiologic tests to determine colonic transit and anorectal dysfunction.

VI. ICD-9 Diagnoses. Constipation; Constipation-drug induced; Constipation-neurogenic; Fecal impaction; Hirschsprung's disease; Hypothyroidism; Intestinal obstruction; Irritable bowel syndrome; Neoplasm (specify site); Rectocele.

VII. Problem Case Diagnosis. Acute small-bowel obstruction due to adhesions from previous surgery.

VIII. Teaching Pearls Question. What is an infectious cause of constipation in South America that may result in diffuse esophageal and bowel dilatation?

IX. Teaching Pearls Answer. Chagas' disease, caused by *Trypanosoma cruzi,* is a common cause of dilated gut, megaesophagus, megaduodenum, and megacolon in South America (Gattuso and Kamm, 1993).

REFERENCES

Gattuso JM, Kamm MA. Review article: The management of constipation in adults. *Aliment Pharmacol Ther* 1993;7:487–500.

Soffer EE. Constipation: An approach to diagnosis, treatment, referral. *Cleve Clin J Med* 1999;66(1):41–46.

Wald A. Constipation. *Med Clin North Am* 2000;84(5):1231–1246.

Wrenn K. Fecal impaction. *New Engl J Med* 1989;321(10):658–662.

19. COUGH IN ADULTS

  I. **Problem:** A 42-year-old nonsmoking female presents complaining of cough for several months. She states the cough is particularly bad at night and is associated with indigestion and a recurrent "bad taste" in her mouth.

II. Immediate Questions

A. Is the airway intact? Always start with airway and breathing. Although cough is an extremely common symptom, do not miss an airway obstruction (eg, foreign body), especially in the pediatric population.

B. What is the duration of the cough? Formulating an appropriate differential diagnosis depends on whether the cough is *acute* or *chronic*.

C. Quality of the cough? Is it productive or nonproductive? If productive, describe the characteristics of the sputum. Is there hemoptysis?

D. Timing of the cough? Is it constant or is there a seasonal component? (Think about allergic symptoms). Is it worse at night/when lying down (CHF) ? After meals (reflux) ? At work (exposures, hypersensitivity) ?

E. Associated symptoms? Fevers/chills, congestion, rhinorrhea/postnasal drip, shortness of breath/wheezing/stridor, orthopnea/PND, indigestion/foul taste in mouth, weight loss.

F. Past medical history? Is the patient a smoker? (how long, how many per day?) History of childhood asthma? Lung disease (asthma, COPD)? Heart disease (CHF)? Atopic history (eczema, food allergies)? Exposures (asbestos, silicon, organic dusts/gases)? Family history (cancers, heart disease, allergies/atopy)? Taking any medications (ACE inhibitors)?

III. Differential Diagnosis

A. Acute Cough (< 3 week's duration)
1. **Viral URI** (most common cause).
2. **Acute bacterial infection.**
   a. Sinusitis.
   b. Pharyngitis.
   c. Bronchitis.
   d. Pneumonia.
3. **Allergic rhinitis.**
4. **Asthma/COPD exacerbation.**
5. **Aspiration of foreign body.**
6. **Pertussis.**

B. Chronic Cough (> 3–8 week's duration)
1. **Smoking'**
2. **ENT disorders'**
   a. Ear-cough (Arnold's reflex)
   b. Postnasal drip.
   c. Neoplasms.
3. **Tracheobronchial disease.**
   a. Chronic bronchitis: smoking, cystic fibrosis
   b. Dysmotile cilia syndrome
   c. Asthma.
   d. Tracheal compression: Vascular ring, neoplasm, lymph node.
   e. Neoplasm: Carcinoma, bronchial adenoma.
4. **Parenchymal lung disease.**
   a. Neoplasms.
   b. Infections: Pneumonia, tuberculosis/fungal (esp. in HIV population).
   c. Diffuse interstitial disease.

     5. Esophageal disease.
       a. Gastroesophageal reflux.
     6. Cardiac disease.
       a. CHF.
       b. Mitral valve disease.
       c. ACE inhibitors.
     7. Neuropsychiatric disorders (psychogenic cough).

IV. Database
A. Physical Exam Key Points
1. **Vital signs.** Febrile? Hypertensive?
2. **Otorhinolaryngeal exam.** Check TM for wax, hair, or foreign body. Assess pharynx for erythema, exudates, or "cobblestoning." Inspect nares for congestion or rhinorrhea.
3. **Sinuses.** Tenderness to palpation, increasing pain when bending over.
4. **Neck.** Check for lymphadenopathy, tracheal asymmetry, or thyromegaly.
5. **Pulmonary.** Start with a general assessment of respiratory status, looking for signs of obvious dyspnea or stridor. Auscultate all lung fields carefully. Listen for wheezes (esp. with forced expiration), rales in lung bases (CHF), or rhonchi/coarse breath sounds.
6. **Cardiac.** Listen for gallops or murmurs.
B. Laboratory Data
1. **CBC with Diff.** Look for signs of infection (high WBCs with large percentage of immature cells) and also check for eosinophilia.
2. **Chest radiograph.** Look for obvious abnormalities (infiltrates, effusions, tumors, or cardiomegaly). Most abnormalities should be considered as the cause.
3. **Sputum examination.** Cytology/cultures, AFB, eosinophilic bronchitis.
4. **Sinus radiographs/CT scans.** Looking for acute or chronic infection, neoplasm.
5. **Peak flow** (and response to bronchodilator therapy), rarely Methacholine challenge test.
6. **GI studies.** EGD, pH monitoring, barium swallow.
7. **Bronchoscopy.**

V. Plan
A. Overall Plan.
Thorough Hx and physical. Most causes can be diagnosed on the basis of Hx and exam alone. Lab studies tend to be supportive of initial impression.
B. Specific Plans
1. **Infections.** Antibiotics for specific cause (See 58. Respiratory Distress, page 174)
2. **Most common causes of cough** (more than 90% of the cases will be attributed to postnasal drip, asthma, reflux, or chronic bronchitis) will be best treated without antibiotics. Beta-agonist and ipratropium nebs for bronchospasm (See 73. Wheezing,

page 216). Cessation of smoking and metered-dose inhaler for chronic bronchitis.

3. **Antitussives/Expectorants.** Avoid unless in dry persistent cough and even then should only be used when work-up for more serious conditions is underway. Oral antihistamine (diphenhydramine) may be tried first. Opioids most effective but may also consider benzonatate (Tessalon, Perles), dextromethorphan, guaifenesin.

VI. ICD-9 Diagnoses. Acute bronchitis; Adverse effect medication-ACE inhibitor; Allergic rhinitis; Asthma; Cardiac asthma (same as CHF); Chronic cough; Cough; Esophageal reflux; Neoplasm; Pertussis; Sinusitis (same as postnasal drip); Smokers cough; Upper respiratory infection.

VII. Problem Case Diagnosis. GERD

VIII. Teaching Pearls Question. What is the most common cause of acute cough?

IX. Teaching Pearls Answer. URI/postnasal drip.

REFERENCES

Irwing R, Madison J. The diagnosis and treatment of cough. *Primary Care* 2000;340; 1715–1721.

Lewis N, Lane T. Cough. In Rakel R, ed. *Conn's Current Therapy.* WB Saunders, 1997:27–30.

Pratter M, Barter T, Akers S, et al. An algorithmic approach to chronic cough. *Ann Intern Med* 1993;119:977–983.

Yu M, Ryu J. Assessment of the patient with chronic cough. *Mayo Clin Proc* 1997;72: 957–959.

20. DECUBITUS ULCER

I. **Problem:** An elderly male is sent to the ED from a nursing home with fever and an ulcer on his sacrum.

II. **Immediate Questions**

A. **What are the vital signs and mental status?** Is the patient tachycardic, hypotensive, or tachypneic (all signs of sepsis)? Is the patient awake and alert or confused? Apply monitors (ECG and pulse oximetry), start IV (NS or RL), apply oxygen (2 L O_2 nasal cannula to start).

B. **Does the patient have any specific complaints?** This can point toward source(s) of fever other than decubitus ulcer. Headache or neck stiffness (ie, meningitis)? Sore throat (ie, group A beta hemolytic strep)? Cough, shortness of breath or pleuritic chest pain (ie, pneumonia, aspiration)? Abdominal pain, vomiting or diarrhea (ie, appendicitis, diverticulitis, cholecystitis, mesenteric ischemia or intra-abdominal infection)? Dysuria, frequency, urgency or flank pain (ie, UTI, prostatitis or pyelonephritis)?

C. **Is the patient ambulatory, wheelchair-bound or bed-confined?** Increasing risk factors for decubitus ulcers.

    D. **Past medical history?** Decubitus ulcers? Cerebral vascular.

    E. **Accident?** Quadriplegia, paraplegia or spinal cord injury? Malnutrition? Peripheral vascular disease? Recent fracture? Urinary or fecal incontinence? DVT? DM?

    F. **What does the ulcer look like?** Location? Depth? Color? Smell? Presence of pus or necrotic tissue? Surrounding erythema?

III. Differential Diagnosis

    A. **Decubitus ulcers.** Chronic debilitated state, confined to bed, spinal cord injury, paraplegia.

    B. **Venous stasis ulcers.** Chronic venous insufficiency, lower extremity edema, skin hyperpigmentation

    C. **Arterial ulcers.** Hx of peripheral vascular disease, claudication, resting pain.

    D. **Cellulitis.** Portal of entry/injury, fever, any location.

    E. **Osteomyelitis.** Long-standing nonhealing ulcer.

IV. Database

    A. **Physical Exam Key Points.** Don't forget other common problems in the chronically ill.

       1. **Mental status.** (See Section IV, 3. Altered Mental Status in the Older Patient, page 301; Appendix, 4. Mini Mental Status Exam, page 656)

       2. **Vital signs.** Abnormal vital signs may be due to infection, sepsis, hypovolemia, or fever.

       3. **Skin exam.**

          a. **Decubitus ulcer.** Usually over bony prominences (most common: sacrum, greater trochanter, ischial tuberosities, heels, and lateral malleoli).

          Classification of decubitus ulcers:

          Grade I. Nonblanchable erythema of intact skin.

          Grade II. Partial-thickness skin loss involving epidermis or dermis.

          Grade III. Full-thickness skin loss involving subcutaneous tissue that may extend to fascia.

          Grade IV. Full-thickness loss extending into muscle or bone.

          Venous stasis ulcer. Most commonly on medial aspect of distal leg and ankles, stocking distribution, skin hyperpigmentation, shallow ulcer movable with skin.

          b. **Arterial ulcer.** Most common over lateral ankles, toes, base of fifth metatarsal, head of first metatarsal, heel and ball of foot. Ulcer usually irregular with rolled border, weak/absent distal pulses.

          c. **Diabetic ulcer.** Usually forefoot and toes, either of ischemic (weak/absent distal pulses) or neurotrophic (ulcers with marginal thickening) origin.

          d. **Cellulitis.** Intact erythematous skin, warm, well demarcated, any location.

B. Laboratory Data. If thorough history and physical exam normal: CBC, bedside glucose (fingerstick). Other studies dictated by Hx and physical exam.

C. Radiographic and Other Studies. Radiographs of all but most superficial ulcers to evaluate for osteomyelitis. Bone scan, CT, MRI all more sensitive. Other studies as suggested by Hx and physical exam: CXR, UA and culture/sensitivity, blood cultures, lumbar puncture, peripheral vascular studies, CT abdomen/pelvis.

V. Plan

A. Overall Plan. Need to admit if severe local or suspected systemic infection, large (> 2 cm), deep (ie, grade III, IV), or multiple ulcers, severe anemia or malnutrition, acute arterial occlusion or DVT, metabolic derangement, or poor social support. Important aspects of general care: improved nutrition, vitamin C supplementation (500 mg PO bid), address urinary/fecal incontinence, relieve pressure from ulcer, frequent dressing changes, and monitoring.

B. Specific Plans

1. For patients with severe local or suspected systemic infection, start intravenous broad-spectrum antibiotics immediately.
2. For patients with grade III, IV ulcers, or large amount of necrotic tissue, surgical debridement.
3. For patients with grade II ulcer, debride necrotic tissue in ED.
4. All ulcers should be irrigated with saline.
5. Wet-to-dry saline dressings for majority of ulcers. Occlusive dressings (ie, hydrocolloid, biodressings) for noninfected superficial (grade II) ulcers.
6. If patient not admitted, must provide strategies for removing pressure from ulcer (ie, frequent patient repositioning, protective padding, special mattresses) and close follow-up.

VI. ICD-9 Diagnoses. Cellulitis; Decubitus ulcer (specify site); Diabetic ulcer; Ischemic ulcer; Osteomyelitis; Stasis dermatitis; Stasis or varicose ulcer; Ulcerative phlebitis.

VII. Problem Case Diagnosis. Grade III decubitus ulcer with sepsis.

VIII. Teaching Pearl Question. Most infected decubitus ulcers are from what organisms?

IX. Teaching Pearl Answer. Polymicrobial.

REFERENCES

Bergstrom N, Bennett MA, Carlson CE, et al. *Clinical Practice Guideline Number 15: Treatment of Pressure Ulcers.*, Rockville, Maryland: US Department of Health and Human Services. Agency for Health Care Policy and Research: 1994. AHCPR publication 95-0652.

Orlando PL. Pressure ulcer management in the geriatric patient. *Ann Pharmacother* 1998;32:1221–1227.

Thomas DR. Issues and dilemmas in the prevention and treatment of pressure ulcers: A review. *J Gerentol Biol Sci Med Sci* 2001;56A(6):M328–M340.

Trott A. Chronic skin ulcers. *Emerg Med Clin North Am* 1992;10(4):823–845.

21. DENTAL PAIN AND INFECTIONS

I. **Problem:** A 31-year-old male presents at 2 AM with severe dental pain that has become progressively worse over the last 36 h.

II. **Immediate Questions**
   A. **Is the airway patent?**
   B. **Is the patient able to tolerate his or her own secretions?**
   C. **Is there trismus?**

III. **Differential Diagnosis**
   A. **Dental Pain**
   B. **MI.** Remember that the pain of an MI can radiate to the lower teeth or jaw. Rarely dental pain occurs without significant chest pain.
   C. **Dental Trauma**
      1. **Contusion.** Trauma to the tooth with injury to the dental ligaments will loosen a tooth. Occasionally there will be a small amount of bleeding.
      2. **Fracture**
         a. **Ellis fractures**
            i. **Ellis I fracture.** Involves only the enamel and is white in appearance.
            ii. **Ellis II fracture.** Involves the dentin and is yellow in color.
            iii. **Ellis III fracture.** Involves the pulp and is pink in color.
         b. **Incomplete avulsion.** Displacement of the teeth typically involves fracture of the alveolar ridge. Early replacement of the teeth to their normal location and splinting often will allow dental salvage.
         c. **Complete avulsion.** Teeth that have left their socket have a poor prognosis. The longer the tooth is out of the socket the poorer the prognosis. If possible, the tooth should be rinsed (not scrubbed which will damage the dental ligament) and replaced in the socket as soon as possible. If the tooth has been out of the socket more than an hour, it is very unlikely that it will survive and should not be replaced. If the patient is unconscious, then the tooth can be transported in milk to the hospital.
      3. **Dental infection.** Closed-space infections surrounding the dental nerve may cause severe dental pain. Occasionally infections at the dental apex may rupture through the alveolar bone and involve local or deep spaces.
      4. **Sinus infection.** The pain of a maxillary sinusitis may cause dental pain in the upper molars.
      5. **TMJ.** Arthritis or repetitive injury to the temporomandibular joint may cause pain that is localized in the region of the mandible.
      6. **TM pathology.** Otitis media, bullous myringitis, or tympanic trauma may be associated with pain that radiates into the mandibular area.
      7. **Facial swelling**

8. **Local infections.** Infections of the gingiva and buccal area are commonly odontogenic in origin. Cellulitis often precedes abscess formation. Incision and drainage of localized abscess is important in preventing spread of infection to deep spaces.
9. **Deep space infections.** May be life-threatening if not appropriately treated. Airway management and prevention of obstruction is key.
10. **Ludwig's angina** (submental space).
11. **Masticator space.**
12. **Pterygomandibular space.**
13. **Lateral pharyngeal space.**
14. **Retropharyngeal space.**

IV. **Database**
   A. **Physical Exam Key Points.**
   1. **Facial appearance.** Do you note any asymmetry or obvious swelling?
   2. **Speech.** Deep space infections in the neck may cause hoarseness or muffled speech.
   3. **Interincisor opening.** The normal opening between upper and lower incisors is > 3 cm. Limitation of opening is called trismus. It implies that there is irritation of the muscles of mastication, often from a deep space infection.
   4. **Occlusion.** How the teeth fit together is an important clue to injury to the teeth, mandible, or TMJ.
   5. **Teeth.** Inspect each tooth for fractures, caries, position, and tenderness. Percussion of the tooth with a tongue blade is a good method of isolating which tooth is tender.
   6. **Gingiva.** Inspect for evidence of gingivitis (redness, swelling, or pus from the gingival recess) or abscess (fluctuant swelling).
   7. **Tongue and submental area.** Note the condition and position of the tongue. Swelling from infection in the submental area will force the tongue up into the mouth. In Ludwig's angina the tongue is forced upward and the submental space has a woody induration.
   8. **Neck.** Observe the neck for asymmetry and palpate for masses, crepitus, or fluctuance.
   9. **TMJ.** Have the patient open and close the mouth while palpating just in front of the tragus or with your fingers in the patient's ears. Clicking, popping, or grinding indicates abnormality of the TMJ.
   A. **Laboratory Data**
   1. **CBC.** It is uncommon that an elevated WBC would help make the diagnosis or help plan treatment in most facial infections.
   2. **Lytes and glucose.** Diabetics may experience elevation of glucose and possibly DKA related to serious dental infections.
   3. **ECG.** In the absence of positive intraoral findings that may explain dental pain, it may be appropriate to obtain an ECG.
   C. **Radiographic and Other Studies**
   1. **Soft tissue radiograph of the neck.** May demonstrate swelling in the prevertebral area. More than 6 mm of swelling anterior to C2 and more than 20 mm of soft tissue anterior to C5 is abnor-

mal and may indicate retropharyngeal infection. Air bubbles in the soft tissues of the neck almost uniformly indicates infection.

2. **CT scan of the neck.** This study provides an excellent evaluation of the extent of deep space infections. It is useful in planning the surgical approach to deep space infections.

V. Plan

A. Overall Plan.
An adequate airway should be ensured. Treat pain as required. Antibiotics are almost always indicated for dental pain. Abscesses should be drained.

B. Specific Plans

1. **Apical abscess or cellulites.** Oral antibiotics (Pen VK, erythromycin, or clindamycin). Drain larger abscesses; follow up with a dentist this week.

2. **Localized facial abscess.** Should be drained in the ED. Oral antibiotics (as in preceding item) should be prescribed and oral rinses with warm saline or half strength peroxide should be done hourly while awake. Follow-up with a dentist should occur within the next 24–48 h.

3. **Deep space infections.** May require oral tracheal intubation or another surgical airway. A CT scan to define the extent of involvement is typically required prior to operation. Intravenous antibiotics such as high-dose penicillin or more commonly clindamycin should be started in the ED. Drainage in the OR is required. Appropriate pain medication, which often includes narcotic analgesics, should be provided.

4. **Dental avulsions.** Should be relocated and splinted as is appropriate for the time delay since injury.

5. **Ellis II fractures.** Should be seen within 48 h by a dental professional.

6. **Ellis III dental fractures.** A dental professional should ideally see patient within 3 h. Oral antibiotics should be started to prevent pulpitis.

VI. ICD-9 diagnoses.
Alveolar (apical) abscess; Dental abscess; Dental infection; Ludwig's angina; Sinusitis; TMJ pain/syndrome; Tooth avulsion.

VII. Problem Case Diagnosis.
Apical dental abscess.

VIII. Teaching Pearl Question.
What is the most common cause of missing teeth?

IX. Teaching Pearl Answer.
Periodontal disease.

REFERENCES

Dale RA. Dentoalveolar trauma. *Emerg Med Clin North Am* 2000;18(3):521–538.
Flynn TR. The swollen face. Severe odontogenic infections. *Emerg Med Clin North Am* -2000;18(3):481–519.
James T. Emergency dental procedures. Amsterdam In: Robert SJ, Hedges J (eds). *Clinical Procedures in Emergency Medicine.* 3rd ed. WB Saunders, 1998:1149–1169.

22. DERMATOLOGIC PROBLEMS

I. **Problem:** A 20-year-old male presents to the ED with a generalized "rash." He has been feeling ill for the past 2 weeks and has some generalized complaints of fevers, deep muscle pains, chills, and nausea. About 3 weeks ago he went on a camping trip with some friends and does not remember a tick exposure. He does not use any medication. The rash is maculopapular, initially appearing around the wrists and ankles, with spread centripetally to the trunk.

II: **Immediate Questions:** (Chief complaint: "rash")
   A. **Duration?** Hours, days, weeks, months, years.
   B. **Quality?** Painful, pruritic, paresthesia, no sensation.
   C. **Progression?** Is it getting better or getting worse? How fast?
   D. **Location?** Where are the lesions? Initially and now at examination.
   E. **Lesion morphology?**
   F. **Associated symptoms?** Fever, chills, nausea, vomiting, myalgias, arthralgias, headache, upper respiratory complaints, weakness, malaise.
   G. **Immunization history?**
   H. **Exposures?** Chemicals including medications, toxins, animals, insects, ill contacts, recent travel, sexual history.
   I. **Medications?** Both prescription and OTC medications.

III: **Differential Diagnosis.** The differential diagnosis of skin diseases is very large. Pattern recognition and lesion morphology are the principle means of diagnosis. The pattern of lesions suggests certain causes.
   A. **Flexor Areas of the Skin.** Atopic dermatitis, candidiasis, eczema, ichthyosis.
   B. **Sun-Exposed Areas.** Sunburn, photosensitive drug eruption, photosensitive dermatitis, SLE, viral exanthem, porphyria.
   C. **Acrodermatitis** (distal extremities). Viral exanthem, atopic/contact dermatitis, eczema, RMSF, gonococcemia
   D. **Pityriasis Rosea** (ant. and post. thorax). Pityriasis rosea, secondary syphilis, drug eruption, atopic/contact dermatitis, psoriasis.
   E. **Clothing-Covered** (thorax distal lower ext.). Contact dermatitis, psoriasis, folliculitis.
   F. **Acneiform** (face and upper thorax). Acne, drug-induced, irritant dermatitis.

IV. **Database**
   A. **Physical Exam Key Points**
      1. **General appearance.** Vital signs, well-appearing or "toxic."
      2. **Skin examination.**
         a. **Type of lesion.** Macule, papule, wheal, nodule, cyst, vesicle-bulla, pustule, ulcer, hyperkeratosis, sclerosis, atrophy, telangiectasia, infarct, purpura, erosion, exudation, scar, scale.
         b. **Color of lesion.**
         c. **Palpation.** Consistency, mobility, tenderness, diascopy (blanches with pressure), estimate depth of lesion.

  d. **Shape of the lesions.** Round, oval, annular (ring-shaped), serpiginous, umbilicated.
  e. **Margination.** Well-defined or not
  f. **Arrangement.** Grouped, disseminated
  g. **Distribution.** Extent, pattern, or characteristic patterns.
  h. **Lesion evolution.** The alteration in lesion appearance due to disease progression (lesion evolution), patient-related change (pruritic rash with excoriations due to "scratching"), and medication effects.
  3. **Hair exam and nail examination.**
  4. **Mucous membrane examination.**
  5. **General medical examination.**
B. **Laboratory Data**
  1. ESR, UA (for active sediment): vasculitis.
  2. Microbiologic studies (cultures of blood, CSF, skin lesions): infectious disease.
  3. Platelet count, PT, PTT, fibrin split products: purpuric/petechial rashes.
C. **Other Studies.** Slide review. Likely unnecessary in most instances.
  1. **KOH preparation.** For suspected molluscum contagiosum, dermatophytosis. Place material on slide, place two (2) drops 20% KOH solution, warm gently. Look for true hyphae (long, branching, green rods, crosses border of epithelial cells). Molluscum bodies (oval discs with homogenous cytoplasm).
  2. **Tzanck smear** (in blistering disorders). Can help diagnose herpes infection. Remove material from the base of the lesion and place on slide. Allow to air dry then stain with Wright's or Giemsa's stain. Characteristic multinucleated giant cells are highly suggestive of herpes infection.

V. **Plan**
A. **Overall Plan.** Diagnose the dermatologic illness and determine the appropriate treatment or refer the patient for immediate or follow-up dermatologic consultation.
B. **Specific Plans**
  1. Be aware of the airway, breathing, circulation (ABCs) (some diseases like angioedema can progress rapidly).
  2. Determine whether this is a severe illness that requires immediate or emergent intervention (ie, IV antibiotics, IV steroids).
  3. Do your best at diagnosing the condition. Use any available textbooks or derm atlas.
  4. If comfortable with the diagnosis, choose the appropriate treatment (ie, curative or symptomatic treatment).
  5. If diagnosis is in question, consider either immediate or follow-up dermatologic consultation.
C. **Admission Criteria**
  1. Most patients complaining of a "rash" will be discharged. Extensive skin involvement, bullae, or palpable purpura suggest the need for immediate consultation.

    2. General medical concerns that warrant admission include cardiorespiratory instability, systemic signs and symptoms, significant comorbidity, patient's age, poor home environment, and the initiation of aggressive medical therapy.

VI. ICD-9 Diagnoses: Dermatitis-allergic/contact; Gonococcemia; Herpes zoster; Lyme disease; Meningococcemia; Pityriasis rosea; Rocky mountain spotted fever; Stevens-Johnson syndrome/Erythema multiforme/TEN; Toxic shock syndrome; Urticaria; Varicella; Viral exanthem.

VII. Problem Case Diagnosis: Rocky Mountain Spotted Fever

VIII: Teaching Pearls Question: What real emergency must be highly considered in a young, menstruating female with fevers, hypotension, vomiting, diarrhea, mental status changes and a diffuse erythematous sunburn-like rash?

IX: Teaching Pearls Answer: Toxic shock syndrome.

REFERENCES

Brady WJ, DeBehnke D. Generalized skin disorders. In: Tintinalli JE, Krome RL, Ruiz E, eds. *Emergency Medicine: A Comprehensive Study Guide.* McGraw-Hill, 1999:1594–1603.

Brady W, DeBehnke D, Crosby D. Dermatologic emergencies. *Am J Emerg Med* 1994;12:217–237.

Brady WJ, Martin ML. Approach to the dermatologic patient in the ED. In Tintinalli JE, Krome RL, Ruiz E, eds. *Emergency Medicine: A Comprehensive Study Guide.* McGraw-Hill, 1999:1571–1576.

Fitzpatrick T, Johnson R, Wolff K. *Color Atlas and Synopsis of Clinical Dermatology, Common and Serious Diseases.* McGraw-Hill, 1997.

23. DIABETIC PROBLEMS

  I. Problem: A young adult male is brought to the ED for altered mental status, a Hx of nausea and vomiting, and decreased strength in his right arm.

  II. Immediate Questions

    A. Is the airway intact? Manage appropriately.

    B. What are the vitals and mental status? Is the patient alert? Are there signs of significant dehydration? Consider fingerstick glucose a vital sign in all diabetic patients. Is the patient hyperglycemic or hypoglycemic?

    C. What brought the patient to the hospital? Altered mental status? Home readings of elevated or depressed blood glucose levels? Signs or symptoms of infection?

    D. What is the history of present illness? Have symptoms developed gradually or suddenly? Does patient have complaints of polydipsia or polyuria? Any change in patient's dietary intake or use of diabetic medications? Ask about associated symptoms (nausea, vomiting, abdominal pain, weight loss, fatigue, sweating).

    E. Any past medical history? Medications/allergies? Does patient have a history of diabetes? Other significant medical problems and medications can affect glucose control, especially in diabetic patients. Patients dependent on insulin are more likely to develop ketoacidosis.

III. Differential Diagnosis
A. Hyperglycemia. DKA; nonketotic hyperosmolar coma; medication or dietary noncompliance; infections including gastroenteritis, UTI, pneumonia, appendicitis and sepsis, pancreatitis, ingestion.

B. Hypoglycemia. Hypoglycemic agent overdose, lack of sufficient caloric intake, sepsis, poisoning/ingestion, neoplasm, hypothyroid, hypopituitarism.

C. Metabolic Acidosis. Alcoholic ketoacidosis, uremia, paraldehyde, INH, lactic acidosis, ethylene glycol, methanol, sepsis, starvation ketoacidosis.

IV. Database
A. Physical Exam Key Points
1. **Mental status.** Is patient awake and alert? Arousable to verbal or painful stimuli?
2. **Vital signs.** Check carefully and continue to monitor. Fingerstick glucose is considered a vital sign in diabetic patients. Note fevers, evidence of dehydration.
3. **Head and neck.** Check mucous membranes for moisture, check ENT for signs of infection, neck for meningismus. Check thyroid for size, tenderness. Any ketotic odor to breath?
4. **Cardiorespiratory.** Note any signs of respiratory infections, tachypnea, Kussmaul respirations, tachycardia.
5. **Abdomen.** Note tenderness, evidence of UTI, appendicitis, pancreatitis.
6. **Neurologic.** Continue to monitor mental status. Any focal motor or sensory deficits?
7. **Skin.** Note turgor, rashes, diaphoresis vs dry skin.

B. Laboratory Data. Close monitoring of blood sugar is essential. Lytes can be significantly altered with volume shifts and hyperglycemia/hypoglycemia and need to be followed. Check BUN and creatinine for renal function or evidence of prerenal state. Check serum osmolarity if blood sugar > 500. If acidosis suspected, consider ABG to evaluate as well as serum ketones. UA for infection and ketones. CBC may show leukocytosis with DKA, but left shift more sensitive for infectious cause. Determining cause may require more extensive work-up, including cardiac enzymes, CSF evaluation, blood and urine cultures.

C. Radiographic and Other Studies. CXR to evaluate for pneumonia, consider head CT in patients with continued altered mental status despite acidosis, fluid, and glucose corrections.

V. Plan
A. Overall Plan. Recognize signs and symptoms of hyperglycemia and hypoglycemia, acidosis, and initiate appropriate management. Include evaluation for possible cause of abnormality, including underlying infection, renal failure, AMI, overdose, etc.

B. Specific Plan

1. **Diabetic Ketoacidosis.** Physical exam findings include evidence of dehydration, may have ketotic or "fruity" odor on breath, Kussmaul respirations, tachypnea, and complain of abdominal pain or nausea/vomiting (Table I–5, p 77).

    a. **Criteria for diagnosis.** Glucose > 300, HCO_3^- < 15, pH < 7.3, ketonemia, ketonuria.

    b. **Treatment**

    i. **Rehydration.** Initially with 0.9% NS, can switch to 0.45% NS after 2 L infused. First liter in initial 30 min, then slow rate to minimize risk of cerebral edema.

    ii. **Insulin.** Initiate infusion of 0.1 units/kg/h IV (5–10 units/h). Consider switching IV fluids to glucose containing when blood glucose falls below 250.

    iii. **Potassium.** Hypokalemia will not be evident until acidosis resolves and volume is replete. Monitor closely and add 20 mEq to each liter IV fluids if adequate renal function and initial serum K < 5.5.

    iv. **Lytes.** Monitor phosphorus and magnesium, replace as indicated.

    v. **Sodium bicarbonate.** Consider use *only* if pH < 6.9, can lead to cerebral edema and paradoxical CSF acidosis.

    vi. **Additional.** Continue evaluation for possible precipitant, eg, pneumonia, UTI, AMI, noncompliance.

    c. **Admission criteria.** ICU if pH < 7, serious concurring illness or associated medical problems, persistent altered mental status or coma, age < 2, > 60. Consider discharge *only* if acidosis resolves, no evidence of concurrent illness/infection, and able to tolerate PO fluids.

2. **Hyperosmolar nonketotic coma.** Presents with Hx of polyuria/polydipsia, dehydration, mental status changes, and neurologic symptoms from weakness or lethargy, to coma, seizures, or focal deficits.

    a. **Criteria for diagnosis.** Serum glucose > 600, absence of ketosis (pH > 7.3), increased serum osmolarity (> 350 Osm/L or > 320 Osm/L *with* mental status changes).

TABLE I–5. SLIDING SCALE OF INSULIN DOSAGE FOR HYPERGLYCEMIA.

Glucose Level	Insulin (Short-Acting/Regular)
<180 mg/dL (10.00 mmol/L)	0 U SC
180–240 mg/dL (10.00–13.34 mmol/L)	3–5 U SC
240–400 mg/dL (13.34–22.23 mmol/L)	8–10 U SC
>400 mg/dL (>22.23 mmol/L)	10–15 U SC[a]

[a]Follow with a stat serum glucose and notify the house officer of result.
SC = subcutaneous.
Reproduced, with permission, from Haist SA, Robbins JB, Gomella LG, eds. *Internal Medicine on Call,* 3rd ed. McGraw-Hill, 2002.

   b. **Treatment**
      i. **Rehydration.** Start with 0.9% NS until hemodynamic stability restored, then switch to 0.45% NS. Goal is to replace 50% of predicted volume deficit in first 12 h. Reassess volume status frequently.
      ii. **Potassium.** Anticipate hypokalemia, begin potassium replacement immediately if patient is producing urine. If K^+ is normal (3.5–5.5 mEq/L) on initial tests, give 20–30 mEq KCl in first liter of fluids, then give 20 mEq/h. If initial K^+ is low (< 3.5), avoid insulin and begin replacement at 40 mEq KCl/h. Recheck K^+ levels every 1–2 h and adjust replacement accordingly.
      iii. **Insulin.** Begin only after patient hemodynamically stable and beginning K^+ replacement. Rapid lowering can lead to hypotension and shock. Goal is to lower glucose approximately 100–200 mg/dL/h.
      iv. **Lytes.** Monitor phosphate and magnesium closely, replace as indicated.
   c. **Admission criteria.** All should be admitted for close monitoring due to potential for arrhythmias and mental status changes. Only patients with mild volume deficits, normal serum osmolarity, normal mental status can be discharged if blood sugar and dehydration corrected.
3. **Hypoglycemia.** Can present with spectrum of symptoms from headache, flushing, diaphoresis, nausea, and hunger to confusion, seizures, and coma. Consider all possible causes including oral hypoglycemic overdose, ethanol abuse, insufficient dietary intake.
   a. **Treatment.** Treat adults initially with D50 (50–100 mL IV), peds with D10 (2 mL/kg IV), repeat as necessary. Monitor blood sugar closely and frequently. Neuroglycopenia can develop if hypoglycemia was sustained resulting to prolonged altered mental status despite correction of blood glucose and may require repeat treatments. Consider laboratory work-up relevant to patient presentation (Lytes, renal function, labs pertinent to overdose or persistent altered mental status).
   b. **Admission criteria.** Hypoglycemia secondary to oral hypoglycemia medications (especially sulfonylurea agents) need to be admitted and continually monitored, consider in patients with long-acting insulin. All intentional overdoses of diabetic medications. Discharge only diabetic patients with accidental hypoglycemia due to short-acting insulin in combination with insufficient dietary intake. Discharge only after 4-h observation, glucose correction, and adequate supervision and follow up.
VI. **ICD-9 Diagnoses:** Diabetes mellitus (state type I or II and controlled or uncontrolled); Diabetic coma (hyperglycemic or hypoglycemic, nonketotic, insulin); Diabetic gastroparesis, Diabetic ketoacidosis; Diabetic nephropathy; Diabetic peripheral neuropathy; Diabetic retinopathy; Diabetic ulcer (state site).

VII. **Problem Case Diagnosis:** New-onset diabetes, with development of hyperglycemic hyperosmolar nonketotic coma.

VIII. **Teaching Pearls Question:** Why does initial serum K$^+$ often register normal or high in patients with DKA?

IX. **Teaching Pearls Answer:** Acidosis drives K$^+$ extracellularly, DKA patients typically have total body K$^+$ depletion that becomes evident as volume deficits and acidosis is corrected.

REFERENCES

Kitabchi AE, Wall BM. Diabetic ketoacidosis. *Med Clin North Am* 1995;79(1):9–37

Pope DW, Dansky D. Hyperosmolar hyperglycemic nonketotic coma. *Emerg Med Clin North Am* 1989;7(4):849–857.

Umpierrez GE, Khajavi M, Kitabchi AE. Review: Diabetic ketoacidosis and hyperglycemic hyperosmolar non-ketotic syndrome. *Am J Med Sci* 1996;310(5):225–233.

24. DIALYSIS PATIENT PROBLEMS

I. **Problem:** 47-year-old patient who receives hemodialysis three times a week presents with fever and weakness.

II. **Immediate Questions**
A. **Is the airway intact?** Manage appropriately.
B. **What are the vitals and mental status?** Is the patient alert and stable? Apply ECG monitor and pulse oximeter, apply oxygen, and attempt to establish IV access. Confused or obtunded? Fever? Hypotension? Heart rate and rhythm? Respiratory distress? Orthostatic changes? Interview the patient if alert and responsive.
C. **Does an obvious source of infection exist?** Productive cough? Dysuria? Flank pain? Tenderness at graft/fistula/PD catheter site? Recent illness?
D. **Is there a concern for a cardiac cause?** Chest pain? Shortness of breath? Syncope? Palpitations?
E. **When was this patient last dialyzed?** Signs of peaked T waves on monitor? Obtain 12-lead ECG and rule out hyperkalemia. Does the patient undergo hemodialysis or peritoneal dialysis? Insidious or acute onset? Recent complications of HD, dialysis schedule, recent missed dialysis sessions, dry weight, average interdialysis weight gain, intradialysis hypotension? Did these symptoms occur while on dialysis? Near the beginning or the end of dialysis?
F. **Other Pertinent History for Patient with ESRD:** Etiology of ESRD, symptoms of uremia, retention of native kidneys.
G. **Other Past Medical History?** Diabetes, HTN, CAD, Medications? Medical Compliance?

III. **Differential Diagnosis.** Patients with ESRD often present with nonspecific complaints. Certain diagnostic possibilities require immediate attention.
A. **Infectious**
1. **Vascular access infection.** Rule out sepsis, often classic signs of infection at graft site are absent.

    2. **Pneumonia.** Productive cough?

    3. **UTI.** Still possible in anuric patient.

    4. **Bacteremia.** Most often *Staphylococcus aureus* from frequent vascular access.

    5. **Wound infection.** Peripheral neuropathy increases likelihood of nonpainful traumatic ulcerations becoming infected.

    6. **Peritonitis.** Common in PD patients. Not as severe as peritonitis from other causes. Send PD fluid for cell count and Diff, and culture.

B. Cardiovascular. Important causes of weakness that may not be related to febrile illness.

    1. **Pericarditis.** Fever, chest pain, pericardial friction rub.

    2. **Hyperkalemia.** Evidence of peaked T waves on monitor or 12-lead ECG. Often asymptomatic. Begin treatment immediately. Tolerated by patients with chronic renal failure better than those with acute renal failure.

    3. **High-output cardiac failure.** Occurs with more than 20% of CO through fistula or graft.

    4. **Volume overload.** Signs of CHF. Due to diet noncompliance or missed HD sessions. Ask patient about his "dry weight." Always consider new ischemia.

    5. **Tamponade.** Beck's triad (JVD, muffled heart tones, hypotension).

C. Neurologic

    1. **Seizure.** Witnessed seizure activity? Can result in fever and postictal state. Focal neuro deficits? Rule out ICH and CNS infection.

D. Hematologic

    1. **Anemia.** Common in ESRD patients secondary to decreased native erythropoietin. Rectal exam to rule out GI bleed. Increased incidence of GI bleeding secondary to blood dyscrasias and heparin use during dialysis.

E. Metabolic

    1. **Uremia.** Syndrome associated with low GFR and ESRD affecting cardiovascular, neurologic, hematologic, and gastrointestinal systems. Increased likelihood of infection secondary to depressed immunity.

IV. Database

    A. Physical Exam Key Points

      1. **Mental status.** Mini mental status exam (See Table A-4, page 656).

      2. **Vitals.** Check orthostatics as well.

      3. **Neck and mouth.** JVD and mucous membrane condition, dry or moist?

      4. **Lungs.** Rales? Local infiltrate? Further evidence of volume overload. (ie, edema).

      5. **Heart.** Tachycardia? Pericardial rub? New murmurs? Muffled heart sounds indicating tamponade? S_3 or S_4? Chest pain that improves with sitting forward.

      6. **Abdomen and rectal.** Check for GI bleeding and perforation, rebound, infection of PD catheter if present and peritonitis.

      7. **Extremities.** Functional vascular access? Check for bruit and thrill. Drop in HR after temporary access occlusion (Branham's sign) erythema, swelling, tenderness, discharge, bleeding, dependent edema? Decubitus ulcers?

      8. **Neurologic.** Check for focal deficits, pupils for equal reactivity (CVA, subdural), peripheral neuropathy.

  B. Laboratory Data. Rapid determination of Lytes, especially life-threatening hyperkalemia, significant increases in BUN/creatinine. Search for infectious cause. CBC with Diff, blood cultures if febrile. CXR and UA with urine culture. CSF studies if indicated. Cardiac enzymes for ischemia.

  C. Radiographic and Other Studies. ECG for hyperkalemia, pericarditis, ischemia. CXR for CHF, pneumonia. Doppler of graft/AV fistula for patency.

V. Plan

  A. Overall Plan. Determine need for emergent dialysis; admit patients with suspected cardiac pathology or infectious process.

  B. Specific Plans

      1. **Infectious.** Identify possible causes including vascular access site as well as routine sources. Treat appropriately. Admit if clinically indicated. If vascular in origin, consult with vascular surgery and nephrology departments to arrange for alternative dialysis options.

      2. **Cardiovascular.** If pericarditis suspected, intensive HD therapy may be beneficial. Rule out tamponade as well as cardiac ischemia, CHF. Low threshold for admission.

      3. **Metabolic.** Determine need for HD, treat appropriately.

      4. **Hematologic.** Rule out GI bleed, drop in Hgb below baseline.

      5. **Neurologic.** Focal neurologic deficits? Deteriorating condition? Rule out ICH and HTN encephalopathy, and CNS infection.

VI. ICD-9 Diagnoses: Acute pulmonary edema; Anemia in ESRD; Electrolyte imbalance (specify type); High-output heart failure; Infection-vascular catheter; Pericarditis-uremic; Sepsis; Uremia.

VII. Problem Case Diagnosis: Vascular access infection.

VIII. Teaching Pearl Question: If a patient has evidence of hyperkalemia and you are unable to obtain prompt IV access, name another treatment option you have?

IX. Teaching Pearl Answer: Nebulized albuterol.

REFERENCES

Hodde, LA, Sandroni S. Emergency department evaluation and management of dialysis patient complications. *Am J Emerg Med* 1992;10:317–334.

Ifudu O. Care of patients undergoing hemodialysis. *N Engl J Med* 1998;339:1054–1062.

25. DIARRHEA

I. **Problem.** A 24-year-old man presents complaining of diarrhea and abdominal cramping of 4-h duration, onset 2 h after eating at a fast food restaurant. He begins to vomit in triage.

II. **Immediate Questions**
   A. **Is the patient dehydrated and in need of IV rehydration?**
   B. **Does the patient have a surgical abdomen?**
   C. **Is the stool watery or bloody, contain mucous, or indicate steatorrhea?**
   D. **Is the patient toxic appearing?**
   E. **Is the diarrhea due to a gastrointestinal infection or something else?**
   F. **Does the patient have any risk factors for infectious diarrhea?** (ingestion of untreated water or contaminated food, foreign travel, exposure to sick humans or pets, day care child or worker, recent antibiotic use, health care worker, or food handler)

III. **Differential Diagnosis**
   A. **Bacteria and Bacterial Preformed Toxins** (Table I–6, p 83.)
   B. **Parasites:** *Giardia lamblia, Ascaris (Anisakis) lumbricoides, Cyclospora cayetensis* (worldwide), *Ancylostoma duodenale, Necator americanus, Cryptosporidium parvum* (Rockies, tropics, Russia), *Trichuris trichiura, Strongyloides stercoralis, Trichinella spiralis, Taenia solium, Taenia saginata, Toxoplasma gondii, Diphyllobothrium latum.*
   C. **Other Dysentery** (bloody-mucus diarrhea and fever): *Clostridium difficile, Entamoeba histolytica, Escherichia coli* (enteroinvasive), *Aeromonas* spp.
   D. **Viruses**
      1. **Rotavirus.** Number 1 cause in < 2 years old; 100% by 4 years old; mostly Oct–Apr; less if breast-fed.
      2. **Norwalk-like.** especially > 12 years old.
      3. **Adenovirus.** Associated respiratory symptoms.
      4. **Other.** Hepatitis A & E, caliciviruses, coronavirus-Like, coxsackie A, herpes, astroviruses.
   E. **Noninfectious Causes**
      1. **Toxins.** Arsenic, lead, mercury, wild mushrooms, MSG.
      2. **Secretory.** Thyrotoxicosis, gastrinoma, carcinoid, secreting villous adenoma, vasoactive intestinal peptide tumor, diabetic dysmotility.
      3. **Inflammatory.** Inflammatory bowel disease, irritable bowel disease, ischemic colitis, lymphoma, cancer, HIV bowel syndrome, appendicitis, diverticular disease, HSP, Hirschsprung's disease, Stevens-Johnson disease, hemolytic uremic syndrome.
      4. **Malabsorption.** Gastrectomy, bowel resection, radiation enteritis, scleroderma, celiac sprue, tropical sprue, Whipple's disease.

TABLE I-6. BACTERIA AND BACTERIAL PREFORMED TOXINS.

	US (cases/year)	Toxin	Incubation	Duration	Other Symptoms	Food Sources
Campylobacter jejuni	2,000,000	–	1–6 days	1–10 days	Dysentery, pain, N/V, Guillain-Barré	Meat, poultry, dairy
Salmonella enteritidis	1,400,200	–	6–48 h	2–7 days	Dysentery, N/V, abc pain	Meat, poultry, eggs
Shigella spp.	450,000	–	12–72 h	1–30 days	Dysentery, N/V, abd pain	Variable
Staphylococci aureus	High	+	1–6 h	1 day	N/V, abd pain	Potato salad, creams, meat
Clostridium perfringens	High	+	4–24 h	1 day	N/V, fever	Meat, poultry
Escherichia coli (travelers)	High	+	16–72 h	3–10 days	N/V, fever, abd pain	Vegetables, fruits
Escherichia coli (O157:H7)	73,000	+	1–8 days	5–10 days	Dysentery, N/V, abd pain, HUS	Ground beef
Bacillus cereus	Moderate	+	1–24 h	1 day	N/V	Meat, poultry, rice, vegetables
Yersinia enterocolitica	Moderate	–	4–10 days	3–14 days	Dysentery, pain, mesenteric adenitis	Dairy, pork
Listeria monocytogenes	2,500	–	3–35 days	Varies	N/V, myalgias, HA, sepsis, meningitis	Dairy
Vibrio cholera	Low	+	12–48 h	2–7 days	Abd pain	Shellfish
Vibrio parahaemolyticus	35	–	5–24 h	1–3 days	Dysentery, N/V	Seafood
Clostridium botulinum	15	+	12–72 h	1–10 days	Paralysis	Canned foods, honey

N/V = nausea and vomiting; HUS = hemolytic uremic syndrome.

   5. Food allergy.
   6. Laxatives. Sorbitol, mannitol, lactulose, PEG, magnesium.
   7. Medicines. Antibiotics, colchicine, cholestyramine, theophylline, digoxin, β-blockers.
   8. Increased mucosal hydrostatic pressure. Portal hypertension, CHF.

IV. Database
A. Stool Studies
   1. Fecal leukocytes (detect with methylene blue).
   2. Guaiac.
   3. Gram stain and C&S for enteric pathogens.
      a. *Salmonella, Shigella, Yersinia enterocolitica, Campylobacter jejuni, Escherichia coli* 0157:H7.
      b. Indications: Dysentery, antibiotic use, day care, fecal leukocytes, 5 day's duration, foreign travel, and/or sick pet.
   4. O&P: *Giardia, Cryptosporidium.*
   5. *Clostridium difficile* toxin.
   6. Rotavirus ELISA or latex fixation test.
B. Sigmoidoscopy: *Shigella, Clostridium difficile, Escherichia coli* 0157:H7, *Campylobacter jejuni,* amoebas.
C. String test. To get duodenal mucus to look for trophozoites.

V. Plan
A. Rehydration: IV NS or oral (avoid hyperosmolar soda and juice).
B. Antidiarrheals
   1. **Loperamide (Imodium AD).** 2 now then 1 after each loose stool (8/day max and 3 days max). May be associated with megacolon and/or *Shigella* sepsis if used w/o antibiotics. Advanced Imodium AD also has simethicone.
   2. **Diphenoxylate + atropine (Lomotil).** 2 tab (or 10 mL) qid.
   3. **Bismuth subsalicylate (Pepto-Bismol).** Two 262-mg tabs (or 30 mL) PO qh × 3 doses.
      a. Turns stools black. Blocks cyclic AMP pump (travelers, *E coli* heat-labile enterotoxin stimulates cAMP pump). Avoid in kids (Reye's syndrome) unless travelers'.
   4. **Adsorbents.** Kaolin-pectin (Kaopectate) & charcoal aren't effective & can adsorb nutrients.
C. Antibiotics
   1. **Empiric.**
      a. Trimethoprim-sulfamethoxazole (TMP/SMX) DS 2 tabs PO now, then 1 tab PO bid × 5 days. Doesn't affect *Campylobacter.*
      b. Ciprofloxacin 1 g PO now, then 500 mg PO bid × 5 days (may stop after 3 days if resolved).
      c. Azithromycin 250 mg PO bid × 3 days.

   2. Specific
   a. *E. coli.* TMP/SMX (high resistance worldwide), azithromycin, ciprofloxacin.
   b. *Shigella.* TMP/SMX, ciprofloxacin, cefixime.
   c. *Salmonella.* TMP/SMX, ciprofloxacin.
   d. *Campylobacter.* Erythro, ciprofloxacin (some resistance in Thailand), azithromycin
   e. *Vibrio cholera.* Cipro, tetracycline.
   f. *Clostridium difficile.* Flagyl, vancomycin.
   g. *Listeria monocytogenes.* Ampicillin.
   h. *Giardia.* Flagyl 250 mg PO tid × 7 days.
   i. Amoeba: Flagyl 750 mg PO tid × 7 days.
   j. *Cyclospora.* TMP/SMX.

VI. **ICD-9 Diagnoses:** Diarrhea; Diarrhea due to (state organism); Enteritis (state organism if known); Gastroenteritis; Pseudomembranous colitis; Regional enteritis (same as Crohn's disease); Travelers' diarrhea; Ulcerative colitis

VII. **Problem Case Diagnosis:** Nonspecific gastroenteritis; improved after IV fluids, IV antiemetic, and oral loperamide.

VIII. **Teaching Pearls Question:** Are most cases of food poisoning due to the most recently eaten meal?

IX. **Teaching Pearls Answer:** No. Most cases of food poisoning are due to a meal 6 h to 6 days prior to the onset of symptoms.

REFERENCES

Kroser JA, Metz DC. Evaluation of the adult patient with diarrhea. *Primary Care* 1996;23: 629–647.

Murphy GS, Bodhidatta L, Echeverria P, Tansuphaswadikul S, Hoge CW, Imlarp S, et al. Ciprofloxacin and loperamide in the treatment of bacillary dysentery. *Ann Intern Med* 1993;118:582–586.

26. DIZZINESS AND VERTIGO

I. **Problem:** 67-year-old female presents with episodic positional vertigo lasting for several seconds. Although she has had no changes in hearing, she has had some "ringing in my ears" and N/V.

II. **Immediate Questions**
   A. **Vertigo vs syncope/near syncope vs lightheadedness/disequilibria?**
   B. **Character of vertigo?** Positional?
   C. **Lasts for how long?** Time course?

    D. Associated symptoms? N/V? Hearing loss? Tinnitus? Cranial nerve/ bulbar complaints?

    E. General medical history? CVA risk factors, connective tissue disease in family history, STD risk? Medications?

III. Differential Diagnosis

    A. Peripheral. Presence of auditory symptoms, absence of CNS symptoms.

    B. Benign paroxysmal positional vertigo. Lasts for seconds, positional, sometimes tinnitus, no hearing loss.

    C. Vestibular neuritis. Lasts for hours, usually a single event not related to position.

    D. Ménière's disease. Lasts for hours, + hearing loss, low-pitched tinnitus.

    E. Migraine. Lasts for minutes.

    F. Acoustic neuroma. + Hearing loss.

    G. Ramsay-Hunt syndrome. + Tinnitus, + hearing loss, often with cranial nerve involvement.

    H. Labyrinthitis. + Hearing loss, + fever.

    I. Perilymphatic fistula. Lasts for minutes.

    J. Labyrinthine trauma.

    K. Autoimmune inner ear disease.

    L. Otosyphilis.

    M. Central. Lessened associated symptoms without auditory symptoms, usually with cranial nerve findings.

    N. TIA/Stroke/vertebrobasilar artery insufficiency cranial nerve findings, drop attacks.

    O. Chiari malformation. In cerebellum.

    P. Head trauma.

    Q. Multiple sclerosis.

    R. Tumors. Cerebellar, cerebellopontine angle.

    S. Global. Systemic processes.

    T. Orthostatic hypotension. Lasts for seconds, positional.

    U. Drugs. Lasix, gentamicin, amiodarone, aspirin.

    V. Anxiety. Lasts for seconds, associated with shortness of breath, chest tightness, paresthesias, sweating.

    W. Multiple systemic diseases with other associated symptoms. DM, HTN, heart disease, connective tissue diseases.

IV. Database

    A. Physical Exam Key Points

        1. **General.** Orthostatic vitals.

            a. **HEENT.** Visual acuity, visual fields, extraocular muscle movements.

            b. **Nystagmus.** Horizontal/rotatory vs vertical. Does nystagmus stop with fixation or fatiguing?

            c. **Neck.** Carotid bruits.

        2. **Cardiovascular.** Murmurs? Irregular heartbeat?

        3. **Neurologic.**

            a. **Cranial nerve.** Full exam, including hearing.

        b. Motor/Sensory. Motor strength, full sensory including proprioception.

        c. Reflexes. DTRs, plantar response.

        d. Cerebellar: Finger to nose, heel to shin, rapid alternating movement.

        e. Gait. Romberg's test, tandem gait.

    5. **Provocative tests** (trying to provoke nystagmus)

        a. Hyperventilation. Nystagmus with vestibular schwannoma, MS, perilymphatic fistula, sometimes with ischemia.

        b. Dix-Hallpike test. Position patient so that head will hang off of bed when lying down, while sitting up turn head 45°, lie patient down with head off of bed at a 45° angle, watch eyes for nystagmus, which may often be delayed by 15–20 s.

        c. Valsalva's maneuver. Nystagmus with perilymphatic fistula, craniocervical junction abnormality (eg, Chiari's malformation).

        d. Vibration of mastoid. Nystagmus with perilymphatic fistula.

B. Laboratory Data: Not useful to do any random screening laboratory testing; all testing should be directed toward suspected diagnosis. Some possible tests for specific suspected disease processes include ESR, rheumatoid factor, syphilis screening, or CBC with Diff.

C. Radiographic and Other Studies: With the exception of a CT scan, which is of little utility, none of the tests will be ordered from the ED.

    1. **CT scan.** Useful if suspecting a CPA tumor.

    2. **MRI/MRA.** Gold standard test to visualize the eighth nerve, good for suspected ischemic event.

    3. **Audiologic studies.** Useful if any hearing abnormality is detected on exam; audiogram, auditory brainstem response.

    4. **Vestibular function tests.** Performed at "dizzy clinics"; electronystagmography, rotational chair, computerized dynamic posturography.

V. Plan

A. Overall Plan

    1. **For days 1–3**

        a. Vestibular suppressants.

        b. Diazepam 2–5 mg tid.

        c. Meclizine 25 mg tid.

        d. Promethazine 25–50 mg tid.

        e. Bed rest.

        f. Radiologic testing if suspected central vertigo.

    2. **After day 3**

        a. Stop vestibular suppressants.

        b. Audiogram if indicated.

        c. Targeted vestibular rehabilitation (for chronic vertigo).

B. Specific Plans

    1. **BPPV.** Canalith repositioning treatment.

        a. Epley maneuvers. Series of maneuvers designed to move canalith out of canal.

        b. Liberatory (Semont/Brisk) maneuvers. Another series of maneuvers.

      c. **Brandt–Daroff treatment (vestibular habituation).** Series of head movements performed repeatedly several times a day until patient is without symptoms for 48 h.
2. **Vestibular neuritis.** Prednisone.
3. **Ménière's disease.** < 2 g/day sodium, decreased tyramine intake; diuretic, acetazolamide, surgery.
4. **Migraine.** < 2 g/day sodium, decreased tyramine intake, other common migraine treatments (eg, phenothiazines, SSRIs).
5. **Ramsay-Hunt syndrome.** Prednisone, acyclovir.
6. **Perilymphatic fistula.** Surgery.
7. **Ischemic disease.** Aspirin, other blood thinner as indicated.
8. **Orthostatic hypotension.** Treat underlying cause.
9. **Drug toxicity.** Stop medication.
10. **Anxiety.** Benzodiazepine.

VI. **ICD-9 Diagnoses:** Acoustic neuroma; Adverse effect medication; Benign positional paroxysmal vertigo; Cerebrovascular disease; Dizziness (coded same as Vertigo); Hypotension-orthostatic; Labyrinthitis; Ménière's disease; Migraine; Ramsay-Hunt syndrome; Vertigo-central origin.

VII. **Problem Case Diagnosis.** Benign paroxysmal positional vertigo.

VIII. **Teaching Pearl Question.** What percentage of patients with BPPV will experience a recurrence of symptoms following canalith repositional therapy?

IX. **Teaching Pearl Answer.** 30–50%.

REFERENCES

Goebel JA. Management options for acute versus chronic vertigo. *Otolaryngol Clin North Am* 2000;33(3):483–493.
Koelliker P, Summers RL, and Hawkins B. Benign paroxysmal positional vertigo: Diagnosis and treatment in the emergency department—A review of the literature and discussion of canalith-repositioning maneuvers. *Ann Emerg Med* 2001;37(4):392–398.
Solomon D. Distinguishing and treating causes of central vertigo. *Otolaryngol Clin North Am* 2000;33(3):579–601.
Tusa RJ. Vertigo. *Neurol Clin* 2001;19(1):23–55.
Walker MF, Zee DS. Bedside vestibular examination. *Otolaryngol Clin North Am* 2000; 33(3):495–506.

27. DROWNING/NEAR-DROWNING

    I. **Problem.** A 9-month-old child, wet and pulseless, is brought in by paramedics.

    II. **Immediate Questions**
      A. **Is the airway intact? Is the patient maintaining adequate tidal volume?** Manage appropriately (See VIII, 15. Rapid Sequence Endotracheal Intubation, page 470).

B. **Is there a pulse?** Treat dysrhythmias according to appropriate ACLS algorithm. (See 11. Bradycardia, page 36, 48. Hypothermia, page 144).

C. **Is trauma a possibility?** (eg, boating, diving, or *any* victim with unknown circumstances.) Secure the cervical spine. Perform a rapid neurologic assessment.

D. **What are the vital signs?** Place on monitor (ECG and pulse ox) and oxygen; establish an IV. Use a rectal thermometer to assess for hypothermia. Recall that hypothermia and the diving reflex may be protective for victims of prolonged submersion.

E. **Altered mental status?** Remember to check the glucose and pulse ox on presentation. Consider intoxications and trauma.

F. **Outcome predictors?** How long was the patient submerged? What was the water temperature? Was the patient in cardiac arrest in the field? In the ED?

G. **Past Medical History?** Does the patient have a seizure disorder? Cardiac disease? Diabetes? Is there a psychiatric history (especially depression)?

III. **Differential Diagnosis.** (The diagnosis is usually self-evident; the cause is often less obvious.)

A. **Depressed or Loss of Consciousness (LOC) as Primary Cause.** (At the water surface, LOC predisposes to going under. Underwater, LOC is rapidly fatal.)

1. **Alcohol/drugs.** Very common, especially in the adolescent and young adult population.

2. **Seizure.** By report or suspected by medical history.

3. **Hypothermia.** Immersion in even mildly cold waters for prolonged periods can cause hypothermia. Especially important in young children.

4. **Trauma.** Often associated with alcohol/drugs, boating, and diving. Use the Hx and any clinical evidence of trauma.

5. **SCUBA-related emergencies.** Consider arterial gas embolism (within minutes of surfacing) and pulmonary overexpansion syndromes (during surfacing).

6. **MI/Dysrhythmia/Syncope.** Older patients; possibly bystander report of chest pain, palpitations, light-headedness, headache.

B. **Other**

1. **Lack of skill/difficult conditions.** Generally in younger children, inexperienced swimmers, or rough waters (eg, rapids or undertows; even buckets or bathtubs for very young children).

2. **Attempted suicide/homicide.** This includes child abuse and neglect.

IV. **Database**

A. **Physical Exam Key Points**

1. **ABCs.** Monitor closely for compromise (inability to maintain airway, tachypnea, hypoventilation, hypoxemia).

2. **Vital signs.** Watch closely for evidence of hypotension. Correct hypothermia.
3. **Lungs.** Rales (pulmonary edema, ARDS).
4. **Cardiovascular.** Check for murmurs, irregular rhythm.
5. **Head and neck.** Check for C-spine tenderness (trauma), jugular venous distention (CHF, pneumothorax), bitten tongue (seizure).
6. **Neurologic.** Check pupils (intracranial lesions, toxidrome) and look for focal deficits (CVA, hyperbaric injuries).
7. **Skin.** Examine thorax for subcutaneous air (trauma or pulmonary overexpansion syndrome). Check for bruising (trauma).

B. **Laboratory Data.** CBC, Lytes, and ABG are appropriate in almost all patients. Alcohol and toxicology screens may be useful. Urine pregnancy test in reproductive-aged women. Pulse oximetry initially.

C. **Radiographic and Other Studies.** ECG in older patients and those in whom a dysrhythmia is considered. CXR is indicated in all patients. If there is suspicion for trauma, obtain C-spine films and head CT, in addition to other clinically indicated films.

V. **Plan**
A. **Overall Plan.** Secure airway if compromised or borderline. Treat but do not overcorrect hypovolemia and acidosis. Only those patients submersed in contaminated water need prophylactic antibiotics. Asymptomatic patients who do not have an oxygen requirement and who are not tachypneic may be sent home with a responsible adult after a period of observation (eg, 6 h). All other patients are admitted for observation or treatment.

B. **Specific Plans**
1. **Hypothermia.** Rewarm patient (begin by removing wet clothing). If pulseless, continue code until euthermic. Admit when hypothermia is significant.
2. **Trauma.** Obtain surgical and subspecialty consultation as needed. Admit for significant or multiple injuries.
3. **Intoxications.** Check carefully for evidence of trauma. Treat intoxications as indicated (eg, naloxone). Hospitalize until alert and appropriate. Observe for withdrawal syndromes.
4. **SCUBA.** Treat pneumothorax. Arrange hyperbaric treatment if arterial gas embolism or decompression illness suspected.
5. **Suspected mistreatment.** Report to the appropriate authorities. Ensure safe environment before discharging patient.

VI. **ICD-9 Diagnoses.** Drowning (synonymous with Adverse effect—submersion and Pulmonary edema—due to near drowning); Hypothermia

VII. **Problem Case Diagnosis.** Neglect—this child drowned in her bathtub.

VIII. **Teaching Pearl Question.** What percent of patients drown because of laryngospasm (so-called "dry-drowners")?

IX. **Teaching Pearl Answer:** 10–15%.

REFERENCES

Modell JH. Drowning. *N Engl J Med* 1993;328(4):253–256.
Sachdeva RC. Near drowning. *Crit Care Clin* 1999;15(2):281–296.
Weinstein MD, Krieger BP. Near-drowning: epidemiology, pathophysiology, and initial treatment. *J Emerg Med* 1996;14(4):461–467.

28. EARACHE

I. **Problem:** A 72-year-old woman presents with severe left ear pain.

II. **Immediate Questions**
   A. **Is the pain primary or referred?**
   B. **Are there other associated symptoms?** URI? Headache? Fever? Dental pain? Neurologic changes? Rash? Auditory changes?
   C. **What is the time course?** Acute? Subacute? Chronic? Recurrent?

III. **Differential Diagnosis**
   A. **Primary causes**
      1. **Bacterial infection.** Consider otitis media, otitis externa, and mastoiditis.
      2. **Viral infection.** Consider herpes zoster oticus (HZO).
      3. **Foreign body.** (See Section VIII. 7. Eye and Nose Procedures, page 451).
   B. **Referred pain**
      1. May occur from infection, trauma, tumor, or other processes involving the proximal cervical region, temporomandibular joint, mandible, teeth, tongue, tonsil, larynx, or cervical esophagus.

IV. **Database**
   A. **Physical Exam Key Points**
      1. **General appearance and mental status.** Is the patient toxic?
      2. **Ears.** Inspect bilaterally to rule out vesicles, infection, foreign bodies, and trauma. Assess hearing.
      3. **Oral/Dental.** Inspect, palpate, and percuss to rule out infection (See 21. Dental Pain and Infections, page 70).
   B. **Laboratory Data.** (Not routinely indicated.)
   C. **Imaging studies and other tests.** (Not routinely indicated unless deep or complicated infections are suspected.)

V. **Plan**
   A. **Overall Plan.** Most cases are managed with outpatient treatment and primary care or ENT follow-up. Some patients may require analgesics.
   B. **Specific Plans**
      1. **Otitis media.** Treat with antibiotics. Assess risk factors for predicting drug-resistant *Streptococcus pneumoniae* (DRSP): age < 2 years, recent antibiotic use, and/or daycare.
         a. **Amoxicillin.** First-line drug in all cases. If at risk for DRSP, use high-dose amoxicillin at 80–90 mg/kg/day PO divided bid–tid.

Otherwise may consider standard dosing at 40–45 mg/kg/day PO divided tid.

b. **Amoxicillin/Clavulanate (Augmentin).** Second-line therapy (ie, recommended for persistent findings after 3 days of amoxicillin). Use 80–90 mg/kg/day of amoxicillin; 6.4 mg/kg/day of clavulanate. Given PO divided bid.

c. **Cefuroxime axetil (Ceftin).** Second-line therapy. Use 30 mg/kg/day PO divided bid.

d. **Ceftriaxone (Rocephin).** Second-line therapy. Also beneficial if noncompliant or unable to tolerate oral medications. Use 50 mg/kg IM once daily for 3 days.

2. **Otitis externa.** Treat with topical Cortisporin otic solution; use the suspension if the TM is perforated or not visualized. Use an ear wick to facilitate instillation into an occluded canal.

3. **Mastoiditis.** May require CT imaging to define the extent and to rule out complications. All patients require parenteral antibiotics, ENT consultation, and admission.

4. **Herpes zoster oticus.** Perform a careful slit lamp exam to rule out ocular involvement. Most patients require analgesics. Oral steroids may reduce the incidence of postherpetic neuralgia. Treat with antiviral medications.

a. **Acyclovir (Zovirax).** 800 mg PO 5 ×/day for 7–10 days.

b. **Famciclovir (Famvir).** 500 mg PO tid for 7 days.

c. **Valacyclovir (Valtrex).** 1000 mg PO tid for 7 days.

5. **Foreign body.** Multiple techniques for removal depending on size, composition, and location. Never dampen any organic foreign body (may cause swelling). Utilize appropriate sedation/restraint.

6. **Referred pain.** Treatment is based on the specific cause. Dental and intraoral causes are most common.

VI. **ICD-9 Diagnoses:** Foreign body in external auditory canal; Otitis externa; Otitis media; Herpes zoster oticus; Mastoiditis

VII. **Problem Case Diagnosis:** Vesicles were identified in the local area. The diagnosis is herpes zoster oticus.

VIII. **Teaching Pearls Question:** What is the Ramsay Hunt syndrome?

IX. **Teaching Pearls Answer:** Bell's palsy occurring with herpes zoster oticus.

REFERENCES

Bentley B II. Otolaryngologic emergencies. In: Cline D, Ma OJ, eds. *Companion Handbook to Emergency Medicine: A Comprehensive Study Guide.* McGraw-Hill,1996:736–743.

Dowell SF, Butler JC, Giebink GS, Jacobs MR, Jernigan D, Musher DM, et al. Acute Otitis Media - Management and Surveillance in an Era of Pneumococcal Resistance: A Report from the Drug-Resistant *Streptococcus pneumoniae* Therapeutic Working Group (DRSPTWG). *Pediatric Infectious Disease Journal* 18:1–9, 1999.

29. EPISTAXIS

I. **Problem.** A 65-year-old male presents with bleeding from his right nostril for the past 2 h. He has a history of hypertension.

II. **Immediate Questions**
   A. **Is the patient's airway intact?** (See Section VIII, 15. Rapid Sequence Endotracheal Intubation, page 470).
   B. **Is the patient hemodynamically stable?** (See 47. Hypotension, page 142, 40. Hemorrhagic Shock, page 122, Section VIII, 7. Eye and Nose Procedures, page 451).
   C. **Does the patient have a coagulopathy or is he taking anticoagulant medications?** (See 10. Bleeding Problems, page 32).

III. **Differential Diagnosis**
   A. **Anterior Bleeding.** Most bleeding is found in Kiesselbach's plexus in the anterior portion of the nasal septum. Mechanical trauma and dry environment are responsible for most bleeding in this area.
   B. **Posterior Bleeding.** Visualization of acute bleeding in this area is difficult or impossible.
   C. **Coagulopathy**

IV. **Database**
   A. **Physical Exam Key Points**
      1. **Vital signs.** HTN is a common finding in epistaxis and is thought to be related to anxiety. Persistent, significant elevations of BP should be treated with antihypertensive agents.
      2. **Intranasal exam.** Gown, gloves, and a full-face shield are essential to protect the physician from blood exposure. Adequate light from a head lamp is key to a good exam. A nasal speculum should be placed in the vestibule and spread in a superior-inferior direction to avoid trauma to the nasal septum. Suction with a Frasier tip is desirable. Inspection should note any acute bleeding sites, trauma, polyps, or masses.
      3. **Oral exam.** Examination of the oral pharynx for blood gives a clue to ongoing bleeding and the possibility of a posterior bleed.
      4. **Skin exam.** Observe for petechiae or ecchymosis from coagulopathy.
   B. **Laboratory Data**
      1. CBC and platelet count will help evaluate the severity of the bleeding, underlying anemia, and presence of thrombocytopenia.
      2. PT and PTT time help make the diagnosis of coagulopathy.
      3. Bleeding time helps determine platelet dysfunction.
      4. T&C should be considered with massive bleeding or in patients who are unable to tolerate significant anemia.
   C. **Radiographic and Other Studies**
      1. Nasal endoscopy may be both diagnostic and therapeutic in patients in whom bleeding is not controlled with standard measures.

      2. Angiography and embolization are also used when standard measures fail.

V. Plan

A. Overall Plan. Unless the site of bleeding is identified and controlled, recurrence of bleeding is common.

B. Specific Plans

  1. Anterior bleeds

    a. Direct pressure on the bleeding site will control the majority of nosebleeds. Having the patient pinch the anterior portion of the nose for a full 5 min without pausing will often control bleeding. If this is not successful then have the patient blow the clots out of the nose and reapply pressure for 10 min. Two tongue blades may be taped together (starting at the end, spiral the tape to just short of half-way) and use as a simple nose clamp (Parkland clamp).

    b. Topical anesthesia and vasoconstrictor use will significantly improve the patient's tolerance to examination and packing. Liberal use may help control profuse bleeding and aid in localization of the bleeding source.

      i. 4% Cocaine

      ii. 2–4% Lidocaine + epinephrine

      iii. 2–4% Lidocaine + phenylephrine (Neo-Synephrine)

    c. Cautery. Silver nitrate sticks may be used for chemical cautery. Bleeding will render the stick useless, so cautery should proceed from superior to inferior and outside to inside in a circular fashion. It should not be left in place more than 15 s or used on both sides of the septum to prevent septal necrosis. To prevent recurrent bleeding, the patient is advised not to bend over or touch the nose in any way. Neo-Synephrine nose spray should be used twice a day for the next 48 h.

    d. Packing

      i. Gauze. Packing the nose with 6 ft of gauze ribbon will allow constant pressure to be applied to the bleeding site. The packing is inserted in an accordion-like fashion from the bottom of the nasal vault until the entire vault is filled. A small gauze dressing is taped over the dressing to absorb any discharge. The patient may change this dressing as needed. This packing is left in place for at least 48 h, and the patient should be placed on oral antibiotics to prevent sinusitis and toxic shock syndrome.

      ii. Tampons. Superabsorbent, expanding sponges are commercially available that are designed to be placed in the nasal cavity. As they absorb moisture they significantly increase in size. These tampons are easier to place and have a high rate of success. The absorbent sponges

have a suture attached that aids in removal. The suture
should be taped to the nose and a small dressing placed
below the nose to absorb any discharge.

2. **Posterior bleeds**
   a. **Posterior packing**
      i. **Gauze.** A tampon of 4×4 gauze pads tied with silk su-
         ture may be passed through the mouth and the ties
         pulled through the nose seating the tampon in the pos-
         terior nasopharynx. Anterior nasal packing should also
         be employed. Because this is time-consuming and un-
         comfortable, the newer balloon devices have essentially
         replaced this method.
      ii. **Balloon.** Commercially available epistaxis balloon de-
         vices have greatly simplified posterior packing. The
         device is fully inserted into the nose and the posterior
         balloon inflated. The device is pulled forward to seat
         the posterior balloon in place and the anterior balloon
         is inflated.
      iii. Patients should be admitted and observed for possible
         airway obstruction.
         (a) **Surgical options.** Arterial embolization and clip-
            ping are reserved for patients who fail standard
            therapy.
         (b) **Coagulopathy** should be managed as is indicated
            by the disorder. Typically the coagulopathy must
            be corrected before epistaxis can be controlled. Di-
            rect pressure should be applied to control bleeding
            until this can be accomplished.

VI. **ICD-9 Diagnoses:** epistaxis

VII. **Problem Case Diagnosis.** Anterior epistaxis.

VIII. **Teaching Pearl Question.** What percentage of epistaxis has a posterior
source?

IX. **Teaching Pearl Answer.** 10%.

REFERENCES

Manthey DE, Harrison BP. Otolaryngologic procedures. In: Roberts J, Hedges J. *Clinical
Procedures in Emergency Medicine*, 3rd ed. WB Saunders, 1998:1137–1145.
Tan LK. Epistaxis. *Med Clin North Am* 1999;83(1):43–56.

30. ETHICAL DILEMMA

I. **Problem.** A woman, approximately 50 years old, arrives by ambulance in
severe respiratory distress. She appears to be chronically ill. She is awake

at present but seems to be deteriorating quickly. You will need to intubate her. You have made the medical decision that intubation will be necessary in the next 10–15 min to save her life. She wants to refuse the procedure. Who makes the decision whether to perform the procedure on this patient? She states that she is not ill and wishes to drive herself home immediately.

II. Immediate Questions
  A. Does this patient retain decision-making capacity sufficient to decide whether and how you should intervene?
  B. If not, are there alternative decision-making sources you should use?

III. Differential Diagnosis
  A. Is this an ethical dilemma?
  B. Does this patient have decision-making capacity?

IV. Database
  A. Ethical Dilemmas. A clinical ethical (or bioethical) dilemma is a problem in which the options all seem equivalent—usually bad. The purpose of bioethics is to find a way through this morass. In medicine, especially in emergency medicine, physicians must make a decision. Indecision often produces an outcome that may not be appropriate or desirable.
  B. Physical Exam Key Points. Aside from an evaluation of the patient's respiratory status, the key issue is whether the patient retains decision-making capacity for this intervention-intubation and ventilation. To determine this, assess the patient's response to three questions:
    1. Do you understand the options?
    2. Do you understand the risks and benefits to you of each option?
    3. Why are you making the decision you did? (The longer version is: Does this decision you made conform to your relatively stable value system?) If the patient fails to respond appropriately (yes, these are subjective interpretations you must make) to any of these questions, then she currently lacks decision-making capacity—although she may regain it at a subsequent point.
  C. Laboratory, Radiographic, and Other Studies. These may be useful in determining the medical decision and may be useful in providing information to the decision maker(s), whether it is the patient or someone else.

V. Plan
  A. Overall Plan. To locate a willing and able decision maker for this patient who has decision-making capacity and give him, her, or them the opportunity to make an informed decision about this patient's treatment.
  B. Specific Plans
    1. If patient retains decision-making capacity, talk with the patient.

2. If the patient lacks decision-making capacity and this is a medical emergency (time-dependent with serious medical consequences), then perform the necessary medical intervention immediately.
3. If the patient lacks decision-making capacity but has completed an advance directive (ie, living will, durable power of attorney for healthcare, etc), use the directive, including any named surrogates.
4. If the patient lacks decision-making capacity but your locale has a statutory or common law surrogate list permitting specific individuals to make healthcare decisions for a patient lacking decision-making capacity. In most jurisdictions, the first person for adult patients is a current spouse not legally separated. Some states have much more extensive lists. Use the surrogate or group of surrogates (eg, adult siblings) that staff can reasonably contact and who are willing to make such decisions.
5. If the patient lacks decision-making capacity and no advance directive or approved surrogates exist, or the patient cannot be identified, perform the necessary medical procedure immediately.

VI. ICD-9 Diagnoses: Counseling NEC.

VII. Problem Case Diagnosis: The patient lacks decision-making capacity because she neither recognizes the options for her treatment nor recognizes the risks or benefits to such treatment.

VIII. Teaching Pearl Question: Does alcohol on the breath mean a patient lacks decision-making capacity?

IX. Teaching Pearl Answer: No. Decision-making capacity is relative to the complexity of the intervention and the seriousness of the consequences. Even significantly inebriated patients may have the capacity to determine whether they wish to have simple procedures with low-risk consequences (eg, whether to suture a small simple laceration) performed.

REFERENCES

Iserson KV. *Grave Words: Notifying Survivors About Unexpected Deaths.* Galen Press, 1999.

Iserson KV. *Pocket Protocols: Notifying Survivors About Sudden Unexpected Deaths.* Galen Press, 1999.

Iserson KV. *The Gravest Words: Notifying Survivors About Sudden, Unexpected Deaths—Video Instruction Guide.* Galen Press, 2000.

Iserson KV. *Death to Dust: What Happens to Dead Bodies?* 2nd ed. Galen Press, 2001.

Iserson KV, Sanders AB, Mathieu DR, eds. *Ethics in Emergency Medicine,* 2nd ed. Galen Press, 1995.

Iserson KV. Bioethics. In: Marx J: *Rosen's Emergency Medicine: Concepts and Clinical Practice,* 5th ed. CV Mosby, 2002:2725–2734.

Iserson KV.: Principles of biomedical ethics. In: Marco CA, Schears RM, eds. Ethical issues in emergency medicine. *Emerg Clin North Am* 1999;17(2):283–306.

Iserson KV. Nonstandard advance directives: A pseudoethical dilemma. *J Trauma* 1998; 44(1):139–42.

31. EYE PAIN/RED EYE

I. **Problem:** 43-year-old male presents with a red painful eye.

II. **Immediate Questions**

A. **Is there a history of toxic exposure?** Is the chemical known? Is the chemical an acid or caustic? Chemical exposures to the eye should be treated immediately with decontamination by high-volume irrigation before proceeding to examination.

B. **Is there a history of trauma?** What is the offending agent? Is it blunt or possibly penetrating trauma? Is a high-energy or high-velocity object involved? Does the patient feel an object is still in the eye?

C. **Is there a significant vision loss?** Is there a segmental vision loss? Does the patient see any "floaters," halos, flashes of light, or other unusual visual phenomena? Segmental vision loss or flashes of light suggest retinal injury.

D. **What are the circumstances surrounding the problem?** Can the patient identify the moment of onset? What was the patient doing at the time (eg, using power tool, entering a darkened area and dilating the pupils)?

E. **What is the quality of the problem?** Is one eye involved or both? Is there a foreign body sensation? Is the pain mild or severe; constant or intermittent? Is the pain more of a deep ache (eg, glaucoma), a burning (infectious conjunctivitis), or a scratchy feeling (allergic conjunctivitis or foreign body)?

F. **Are there other symptoms?** Is there a purulent or watery discharge from the eye (eg, infectious or allergic causes)? Has the patient had a recent illness such as URI with accompanying viral conjunctivitis?

G. **Has the patient had any previous similar episodes or underlying eye problems?** Is there a history or family history of glaucoma? Does the patient have an autoimmune disorder such as Reiter's syndrome (with accompanying conjunctivitis)? Does the patient wear corrective lenses (glasses or contacts)?

III. **Differential Diagnosis**

A. **Infections**

1. **Conjunctivitis.** Bacterial and simple viral. Specific infections such as chlamydia, gonorrhea, and conjunctivitis neonatorum may require specific treatment.

2. **Keratitis, iritis/uveitis, and infected corneal ulcer.** Involve deeper structures. Consider specific causes such as herpes simplex (characteristic dendritic ulcer), herpes zoster, and *Pseudomonas* (may be associated with contact lens use).

3. **Blepharitis, stye, and chalazion.** Lid infections may still produce eye redness and pain. Also periorbital (preseptal) and orbital cellulitis.

B. **Inflammatory, Allergic, and Autoimmune Problems.** Allergic conjunctivitis, Reiter's syndrome, JRA. Chronic corneal dryness and ulceration may occur with hypervitaminosis A, corneal dystrophy (Coggan's).

C. **Elevated Intraocular Pressure.** Acute angle closure glaucoma, chronic glaucoma exacerbation, space-occupying lesions within the orbit, eg, abscess, hematoma, tumor.

D. **Trauma**
1. **Corneal injury.** Corneal abrasion, foreign body. Suspect foreign body trapped beneath a lid with multiple linear corneal abrasions (ice-rink appearance).
2. **Blunt globe injury.** Traumatic iritis, lens dislocation, retinal tear or detachment.
3. **Penetrating globe injury.** Be suspicious of high-velocity injury. Look for aqueous humor leakage, and secondary signs such as flattening of the anterior chamber or pupil irregularities.
4. **Chemical exposure.** Acid, alkali, other irritants. Remember that exposure to fumes alone may be sufficient to cause symptoms.

IV. **Database**
A. **Physical Exam Key Points**
1. **Visual acuities**—"vital sign of the eye." Use Snellen charts, hand-held charts, newsprint, finger counting, or light perception. Topical anesthetic may be helpful if the patient is in too much pain to do a proper examination.
2. **Inspect the eye and surrounding structures.** Is there obvious trauma, swelling, redness, drainage, or foreign body? Do gross inspection of the conjunctivae and cornea. Evert the eyelids to inspect the cul-de-sac and undersurface of the lids.
3. **Check pupillary responses.** Direct and consensual responses. Note any irregularity of pupil shape.
4. **Assess extraocular muscle function and visual fields.** Ask about diplopia occurring during exam of extraocular muscles. Confrontation method commonly used in ED for detecting field defects.
5. **Funduscopic examination.** Difficult to do thoroughly without dilation of pupil—use short-acting mydriatic if elect to do this exam. Look for changes in the appearance of the disk, retinal hemorrhage in case of trauma.
6. **Measure intraocular pressure.** Various methods include hand-held Schiötz tonometer, Tono-Pen, or applanation tonometer. Use a method with which you are familiar to ensure reliable results. Normal range is up to 20 mm Hg.
7. **Slit lamp examination.** Examine cornea, iris, anterior chamber. Look for signs of trauma, eg, foreign body, corneal abrasion, or hyphema. Look for signs of infection, eg, hypopyon (pus in anterior chamber) or cell and flare. Can estimate anterior chamber angle by looking at the most peripheral portion of the clear cornea and angling a narrow slit of light 60° out from the observer angle. If the distance between the endothelium and iris is less than 1/4th the corneal cross-section's width, then the angle is narrow.

        8. Fluorescein dye. Collects in corneal defects, will fluoresce under short-wave blue (slit lamp cobalt filter) or ultraviolet light. Hand-held Wood's lamp (ultraviolet) may be used in patients who are unable to cooperate with slit-lamp examination. Continued streaming of stain away from a corneal defect suggests penetration of the globe.

  B. Laboratory Data. Usually not useful except in special cases.

      1. Cultures may be done for suspected special infections. For example herpes, *Chlamydia,* or *Pseudomonas* infection.

      2. Measuring ocular pH with nitrazine paper may help assess efficacy of irrigation treatment.

  C. Radiographic and Other Studies

      1. Plain x-ray films of orbits. Useful to detect fractures of the orbit. Radiopaque foreign bodies include metal and most glass larger than 1 mm. If using plain film to screen for intraocular foreign body, then specify in the order so that proper exposure window is used.

      2. CT scan of orbits. Specify thin cuts. Can identify orbital fractures, intraorbital hematoma and abscess, and foreign bodies. Can often assess damage to ocular structures. In cases of ocular foreign body, 3-D reconstructions or reconstruction in the coronal as well as axial planes will help localize the item and define damage done.

V. Plan

  A. Overall Plan. The primary consideration in all cases must be preservation of sight. When in doubt about potential seriousness of a situation, obtain ophthalmology consultation.

  B. Specific Plans

      1. Simple infections of the conjunctiva and lid are managed with topical antibiotic drops or ointment, eg, sodium Sulamyd, gentamycin, or ofloxacin. Suspected specific infectious agents should be treated with appropriate antibiotics, eg, tobramycin or ofloxacin for suspected *Pseudomonas.* Patients with eye discharge should be instructed to carefully clean the purulence away from the eyelids and lashes with a clean washcloth and should be warned about the potential for spreading the infection by contact with the cloth or hands. Warm compresses several times a day will help with lid abscess problems (stye, chalazion).

      2. Suspected deeper or more complex infections should be managed in consultation with an ophthalmologist, who should also provide urgent follow up care.

         a. Potential pitfalls. Do not use topical steroids in the eye without ophthalmologic consult because of the potential for exacerbating infectious such as herpes simplex ulcers. Eye patching for simple abrasions is probably not useful in any case and should never be done when *Pseudomonas* contamination of the abrasion is at issue, eg, in abrasions from contact lenses.

      3. Allergic rhinitis may respond to systemic antihistamines or topical decongestants/vasoconstrictors. Chronic dryness may respond to artificial tears but should be referred to an eye specialist if causing ulceration of the cornea.

4. **Autoimmune disorders** manifesting eye symptoms should be managed in conjunction with the appropriate specialist and possibly ophthalmologic referral.

5. **Acute glaucoma** is treated with topical pilocarpine 2% every 5 min for 3 doses, topical timolol 0.5% single dose, and acetazolamide 500 mg PO or IV. Recheck pressure every 15 min during treatment. The patient should also have an emergent ophthalmology consult.

6. **Simple corneal abrasions** with or without foreign body can be managed without specialist consultation, provided that the foreign body can be completely removed using a slit lamp or hand lens and needle or ophthalmic burr tool. Prescribe topical antibiotics and daily follow-up until lesion is healed. Give tetanus prophylaxis and pain control as appropriate.

   a. Metallic objects will usually leave a rust stain, which can be removed acutely using the burr, if small and superficial, or removed by an ophthalmologist at follow-up in several days.

7. **Blunt trauma** with pupil abnormalities, hyphema, or visual field defects should be managed with emergent eye specialist consultation.

8. **Globe penetration or lachrymal duct injury** will require immediate ophthalmologic consultation. Penetrating eye injuries should be protected by an eye shield, which does not put pressure on the eye. Again, give tetanus prophylaxis and pain control as appropriate.

   a. Damage to the lid margins may require plastic surgical or ophthalmologist repair to ensure maintenance of complete eye coverage on closing.

9. **Chemical exposure** should be treated with immediate irrigation with saline or clean water for at least 15–20 min before any further examination or assessment is performed. Attempt to identify chemical, and contact a poison control center for potential effects. Efficacy of irrigation in acid or alkali burns can be assessed with nitrazine paper testing of the eye. Pain control and tetanus prophylaxis may again be needed.

   a. Do not attempt to neutralize an acid with an alkaline irrigation solution or vice versa, as an exothermic reaction will occur and may worsen the damage.

   b. If there is evidence of corneal injury on examination after decontamination, obtain emergency ophthalmology consultation.

VI. **ICD-9 Diagnoses:** Acute conjunctivitis; Acute glaucoma; Acute iritis; Allergic conjunctivitis; Central retinal artery/vein occlusion; Chemical conjunctivitis; Corneal abrasion; Corneal foreign body; Herpes zoster ophthalmicus; Viral conjunctivitis

VII. Problem Case Diagnosis: Corneal abrasion with embedded metallic foreign body.

VIII. Teaching Pearl Question: Which type of chemical exposure to the eye tends to penetrate and damage the eye more deeply, acid or alkali? Why?

IX. Teaching Pearl Answer: Alkali burns. Alkaline chemicals will cause a liquefaction necrosis of tissue and so will continue to penetrate until neutralized. Acid solutions tend to cause a coagulation of protein and so be self-limiting. Exceptions include hydrofluoric acid and heavy metals, which can penetrate the cornea (Knoop and Trott, ref 2).

REFERENCES

Juang PS, Rosen P. Ocular examination techniques for the emergency department. *J Emerg Med* 1997;15(6):793-810.

Knoop K, Trott A. Ophthalmologic procedures in the emergency department—Part I: Immediate sight-saving procedures. *Acad Emerg Med* 1994;1(4):408–412.

Knoop K, Trott A: Ophthalmologic procedures in the emergency department—Part II: Routine evaluation procedure. *Acad Emerg Med* 1995;2(2):144–150.

Knoop K, Trott A: Ophthalmologic procedures in the emergency department—Part III: Slit lamp use and foreign bodies. *Acad Emerg Med* 1995;2(3):224–230.

Trobe JD. *The Physician's Guide to Eye Care.* American Academy of Ophthalmology, 1993.

32. FEVER IN ADULTS

I. Problem. A 50-year-old male presents with a decreased LOC, abdominal pain, fever of 100.6°F, tachycardia, hypotension, and a history of severe persistent asthma.

II. Immediate Questions

    A. What are the vitals and mental status? ABCs. What are the mental status and vitals? Apply cardiac monitor, pulse ox, IV and O_2 as indicated.

    B. Does the patient have an objective fever? Fever is considered > 100.4°F. In high-risk patients (eg, postsplenectomy, neutropenia, immunocompromised, recent invasive procedure, or indwelling device) even a history of fever should be taken seriously. Ask about duration and periodicity.

    C. Any other complaints? A thorough HPI and ROS are important.

    D. PMH, PSH, SH, FH? Especially important in fevers with no clear cause. Ask about DM, depression (and history of suicide attempt), CAD, PUD, pancreatitis or alcohol use, malignancy, HIV, immunocompromised state (including organ transplant recipients or neutropenic), endocarditis risk factors, DVT, PE, and rheumatologic disorders. Remember to ask about exposures, ingestions, recent travel, medications (including new or recently discontinued, sick contacts, recent surgery (or other invasive procedure), hemodialysis, and employment.

III. Differential Diagnosis

A. Infections. Immunocompromised patients, consider *ALL* common infections *AND:*

1. **Neutropenic fever.** ANC < 500/mm^3. Fungemia (if already on antibiotics > 1 week), mucositis, herpes, pseudomembranous colitis, cecitis, bacteremia.

2. **HIV or transplant.** Consider CMV infections, including pneumonia, colitis, retinitis, hepatitis, esophagitis, or pancreatitis. Also toxoplasmosis, cryptococcosis, histoplasmosis, MAC, candidiasis, cryptosporidiosis, TB, and PCP.

3. **Diabetic.** Cellulitis, abscesses, mucormycosis.

4. **Asplenic.** (Surgically or secondary to sickle cell) Risk of overwhelming sepsis from encapsulated organisms.

5. **Inherited or congenital immunodeficiency**

B. Infections, common: Recently hospitalized, instrumented, or indwelling device present.

1. **Nosocomial infection.** Pneumonia, UTI, line infection, MRSA.

2. **Recent OB procedure/delivery.** Endometritis/myometritis, DIC, uterine/vaginal perforation, fat emboli syndrome.

3. **Indwelling device** (including hemodialysis patients). Line infection and/or bacteremia. (See 49. Indwelling Catheter Problems, page 146)

4. **Surgery.** The 5 "W"s: **W**ind (pneumonia), **W**ater (UTI), **W**ound, **W**alking (thromboembolism), **W**onder drugs (drug fever)

5. **Bronchoscopy, endoscopy, ERCP.** Peritonitis, mediastinitis, cholangitis.

C. Infections, Common. Any patient.

1. Pneumonia, UTI, sinusitis, viral syndrome, pharyngitis, Otitis, enterocolitis, gastroenteritis, EBV, PID (including tuboovarian abscess), appendicitis (and other causes of intraabdominal abscess or peritonitis), cholecystitis, periodontal infection, diverticulitis, hepatitis, cellulitis (and other skin or soft-tissue infections), allergic reaction (including anaphylaxis), meningitis.

D. Infections, Uncommon

1. TB, malaria, syphilis, toxic shock syndrome, acute HIV infection, rabies, viral hemorrhagic fevers (Dengue, Rift Valley Fever, etc), encephalitis, systemic or pulmonary zoonotic infections (*Yersinia,* Q Fever, anthrax, tick fevers, etc), parasitic infections (See 61. Sepsis, page 183).

E. Noninfectious

1. **Collagen vascular or immune-mediated disease.** Giant-cell arteritis, SLE, rheumatic fever, PAN, RA, erythema multiforme, inflammatory bowel disease, sarcoidosis.

2. **Toxic ingestions or poisonings.** Especially in the patients with unexplained neurologic deficits or decreased LOC. Alcohol withdrawal, serotonin syndrome, neuroleptic malignant syndrome, amphetamine, cocaine use, stimulants, phencyclidine, LSD,

psilocybin, hydrocarbons, organophosphates, anticholinergics, cyanide, carbon monoxide poisoning, MAOI, salicylate, TCA, antipsychotic (see Section V, page 316)

3. **Environmental.** Heat stroke.
4. **Miscellaneous.** MI, ectopic pregnancy, subarachnoid hemorrhage, CVA (hypothalamic), malignancy, pancreatitis.

IV. Database
  A. **Physical Exam Key Points**
    1. **Mental status.** Mini mental status? (See Table A-4, page 658)
    2. **Vitals.** Are there signs of shock? Check pulse ox.
    3. **HEENT.** The more nonfocal the history, the more thorough the exam. Conduct thorough eye exam including funduscopy in IV drug users, patients with prosthetic valves or valvular heart disease, and other immunocompromised patients. Also assess adenopathy, meningismus, evidence of a toxidrome, any physical findings consistent with complaints or suspicions.
    4. **Pulmonary and cardiac.** Lung sounds, murmurs, evidence of respiratory distress.
    5. **Abdomen, Rectal, and Pelvic.** Bowel sounds, hepatosplenomegaly, peritoneal signs, tenderness?
    6. **Skin.** Rash, petechiae.
    7. **Neurologic.** Indicated in all patients with fever and headache with no other causative finding or complaint.
  B. **Laboratory and Radiographic and Other Studies.** Depend on history and exam. Patients who are not ill and have symptoms that point to a cause with no comorbid conditions do not warrant laboratory analysis unless it will change disposition, treatment, or follow-up. Immunocompetent patients should have laboratory and radiologic evaluation directed by history and symptoms. Immunocompromised patients should have a CBC, UA (and culture), CXR, and blood cultures. Lytes, renal function tests, cardiac enzymes, DIC panel, ECG, CT scans, LFTs, ABGs, and other studies should be dictated by history and exam.

V. Plan
  A. **Overall Plan.** Immunocompromised patients should be considered for admission. Patients with significant underlying comorbidity or functional decline should also be strongly considered for admission. Consider other patients based on specific cause.
  B. **Specific Plan**
    1. **Neutropenia or postsplenectomy.** Admission with intravenous broad-spectrum antibiotic (imipenem, ceftazidine, ticarcillin/clavulanate, etc) if high-risk (defined as neutropenia expected to persist longer than 10 days, hemodynamic instability, abdominal pain, nausea and vomiting, diarrhea > 6 ×/day, suspicion of catheter-associated infection, neurologic or mental status

changes, or a new pulmonary infiltrate). If low-risk, may consider admission or discharge with close follow-up on broad-spectrum oral antibiotics (ciprofloxacin plus amoxicillin/clavulanate).

2. **Sepsis.** Start broad-spectrum antibiotics and hemodynamic support, as indicated. See 61. Sepsis, page 183.

3. **Other infections.** Disposition and treatment should be based on the most likely and life-threatening specific cause or causes considered. See specific problems. Patients with most simple infections can go home if the patient has few or no comorbidities and is able to tolerate oral intake.

4. **Endocrine.** Err in favor of treating patients with a risk of Addison's disease presumptively if symptoms are suggestive. See specific problem.

5. **Toxic ingestion.** Treat ingestion. See specific problem. In the absence of GI pathology and aspiration risk, presumptive treatment with activated charcoal carries little risk.

VI **ICD-9 Diagnoses:** Fever (include source if known); Fever unknown origin; Neutropenic fever; Postoperative fever.

VII. **Problem Case Diagnosis:** Adrenal crisis.

VIII. **Teaching Pearls Question:** What is the classic triad of *Pneumocystis carinii* pneumonia?

IX. **Teaching Pearls Answer:** Fever, nonproductive cough, and exertional dyspnea.

REFERENCES

Freifeld A, Marchigiani D, Walsh T, Chanock S, Lewis L, Hiemenz J, et al: A double-blind comparison of empirical oral and intravenous antibiotic. Cancer chemotherapy. *N Engl J Med* 1999;341(5):305–311.

Pizzo PA. Fever in Immunocompromised patients. *N Engl J Med* 1999;341(12):893–900.

Pizzo PA. Drug therapy: Management of fever in patients with cancer and treatment induced neutropenia. *N Engl J Med* 1993;328(18):1323–1332.

33. FOREIGN BODY IN RECTUM

I. **Problem.** A 22-year-old male presents with a broomstick handle in his rectum. The patient also notes abdominal pain and rectal bleeding.

II. **Immediate Questions**
   A. **What are the vital signs?** Fever, tachycardia, and hypotension all indicated a serious complication (perforation, peritonitis, sepsis, blood loss). Place an IV(s) and begin appropriate resuscitation.
   B. **What is the nature of the foreign body?** The spectrum of rectal foreign bodies is wide. Is the object sharp, glass, breakable, or friable?

Such characteristics make removal difficult, increase complications, and place the examiner/patient at risk.

C. **What attempts have been made at removal?** Often patients have delayed presentation (> 24 h) because of embarrassment or hopes of spontaneous passage. Assume numerous attempts at removal have been made and determine if the patient used any instrumentation (potentially traumatic).

D. **Was the patient a victim of assault?** The causes of rectal foreign bodies include (1) autoerotic (most common) (2) iatrogenic, (3) assault, (4) self-administered treatment (prostatic massage), and (5) ingestion. Identifying assault and circumstances of traumatic insertion is very important because of increased risk of complications. Refrain from comical or disparaging comments and gain the patient's trust.

E. **Does the patient have symptoms of concern?** Symptoms such as abdominal pain, fever, vomiting, and profuse rectal bleeding signify complications needing prompt diagnosis and treatment. Maintain a high index of suspicion for rectal foreign bodies in prisoners or psych patients presenting with rectal pain or bleeding.

III. **Differential Diagnosis**

A. **Inserted vs Ingested.** Most objects are inserted into the rectum and this fact is easily determined by history alone. Small objects such as bones, sunflower seeds, and toothpicks when ingested may lodge in the rectum or anal crypts. Such patients are often unaware of the foreign body and present with fever, anal discharge, pruritus, or bleeding.

B. **Object Location.** Rectal foreign bodies can be classified as high-lying or low-lying. Those distal to the rectosigmoid junction are low-lying, and those proximal are high-lying. This distinction is important because high-lying rectal foreign bodies are difficult to visualize and remove, even with a rigid proctosigmoidoscope.

C. **Complications.** Potential complications of rectal foreign bodies include intraperitoneal rectal perforation, extraperitoneal rectal perforation, peritonitis, bowel obstruction, rectal abscess, and sepsis. Identifying patients at risk and performing appropriate evaluation are essential in reducing morbidity.

IV. **Database**

A. **Physical Exam Key Points.** Fever indicates potential complication from infection. Intraperitoneal perforation with peritonitis, extraperitoneal perforation with abscess, and sepsis must all be considered. Abdominal tenderness, rebound, or rigidity all suggest potential perforation. Consider deferring rectal exam until after plain films (dangerous objects?). Look for blood on rectal exam (rectal tear) and palpation of foreign object.

B. **Laboratory Data.** Most lab tests are of limited value. Consider hematocrit if concerned about significant hemorrhage and WBC if concerned about infectious complications.

    C. Radiographic and Other Studies. Plain films can be very helpful in both characterizing the foreign body and determining its location (low- or high-lying). Also useful in identifying free air secondary to perforation and signs of bowel obstruction.

V. Plan

    A. Removal. Most low-lying rectal foreign bodies can be safely removed in the ED. Adequate visualization (Park's retractor or vaginal speculum) and sedation are essential. Ring forceps or tenaculum forceps have been used effectively. Be careful of friable or breakable objects. Foley catheters are effective in breaking vacuum suction of rectal mucosa. Some authors advocate mandatory proctoscopy after foreign body removal to evaluate for rectal injury. Consider contrast enema if high-risk injury (assault) or high clinical suspicion for rectal tear/perforation.

    B. Admission. Patients with high-lying rectal foreign bodies, signs of perforation, or objects refractory to ED removal are candidates for admission and surgical consultation. Free air and peritonitis are clearly an indication for emergent surgical consultation.

    C. Disposition. Most patients with uncomplicated foreign body removal can be safely discharged from the ED. Discharge instructions regarding the signs of infection and perforation are mandatory. Surgery follow-up or ED reexamination in 24 h may be useful in diagnosing occult rectal injury.

VI. ICD-9 Diagnoses: Rectal foreign body.

VII. Problem Case Diagnosis: Traumatic insertion with extraperitoneal rectal perforation identified with contrast enema. Patient underwent ED foreign body removal, anoscopy and rigid proctoscopy (all normal). The enema was performed because of the high-risk mechanism.

VIII. Teaching Pearls Question: True or false? Rectal foreign bodies are seen equally among men and women.

IX. Teaching Pearls Answer: False. Rectal foreign bodies are seen 28 times more common in men than women (28:1) and the incidence is increasing (Busch and Starling).

REFERENCES

Barone J, Sohn N, Nealon T. Perforations and foreign bodies of the rectum. *Ann Surg* 1976;184:601–604.

Bloom RR, Nakano PH, Gray SW, Skandalakis JE. Foreign bodies of the gastrointestinal tract. *Am Surg* 1986;52:618–621.

Busch D, Starling J. Rectal foreign bodies: Case reports and a comprehensive review of the world's literature. *Surgery* 1986;100:512–519.

Losanoff J, Kjossev K. Rectal "oven mitt": The importance of considering a serious underlying injury. *J Emerg Med* 1999;17:31–33.

34. GASTROINTESTINAL BLEEDING

I. **Problem:** A 42-year-old alcoholic male presents with a history of profuse vomiting of bright red blood.

II. **Immediate Questions**
   A. **Is the airway intact?** Significant hematemesis may lead to aspiration or airway obstruction and require endotracheal intubation.
   B. **What are the vital signs, and how is the patient's perfusion?** Orthostatic vital signs may reveal evidence of hypovolemia missed by resting vitals.
   C. **Is the source of bleeding the upper or lower GI tract?** Melena, "coffee-ground" emesis, and/or hematemesis usually suggest an upper source. Hematochezia usually signifies a lower source; however, may be present in UGIB with rapid transit through the bowel.
   D. **What are the risk factors for GI bleeding?** A history of previous GIB may reveal source (varices, diverticula). NSAIDs may cause bleeding from peptic ulcer disease and colonic diverticula. A history of alcohol abuse and/or hepatitis may suggest cirrhosis, portal hypertension, and varices. A history of abdominal aortic surgery or trauma predisposes to aortoenteric fistulae. A history of constipation or hard stools suggests hemorrhoids, anal tears, or rectal ulcers. Aortic stenosis, chronic renal disease, collagen vascular disease, COPD, cirrhosis, and atherosclerotic heart disease are all associated with GI angiodysplasia. Anticoagulation therapy may cause spontaneous GIB. A history of preceding vomiting, coughing, or straining may indicate the presence of a Mallory-Weiss tear.
   E. **What is the other medical history?** Determine presence of bleeding disorders, liver and renal disease, and other comorbidities (history of angina, MI, CHF, or peripheral vascular disease significantly increases associated mortality).
   F. **What is the natural history of the disease?** Mortality associated with UGIB is related to degree of initial bleeding, rebleeding after initial therapy, age of the patient, and presence of significant comorbid diseases and is as high as 10% (greater than 30% for variceal bleeding). Most cases of LGIB will stop spontaneously and LGIB carries a low mortality.

III. **Differential Diagnosis**
   A. **Upper GI Hemorrhage (proximal to ligament of Treitz).**
      Peptic ulcer disease (50% of cases of UGIB); gastritis; esophagitis; esophageal or gastric varices; Mallory-Weiss tears; A-V malformations; aortoenteric fistula; malignancy
   B. **Lower GI Hemorrhage (distal to ligament of Treitz).**
      Diverticulosis; angiodysplasia; inflammatory bowel disease; ischemic colitis; rectal ulcers; NSAID-induced colonic ulceration; acute infectious colitis; pseudomembranous colitis; Meckel's diverticulum; malignancy; radiation colitis.

IV. Database

A. **Physical Exam Key Points.** Ascites, cutaneous spider angiomas, gynecomastia, palmar erythema, and splenomegaly are signs of possible cirrhosis. Rectal exam will show stool color and rule out rectal/anal malignancies. Anoscopy may identify anal and distal rectal lesions.

B. **Nasogastric Aspiration.** If positive, confirms bleeding source as upper (may be negative in the setting of even large duodenal hemorrhage). Aspiration of fresh blood and failure to clear with lavage indicate active bleeding.

C. **Laboratory Data.** CBC, T&C, PT, and PTT should be obtained emergently. Thrombocytopenia, elevated PT, and hypoalbuminemia are suggestive of portal HTN. A BUN to creatinine ratio of ≥36 without renal failure is suggestive of UGIB.

V. Plan

A. **Control Airway.** Massive UGIB can compromise airway and lead to fatal aspiration.

B. **Resuscitate with Fluids and Blood as Needed.** Establish large-bore IV access and administer warm NS bolus. Blood transfusion should be considered in patients with hematocrit of ≤21, evidence of ongoing massive bleeding, or hematocrit of < 30 and presence of significant cardiovascular disease or worrisome symptoms such as angina.

C. **Correct Coagulopathy.** Replace platelets as dictated by CBC (each unit of random donor platelets will raise the platelet count by approximately 10,000. Use FFP for elevations of PT and PTT (initial dose is 10–15 mL/kg). Vitamin K of little benefit in clotting disorders secondary to liver disease.

D. **Medical Management.** Administration of proton pump inhibitors in patients with UGIB from peptic ulcer disease has been shown to reduce the incidence of rebleeding and the need for surgery. Administration of H_2-blockers has not been found to be effective. Octreotide (somatostatin analog) decreases splanchnic and hepatic blood flow and variceal pressure and has been found as effective as endoscopic therapy in controlling variceal hemorrhage. Acid suppression has no effect on variceal bleeding.

E. **Endoscopy.** Hemostasis may be achieved in more than 90% of UGIB. Injection therapy and coagulation are used for bleeding ulcers. Injection therapy and band ligation may be used for varices and Mallory-Weiss tears. Emergent endoscopy in indicated in patients with UGIB and hemodynamic compromise, high transfusion requirement, and exsanguination.

F. **Esophageal Balloon Tamponade.** May be life-saving in cases of exsanguinating UGIB secondary to varices. Requires endotracheal intubation for protection of airway.

G. **Colonoscopy.** Diagnostic yield for acute LGIB is between 48 and 90%. Use of cautery may be therapeutic.

H. Radionuclide Scans. Technetium 99m-labeled RBC extravasation into the intestinal lumen can be identified by gamma camera scanning if the rate of bleeding is 0.1 mL/min or greater and may be used to identify need for angiography and select site for surgery.

I. Angiography. May accurately identify bleeding site and selective vasopressin infusion and transcatheter arterial embolization. Can be used in both upper and lower bleeds to control bleeding in 80% of cases in which endoscopic control has failed.

J. Surgery. Due to advances in therapeutic endoscopy, surgical management of UGIB is rarely needed. Massive LGIB may require partial or total colectomy for control of hemorrhage. If hemodynamic status permits, preoperative localization of bleeding site improves postoperative morbidity and mortality. Aortoenteric fistulas require emergent surgical correction. Portocaval shunts decompress the portal circulation and can help stop variceal bleeding.

K. Disposition—UGIB. Patients with a history of minimal bleeding, stable vital signs, normal hematocrit, no evidence of active bleeding on gastric aspirate, and no significant comorbid diseases may be discharged with gastroenterology follow-up. All others should be admitted following gastroenterology consultation. Timing of endoscopy, use of ancillary testing, and need for ICU admission are dictated by the clinical scenario.

L. Disposition—LGIB. The majority of patients will have spontaneous bleeding cessation and may discharged with planned, outpatient gastroenterology follow-up. Hemodynamic instability, significant anemia, history of massive bleeding, and the presence of significant comorbid disease necessitate admission.

VI. ICD-9 Diagnoses: Acute gastritis with hemorrhage; Anal fissure; Duodenal ulcer (with hemorrhage, perforation); Gastrointestinal bleeding; Hemorrhoids (internal, external, bleeding, thrombosed); Neoplasm; Peptic acid disease; Rectal bleeding; Reflux esophagitis.

VII. Problem Case Diagnosis: Both peptic ulcer disease and variceal hemorrhage should be suspected.

VIII. Teaching Pearl Questions
    A. In a patient with know portal hypertension, what is the most common cause of UGIB?
    B. What are the causes of a falsely positive and falsely negative fecal occult blood testing?

IX. Teaching Pearl Answer
    A. Peptic ulcer disease.
    B. **False positives.** Red meat; aspirin and NSAIDs; steroids, antimetabolites (iron supplements and bismuth can simulate melena, but fecal occult blood testing will be negative).
    False negatives. Vitamin C in excess of 250 mg/day.

REFERENCES

Fallah MA, Prakash C, Edmundowicz S. Acute gastrointestinal bleeding. *Med Clin North Am* 2000;85(5):1183–1208.

Mallory S, Van Dam J. Advances in diagnostic and therapeutic endoscopy. *Med Clin North Am* 2000;85(5):1059–1083.

Maltz GS, Siegel JE, Carson JL. Hematologic management of gastrointestinal bleeding. *Gastroenterol Clin North Am* 2000;29(1):169–187.

Peter DJ, Dougherty JM. Evaluation of the patient with gastrointestinal bleeding: An evidence based approach. *Emerg Med Clin North Am* 1999;17(1):239–261.

Stabile BE, Stamos MJ. Surgical management of gastrointestinal bleeding. *Gastroenterol Clin North Am* 2000;29(1):189–222.

35. GASTROINTESTINAL CATHETER PROBLEMS

I. **Problems**
   A. A middle-aged man with PMH of severe stroke and status-post percutaneous endoscopic gastrostomy (PEG) tube placement presents because his PEG tube seems clogged and his caregivers "cannot feed him his tube feeds."
   B. A young girl presents after a suicide attempt by overdose. She had an NG tube placed for charcoal administration and now is in respiratory distress.

II. **Immediate Questions**
   A. **What is the general appearance of the patient and vital signs?** Is the patient hemodynamically stable and alert? Provide supportive measures as needed (attention to airway and breathing, IV access with fluids if needed, cardiac and BP monitoring, pulse oximetry).
   B. **Is there any history of trauma or difficult insertion of the catheter?** Tube dislodgement or kinking is a common presenting problem.
   C. **Has a long-standing PEG tube been removed?** If the tube has a mature fistula, prepare to place a Foley catheter or more permanent replacement tube through the stoma. Time is key as the stoma may close completely within 24 h.

III. **Differential Diagnosis**
   A. **Catheter Obstruction.** May be caused by intraluminal contents, catheter malposition, or kinking of the tube.
   B. **Tube Migration.** Can be associated with infection, rupture of viscous or pulmonary complications/aspiration.
   C. **Gastroesophageal Reflux/Aspiration of Tube Contents.** May cause severe pneumonitis or pneumonia.
   D. **Tension Pneumothorax or Pneumomediastinum.** May result from NG tube or PEG tube placement.
   E. **Bowel Obstruction.** May result from the catheter balloon or kinking of the tube.

    F. Peritonitis. May result from repeated (aggressive) attempts at replacing tube causing rupture of track and spillage of intestinal fluids into peritoneum.

IV. Database
A. Physical Exam Key Points
1. **Review vital signs and mental status.** Provide airway and circulatory support if indicated.
2. **HEENT.** If NG tube, evaluate tube position and oropharyngeal exam.
3. **Abdomen.** If PEG tube, examine for tenderness, peritoneal signs, distention, or masses (may signify bowel or gastric obstruction or perforation), as well as for signs of infection or irritation in skin surrounding catheter. Check for drainage/bleeding around catheter.
4. **Lungs.** Especially if aspiration is suspected.

B. Laboratory Data.
Generally not indicated for uncomplicated cases. If respiratory compromise/aspiration/vomiting, consider ABG and possibly Lytes.

C. Radiographic and Other Studies
1. **CXR.** Evaluate for signs of aspiration/pneumonitis, pneumonia, pulmonary malposition of tube, free air under diaphragm, PTX, pneumomediastinum.
2. **Abdominal x-ray films (acute abdominal series).** Evaluate position of tube and for evidence of obstruction.

V. Plan
A. Overall Plan
1. Uncomplicated PEG or NG tube occlusion or malfunction can usually be managed by replacing the tube and confirming position, with subsequent discharge.
2. Patients with pulmonary complications, viscous perforation, bowel obstruction, or serious infection require admission with medical/GI or surgical consultation as indicated.

B. Specific Plans
1. For PEG tube occlusion (presumed to be intraluminal) with mature fistula tract:
   a. Try simple flushing or instillation of carbonated beverage.
   b. Usually requires removal of tube and placement of either temporary
   c. Foley catheter (to maintain patency of stoma), or appropriate permanent replacement tube.
   d. Obtain water-soluble contrast study through the tube to confirm position.
2. For PEG tube with immature fistula tract and apparent occlusion:
   a. May attempt brief trial at flushing, etc if no history or suggestion of tube migration or malposition.

        b. Usually best managed via endoscopic or operative management and requires consultation of surgeon or GI physician who placed catheter.
3. For NG tube malposition.
    a. Remove tube if pulmonary position.
    b. May replace tube if no obvious complications.
    c. Treat pulmonary/other complications (aspiration, intracranial placement etc as situation dictates).

VI. ICD-9 Diagnoses: Gastrostomy, Jejunostomy, or Colostomy infection or mechanical complication; Can also state "Attention to jejunostomy tube"—includes removal, cleaning, replacing, adjusting-coded as a V code.

VII. Problem Case Diagnoses
  A. Obstructed (intraluminal) PEG tube.
  B. Intrapulmonary tube placement with direct charcoal instillation into lung.

VIII. Teaching Pearl Question: How long after PEG tube placement does it usually take for tract maturation, allowing safe replacement of tube without endoscopic or surgical assistance (ie, can be replaced in the ED)?

IX. Teaching Pearl Answer: Although some clinicians believe 2 weeks is adequate, full tract maturation may take up to *3 months,* and this is generally viewed as a safe time frame to replace tubes.

REFERENCES

Freij RM, Mullett ST. Inadvertent intracranial insertion of a nasogastric tube in a non-trauma patient. *J Accid Emerg Med* 1997;14(1):45–47.
Sabga E, Sabga E, Dick A, Lertzman M, Tenenbein M. Direct administration of charcoal into the lung and pleural cavity. *Ann Emerg Med* 1997;30(5):695–697.
Willwerth BM. PEG or skin-level gastrostomy tube replacement. *Pediatr Emerg Care* 2001;17(1):55–58.

36. GENITOURINARY CATHETER PROBLEMS

I. Problems
  A. An elderly man with a chronic indwelling urinary catheter presents with lower abdominal pain, altered mental status, and decreased urinary output.
  B. An elderly man presents with gross hematuria and now sudden decrease in urinary output.
  C. A middle-aged female presents after placement of a ureteral stent with worsening right flank pain and gross hematuria.

II. Immediate Questions
  A. What is the general appearance of the patient and vital signs? Is the patient hemodynamically stable and alert? Provide supportive

measures as needed (attention to airway and breathing, IV access with fluids or blood if needed, cardiac and BP monitoring, etc). Look for signs of infection (fever, tachycardia, mental status changes, vomiting, etc).

B. Is there any urine output currently? Is there ongoing bleeding through the catheter? This may provide clues as to mechanical complications (postrenal) vs medical (renal or prerenal)

C. Is there any history of trauma? This may require urologic consultation if severe.

III. Differential Diagnosis

A. Infection. UTI or urosepsis is common and may require aggressive fluid, antibiotic, and other management. Fungal infections or periurethral abscess are possible as well.

B. Hematologic Disorder. Warfarin or heparin anticoagulation therapy, aspirin or other antiplatelet medication, thrombocytopenia or other coagulopathy may be present.

C. Mechanical Complications. Encrustation of the catheter with obstruction by crystalline deposits inside the lumen, kinking of the catheter, or clotted blood may be present. Bladder perforation, urethral erosion, or bladder stones may contribute.

D. Ureteral Stent Complications include obstruction, migration, and infection.

IV. Database

A. Physical Exam Key Points

1. **Review vital signs and mental status.** Look for evidence of infection.
2. **Abdomen.** Check for abdominal tenderness, masses, and distention. CVA tenderness (pyelonephritis/hydronephrosis).
3. **Genitourinary.** Look for signs of local trauma or infection, or for blood leaking around the catheter.

B. Laboratory Data. Most cases require UA with urine culture, especially if suspecting infection/sepsis. Possibly: BUN and creatinine (if suspecting renal dysfunction or postrenal failure), CBC (platelets, H/H for bleeding; WBC with infection), coagulation studies (continued bleeding, warfarin/heparin therapy).

C. Radiographic and Other Studies. Usually none required in uncomplicated cases. If ureteral stent problem, consider ultrasound, KUB, IVP, renal scan, or contrast CT.

V. Plan

A. Overall Plan. Simple catheter obstruction may only need irrigation with likely catheter replacement and allow discharge home. Significant infection or continued GU bleeding will need admitted.

B. Specific Plans

1. Remove and replace catheter if uncomplicated.
2. Evaluate and treat for infection/urosepsis as indicated by clinical/lab findings.

3. Evaluate for cause of continued bleeding as indicated. Reversal of anticoagulation, platelet, or PRBC transfusion may be needed. Consider bladder irrigation.
4. Consider suprapubic catheter and/or urologic consultation if unable to place urethral catheter.
5. Obtain imaging study and urologic consultation if stent complication.

VI. **ICD-9 Diagnoses:** Infection, inflammation, or mechanical complication due to indwelling urinary catheter or intrauterine contraceptive device (then also state type of infection, eg, cystitis)

VII. **Problem Cases Diagnoses**
   A. UTI with urosepsis.
   B. Catheter obstructed by clotted blood.
   C. Stent migration.

VIII. **Teaching Pearl Question:** What organism is the most common cause of UTI in patients with indwelling urinary catheters?

IX. **Teaching Pearl Answer:** Gram-negative organisms (*E. coli, Protous mirabilis, Pseudomonas aeruginosa, Providencia stuartii*), followed by enterococci (Nicolle).

REFERENCES

Farraye MJ, Scaberg D. Indwelling Foley catheter causing extraperitoneal bladder perforation. *Am J Emerg Med* 2000;18(4):497–500.
Nicolle LE. The chronic indwelling catheter and urinary infection in long-term-care facility residents. *Infect Control Hosp Epidemiol* 2001;22(5):316–321.

37. HEADACHE

I. **Problem.** A 17-year-old female comes to the ED complaining of a severe headache and worsening fever for 3 days. Is on amoxicillin for sinusitis.

II. **Immediate Questions**
   A. Is the patient urgent or emergent? Are the ABCs intact? Is the patient in extremes? Are the vital signs normal? Is the patient conscious?
   B. What is the mental status and neurologic exam? Is the patient awake and alert? Is the patient responding appropriately to questions? Is there slowness of speech or inappropriate words? Any confusion? Did the patient walk in or was she brought in? Does she have normal strength and sensation in the extremities?
   C. What is the level of pain? Is the pain significant enough that it should be treated immediately? If you are treating immediately, have you discussed the possible course of action, diagnostic tests, and risks of each (including lumbar puncture).

    D. PQRST (Palliation, Provocation, Quality, Radiation, Severity, Timing). Did this start suddenly or gradually? Any trauma? Was there any activity just prior to the event (sex is sometimes a precipitating factor in SAH)? Does leaning over make it worse? Is there any evidence of sinus infection/congestion/drainage? Is the pain stabbing, aching, one-sided, or generalized? Does the pain extend down the neck? Is this the worst headache of your life? Is the pain constant or have you had an episode of it each day?

    E. Past History. Is there a history of headaches? Is this headache like others? Any recent new/mild headache? Any chance of immunocompromise? Does the family have a history of headaches or aneurysms? Any recent use of medications, drugs, or alcohol?

III. Differential Diagnosis

    A. Disaster. Subarachnoid hemorrhage, subdural hematoma, epidural hematoma, meningitis, encephalitis, neoplasm, glaucoma, hypertensive emergency.

    B. Discomfort. Tension, migraine, cluster, sinusitis, pharyngitis.

IV. Database

    A. Physical Exam Key Points

        1. Neurologic. Mini mental status exam (see Table A-4, page 656), cranial nerves, motor, sensory, and proprioception (Can the patient walk normally and stand with her eyes closed?). CNS tumors often affect small areas that are ignored by patient (eg, a gaze paralysis, slowly reacting pupil, or visual field defect).

        2. HEENT. Look for evidence of trauma. Is there any discoloration of the cornea or irregularity in the reactivity of the pupils? A funduscopic exam can predict the outcome of the CT if there is blurring of the disc margins. Always look in the nose. Tumors sometimes have delayed diagnosis while treated as chronic sinusitis. Strep throat often causes significant headache.

        3. Neck. Feel for lymphadenopathy. Check for evidence of meningitis.

    B. Laboratory Data

        1. Blood work. Rarely useful except in immunocompromised or coagulopathic patients where a CBC and PT/PTT are indicated.

        2. CSF. If meningeal signs are present (neck stiffness, and pain with movement, new onset headache) and no other clear cause, then a spinal tap is mandatory. Temperature at presentation is irrelevant due to frequent use of antipyretics. Believe the history. It is not uncommon to find meningitis a few days after symptoms begin and have been "treated" by a primary care physician.

    C. Radiographic and Other Studies. CT scan should be used liberally in the ED. Although 90% of headaches in the ED do not have a significant cause, the 10% with potentially disastrous causes can be difficult to rule out by history and physical alone.

V. Plan

A. Overall Plan. The main duty is to rule out the 5–10% of headaches that are caused by serious pathology. This might be accomplished by history and physical alone, but often requires a CT scan and spinal tap to be certain. The other important duty is to make the patient feel better. Don't make the patient wait for test results before you start treating the pain.

B. Specific Plans

1. **Disasters (the 10%)**—ABCs, minimize the disaster and get definitive care emergently. Elevate the head of the bed. Intubate not just for airway control but to hyperventilate. Correct coagulopathies early with FFP. Treat presumptively with antibiotics. Contact the neurosurgeon and the OR when you think you of a patient with one of the 5% causes of headaches.

2. **Discomfort (the 90%)**—Control the symptoms

   a. **5-HT₁ Serotonin receptor agonist (sumatriptan succinate: Imitrex)**—suppresses inflammation of cranial arteries associated with migraines.

   b. **Ergot alkaloids (ergotamine: Cafergot)**—Has α-adrenergic antagonist and serotonin antagonist effects. Constricto peripheral and cranial blood vessels.

   c. **Antiemetics** (Prochlorperazine/droperidol/metoclopramide/promethazine: Phenergan)—stops vomiting and sometimes the headache.

   d. **Analgesics (Tylenol to morphine)**—type dependent on severity and response.

VI. ICD-9 Diagnoses:
Acute glaucoma; Acute sinusitis; Brain neoplasm; Cluster headache; Headache; Lumbar puncture headache; Meningitis (aseptic, bacterial); Migraine headache; Temporal arteritis; Tension headache

VII. Problem Case Diagnosis:
Bacterial meningitis.

VIII. Teaching Pearl Question:
What percent of subarachnoid hemorrhages are missed on CT scan?

IX. Teaching Pearl Answer.
3–5%.

REFERENCES

Blanda M, Wright J. Headache, migraine. *eMedicine.com* 2001;2:11. Available at: http://www.emedicine.com/emerg/topic230.htm

Caesar R. Acute headache management: The challenge of deciphering etiologies to guide assessment and treatment. *Emerg Med Rep* 1995;16:13.

Clinical Policy for the Initial Approach to Adolescents and Adults Presenting to the Emergency Department With a Chief Complaint of Headache: *Ann Emerg Med* 1996;27: 821–844.

Morgenstern LB, Luna-Gonzales H, Huber JC Jr, Wong SS, Uthman MO, Gurian JH, et al. Worst headache and subarachnoid hemorrhage: Prospective, modern computed tomography and spinal fluid analysis. *Ann Emerg Med* 1998;32:297–304.

38. HEART MURMUR

I. **Problem.** A 47-year-old male with acute SOB and a new IV/VI systolic murmur.

II. **Immediate Questions**
   A. **Is the airway intact?** Will he require intubation? Manage appropriately. (See Section VIII, 15. Rapid Endotracheal Intubation, p 470.)
   B. **What are the vital signs and mental status?** Febrile? Stable and alert? Apply monitors (ECG and pulse oximetry) and oxygen. Start IV. Stat PA and lateral CXR if stable (otherwise stat portable CXR).
   C. **Is the patient having chest pain?** Character, onset, radiation to other areas?
   D. **Fever?** Shaking chills? Sweats?
   E. **Past history?** Prior MI, CHF, pulmonary edema, rheumatic fever, cardiac surgery (including valves). IV drug use? DVT or PE? Last echocardiogram? Changed or missed medications (especially diuretic)? Marfan's syndrome? Known MVP?

III. **Differential Diagnosis**
   A. **Systolic Murmur** (mitral regurgitation = MR).
      1. Chordae tendinea rupture. Myxomatous degeneration, infective endocarditis (fever, IV drug use), trauma.
      2. Papillary muscle dysfunction or rupture. Ischemia may cause dysfunction. Past infarction predisposes to rupture. Trauma.
      3. Mitral valve perforation. Infective endocarditis (fever, IV drug use).
      4. Degeneration of artificial valve. Usually infectious.
      5. Chronic mitral regurgitation. Dilated LV, Marfan's syndrome, rheumatic fever, mitral valve prolapse.
      6. Dilatation of mitral annulus. Marfan's syndrome.
   B. **Systolic Murmur** (aortic stenosis = AS).
      1. Fibrous or calcific aortic stenosis.
      2. Bicuspid aortic valve.
   C. **Diastolic Murmur** (aortic regurgitation = AR).
      1. Aortic valve perforation. Infective endocarditis, rheumatic fever.
      2. Degeneration of artificial valve. Usually infectious.
      3. Dilation of aortic root. Aortic dissection, Marfan's syndrome.
      4. Diastolic murmur (mitral stenosis = MS).
      5. Scarring of mitral valve. Rheumatic fever, calcification.

IV. **Database**
   A. **Physical Exam Key Points**
      1. **Vital signs.** Febrile (think endocarditis), widened pulse pressure (AR).
      2. **Vascular.** Check JVD (CHF), carotid bruits (transmitted AS murmur), palpate carotid upstroke (decreased = AS, bounding = AR). Peripheral pulses unequal (aortic dissection).
      3. **Location of maximal heart sounds.** Apex (mitral). Right second interspace (aortic).

      4. Timing of heart sounds. Murmur ending before S_2 (AS). With S_2 (MR). Diastolic (AR).

      5. Duration of heart sounds. Holosystolic in MR but acute MR may be louder in early and mid systole. Crescendo-decrescendo (AS).

      6. Character of heart sounds. Blowing like "whooooo" (MR). Harsh like "shshshsh" (AS).

      7. Radiation of heart sounds. To left axilla (MR). To carotids (AS).

      8. Other sounds? S_3, S_4 (MI, CHF, acute MR).

      9. Pulmonary exam. Diffuse rales (pulmonary edema, CHF, acute MR). Normal (MI, PE).

  B. Laboratory Data. If infection suspected then CBC, blood cultures, possibly ESR or CRP. BMP for lytes if CHF or on diuretics. D-dimer if suspect PE. Cardiac enzymes if suspect MI.

  C. Radiographic and Other Studies. CXR and ECG. If stable and PE possible, consider CT or V/Q. If aortic dissection possible, get chest CT with contrast. Bedside TTE will show cardiac function, valve integrity, and tamponade. TEE is best for visualizing valves and vegetations.

V. Plan

  A. Overall Plan. A new systolic murmur with symptoms at rest or a diastolic murmur should be referred to a cardiologist for admission and echocardiogram. If the new systolic murmur is without symptoms, refer to cardiologist or primary physician.

  B. Specific Plans

      1. Febrile, suspect infection. IV Nafcillin + IV gentamycin + PO rifampin **or** IV vancomycin + IV gentamycin + PO rifampin if PCN allergic. Consult cardiothoracic surgeon immediately, especially if prosthetic valve. (Also see Problem 61. Sepsis, page 183)

      2. Aortic dissection or valve rupture. Immediately consult cardiothoracic surgeon. Goal systolic BP of 100–120 and HR 60–80 with IV labetalol, metoprolol, or esmolol. Control pain with IV opiates. Small (250–500 mL) crystalloid boluses if hypotensive. Stat T&C 10–15 units of blood. (Also see 13. Cardiac Arrest, page 41)

      3. Ongoing MI. (See Problem 15. Chest Pain, page 51)

        a. Cardiogenic shock. (See 13. Cardiac Arrest, page 41)

      4. CHF with pulmonary edema. (See Problem 16. CHF/Pulmonary Edema, page 54)

VI. ICD-9 Diagnoses: Acute endocarditis; Aortic stenosis; Aortic insufficiency; Atrial septal defect; Heart murmur; Mitral stenosis; Mitral insufficiency; Papillary muscle rupture; Patent ductus arteriosus; Pulmonary stenosis; Ventricular septal defect

VII. Problem Case Diagnosis: Papillary muscle rupture from old MI.

VIII. Teaching Pearl Question: Ischemia/infarction of which wall of the heart would most likely be the cause of papillary muscle dysfunction/rupture?

IX. Teaching Pearl Answer: Inferior wall. (Tintinalli, et al).

REFERENCES

Carabello BA, Crawford FA. Valvular heart disease. *N Engl J Med* 1997;337(1):32–41.
Mylonakis E, Calderwood SB. Infective endocarditis in adults. *N Engl J Med* 2001;345(18):
    318–1330.
Schlant RC, Alexander RW, O'Rourke RA, Roberts R, Sonnenblick EH, eds. *The Heart,*
    8th ed. McGraw-Hill, 1994.
Tintinalli JE, Kelen GD, Stapczynski JS, eds. *Emergency Medicine: A Comprehensive
    Study Guide,* 5th ed. McGraw-Hill, 2000.

39. HEMOPTYSIS

I. **Problem.** A homeless, intravenous drug user presents with 2 weeks of weight loss and nonproductive cough and 1 day of bloody sputum.

II. **Immediate Questions**

   A. **Is the airway intact?** Massive hemoptysis can lead to airway compromise. When intubation is required, a large ETT is preferred to allow for better suctioning. Selective mainstem intubation should be considered to allow ventilation of the unaffected lung and to minimize the spread of blood from the affected lung. To accomplish right mainstem intubation, simply advance the ETT 4–5 cm beyond its usual position. For left mainstem intubation, rotate the ETT 90° to the left while positioning the concavity of the tube to the left during intubation. If available, a double-lumen ETT can be used for selective mainstem intubation. (See Section VIII, 15. Rapid Endotracheal Intubation, p 470.)

   B. **Are oxygenation and ventilation adequate?** What is the pulse oximeter reading? Does the patient show signs of respiratory distress? Apply oxygen as needed. If one side of the lung is suspected to be the source of bleeding (eg, left or right lung), position the patient with the affected side down.

   C. **Is blood coming from the respiratory tract?** Hemoptysis involves expectoration of blood from below the level of the vocal cords. This must be differentiated from nasopharyngeal bleeding (eg, epistaxis) and gastrointestinal bleeding (hematemesis).

   D. **What is the degree of hemoptysis?** Classically, massive hemoptysis is greater than 600 mL/day or 100 mL/h. From a practical standpoint, it is most helpful to determine if the patient is experiencing large amounts of hemoptysis, only blood-tinged sputum, or somewhere in between. Cardiac monitoring and IV access should be initiated for patients with anything but very minor hemoptysis, as their condition may deteriorate rapidly.

   E. **Any past medical history?** Tuberculosis, pneumonia, CHF, mitral stenosis, lung cancer, PE or DVT, anticoagulant use?

   F. **Any associated symptoms?** Cough, fever, weight loss, night sweats, chest pain, leg pain, or swelling?

III. Differential Diagnosis

A. Infectious or Inflammatory. Bronchitis, bronchiectasis, pneumonia (bacterial, viral, fungal), TB, pulmonary abscess, parasitic (paragonimiasis, schistosomiasis, ascariasis).

B. Neoplastic. Bronchogenic carcinoma, bronchial adenoma, metastatic malignancy (breast, colon, melanoma, renal, others), Kaposi's sarcoma, hamartoma.

C. Cardiovascular. CHF, PE, mitral stenosis, primary pulmonary hypertension, A-V malformation, aortic aneurysm or dissection.

D. Immunologic/Systemic Illness. Collagen vascular diseases (lupus), Goodpasture's syndrome, vasculitis, sarcoid, Wegener's granulomatosis.

E. Others. CF, trauma, coagulopathy (anticoagulants, thrombolytics, thrombocytopenia, hemophilia).

IV. Database

A. Physical Exam Key Points

1. **General appearance.** Pale skin (anemia), cachexia (TB, malignancy), respiratory effort.
2. **Vital signs.** Check carefully and repeat during evaluation. Count the respiratory rate yourself. Fever suggests pulmonary infection, but low-grade fever may be present with PE.
3. **Head and neck.** Pale conjunctiva (anemia). Check to rule out epistaxis or oral bleeding. Adenopathy (TB, malignancy), JVD (CHF).
4. **Lungs.** Diffuse rales (CHF), focal abnormalities (pneumonia, malignancy).
5. **Heart sounds.** Mitral stenosis murmur is usually low-pitched and diastolic, and may be preceded by an opening snap. S_3 suggests CHF.
6. **Extremities.** Symmetric pitting edema suggests CHF. Unilateral leg swelling, local tenderness, and presence of a palpable cord suggest DVT (causing PE). Cyanosis may be present from severe hypoxia or congenital heart disease (VSD, tetralogy of Fallot, transposition of great arteries). Clubbing suggests long-standing cardiopulmonary disease (cyanotic heart disease, malignancy, lung abscess).

B. Laboratory Data. Order CBC for most patients. For patients with minimal amounts of hemoptysis (faint blood-tinged sputum) who clinically are not significantly anemic (normal skin color, pink conjunctiva, no symptoms of anemia) and when a benign cause is suspected (bronchitis), lab testing may be omitted. Other studies if risk factors uncovered in history and physical. Type and screen or T&C if nontrivial hemoptysis.

C. Radiographic and Other Studies. CXR should be obtained on almost all patients. An exception would be a young, healthy patient, with an otherwise normal history and physical exam, without risk factors for pulmonary TB, when acute bronchitis is clinically suspected.

The CXR is the most helpful study for determining the cause of he-moptysis. Other specific tests may be obtained, depending on the suspected cause (eg, chest CT for malignancy, V/Q scan or helical CT for PE, echocardiogram for valvular disease for CHF, mycobac-terial sputum stains, and cultures for TB).

V. Plan

A. Overall Plan. Support ABCs. Correct anemia, thrombocytopenia, and coagulopathy. Treat the underlying cause of hemoptysis. Consider consultation for localization and control of bleeding (pulmonary con-sult for bronchoscopy, angiography consult for embolization, cardio-thoracic surgery consult for lung resection). Patients can generally be discharged if they have a minor degree of hemoptysis, normal vital signs, a near-normal hematocrit, no significant hemoptysis over 1–3 h of observation, and no other acute condition requiring hospitalization (eg, CHF, PE, pneumonia). Discharged patients should be instructed to follow up with a primary care physician, and to return to the ED if wors-ening symptoms. Patients with unstable vital signs, life-threatening he-moptysis, or potential respiratory compromise should generally be admitted to an ICU.

B. Specific Plans. Treat underlying conditions as appropriate (eg, nitrates and diuretics for CHF, antibiotics for pneumonia, anticoagulation for PE). See list of problems for specific diseases.

VI. ICD-9 Diagnoses: Acute bronchitis; Bronchiectasis; Churg-Strauss syn-drome; Cystic fibrosis; Hemoptysis; Pneumonia; Pulmonary neoplasm; Pul-monary tuberculosis; Pulmonary embolus; Pulmonary coccidioidomycosis.

VII. Problem Case Diagnosis: Pulmonary tuberculosis.

VIII. Teaching Pearl Question. What is the usual cause of death in a patient with hemoptysis?

IX. Teaching Pearl Answer: Suffocation, not exsanguination.

REFERENCES

Dweik RA, Stoller JK. Role of bronchoscopy in massive hemoptysis. *Clin Chest Med* 1999;20(1):89–105.

Glauser J, D'Amore JZ. Clinicopathological conference: A previously healthy 40-year-old woman with hemoptysis. *Acad Emerg Med* 2001;8(4):374–381.

Herth F, Ernst A, Becker HD. Long-term outcome and lung cancer incidence in patients with hemoptysis of unknown origin. *Chest* 2001;120(5):1592–1594.

Jean-Baptiste E. Clinical assessment and management of massive hemoptysis. *Crit Care Med* 2000;28(5):1642–1647.

40. HEMORRHAGIC SHOCK

I. Problem. Young woman presents with confusion, hypotension, cool, mottled extremities and history of syncope after 1 day of progressive lower abdominal pain.

II. Immediate Questions

A. Primary Survey. ABCs? Are there diminished pulses or other signs of poor peripheral perfusion?

B. What are the vitals and mental status? Is the patient stable and alert? Apply monitors (ECG and pulse ox), start IV, apply oxygen. Confusion, orthostatic changes, heart rate and rhythm, and BP discrepancy between arms may offer clues to cause.

C. Was there any history of trauma? Interview any witnesses, EMS personnel, family members.

  1. If yes, then what was the mechanism of trauma? Blunt or penetrating trauma? If MVA, was the patient belted or unbelted? If a fall occurred, then how far? Self-inflicted? Consider location for hidden blood—chest, abdomen, pelvis, upper legs.

  2. If no, then consider other medical sources for hemorrhage. Ask about pregnancy, GI sources, aortic aneurysm, epistaxis, hemoptysis, fevers.

D. Any past medical history? Heart disease, hypertension, aortic disease, coagulopathies, liver disease, peptic ulcers, history of PID or ectopic pregnancies, thoracic tumors or infections, Marfan's syndrome?

E. Medications? Anticoagulants, NSAIDS, corticosteroids or other medications that may precipitate a bleed. Beta-blockers or calcium channel blockers that may mask worsening shock symptoms?

F. Social history? Alcohol, drugs, domestic abuse.

III. Differential Diagnosis

A. Blunt Trauma
  1. Hemothorax.
  2. Traumatic aortic injury.
  3. Hemoperitoneum.
  4. Retroperitoneal bleeding.
  5. Pelvic fracture.
  6. Thigh hematomas from femur fracture.

B. Penetrating Trauma
  1. Hemothorax and cardiac injury.
  2. Hemoperitoneum.
  3. Retroperitoneal bleeding.
  4. Vascular injury.
  5. Severe scalp injury.

C. Gastrointestinal Bleeding
  1. Upper GI bleeding; PUD, esophageal varices.
  2. Lower GI bleeding; diverticula.
  3. Hemorrhagic pancreatitis.

D. Ruptured Aortic Aneurysm

E. Massive Hemoptysis
  1. Infectious.
    a. TB.
    b. Abscess.
    c. Fungal (ie, aspergillosis).
  2. Neoplasms.

F. Gynecologic Bleeding
1. Early complications of pregnancy.
   a. Ectopic pregnancy.
   b. Bleeding secondary to spontaneous or surgical abortion.
2. Late complications of pregnancy.
   a. Placenta previa.
   b. Placental abruption.
   c. Postpartum bleeding.
3. Hemorrhagic ovarian cyst.

G. Epistaxis
1. Usually a posterior bleed

H. Infectious
1. Viral hemorrhagic fevers.
2. Mononucleosis related splenic rupture.

IV. Database
A. Physical Exam Key Points (Table I–7, p 124)
1. **Mental status.** Mini mental status exam (See Table A-4, page 656). Changes range from anxiety to coma as shock progresses.
2. **Vital signs.** Check carefully and repeat during evaluation.
3. **Skin.** Cool, mottled or dusky skin. Increased capillary refill time. Active bleeding, large lacerations, entrance/exit penetration wounds.
4. **HEENT.** Epistaxis or severe facial bleeding.
5. **Chest.** Diminished breath sounds, dullness to percussion, crepitus, subcutaneous air, ecchymosis, seat belt sign, entrance/exit penetrating wounds.
6. **Cardiac.** Tachycardia, faint pulses, pulsatile bleeding. Progressive hypotension.

TABLE I–7. CLASSES OF SHOCK.

	Class I	Class II	Class III	Class IV
Blood loss (mL)	< 750	750–1500	1500–2000	> 2000
Blood loss (% blood volume)	> 15%	15–30%	30–40%	> 40%
Pulse rate	> 100	> 100	> 120	> 140
Blood pressure	Normal	Normal	Decreased	Decreased
Pulse pressure	Normal or increased	Decreased	Decreased	Decreased
Respiratory rate	14–20	20–30	30–40	> 35
Urine output (mL/h)	> 30	20–30	5–15	Negligible
CNS/Mental status	Slight anxiety	Moderate anxiety	Anxious and confused	Confused and lethargic

Reproduced, with permission, from *Advanced Trauma Life Support Manual,* 1997.

   7. **Abdomen, rectal and pelvic.** Check for distension, tenderness, ecchymosis of flanks or umbilicus. Document location of all entrance and exit penetrating wounds. Check for pulsatile abdominal mass (AAA). Check vagina and stool for blood. Pelvic exam for pregnancy or asymmetric tenderness (ectopic).
   8. **Neurologic exam.** Monitor mental status.
B. **Laboratory Data.** T&C is the single most important lab test. CBC, Lytes may be normal in early hemorrhagic shock, ABG will often give clue to inadequate tissue perfusion. Pregnancy test in women.
C. **Radiographic and Other Studies**
   1. Chest and pelvis films with trauma, femur film if suspected fracture.
   2. FAST abdominal ultrasound for blunt abdominal (See Figure VIII–5, p 426.) or chest trauma in stable or unstable patient. Pelvic ultrasound for suspected ectopic pregnancy or other gynecologic cause. Bedside ultrasound for unstable patient with suspected aortic aneurysm.
   3. Abdominal CT for abdominal and chest trauma in initially stable patient. May also evaluate for retroperitoneal bleeding and bleeding aortic aneurysm.
   4. Diagnostic peritoneal lavage in unstable trauma patient or in penetrating trauma of the abdomen.
   5. Endoscopy to identify sources of GI bleeding.

V. Plan
A. **Overall Plan**
   1. Identify location and source of hemorrhage.
   2. Maintain intravascular volume until source of active hemorrhage can be addressed.
B. **Specific Plans**
   1. Initial IV bolus for adults is 1–2 L of NS or RL and 20 mL/kg for children. Warmed IV fluids and blood are preferred.
      a. Patients who rapidly normalize their vitals and remain hemodynamically stable after the initial fluid bolus can be placed on maintenance fluids while sources of bleeding are identified. Assume < 20% blood loss
      b. Patients who initially respond and then show signs of deterioration generally have active hemorrhage or inadequate resuscitation. They will need continued fluids and blood products in a 3:1 ratio and urgent identification of sources of bleeding. Assume 20–40% blood loss.
      c. Patients who show no response at all to the initial fluid challenge will generally need aggressive fluid and blood administration as well as emergent surgical intervention to control life-threatening hemorrhage. Assume > 40% loss of blood volume.

2. Choice of blood products determined by how urgently they are needed
   a. Type O blood (O– in women): immediate.
   b. Type specific blood : 10 min.
   c. Fully cross matched: 1 h.
3. For patients with complicated medical issues such as heart disease, invasive cardiac monitoring may be needed to guide fluid administration.

VI. ICD-9 Diagnoses: Hemorrhagic shock (state due to disease, surgery, or trauma).

VII. Problem Case Diagnosis: Ectopic pregnancy.

VIII. Teaching Pearl Question: What are the first signs of hemorrhagic shock?

IX. Teaching Pearl Answer: Tachycardia and cutaneous vasoconstriction?

REFERENCES

Bellamy FR, Maningas PA, Wenger BA. Current shock models and clinical correlations. *Ann Emerg Med* 1986;12:1392–1395.

Dronen SC, Bobek EMK. Fluid and blood resuscitation. In: Tintinalli JE, Kelen GD, Stapczynski JS, eds. *Emergency Medicine: A Comprehensive Study Guide,* 5th ed. McGraw-Hill, 2000.

Spaite DW, Valenzuela TC, Criss EA, Meislin HW, Hinsberg P. A prospective in-field comparison of intravenous line placement by urban and non-urban emergency medical personnel. *Ann Emerg Med* 1994;24:209–214.

41. HERNIA

I. Problem: A young man develops a bulge and pain in his groin while lifting a heavy box.

II. Immediate Questions
   A. Is the hernia incarcerated or strangulated? Has the hernia caused an intestinal obstruction? Is there a fever or tachycardia? Is the patient vomiting? Is there diffuse abdominal pain?

III. Differential Diagnosis
   A. Genitourinary
      1. Testicular torsion.
      2. Epididymitis.
      3. Testicular tumor.
      4. Hydrocele.
      5. Varicocele
      6. Undescended testis.
      7. Urinary tract infection.
      8. Prostatitis.
      9. Sexually transmitted disease.

B. Abdominal
   1. Appendicitis.
C. Pelvic
   1. Ectopic pregnancy.
   2. Tuboovarian abscess.
   3. Ovarian cysts.
D. Lymphatic
   1. Lymphadenitis
E. Vascular
   1. Femoral artery bypass graft abscess.
   2. Femoral artery bypass graft hematoma.
   3. Femoral artery pseudoaneurysm secondary to instrumentation.

IV. Database.
   A. Physical Exam Key Points
      1. **Vital Signs.** Likely abnormal with incarcerated and strangulated hernias.
      2. **Abdomen.** Check for presence of bowel sounds and tenderness to palpation. Check internal ring for presence of hernia sac.
      3. **Genitourinary.** Check for swelling and bulge in the scrotum. Check for testicular masses.
   B. Laboratory Data. CBC will likely reveal leukocytosis if hernia is strangulated. Lytes may be decreased with protracted vomiting.
   C. Radiographic and Other Studies. Acute abdominal series will show an obstructive pattern if incarcerated or strangulated. Ultrasound can identify a testicular source of scrotal swelling.

V. Plan
   A. Overall Plan. Attempts to manually reduce hernia. Strangulated hernias require immediate surgical intervention. Incarcerated hernias require admission for urgent surgical intervention. IV hydration.
   B. Specific Plan
      1. **Reduction.** If patient is in severe pain, IV analgesia and/or sedation may be required. Patient is placed in Trendelenburg's position for 20 min for possible spontaneous reduction. If this fails, manual reduction should be attempted by placing constant, gentle pressure on the hernia (*Note:* Contraindications to reduction include fever and leukocytosis).
      2. **Incarcerated and strangulated hernias.** NPO, IV fluid, NG tube, surgical consultation, preoperative antibiotics for strangulated hernias.

VI. **ICD-9 Diagnoses:** Hernia (for all, specify location, obstruction/incarceration, gangrene as applicable); Femoral hernia; Hiatal hernia; Inguinal hernia (specify unilateral or bilateral and recurrent as applicable); Umbilical hernia; Ventral hernia.

VII. **Problem Case Diagnosis:** Indirect inguinal hernia.

VIII. **Teaching Pearls Question:** What is the most common hernia?

IX. **Teaching Pearls Answer:** Indirect inguinal hernia, caused by a failure of obliteration of the processus vaginalis.

REFERENCE

Mensching JJ, Musielewicz AJ. Abdominal wall hernias. *Emerg Med Clin North Am* 1996;14(4);739–756.

42. HICCUPS

I. **Problem.** A 44-year-old woman presents with 9 days of persistent hiccups and blurry vision in her right eye.

II. **Immediate Questions**
   A. **What is the time course of the hiccups?** Longer episodes (> 48 h) may signal occult organic disease.
   B. **What other symptoms are present?** Headache? Neurologic changes? Abdominal pain? Ear or throat pain? Pulmonary symptoms? Weight loss?
   C. **Is the patient taking drugs that may causes hiccups?** Steroids? Benzodiazepines?

III. **Differential Diagnosis**
   A. **Neurologic.** MS, stroke, CNS tumors, Parkinson's disease.
   B. **HEENT.** Tympanic irritation, pharyngeal or laryngeal disease.
   C. **Intrathoracic.** Aortic aneurysm, pulmonary lesions/infection.
   D. **Diaphragmatic Irritation.** Secondary to pericarditis, tumor, peritonitis, hepatic disease, or splenic disease.
   E. **Gastroenterologic.** Esophageal lesions, gastric distention, excessive alcohol intake, hepatitis, pancreatitis, biliary disease, inflammatory bowel disease, appendicitis. May also follow abdominal surgery.
   F. **Metabolic.** Hyponatremia, uremia (often secondary to chronic renal failure), DM.
   G. **Drug-Induced.** Dexamethasone, methylprednisolone, benzodiazepines, barbiturates.
   H. **Psychogenic**
   I. **Idiopathic**

IV. **Database**
   A. **Physical Exam Key Points**
      1. **HEENT.** Check for tympanic membrane and pharyngeal lesions. Palpate the throat and assess voice quality.
      2. **Chest.** Examine for evidence of intrathoracic disease.
      3. **Abdomen.** Examine for evidence of peritonitis, organomegaly, or distention.
      4. **Neurologic.** Examine for focal neurologic deficits that might suggest stroke, MS, or tumors.

   B. Laboratory Data. Patients with a brief episode of hiccups do not require testing. Persistent hiccups (> 48 h) require evaluation. Entities in the differential diagnosis should be systematically ruled out. A basic metabolic panel will rule out uremia, DM, and hyponatremia.

   C. Imaging tests and other studies. CXR is a useful starting point. May also need to consider CT imaging of the chest and/or abdomen. MRI of the head may aid in the diagnosis of stroke, MS, and other CNS lesions.

V. Plan

   A. Overall Plan. Rule out underlying causes of hiccups while treating the symptoms.

   B. Specific Plans

     1. Treat any identified underlying illness.

     2. Try nonpharmacologic treatment first.

       a. Press firmly on soft palate with a cold spoon.

       b. Swallow granular sugar or peanut butter.

       c. Tongue traction.

       d. Drink from the far side of a cup.

     3. Pharmacologic treatment

       a. Lioresal (Baclofen), 5–10 mg PO tid PRN.

       b. Chlorpromazine (Thorazine), 25–50 mg IV followed by 25 mg PO tid PRN.

       c. Metoclopramide (Reglan), 10 mg IV followed by 10 mg PO tid PRN.

       d. Phenytoin (Dilantin), 200 mg IV, then 100 mg PO qid PRN.

     4. Consultation. Consult a neurologist and/or gastroenterologist in refractory cases.

VI. ICD-9 Diagnoses: Hiccups, NOS.

VII. Problem Case Diagnosis: MS with associated optic neuritis.

VIII. Teaching Pearl Question: What percentage of men has an organic basis for hiccups?

IX. Teaching Pearl Answer: 90% of men have an organic basis for hiccups. In women, psychogenic causes predominate.

REFERENCES

Lewis JH. Hiccups: Causes and cures. *J Clin Gastroenterol* 1985;7(6):539–552.

Ramirez FC, Graham DY. Treatment of intractable hiccup with baclofen: Results of a double blind randomized, controlled, crossover study. *Am J Gastroenterol* 1992; 87(12):1789–1791.

43. HIV PROBLEMS

   I. Problem: A 35-year-old male with HIV presents to the ED having a generalized seizure. Friend states patient has been complaining of headache intermittently over last 2 weeks. In a hurry the nurse rushes to establish an IV. Although successful, the nurse accidentally drives the contaminated needle into her hand.

II. Immediate Questions
A. ABCs.

B. Is the patient febrile?

C. Does the patient have a history of seizures?

D. Is the patient on any medications? Especially antiretroviral, antidepressants.

E. What is the last CD4 count or viral load? CD4 < 200 or viral load > 7000 copies associated with increased risk for opportunistic infections.

F. Any history of opportunistic infections?

G. Recent illness? Any diarrhea, dyspnea, chest pain, visual changes, weakness (general or focal)?

H. Any history of depression or suicidal ideation?

III. Differential Diagnosis
A. Infectious. Bacterial meningitis, toxoplasmosis, cryptococcal meningoencephalitis, CMV, herpes, TB, syphilis, HIV encephalitis, or systemic sepsis.

B. Neoplastic. Kaposi's sarcoma, lymphoma.

C. Metabolic: Electrolyte abnormalities, drug toxicity or overdose, ECVD, hypoglycemia.

D. Structural. Seizure disorder, white matter disease.

E. Cardiovascular. Dysrhythmia.

F. Respiratory. Hypoxia, community acquired pneumonia, PCP.

IV. Database
A. Physical Exam Key Points
1. **General/Vitals.** Body habitus, temporal wasting, alopecia, fever, tachycardia, low oxygen saturation.
2. **HEENT.** Pupils unequal, fundi (CMV retinitis, papilledema), hairy leukoplakia, Kaposi's sarcoma, oral thrush, aphthous ulcers.
3. **Neck.** Lymphadenopathy, nuchal rigidity.
4. **Chest.** Respiratory effort, rales, egophony, dullness to percussion.
5. **CV.** Murmurs.
6. **GI.** Hepatosplenomegaly.
7. **GU.** Active herpes, genital candidiasis, cervical lesions.
8. **Neurologic.** level of consciousness, decreased sensation or paresthesia, focal weakness (mass lesion or meningoencephalitis)
9. **Skin.** Kaposi's sarcoma, fungal infections, molluscum contagiosum, ichthyosis.

B. Laboratory Data
1. **Chemistries.** Fingerstick glucose, Lytes, BUN, CrCl, amylase, lipase, others, eg, LFTs as clinical situation dictates.
2. **CBC.** Looking for high or low WBC with immature forms, platelets, pancytopenia (**Caution:** AIDS patients may not mount appropriate WBC response to overwhelming infections). Consider CD4 count if rapidly available.

3. **ABG.** To assess oxygenation and ventilation and determine acid-base status.
4. **EKG.** To assess dysrhythmias, severe electrolyte imbalance, may be useful in certain overdoses (TCA, anticonvulsants, antifungals).
5. **Cultures.** Blood, urine, CSF (bacterial, viral, cryptococcal antigen, and fungal), sputum for Gram's stain, C&S, AFB smear and culture, serum cryptococcal antigen.
6. **Other.** Drug levels, UA, urine drug screen as appropriate (antiepileptics).

C. Radiographic and Other Studies
1. **CXR.** Diffuse patchy perihilar infiltrate with PCP pneumonia, infiltrate, effusion, cardiomegaly, pericardial effusion, pneumothorax (**Caution:** Active TB may have any appearance on CXR in AIDS).
2. **CT.** All focal neurologic deficits, new mental status, seizures.
3. **MRI.** Definitive for toxoplasmosis, white matter degeneration.

V. Plan
A. Overall Plan
1. **ABC issues.** Control airway with rapid sequence intubation as needed for hypoxia, hypoventilation, depressed mental status, status epilepticus, obtain secure IV access. (See Section VIII, 15. Rapid Endotracheal Intubation, p 470.)
2. **Address easily treatable conditions.** Consider glucose, thiamine, naloxone.
3. **Stop seizure.** IV benzodiazepines, fosphenytoin/phenytoin, barbiturate, paralysis.
4. **Look for causes.** Systemic approach to complications/opportunistic infections.
5. **Prompt antibiotics/antifungals as indicated.** (**Caution:** With seizure, cover for viral (acyclovir) and fungal (amphotericin B) causes empirically in addition to bacterial (3rd-generation cephalosporin).
6. **Consultation/disposition.** Internal medicine, infectious diseases, neurology consult and admission to monitored bed.

B. Specific Plans
1. **CNS infections.** Toxoplasmosis: pyrimethamine, sulfadiazine. Cryptococcus: fluconazole, amphotericin B. Bacterial: 3rd-generation cephalosporin. Viral: herpes (acyclovir)
2. **Ocular.** CMV (ganciclovir).
3. **Oral/Esophageal.** Candidiasis (fluconazole); herpes (acyclovir)
4. **Pulmonary.** Pneumocystis: SMX/TMP preferred, pentamidine, dapsone. CAP: varies by disposition and organism. TB: four drug therapy.
5. **Cardiovascular.** Treat specific dysrhythmias, sodium bicarbonate for TCA OD.
6. **Metabolic.** Treat electrolyte abnormalities, check toxicology screen and drug levels.
7. **GI.** Diarrhea treatment specific to agent. (**Caution:** Beware of possibility of *Clostridium difficile* in patients on chronic suppres-

sive antibiotics.) Treat pancreatitis with NPO and discontinuing precipitating medication. (**Caution:** Antiretrovirals are notorious causes of pancreatitis.)
8. **Psychiatric.** Evaluate for suicidal ideation or drug ingestion.
9. **Healthcare worker exposure**/prophylaxis issues (also see Section III. 12. Needlestick, page 287)
   a. **Needlestick**
      i. Hollow or solid needle? Contaminated or clean?
      ii. Scalpel or sharp instrument? Contaminated or clean?
      iii. Was there blood on the needle?
      iv. Was the healthcare worker wearing gloves?
      v. Was the wound immediately recognized cleaned?
   b. **Risk stratify the exposure**
      i. Blood/body fluid on intact skin or mucus membrane is a lower risk, low inoculum exposure.
      ii. Solid needle or scratch is moderate inoculum: lower risk HIV, high risk hepatitis B & C.
      iii. Percutaneous injuries with hollow needles or lacerations with contaminated blades/instruments are large inoculum exposures.
      iv. Determine the HIV, HBV, HCV status of the source and healthcare worker (No effective prophylaxis against hepatitis C).
      v. Administer HBIG and begin Heptavax if healthcare worker has not been vaccinated for hepatitis B.
   c. **Postexposure prophylaxis regimen for HIV.** Start ASAP (most effective when started within 24–36 h after exposure) and continue 4 weeks.
      i. ZDV 600 mg/d.
      ii. Lamivudine 150 mg bid.
      iii. Combivir includes both of these meds in same pill and can be taken twice daily as an alternative.
      iv. Use for unknown, low to moderate exposures, with known low HIV viral titers in the source patient (< 1500 copies).
      v. Draw baseline CBC and LFTs.
   d. **Extended postexposure prophylaxis regimen.** (Use with high risk, large inoculum exposures)
      i. Indinavir 800 mg orally tid or
      ii. Nelfinavir 750 mg tid
      iii. Need to be tested for HIV at time of exposure, 6 weeks, 12 weeks, 6 months.
C. **Side Effects of Antiretrovirals**
   1. **Nucleoside reverse transcriptase inhibitors (NRTIs).** Peripheral neuropathy, hepatic steatosis, lactic acidosis, pancreatitis, marrow suppression.
   2. **Nonnucleoside reverse transcriptase inhibitors (NNRTI).** Self-limited maculopapular rash, rarely Stevens-Johnson syndrome, pancreatitis.

3. **Protease inhibitors.** Fat redistribution, lose fat in arms leg and face, fat is deposited in abdomen, base of neck, and mesentery "protease paunch." Easy bleeding, nephrolithiasis are also frequent.
4. Drug interactions are frequent sometimes serious and can effect metabolism, drug absorption, elimination.
5. Side effect symptoms vary and commonly include nausea, vomiting, headache, and fatigue.

VI. ICD-9 Diagnoses: Probable or possible HIV will not be coded; HIV disease (if HIV-related illness); HIV infection (a V code for asymptomatic infection); Cryptococcosis; Cryptosporidiosis; Kaposi's sarcoma; Oral candidiasis; *Pneumocystis carinii* pneumonia; Toxoplasmosis.

VII. Problem Case Diagnosis: Toxoplasmosis infection of the brain. Nurse was placed on high-risk prophylaxis regimen and remained HIV-, HepB-, and HepC-negative at 1-year after exposure.

VIII. Teaching Pearl Question: At what viral load or CD4 count does a patient become at high risk for opportunistic infections?

IX. Teaching Pearl Answer: CD4 count of 200/µL, viral load of ≤ 7000 copies/mL (4).

REFERENCES

Centers for Disease Control. Updated US Public Health Service guidelines for the management of occupational exposures to HBV, HCV, and HIV and recommendations for post-exposure prophylaxis. *MMWR* 2001;50(RR11):1–42. Recommendations for Postexposure Prophylaxis" *MMWR.* Vol 47: May 15, 1998.

Kaplan JE, Hanson DL, Jones JL, Dworkin MS. Viral load as an independent risk factor for opportunistic infections in HIV-infected adults and adolescents. *AIDS* 2001;15: 1831–1836.

Pascual-Sedano B, Iranzo A, Marti-Fabregas J, Domingo P, Escartin A, Fuster M, et al. Prospective study of new-onset seizures in patients with human immunodeficiency virus infection: Etiologic and clinical aspects. *Arch Neurol* 1999;56:609–612.

Piscitelli SC, Gallicano KD. Drug therapy: Interactions among drugs for HIV and opportunistic infections. *N Engl J Med.* 2001;344:984–996.

44. HOSTILE PATIENT

I. **Problem.** A 28 year-old male in the ED for vomiting and diarrhea leaves his room 5 min after arrival and starts yells at nursing and physician staff about the long wait. He is belligerent and aggressive.

II. **Immediate Questions**
   A. **Does the patient pose an immediate threat to yourself, the staff, or other patients?** Does he have a weapon? Does he appear to be truly threatening?
   B. **Is the patient stable?** Airway intact? Manage appropriately. (see Section VIII, 15. Rapid Endotracheal Intubation, p 470.)

    C. What are the vital signs and mental status? Is he acting inappropriately due to hypoxemia? (Check pulse oximetry.) Is the patient confused due to head injury or neurologic problem? (Neurologic examination.)

    D. What was the patient's mental status upon arrival in the emergency department? Was he agitated, confused, belligerent?

    E. Is there a serious medical problem causing a change in behavior? Does he have a history of thyroid disorder, seizures, or other neurologic disease?

    F. Is there a history of psychiatric disorder? Is there a history of drug or alcohol abuse? Is he withdrawing from sedative-hypnotics or alcohol?

III. Differential Diagnosis

    A. Situational. (Most common) Is the patient in pain? Has he/she waited long? Is the patient concerned about others who may be ill or injured? Was there miscommunication? Is there a gap between expectations and reality?

    B. Psychiatric Disorders. (Very common) Underlying/comorbid state.
        1. Schizophrenia. Particularly with paranoid type.
        2. Personality disorders. Borderline and antisocial.

    C. Neurologic
        1. Seizures. Postictal confusional state, temporal lobe epilepsy.
        2. CNS Infections. Encephalitis, meningitis.
        3. Organic. Delirium, dementia.
        4. Other. CNS malignancies, ICH, malignant hypertension.

    D. Respiratory. Hypoxemia from any cause.

    E. Trauma. CNS trauma or hypoxia or hypotension due to systemic trauma.

    F. Endocrine Disorders. Hyperthyroidism, hypoglycemia, steroid-induced psychosis.

    G. Electrolyte Disturbances. Hypocalcemia, hypercalcemia, hyperkalemia.

    H. Environmental. Hyperthermia, hypothermia.

    I. Substance abuse
        1. Intoxication: Phencyclidine, cocaine, amphetamines, aromatic hydrocarbons, alcohol, LSD.
        2. Withdrawal. Alcohol, sedative-hypnotics, narcotics.
        3. Unanticipated reaction to prescribed or OTC medications. More common in the elderly or patients with brain injury or organic brain syndromes.

IV. Database

    A. Physical Exam Key Points
        1. Mental status. (See Table A-4. Mini-Mental Status Exam.)
        2. General examination. Body posture. Are the hands clenched? Does he have a threatening stance? Is he staring you down?

3. **Vital signs.** Look for hypotension, tachycardia or bradycardia, tachypnea or bradypnea. Is the patient cold or hot? Repeat VS often.
4. **HEENT.** Look for signs of trauma. Look for nystagmus, pupillary abnormalities consistent with drug abuse or withdrawal.
5. **Cardiovascular.** Tachycardia or bradycardia.
6. **Respiratory.** Evidence or hyperventilation, cyanosis.
7. **Neurologic examination.** Pupil reactivity, fundi for evidence of papilledema or hemorrhage, focal neurologic deficits and confusion.
8. **Psychiatric disorder.** Is there a thought disorder? Rational or irrational reasons for being upset?

B. **Laboratory Data.** If physical examination and history do not point to a particular cause, check blood sugar and pulse oximetry at a minimum.

C. **Radiographic and Other Studies.** Check specific labs and radiologic studies based on history and physical examination.
1. CT of head if suspected head injury or CNS mass/bleed.
2. Thyroid function tests, drug screens, Lytes as indicated.
3. ECG for heart rate/rhythm abnormalities.
4. Lumbar puncture if CNS infection or occult bleeding suspected.
5. **Key point: Check old medical records for clues to current episode!**

V. **Plan**

A. **Overall Plan**
1. **Defuse the situation.** Treat the underlying illness. Avoid escalation from hostility to violence. If unreasonable or a threat, restrain patient by show of force, chemically or physically to maintain a safe environment for the patient, other patients, and staff. Ensure that trained security personnel are available to restrain patient and search for/remove weapons.

B. **Specific Plans**
1. **Situational.** Reason with patient. Attend to reasonable needs. Treat pain, feed patient, evaluate patient who is angry due to wait. Remove patient from situation and people exacerbating hostility.
2. **Hypoxemia.** Start O_2 therapy, determine cause of hypoxia (PE, pneumonia) and treat appropriately.
3. **Hypoglycemia and other endocrine/electrolyte abnormalities.** Diagnose and treat appropriately.
4. **Substance abuse**
   a. Treat alcohol withdrawal with benzodiazepines and admit.
   b. Treat amphetamine/cocaine intoxication with benzodiazepines and observe/admit if symptoms persist.
   c. **Narcotic withdrawal.** Treat patient symptomatically for nausea and vomiting. Hydrate patient. Small doses of narcotics may alleviate symptoms and hostility.

5. **CNS Trauma/diseases.** Diagnose and treat appropriately.
6. **Psychiatric disorders.** Treat psychotic symptoms with neuro-leptics (haloperidol, droperidol). Addition of antihistamines (diphen-hydramine, benztropine) may help by sedating patient and pre-venting dystonia.

VI. **ICD-9 Diagnoses:** Acute delirium; Electrolyte imbalance; Hypoxia; Intox-ication (state substance); Acute drug-induced psychosis; Meningitis; Schizophrenia.

VII. **Problem Case Diagnosis:** Narcotic withdrawal. A weapon was removed from patient.

VIII. **Teaching Pearl Question:** What percent of major trauma patients seen in an inner city ED are found to be carrying weapons?

IX. **Teaching Pearl Answer:** 26.7% in one study. (Ordog).

REFERENCES

Lavoie FW. Violence in emergency facilities. *Acad Emerg Med* 1994;1(2):166–168.
Ordog JG, Wasserberger J, Ordog C, Ackroyd G, Atluri S. Weapon carriage among major trauma victims in the emergency department. *Acad Emerg Med* 1995;2:109–114.
Oster A, Bernbaum S, Patten S. Determinants of violence in the psychiatric emergency service. *CMAJ* 2001;164(1):32–33.

45. HYPERTENSION

I. **Problem.** A 48-year-old female presents to the ED confused and com-bative with a BP of 225/130.

II. **Immediate Questions**
A. **Is the airway intact?**
B. **What are the vitals and the mental status?** Apply cardiac monitor, pulse ox, IV, and oxygen. Check BP discrepancy between all ex-tremities to evaluate possibility of aortic dissection. Perform a quick neurologic exam.
C. **Are there signs of end-organ damage?** Chest pain may reveal signs of acute MI or unstable angina; mental status changes may re-veal signs of encephalopathy or intracranial hemorrhage; poor oxy-genation may indicate acute pulmonary edema secondary to LV fail-ure; peripheral edema may indicate renal insufficiency; abdominal pain/back pain may indicate aortic dissection/aneurysm or possible HELLP syndrome if pregnant.
D. **Is the patient pregnant?** Preeclampsia.
E. **Is the patient taking MAO inhibitors?** Tyramine interactions lead-ing to catecholamine excess and hypertensive crisis may occur if pa-tient eats chocolate, beer, wine, cheese, citrus, coffee, snails, broad beans, chicken liver, or pickled herring.

    F. Paroxysms of hypertension? Also associated with palpitations, sweating, tachycardia, and apprehension? History of von Recklinghausen's disease? Consider pheochromocytoma.

    G. History of cocaine/amphetamine/PCP use?

    H. Past medical history? Medications? Long-standing HTN (controlled or uncontrolled)? History of alpha$_2$-agonist use? (When discontinued suddenly can cause rebound hypertension). Cardiac history? History of depression? On dialysis or history of renal impairment? Drugs such as the oral contraceptive pill, NSAIDS, and OTC decongestants can decrease the efficacy of antihypertensive medication.

III. Differential Diagnosis

    A. Hypertensive Emergency. Defined as elevated blood pressure with evidence of end-organ damage.

        1. This is a *clinical* diagnosis based on evidence of target organ damage to the heart, kidneys, or brain; there are no numeric criteria.

        2. Affects less than 1% of hypertensive patients.

        3. Treatment aimed at reducing BP by 25% over first 2 h then gradually toward 160/100 over 2–6 h, avoiding excessive falls in pressure that may lead to renal, cerebral, or coronary ischemia.

    B. Hypertensive Urgency. Defined as elevated blood pressure with a diastolic greater that 110 mm Hg and/or systolic greater than 180 mm Hg *without* signs of end-organ damage.

        1. May be associated with headache and/or optic disc edema but without mental status changes.

        2. Treatment aimed at reducing blood pressure gradually over 24–48 h.

    C. Mild Hypertension. Defined as a diastolic pressure between 90–110 mm Hg.

        1. May be related to anxiety, pain, or urinary retention.

        2. Treatment usually initiated in outpatient setting.

IV. Database

    A. Physical Exam Key Points. Look for signs of end-organ damage.

        1. Mental status. Perform mini mental status exam (See Table A-4, page 656).

        2. Vital signs. Should be repeated at least every 15 min. Blood pressure discrepancy between extremities may indicate aortic dissection.

        3. Cardiovascular. Check for diastolic murmur. (aortic regurgitation in aortic dissection). S_3 or S_4 (MI, CHF). Check for JVD (LV failure).

        4. Pulmonary. Rales may indicate pulmonary edema.

        5. Abdomen. Check for pregnancy and pulsatile masses (AAA).

        6. Neurologic exam. Fundi for edema, focal deficit may indicate ICH. Clonus and hyperreflexia in pregnant women.

    B. Laboratory Data. UA, Lytes, BUN, creatinine, and ECG. Consider cardiac enzymes, CBC, LFTs, and uric acid based on clinical picture.

   C. Radiographic and Other Studies. Consider CXR, head/chest CT
   based on clinical picture.

V. Plan
   A. Overall Plan
      1. **Hypertensive emergencies.** Should be admitted to ICU for mon-
         itoring and parenteral treatment. Treat possible MI, ICH, pulmonary
         edema, and/or eclampsia appropriately.
      2. **Hypertensive urgencies.** Should be discharged with close fol-
         low-up within 24–48 h. Consider initiating treatment in ED.
      3. **Mild hypertension.** Treat underlying pain/anxiety/urinary reten-
         tion. Follow-up with primary care physician 1–2 weeks for blood
         pressure recheck.
   B. Specific Plans
      1. **Hypertensive emergency**
         a. Vasodilators
            i. **Sodium nitroprusside.** (0.25–10 µg/kg/min IV) Can be
               used with most hypertensive emergencies but caution
               with high ICP or azotemia. Watch for cyanide toxicity.
            ii. **Nitroglycerin.** (5–100 µg/min IV). Use with coronary
               ischemia.
            iii. **Nicardipine.** (5–15 mg/h IV). Caution if underlying heart
               failure or coronary ischemia. May use for eclampsia.
            iv. **Fenoldopam.** (0.1–1.6 µg/kg/min IV). Caution if under-
               lying glaucoma.
            v. **Hydralazine.** (10–20 mg IV). Use with eclampsia. Cau-
               tion as precipitous drop in BP may occur, lasting as long
               as 12 h.
         b. Adrenergic inhibitors
            i. **Labetalol.** (20–80 mg IV bolus every 10 min or 0.5–2
               mg/min IV infusion. Max dose 300 mg/24 h.). Can be
               used with most hypertensive emergencies including
               eclampsia except with heart failure.
            ii. **Esmolol.** (250–500 µg/kg/min for 1 min then increase
               by 50–100 µg/kg/min). Use for aortic dissection.
            iii. **Phentolamine.** (5–15 mg IV up to a max dose of 15 mg).
               Use for catecholamine excess.
      2. **Hypertensive urgency**
         a. Sublingual *fast-acting* nifedipine. Avoid use as the inability
            to control the rate and degree of fall of the BP has been asso-
            ciated with coronary and cerebral ischemia.
         **b. Consider α_2-agonists, loop diuretics, ACE inhibitors or
            calcium channel blockers.**

VI. ICD-9 Diagnoses: Elevated blood pressure; Hypertension (specify benign,
malignant where applicable); Hypertension—controlled or uncontrolled;
Secondary hypertension; Transient hypertension.

VII. Problem Case Diagnosis: Intracerebral hemorrhage.

VIII. Teaching Pearl Question: What percent of patients have elevated BP in the ED but normal BP when measured at home? (A.K.A. "white coat hypertension")

 IX. Teaching Pearl Answer: About 15%. (Calvert).

REFERENCES

Elliott WJ. Hypertensive emergencies. *Crit Care Clin* 2001;17(2):435–451.
Sixth Report of the Joint National Committee on the Prevention, Detection, Evaluation, and Treatment of High Blood Pressure. *Arch Inter Med* 1997;157:2413–2446.
Varon J, PE Marik. The diagnosis and management of hypertensive crises. *Chest* 2000;118(1):214–217.

46. HYPERTHERMIA

 I. Problem. An elderly "frequent flyer" to the ED presents obtunded after EMS found him alone in his Midwestern US apartment on an afternoon in mid-July.

 II. Immediate Questions
   A. Are the ABCs intact?
   B. What are the vital signs and mental status? Does the patient feel hot? Diaphoresis? The presence of confusion/lethargy/coma, fever, tachycardia, hypotension should direct further search for causes.
   C. What is the temperature? Temperature is critical in defining as well as risk stratification. Heat exhaustion often demonstrates a normal temperature and if elevated often below < 40°C. Heat stroke usually > 40.5°C
   D. When did others last see the patient? How was he behaving? How was patient found? Were there any findings at the scene that could offer clues to presentation? Seizure activity, medication bottles, apartment temperature.
   E. Past medical history? Past episodes, history of depression, suicide attempts? Medications or drugs such as TCAs, antihistamines, antipsychotics, methamphetamine, or cocaine. Diseases such as scleroderma, CF, hyperthyroidism.

 III. Differential Diagnosis
   A. Febrile Illness. (See Problem 32. Fever and remember infectious problems may accompany noninfectious febrile conditions)
   B. Environmental Hyperthermia
     1. Minor heat illness. Heat cramps in large muscle groups. First few days of strenuous work in hot climates. Salt deficiency plays a role. Highest risk is to athletes, roofers, field workers, steel workers, coal miners, and boiler room operators.

2. **Heat syncope.** Syncope related to physiologic adaptations to hot, humid climates. Peripheral vasodilation depletes thoracic intravascular volume. Cardiac output drops, w/decreased cerebral perfusion. Elderly, people standing for long periods of time most at risk.

3. **Heat exhaustion.** Formerly called heat prostration. Two subtypes. Water depletion and salt depletion. Both types have nonspecific symptoms including generalized weakness, headaches, nausea and vomiting, impaired judgment ability. Core temp. usually < 40°C. Water depletion affects those working in heat w/o adequate fluid replacement. Sweating losses exceed intake. Most at risk are military, laborers, athletes, nursing home patients. Salt depletion occurs w/copious sweating, replacement w/water, but insufficient salt. Workers drinking only water.

4. **Heat stroke.** Life-threatening. On a continuum with heat exhaustion. Failure of central thermoregulatory mechanisms. Temps > 40.5°C. Leads to multisystem organ dysfunction and failure. Neurologic changes (often with cerebral edema). Divided into two forms:

   a. **Classic heat stroke.** Protracted elevation in environmental temp. High humidity. Body's ability to rid heat is impeded. Usually affects poor, debilitated, and elderly. Often no sweating. Affects those with illnesses predisposing to heat-related illness (alcoholism, schizophrenia).

   b. **Exertional heat stroke.** Acute exposure to elevated temp AND high levels of physical activity. Usually affects young athletes and military recruits. Body's ability to decrease heat load is overwhelmed.

C. **Medication-Related Hyperthermia**

1. **Neuroleptic malignant syndrome.** Caused by use of antipsychotic medications. Develops with administration of neuroleptic drugs and/or withdrawal of dopaminergic agents. Triad of symptoms is hyperthermia, encephalopathy, and skeletal muscle rigidity.

2. **Serotonin syndrome.** Characterized by autonomic and neuromuscular manifestations. Mental status changes often seen. Thought related to hyperstimulation of 5-HT1$_A$ receptors in brain and spinal cord. Symptoms generally require two or more implicated medications to be taken simultaneously, (eg, SSRI + MAOI). Frequently noted with change of medication or dosing.

3. **Malignant hyperthermia.** Very rare. Associated with disturbance of Ca^{2+} regulation in striated muscle. Severe muscle rigidity, hyperthermia, and recent anesthetic use. Reported with exposure to general anesthetics, and depolarizing muscle relaxants. Rarely seen in outpatient setting. Usually associated with anesthesia.

IV. Database

A. Physical Exam Key Points.
Always consider febrile illness, as well as hyperthermia.

1. **ABCs**
2. **Mental status**
3. **Vital signs.** Is temp < or > 40.5°C? Use indwelling thermometer if possible. Is patient hypotensive, tachycardic?
4. **HEENT.** Diaphoresis, temperature, skin turgor, pupil size and response (miosis in majority with heat stroke mydriatic with anticholinergics), scleral icterus, pale conjunctivae, dry mucus membranes.
5. **Neck.** Thyroid palpable? Large or nodular?
6. **Cardiovascular.** Tachycardia? Check peripheral pulses.
7. **Lungs.** Observe rate and depth for hints regarding acid-base status.
8. **Abdominal.** Nausea, vomiting may indicate splanchnic vasoconstriction and/or irritation.
9. **Genitourinary.** Once urinary catheter is placed, watch for adequacy of urine output.
10. **Musculoskeletal.** Observe for tetany, rigidity
11. **Neurologic.** Mental status, behavior, hallucinations, posturing (usually decerebrate), cerebellar dysfunction, opisthotonos. Patient may exhibit coarse tremors, dystonic movements, seizures.

B. Laboratory Data.
CBC, Lytes, BUN, creatinine. UA (casts, myoglobinuria, possibly WBCs or bacteria). If heat stroke is a consideration, LFTs and PT/PTT/DIC panels give indication of hepatic involvement, and potential coagulopathy. Consider TSH if febrile/tachycardic, or known history. Obtain levels for any agents that may precipitate hyperthermia (aspirin, drugs of abuse panel).

C. Radiographic and Other Studies.
CT for persistent altered mental status or evidence of head trauma. EKG for those with cardiac risk /elderly/ingestions. CXR if considering aspiration pneumonia/ARDS. Later, EEGs may reveal diffuse flattening but delayed recovery still possible.

V. Plan

A. Overall Plan.
Temperature > 40°C? If so, begin immediate interventions to rapidly cool. Attempt to identify circumstances, illnesses, or toxins that may play causative role. Direct treatment accordingly.

B. Specific Plans

1. **Rapid cooling.** Remove patient from any obvious heat sources (sunlight, confined space, etc), disrobe, monitor temp w/rectal or bladder probe. Evaporative cooling (most effective practical plan) by spraying patient with mist of water while fanned. Conductive cooling (cold-water immersion) can rapidly reduce temp to 37–38°C in 10–40 min. May also use ice packs applied to neck,

axilla, groin (areas where large vessels are superficially located). Other techniques include peritoneal, rectal, and gastric lavage with cold fluids, as well as cardiopulmonary bypass. Almost never needed if aggressive evaporative cooling pursued.

2. **Avoid hypothermic overshoot.** Constantly monitor core temp. When temp reaches 39°C, remove cooling measures to avoid continuous drop of core temp.

3. **Provide additional support.** Rehydration with 0.9% NS 0.5–1 L. Consider glucose, thiamine, naloxone in any patient who is altered. Address other issues (seizures, vomiting) as they arise in conventional fashion.

VI. **ICD-9 Diagnoses:** Fever; Heat cramps; Heat exhaustion; Heat Edema; Heat syncope; Heat stroke; Hyperthermia/pyrexia; Malignant hyperthermia; Hyperthermia; Salicylism.

VII. **Problem Case Diagnosis:** Heat stroke.

VIII. **Teaching Pearl Question:** What is the ancient Greek name for heat stroke?

IX. **Teaching Pearl Answer:** Siriasis, named after the dog star Sirius, which accompanied the midsummer sun.

REFERENCES

Carbone JR. The neuroleptic malignant and serotonin syndromes. *Emerg Med Clin North Am* 2001;18(2):317–325.

Vassallo S, Delaney K. Thermoregulatory principles. In : *Goldfrank's Toxicologic Emergencies,* 7th ed. Appleton and Lange, 2002:261–281.

Yarbrough B, Vicario S. Heat illness. In Marx J: *Rosen's Emergency Medicine Concepts and Clinical Practice,* 5th ed. Mosby, 2001:1997–2009.

47. HYPOTENSION

I. **Problem:** Medics bring in a 67-year-old man with weak pulses and diaphoresis after being found by his wife on their bathroom floor.

II. **Immediate Questions**
   A. What are his vital signs, pulse oximetry, capillary blood sugar, and Glasgow Coma Scale score?
   B. Does he have a heart murmur, abnormal breath sounds, pulsatile abdominal mass, trauma, bloody stool, or insect bite?
   C. Does he use cardiac, diabetic, or corticosteroid drugs?
   D. What does his ECG show?

III. **Differential Diagnosis: "SHOCKE"**
   A. **Spinal (neurogenic).** Spinal cord injury, hypothalamus/brainstem trauma, anesthesia.

    B. Hypovolemic. Trauma, GI bleed, ruptured AAA, ruptured ectopic pregnancy, surgery, etc. *Nonhemorrhagic:* Burns, diarrhea, vomiting, diuretics, diabetes insipidus, DKA, nonketotic hyperglycemic hyperosmolar coma, severe diaphoresis, poor oral intake, exfoliative dermatitis, etc.

    C. Obstructive. Tension pneumothorax, cardiac tamponade, massive PE, inferior vena cava occlusion.

    D. Cardiogenic. MI, valvular heart disease, CHF, asystole, dysrhythmias, cardiac contusion, drug toxicity.

    E. Kinetic (vasogenic or distributive). Anaphylaxis, sepsis, toxic shock syndrome, pit viper envenomation, vasodilator drug toxicity.

    F. Endocrine. Adrenocortical insufficiency/crisis, myxedema coma, pheochromocytoma.

IV. Database

  A. Physical Exam Key Points

    1. **Cardiovascular.** Hypotension, tachycardia (may have bradycardia in spinal shock or if taking β-blockers), hypoxia, weak pulses, and/or prolonged capillary refill. New or different murmur in cardiogenic shock due to valvular heart disease.

    2. **HEENT.** Dry mucous membranes in hypovolemic shock.

    3. **Neck.** JVD in cardiogenic and obstructive shock.

    4. **Skin.** Cyanosis, diaphoresis, pallor, and/or cold (warm in spinal/kinetic shock).

    5. **CNS.** Confused, disoriented, agitated, obtunded, and/or comatose.

    6. **Abdomen/pelvic.** Distension, tenderness, pulsatile masses, obvious bleeding.

    7. **Renal.** Oliguria or anuria.

  B. Laboratory Data. CBC, Lytes, glucose, BUN, creatinine, LFTs, PT/PTT, HCG, ABG, T&C, cardiac enzymes, and/or blood culture.

  C. Radiographic and Other Studies. CXR and ECG are essential. Echocardiogram, chest/abdominal CT, and/or abdominal US may be needed depending on case. Continuous cardiopulmonary monitor, pulse oximeter, arterial line, Foley catheter, and/or Swan-Ganz catheter.

V. Plan

  A. Overall Plan. At least two large bore IVs, IV fluid (NS or LR), 100% O_2, and Trendelenburg's position.

  B. Specific Plans

    1. **Spinal.** Neurosurgery, pressors (phenylephrine), and/or steroids.

    2. **Hemorrhagic.** Blood products, surgery, and/or MAST.

    3. **Obstructive.** Chest tube, pericardiocentesis, pressors, and/or thrombolytic.

    4. **Cardiogenic.** ACLS, pressors (dopamine), thrombolytic, valve surgery, and/or intraaortic balloon pump.

VI. ICD-9 Diagnoses: Chronic hypotension; Hypotension; Orthostatic hypotension; Transient hypotension.

VII. **Problem Case Diagnosis:** Ruptured AAA.

VIII. **Teaching Pearl Question:** How low does the systolic blood pressure have to be before the term *shock* is applicable?

IX. **Teaching Pearl Answer:** The definition of shock is generalized inadequate tissue perfusion. Blood pressure and/or heart rate are not included in the definition of shock.

REFERENCE

Rivers EP, Rady MY, Bilkovski R. Approach to the patient in shock. In Tintinalli: *Emergency Medicine: A Comprehensive Study Guide.* McGraw-Hill, 2000:215–222.

48. HYPOTHERMIA

I. **Problem.** A middle-aged male is found lying on the street with no evidence of trauma (ambient temperature = 45°F or 7°C).

II. **Immediate Questions**
   A. **Is the patient responsive? If yes, is the patient shivering?** If yes, is core temperature > 32°C?
   B. **What are the vital signs?** Apply monitors (ECG and pulse ox). Ventilate with oxygen, start IV. If unable to obtain VS, assess breathing and pulse for 30–45 s to confirm respiratory and pulseless cardiac arrest. (See specific plan for hypothermic cardiac arrest and Problem 13. Cardiac Arrest, page 41).
   C. **What is the core temperature?** Measure esophageal or rectal temperature.
   D. **What was the exposure?** Duration? Environmental conditions?
   E. **Any past medical history?** Predisposing conditions may contribute to hypothermia through decreased heat production (endocrine disorders, malnutrition, immobility), increased heat loss (vasodilation from ethanol, burns, sepsis), or impaired thermoregulation (CNS trauma, CVA, infection, drugs).
   F. **Are there other reasons for altered mental status?** (See Problem 3. Altered Mental Status, page 11). Check glucose, consider naloxone.

III. **Differential Diagnosis:** May be confused with any condition causing altered mental status. (See Problem 3. Altered Mental Status, page 11). Must rule out predisposing pathology to distinguish between primary and secondary hypothermia.
   A. **Drugs.** Consider alcohol, sedatives, phenothiazines.
   B. **Endocrine.** Consider hypoglycemia (may be precipitated by shivering and exhaustion), myxedema, adrenal crisis.
   C. **Metabolic.** Consider hepatic failure, uremia.
   D. **Trauma/Structural Lesions.** Consider intracranial hematoma or hemorrhage, CVA.
   E. **Infection.** Consider meningitis, encephalopathy.

IV. **Database**
   A. **Physical Exam Key Points**
      1. **Mental status.** Assess for apathy, confusion, slurred speech.
      2. **Vital signs.** Heart rate and blood pressure gradually decrease with lower temperature. Respiration is initially stimulated, then decreases progressively.
      3. **Heart rhythm.** May be in atrial fibrillation or other arrhythmia below 30°C.
      4. **Lungs.** Assess for wheezes, rhonchi.
      5. **Neurologic.** Dilated pupils. Hyperreflexia, then hyporeflexia with decreasing temperature.
   B. **Laboratory Data.** Bedside glucose (hypoglycemia may be precipitated by shivering and exhaustion), ABG, CBC (Hct should be high due to decreased plasma volume), Lytes (hyperkalemia), coagulation panel (PT, PTT may be normal despite clinical coagulopathy. Leukopenia, thrombocytopenia, and coagulopathy generally reverse with rewarming). Consider cardiac enzymes, blood cultures, thyroid and cortisol tests, tox screen, as indicated.
   C. **Radiographic and Other Studies.** CXR, ECG (look for Osborne "J" waves, sinus bradycardia or junctional bradycardia, AF, sinus tachycardia, prolonged QTC intervals).

V. **Plan**
   A. **Overall Plan.** Handle patient gently, but do not withhold interventions such as intubation or central line placement if indicated (associated with development of VF in few case reports, but not in several larger studies). Prevent further heat loss by removing wet clothing and insulating the victim from the environment. Monitor cardiac rhythm, oxygen saturation, and core temperature. Most patients will require volume expansion with warmed intravenous fluids (NS) as vasodilation occurs with rewarming. Monitor for hyperkalemia during rewarming.
   B. **Specific Plans**
      1. **Mild hypothermia** (core temp > 34°). Passive (exogenous external) rewarming with warm blankets, warm room, heat packs to truncal areas—provide same rate of warming as shivering.
      2. **Moderate hypothermia** (30° < T < 34°). Exogenous external rewarming as already described. Forced air rewarming. Warm IV fluids (43°C) and warm humidified oxygen (42°–46°C).
      3. **Severe hypothermia** (T < 30°C). Active internal rewarming (extracorporeal blood rewarming, peritoneal lavage, pleural lavage, esophageal rewarming tube).
      4. **Hypothermic cardiac arrest** (See Problem 13. Cardiac Arrest, page 41).
         a. **Start CPR.** The hypothermic heart may be unresponsive to defibrillation and medications.
         b. **Defibrillate VF/pulseless VT** up to a maximum of three shocks (200 J, 300J, 360 J) if temperature less than 30°C. Repeat defibrillation as core temperature rises.

    c. **Intubate.** Ventilate with warm, humidified oxygen (42–46°C).
    d. **Establish IV.** Infuse NS (43°C).
    e. **Hold IV medications** until T > 30°C, then increase dosing intervals.
    f. **Initiate active internal rewarming** (extracorporeal rewarming is preferred).

VI. **ICD-9 Diagnoses:** Chillblains; Frostbite (specify location); Hypothermia; Hypothermia not associated with low environmental temperature; Trench foot.

VII. **Problem Case Diagnosis:** Alcohol intoxication with secondary hypothermia.

VIII. **Teaching Pearl Question:** What is the lowest reported temperature in a survivor of accidental hypothermia?

IX. **Teaching Pearl Answer:** 13.7°C (Gilbert).

REFERENCES

Giesbrecht G. Cold stress, near drowning and accidental hypothermia: A review. *Aviat Space Environ Med* 2000;71:733–752.

Gilbert M, Busund R, Skagseth A, Nilsen P, Solbo J. Resuscitation from accidental hypothermia of 13.7°C with circulatory arrest. *Lancet* 2000;355:375–376.

Graham CA, McNaughton GW, Wyatt JP. The electrocardiogram in hypothermia. *Wilderness Environ Med* 2001;12:232–235.

49. INDWELLING CATHETER PROBLEMS

I. **Problem:** A 43-year-old female hemodialysis patient complains of a painful swollen left arm.

II. **Immediate Questions**
    A. **Are the vital signs (including temperature) stable?** Fever, tachycardia, hypotension may indicate sepsis. Place on monitor. Start IV. Administer fluid bolus if hypotensive.
    B. **What is the neurovascular status of the extremity?** Diminished or absent pulses? Delayed capillary refill? Pallor? Cyanosis? Cold?
    C. **What type of device is in place?** Catheter with external port (Hickman, Broviac, Groshong, PICC). SQ infusion port (Infusaport, Mediport). Subcutaneous A-V fistula (dialysis access).
    D. **What is given through the device?** Dialysis, antibiotics, TPN, chemotherapy).

III. **Differential Diagnosis**
    A. **Infection**
        1. **Local.** Exit site infection. Symptoms at site only.
        2. **Regional.** Tunnel/port pocket infection. Symptoms along SQ course of catheter.
        3. **Systemic.** Systemic symptoms. May have no localizing signs.

    B. Occlusion
1. **Complete.** Clot in lumen. Precipitate in lumen. Mechanical obstruction.
2. **Withdrawal** (can infuse; cannot aspirate). Catheter against vessel wall. Fibrin sheath at tip. Ball valve/mural thrombus. Subclavian vein thrombosis.
3. **Intermittent complete/withdrawal occlusion.** Pinch-off syndrome (between clavicle and first rib).

    C. Hemorrhage. Around catheter site or thorough last puncture site.
    D. Extravasation/Leakage. SQ or external.
    E. Dislodgement. Accidental displacement from vessel.
    F. Catheter Embolus. Broken piece of catheter embolizes.

IV. Database
  A. Physical Exam Key Points
1. **Vital signs.** Fever. Tachycardia. Hypotension.
2. **Local inspection.** Erythema at site or tracking along catheter. Warmth. Tenderness. Drainage at site. Integrity of catheter.
3. **Systemic symptoms.** Fever. Chills. Chest pain. Dyspnea. Vomiting.

  B. Laboratory Data. CBC. Culture drainage. Two blood cultures (one peripheral, one via catheter).
  C. Radiographic and Other Studies. CXR if suspected catheter embolus, occlusion, or rupture. Duplex US ± venogram if suspected venous thrombus.

V. Plan
  A. Overall Plan. Admit if systemically ill, unstable vital signs, vascular compromise of extremity, or continuous use of device is essential.
  B. Specific Plans
1. **Infection.** Early administration of broad-spectrum antibiotics. Cover *Staphylococcus epidermidis, S. aureus* and others if patient is immunocompromised. Consider removal of device after other IV access is obtained. Consult primary care physician or specialist.
2. **Occlusion.** Consider urokinase if clot in lumen is suspected. Consider subclavian vein thrombosis if unresponsive to declotting attempts.
3. **Hemorrhage.** Direct pressure. Pressure bandage. Rule out coagulopathy.

VI. ICD-9 Diagnoses: Infection/inflammation reaction due to indwelling catheter; Mechanical complication of indwelling catheter (breakdown, displacement, leakage, obstruction, protrusion); Other complication due to indwelling catheter (pain, hemorrhage, stenosis, fibrosis, thrombosis).

VII. Problem Case Diagnosis: Thrombosed A-V fistula.

VIII. Teaching Pearls Question: What is the most common complication of a subcutaneous A-V fistula?

IX. Teaching Pearls Answer: Thrombosis.

REFERENCES

Aufderheide TP. Peripheral arteriovascular disease. In: Marx J. *Rosen's Emergency Medicine: Concepts and Clinical Practice.* 5th ed. Mosby, 2002:1187–1209.

Johnson JC. Complications of vascular access devices. *Emerg Med Clin North Am* 1994;12(3):691–705.

Massorli S. Managing complications of central venous access devices. *Nursing* 1997; 27(8):59–63.

Whitman ED. Complications associated with the use of central venous access devices. *Curr Probl Surg* 1996;33(4):309–378.

50. JAUNDICE

I. **Problem.** A 43-year-old female presents complaining of nausea and decreased appetite for 1 week. She describes a constant "ache" in her upper abdomen and intermittent chills. Her physical exam reveals a thin, moderately ill female with yellowish tinge to her skin and sclera.

II. **Immediate Questions**

   A. **What are the patient's vital signs?** Is she febrile, tachycardic, or hypotensive, suggesting infectious or toxic/metabolic causes of illness?

   B. **What is the patient's mental status?** Is the patient alert and oriented, or is she confused and/or somnolent, which would suggest encephalopathy, hypoglycemia, or drug ingestion?

   C. **Are there constitutional symptoms,** suggestive of malignancy or HIV? Ask the patient about fevers, weight loss, night sweats, or recent illnesses.

   D. **Is the patient complaining of pain?**
      1. Colicky right upper quadrant pain—consider cholecystitis.
      2. Back or epigastric pain—consider pancreatitis.
      3. Diffuse joint pain—consider sickle cell crisis.

   E. **Does the patient complain of dark urine or acholic (clay-colored) stool?**

   F. **Does the patient have risk factors for infectious causes of jaundice?**
      1. Does the patient have multiple sexual partners or exposure to a person with hepatitis?
      2. Does the patient use IV drugs?

   G. **Has the patient been exposed to drugs or toxins?**
      1. Is there an exposure to acetaminophen or sulfa drugs?
      2. Does the patient use excessive amounts of alcohol?
      3. Is the patient depressed? Is there concern about intentional overdose?

   H. **Is the patient C/O dyspnea and fatigue?** Does she have a history of erythrocyte, enzyme/hemoglobin, or membrane defect that would put her at risk for hemolysis? (sickle cell disease the most common)

III. Differential Diagnosis

A. Prehepatic. Intravascular hemolysis or failure of hepatic conjugation

   1. **Hemolysis.** Sickle cell disease, G6PD deficiency, drug-induced: penicillin, quinine, methyldopa, autoimmune hemolytic anemia.
   2. **Decreased hepatic uptake.** Drugs, fasting, sepsis.
   3. **Decreased conjugation of bilirubin.** Gilbert's syndrome, Crigler-Najjar disease, neonatal jaundice, sepsis, drug inhibition: chloramphenicol.

B. Hepatocellular Dysfunction

   1. **Hepatitis**
      a. **Infectious.** Viral causes are most common.
      b. **Alcoholic.** Both acute hepatitis and secondary cirrhosis.
      c. **Toxin-induced.** Mushroom, carbon tetrachloride, recent halothane exposure.
      d. **Drug-induced.** Acetaminophen, sulfa drugs.
   2. **Sepsis**
   3. **Chronic hepatocellular disease.** Wilson's disease, hemochromatosis.

C. Intrahepatic Cholestasis

   1. **Pregnancy.** Most commonly seen in the third trimester.
   2. **Drugs.** Oral contraceptives, anabolic steroids, chlorpromazine, erythromycin.
   3. **TPN.**
   4. **Acquired disorders of the bile ductules** such as primary biliary cirrhosis.
   5. **Postoperative jaundice.**

D. Extrahepatic Obstruction

   1. **Cholelithiasis** and choledocholithiasis.
   2. **Pancreatitis.**
   3. **Primary or metastatic carcinomas** of the liver, gall bladder, or pancreas.
   4. **Biliary stricture** secondary to infectious or neoplastic causes.

IV. Database

A. Physical Exam Key Points

   1. **General appearance.** Is the patient cachectic, which could suggest malignancy, HIV, or prolonged alcohol/IV drug abuse?
   2. **Skin.** Are there stigmata of cirrhosis? Note evidence of IV drug abuse—needle tracks, ulcers.
   3. **Abdominal exam**
      a. Note the presence of right upper quadrant/midepigastric tenderness, suggesting gallbladder disease or pancreatitis.
      b. Note the presence of abdominal masses, suggesting a malignancy (GI or lymphoma).
      c. Look for signs of ascites that would indicate advanced liver disease.
      d. Is the liver enlarged, as seen in infectious hepatitis?

      e. Is there splenomegaly, which may be due to portal hypertension, EBV infection, or RBC sequestration in hemolysis?

      f. Is the stool clay-colored, suggesting biliary obstruction?

   4. Neurologic. Note presence of lethargy, asterixis, and encephalopathy

B. Laboratory Data. First must determine whether the jaundice is due to conjugated or unconjugated bilirubin—check the urine first!

   1. Absence of bile in the urine suggests unconjugated hyperbilirubinemia (not filtered by glomerulus) or hemolytic jaundice. Bilirubin rarely exceeds 3–4 mg/dL. Order a CBC and peripheral smear, LDH, and reticulocyte count.

   2. Presence of bile in urine indicates either hepatocellular jaundice or obstructive jaundice. Total indirect (unconjugated) and direct (conjugated) bilirubin

      a. Alkaline phosphatase. Markedly elevated in obstructive (intrahepatic or posthepatic) jaundice.

      b. SGOT/SGPT. Significant elevations seen in hepatocellular disease; moderate elevations seen in posthepatic disease.

      c. G-GTP. Increased in extrahepatic obstruction.

      d. 5'-Nucleotidase. Elevated in intrahepatic cholestasis and confirms hepatic origin of alkaline phosphatase.

      e. Albumin. Decreased levels associated with severe hepatic disease.

      f. PT. Prolongation indicates severe hepatic disease.

      g. Lipase. Specific for pancreatic disease/inflammation.

      h. Viral hepatitis panel for suspected hepatitis A, B, or C infection.

      i. Serum glucose. Decreased in severe liver disease due to reduced glycogen stores.

      j. Urine and or serum drug screens for suspected toxic or drug exposures. Serum acetaminophen strongly suggested for hepatitis of unclear origin.

C. Radiographic and Other Studies

   1. US. Preferred test for delineating biliary tract anatomy. Reliably demonstrates gallbladder and biliary tree pathology (obstruction, stones, inflammation). Masses in liver or pancreatic head may be detected

   2. CT scan. Superior to US for identification of both retroperitoneal (pancreatic) and intraabdominal masses

   3. HIDA/DISIDA. Depicts biliary tree and gallbladder function. Study of choice for identification of acute biliary tract obstruction, cholecystitis. Test may be unreliable when bilirubin levels are significantly elevated.

   4. ERCP. Indicated for patients with suspected acute cholangitis.

V. Plan

A. Overall Plan. Stabilize the patient! IV fluids and/or antibiotics if patient is hemodynamically unstable. Fingerstick blood sugar, pulse oximetry, and drug screen if mental status is altered.

B. **Specific Plans.** The initial work-up should focus on identifying whether the cause of the jaundice is pre-, intra- or posthepatic. Test ordering should be prioritized to identify those patients requiring urgent intervention or at risk for clinical deterioration. These include patients suspected of having any of the following:

1. **Ascending cholangitis, cholecystitis.** IV antibiotics, surgical, and/or GI consultation.
2. **Fulminant hepatitis.** Patients with altered mental status, coagulopathy, hypoglycemia and/or markedly elevated bilirubin should be admitted with GI consultation.
3. **Hemolytic anemia.** Usually require consultation with a hematologist if this is a new condition.

C. **Admission Criteria**
1. Any of the preceding three high-risk diagnoses.
2. Intractable pain.
3. Intractable emesis.
4. Associated pancreatitis.
5. Evidence of severe liver dysfunction: Encephalopathy, prolonged PT, impaired glucose metabolism, albumin level < 2.5 g/dL.
6. Pregnant patients.
7. Immunocompromised patients.
8. Patients with toxic hepatitis.
   The management for the remainder of patients depends on the ability to create a safe program of follow-up and outpatient consultation.

VI. **ICD-9 Diagnoses:** Acute hepatitis; Alcoholic hepatitis; Benign cholestatic jaundice; Cholangitis; Choledocholithiasis; Hemolytic jaundice; Jaundice; Liver cirrhosis (with or without alcoholism); Neoplasm.

VII. **Problem Case Diagnosis:** Hepatitis B.

VIII. **Teaching Pearls Question:** At what serum bilirubin level can jaundice be reliably detected on physical exam?

IX. **Teaching Pearls Answer:** 2.0–2.5 mg/dL (Harrison's).

REFERENCES

Chang A. Jaundice. In Rosen P, Barkin RM, Hayden SR, Schaider J, Wolfe R, eds. *The 5 Minute Emergency Medicine Consult.* Lippincott, Williams & Wilkins, 1999: 614–615.

Scott BC, Falk JL. Surgical causes of jaundice. In Harwood-Nuss A, ed. *The Clinical Practice of Emergency Medicine.* 3d ed. Lippincott, Williams & Wilkins, 2001: 179–180.

Kaplan L, Isselbacher K. Jaundice. In Braunwald E, Fauci AS, Kasper DL, Hauser SL, Longo, DL, Jameson, JL, eds. *Harrison's Principles of Internal Medicine.* 14th ed. McGraw-Hill, 1998:249–254.

Shields RO, Jr. Jaundice. In Tintinalli JE, Kelen GD, Stapczynski JS, eds. *Emergency Medicine, A Comprehensive Study Guide.* 5th ed. McGraw-Hill, 2000:574–576.

51. JOINT SWELLING

I. **Problem.** A middle-aged male presents with a swollen, painful knee.

II. **Immediate Questions**
  A. **History of trauma?**
  B. **Presence of constitutional symptoms?** Fever or chills?
  C. **Number of joints involved?** Monarthritis, oligoarthritis, polyarthritis.
  D. **History of IV drug abuse?**
  E. **History of prosthetic surgery?**
  F. **Any past medical history? Diabetes? Gout? Rheumatoid or osteoarthritis? HIV?**
  G. **Medications?** Steroids, anti-inflammatories.
  H. **Exposure to ticks?**

III. **Differential Diagnosis**
  A. **Infection.** Bacterial (medical emergency)—gonococcal (most common cause of septic joint in young adults) vs nongonococcal (hematogenous spread, migration of bacteria from overlying skin infection, direct inoculation), IV drug abuse, prosthetic joint, viral, granulomatous.
  B. **Crystal-Induced Gout, or Pseudogout.** Middle-aged to elderly patients. Develop acutely over hours (gout) to a day (pseudogout), may be precipitated by trauma, illness, major surgery, or change in medication. Risk factors—obesity or weight gain as young adult, hypertension, DM, heavy alcohol use (can follow a binge), lead exposure, use of proximal loop diuretics.
  C. **Trauma.** Can have associated ligamentous injury and intraarticular fracture. Remember to assess ABCs and for neurologic injury.
  D. **Inflammatory**
    1. **Rheumatoid arthritis.** Symmetric, polyarticular, spares the DIP. Morning stiffness, generalized malaise, fatigue, depression.
    2. **Lyme disease.** Monoarticular or oligoarticular, symmetric, migratory pattern, may give history of tick bite or rash.
    3. **Reiter's syndrome.** Asymmetric, oligoarthritis, preceded by infectious illness—diarrheal, urethritis. Classic presentation, conjunctivitis/iritis/uveitis, urethritis, arthritis "Can't see, can't pee, can't dance with me."
    4. **Ankylosing spondylitis.** Pain in spine and pelvis, multisystem involvement, associated with HLA-B2. Radiograph shows "bamboo spine," a squaring of the vertebral bodies." SLE.
  E. **Degenerative Osteoarthritis.** Avascular necrosis.

IV. **Database**
  A. **Physical Exam Key Points**
    1. **HEENT.** Eyes, iritis, uveitis (Reiter's syndrome), Oral mucosa, ulcers (SLE, Reiter's syndrome)
    2. **Cardiac.** Murmur (endocarditis), rub (SLE, rheumatoid arthritis).

    3. **Lungs.** Pleuritis (SLE, rheumatoid arthritis).
    4. **Genitourinary.** Lesions, urethral discharge, cervicitis (Reiter's syndrome, gonococcal infection).
    5. **Skin.** Rash (psoriasis), pustular lesions (gonococcal infection), tophi (gout), Heberden's nodules (osteoarthritis), Erythema chronicum migrans (Lyme disease), Track marks (IVDA), sausage digits (Reiter's syndrome).
    6. **Joints.** Inspect for signs of trauma; palpate for crepitance, joint effusion; test range of motion, muscle strength, ligament stability, swan neck deformity (rheumatoid arthritis).
    7. **Vitals.** Look for a fever.
  B. **Laboratory Data**
    1. **Joint fluid analysis.** Leukocyte count with Diff, crystal analysis, Gram's stain, and culture.
      a. **Normal.** WBC < 200, PMNs < 25, no crystals, no organisms.
      b. **NonInflammatory** (osteoarthritis, trauma). WBC < 200–2000, PMNs < 25, no crystals, no organisms.
      c. **Inflammatory** (gout, pseudogout, rheumatoid arthritis, Lyme disease, SLE). WBC 200–50,000; PMNs > 50%; positive crystals; no organisms.
      d. **Septic** (gonococcal and nongonococcal). WBC > 50,000; PMNs > 50%; no crystals; positive culture.
    2. **ESR.** Notoriously low in sensitivity but makes the consultants happy, can be useful for following the disease process.
    3. **CBC with Diff.** If suspect septic joint.
    4. **Uric acid level.** Does NOT check for gout, level does not correlate with an acute attack.
    5. **Blood cultures.** If suspect septic joint.
    6. **Gonococcal cultures.** Mouth, cervix, urethra, rectum, skin lesions in addition to joint fluid to improve probability of positive culture (joint fluid culture positive only 25–50%).
  C. **Radiographic and Other Studies.** Plain films to evaluate for foreign body, fracture, effusion, osteoporosis, osteomyelitis, osteoarthritis, aseptic necrosis, cartilaginous stippling (pseudogout), calcifications, joint space narrowing.

V. **Plan**
  A. **Overall Plan.** Plain film of affected joint, check appropriate labs, arthrocentesis, consider admission in debilitated or immunocompromised patient, or if cannot rule out septic joint based on initial evaluation.
  B. **Specific Plans**
    1. **Trauma.** Consider aspirating joint for relief if large effusion. Standard: rest, ice, elevate, crutches if unable to weight bear.
    2. **Septic arthritis.** Admit for IV antibiotics. Orthopedic consult: incision and drainage, irrigation. Treat for *S. aureus* if trauma, skin infection is cause. Infants at risk for *Escherichia coli. Salmonella* in sickle cell/SLE. IV drug abuse, MRSA, and gram-negative

Pseudomonas, Klebsiella, Serratia. Prosthetic joints, cover for *Staphylococcus epidermidis.*

3. **Crystal-induced.** Treat acute attack of gout (negative birefringent crystals) with colchicine (0.6 mg PO qh until pain is relieved or side effects emerge) and NSAIDs (indomethacin). May need long-term therapy (allopurinol) to reduce uric acid level.

4. **Pseudogout** (positive birefringent crystals). Treat with NSAIDs or colchicine. Not as effective as in gout.

5. **Inflammatory.** *Rheumatoid arthritis:* Initially rest the joint as movement increases inflammation, NSAIDs, prednisone, gold, penicillamine, methotrexate. *Lyme disease* (assess for neurologic, cardiac manifestations): Treat with doxycycline, amoxicillin as outpatient. More severe cases, use IV penicillin or ceftriaxone. *Reiter's syndrome:* Treat with NSAIDs. *Ankylosing spondylitis:* NSAIDs, strengthening exercise.

6. **Degenerative.** NSAIDs or acetaminophen for pain, exercise to strengthen muscle, long term may require joint replacement.

VI. **ICD-9 Diagnoses:** Acute gouty arthritis; Arthritis (state site); Arthritis due to crystals; Gonococcal arthritis; Hemarthrosis; Joint effusion; Septic arthritis; Sprain; Synovitis.

VII. **Problem Case Diagnosis:** Gouty arthritis—joint fluid analysis showed needle-shaped negatively birefringent crystals. Patient started on indomethacin and colchicine.

VIII. **Teaching Pearl Question:** What clinical entities are in the differential of a polyarticular arthritis?

IX. **Teaching Pearl Answer:** Viral syndrome (periarthralgias), early hepatitis, rheumatic fever, collagen vascular disease, Goodpasture's syndrome (immune complex disease), chronic osteoarthritis, Lyme disease, rheumatoid arthritis, ankylosing spondylitis, Reiter's syndrome.

REFERENCES

Dearborn JT, Jergesen HE. The evaluation and initial management of arthritis. *Prim Care* 1996;23:215–240.

Pittman JR, Bross MH. Diagnosis and management of gout. *Am Fam Physician* 1999;59:1799–1806.

52. PACEMAKER PROBLEMS

I. **Problem:** A man comes to the ED saying, "My pacemaker has fired twice. Bang. There it goes again."

II. **Immediate Questions**
   A. **ABCs? Vital signs stable?**
   B. **Oxygen, ECG, IV access underway?**

C. ECG. Underlying rhythm, pacing spikes visible? Pacing capture (consistent QRS following spikes) visible?

D. Chest pain? History of recent chest pain? Characterize pain and evaluate for cardiac if present.

E. Shortness of breath? Similarly, consider as cardiac symptom?

F. Device? What type? When placed? Where? Who's his cardiologist? Patient should be carrying identification card in pocket with device info.

    1. AICD/ICD. Often have integrated pacemakers.

    2. Pacemaker codes

        Position I: Chamber paced.

        Position II: Chamber sensed.

        Position III: Mode.

        Position IV: Programmable functions.

        Position V: Antitachycardia functions.

        Typical codes: V = ventricle, A = atrium, D = dual, O = none, I = inhibited, T = triggered, P= simple programmable, M = multiprogrammable, C = communicating.

III. Differential Diagnosis: What is going on with device?

A. Specific to AICDs

    1. Appropriate action? Patient experiencing runs of VT/VF?

    2. Sensing problems? Device will not sense VT below a threshold cut-off rate. Slow VT may produce poor blood pressure, yet not trigger cardioversion.

    3. Inappropriate firing? Similarly, atrial fibrillation with a rapid ventricular response can be mistaken for VT and can cause inappropriate cardioversion.

    4. Failure to cardiovert? Caused by failure to sense (lead migration or fracture), electrical interference, device failure.

    5. Ineffective cardioversion? Poor energy output, displaced leads, medications causing increase in defibrillation threshold, lead fracture or dislodging, or MI.

B. Failure Modes Also Found in Regular Pacemakers

    1. Failure to output? Absent pacing spike due to battery failure, lead failure, inhibited output due to decreased sensing threshold, or interference between ventricular and atrial leads.

    2. Hysteresis? Irregular rate caused when sensor set lower than lowest pacing rate. Brief periods of pacing at the lowest rate will be interspersed with periods when the rate "wanders" back down to the threshold required to trigger pacing again, which again is sensed as a normal rate and so shuts off pacing.

    3. Failure to capture? Pacing spike is not followed by a QRS. Caused by lead problems, tissue damage/infarction at tip, medications, metabolic abnormalities, or improper pacer settings (Figure I–4).

    4. Oversensing? Pacemaker may sense muscular activity and fail to pace correctly, causing a bradycardia.

Figure I–4. Failure to capture. The rhythm is a nodal rhythm at 40 bpm. The pacemaker spikes occur at 72 bpm. The pacemaker spikes are not associated with the ventricular depolarizations. (Reproduced, with permission, from Haist SA, Robbins JB, Gomella, LG, eds. *Internal Medicine on Call,* 3rd ed. McGraw-Hill, 2002.

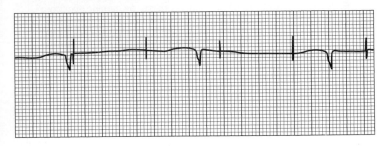

    5. Undersensing? Depolarization not sensed, causing inappropriate firing. May be due to lead problems, low battery, and localized tissue damage/infarction (Figure I–5).

IV. Database
  A. Physical Exam Key Points. Vital signs, level of consciousness, others specific to cardiac function following pacemaker malfunction.
  B. Laboratory Data. None pertinent to pacemaker, however, consider myocardial damage following pacemaker-induced tachycardias, or prolonged bradycardias or other stressful arrhythmias from pacemaker malfunction.
  C. Radiographic and Other Studies. Certain lead fractures causing failure to capture may be visible on CXR, as may displaced leads.

Figure I–5. Failure to sense. A pacemaker spike is seen immediately after the 3rd, 4th, 5th, and 6th QRS complexes. The pacemaker should have been inhibited by the QRS complexes. (Photograph courtesy of Alberto Mazzoleni, MD.)

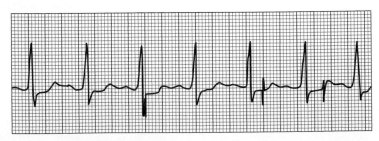

The study should be performed; however, the findings are not likely to change immediate clinical management of the consequences of the failure.

V. Plan
   A. **Overall Plan.** Treat cardiovascular consequences of pacer malfunction. Consider external pacer to support a consequent bradycardia. Consider cardioversion or defibrillation to treat an ineffective device. Consider evaluating for cardiac damage.
   B. **Specific Plans.** Consider inhibiting pacer or AICD with magnet, which will trigger a constant, intrinsic rate of device, which may have diagnostic potential. Different rates will indicate full battery, elective replacement time, and empty battery. These rates will be on info card.

VI. ICD-9 Diagnoses:
Cardiac pacemaker reprogramming (a V code); Infection/inflammation due to cardiac device; Mechanical complication of cardiac device (breakdown, displacement, perforation, protrusion), Other complication of cardiac device (fibrosis, hemorrhage, pain, stenosis); Pacemaker malfunction.

VII. Problem Case Diagnosis:
New-onset AF, causing inappropriate firing of the patient's AICD.

VIII. Teaching Pearl Question:
What is the simplest common pacemaker, how many wires does it use, and what does the "I" stand for? Extra credit: What happens when you hold a magnet to it?

IX. Teaching Pearl Answer:
The VVI pacer is a single-wire pacer that senses and paces the ventricle. A ventricular depolarization within the expected interval inhibits (the "I") the pacer from firing, allowing the heart to maintain a normal rhythm. Holding a magnet to it activates an internal switch and causes the pacemaker to fire at a steady rate.

REFERENCES

Cardall TY, Brady WJ, Chan TC, Perry JC, Vilke GM, Rosen P. Permanent cardiac pacemakers: Issues relevant to the emergency physician, part II. *J Emerg Med* 1999;17(4):697–709.

Cardall TY, Chan TC, Brady WJ, Perry JC, Vilke GM, Rosen P. Permanent cardiac pacemakers: Issues relevant to the emergency physician, part I. *J Emerg Med* 1999; 17(3):479–89.

Shan PM, Ellenbogen KA. Life after pacemaker implantation: Management of common problems and environmental interactions. *Cardiol Rev* 2001;9(4):193–201.

Weinberger BM, Brilliant LC. Pacemaker and automatic internal cardiac defibrillator. *eMed J* [serial online]. July 25 2001;2(7). Available at: http://www.emedicine.com/emerg/topic805.htm

53. PALPITATIONS

   I. **Problem:** Middle-aged female complains that she feels her heart "fluttering" intermittently.

158

II. Immediate Questions

A. **Is the patient hemodynamically stable?** What are the vital signs and mental status? Cardiac monitoring for heart rate and rhythm.

B. **What is the underlying cardiac substrate?** Is there CAD, known arrhythmia or conduction block or structural abnormality? ECG to rule out AMI or arrhythmia.

C. **What other symptoms are associated?** Does the patient experience concomitant syncope, lightheadedness, chest pain, or shortness of breath?

D. **Is the patient currently symptomatic?** Does the monitor show any irregularities that correlate with patient's symptoms?

E. **Any past medical history?** Cardiac disease, thyroid disease, anemia?

F. **Drugs or medications?** Cocaine, amphetamines, nicotine, or caffeine? Thyroid replacement, atropine, monoamine oxidase inhibitors, ephedrine, diet pills?

III. Differential Diagnosis

A. **Tachycardias**

1. **Atrial.** Fibrillation or flutter. Usually abrupt onset and end. May be constant or last minutes to hours. Fibrillation is irregular and rapid. Flutter more regular, often rate is approx. 150 bpm. Both are independent of exertion or mental state.

2. **Ventricular.** May cause lightheadedness, syncope. Rare without underlying cardiac disease.

3. **Sinus.** Consider PE, fever, thyrotoxicosis, anemia, drug use (see Immediate Question F) if clinical picture is consistent. Anxiety may cause rapid HR or sensation of rapid rate with documented normal rate/rhythm.

B. **Bradycardias**

Consider AV block or SA node pathology.

C. **Individual Beats**

Patients may describe "skipped beats" or "flip flopping." Usually corresponds to premature atrial or ventricular contractions with compensatory pause. Common and benign in normal hearts but may increase risk of death if occurring after MI.

IV. Database

A. **Physical Exam Key Points**

1. **Mental status.** Assess perfusion to brain, anxiety.

2. **Vital signs.** Temperature, HR, BP.

3. **HEENT.** Proptosis, thyroid exam (thyroid disease), pale conjunctiva (anemia).

4. **CV.** Murmur, rhythm, hyperdynamic precordium.

5. **Lungs.** Dyspnea, rales (fluid overload).

6. **Neurologic.** Nystagmus, agitation, pupil size (drug use).

7. **Skin.** Diaphoresis (drug use, ischemia), needle tracks.

8. **Extremities.** Edema (heart failure, DVT), peripheral pulses.

    B. Laboratory Data. TSH, Hgb/Hct, Lytes. Consider PT/PTT if patient on warfarin (Coumadin) for AF. Pregnancy test if applicable. Cardiac enzymes if history suggests ischemia

    C. Radiographic and Other Studies. ECG immediately. May arrange ambulatory monitoring if patient has hemodynamic instability or significant symptoms without a diagnosis. Consider echocardiogram in patients with AF/flutter, evidence of heart disease, or heart failure.

V. Plan

    A. Overall Plan. Evaluate for hemodynamic stability and for underlying cardiac ischemia or arrhythmia. Admit patients as appropriate for cardiac work-up (associated syncope, chest pain, shortness of breath). If no cardiac pathology suspected, initiate work-up for other causes and arrange follow-up.

    B. Specific Plans

        1. Cardiac. Treat ischemia if suspected (oxygen, aspirin, nitro, heparin, β-blocker). Treat dysrhythmias accordingly. Admit if signs of ischemia or hemodynamic instability (syncope).

        2. Medication or drugs. Supportive care. Discharge home with advice to avoid precipitating substance in future.

        3. Thyroid disease. If signs of thyroid storm, treat accordingly. Otherwise, initiate lab work-up and refer for follow-up.

        4. Pregnancy. Reassurance and follow-up if normal ECG, monitor. May arrange ambulatory monitoring if symptoms severe or persistent.

        5. Other. PVC or PACs without other pathology are usually benign. May refer for ambulatory monitoring. Discharge with reassurance.

VI. ICD-9 Diagnoses: Adverse effect of drug (state drug); Hyperthyroidism; Palpitations; Paroxysmal tachycardia (atrial or ventricular); Supraventricular tachycardia; WPW.

VII. Problem Case Diagnosis: Benign PVCs

VIII. Teaching Pearls Question: Characterize the palpitation patient with hyperkinetic heart syndrome.

IX. Teaching Pearls Answer: Hyperkinetic heart syndrome is a condition found in young adult patients, with or without precipitating anxiety, that develop volatile and exercise-related β-adrenergic-mediated palpitations. This entity is often treated with β-blockers after other organic causes of palpitations are excluded.

REFERENCES

Barsky AJ. Palpitations, arrhythmias, and awareness of cardiac activity. *Ann Intern Med* 2001;134 (9 Pt 2):832–837

Frohlich ED, Tarazi RC, Dustan HP. Hyperdynamic beta adrenergic circulatory state. *Arch Intern Me,* 1969;123:1–7.

54. PARESTHESIAS

I. **Problem:** A 55-year-old woman with a history of breast cancer presents complaining of a 3-week history of worsening numbness and tingling of her right leg.

II. **Immediate Questions**
  A. **Is there arterial insufficiency?** Check for warmth, capillary refill, and pulse (palpable or Doppler) in the affected extremity. High flow O_2, vascular access, emergent vascular surgery consult.
  B. **Is there venous insufficiency?** Is there associated pain, pallor; poikilothermia; paralysis, suggesting a compartment syndrome? This requires O_2, vascular access, emergent orthopedic consultation. Are there risk factors for DVT (cancer, recent trauma or surgery, prior history etc)? O_2, vascular access, consider anticoagulation.
  C. **Is this posttraumatic?** Consider spinal cord injury. Initiate full spine precautions.
  D. **Are there associated neurologic deficits?** Consider TIA or acute cerebrovascular accident.

III. **Differential Diagnosis**
  A. **Vascular**
    1. **Arterial insufficiency.** Acute or acute on chronic arterial obstruction, traumatic arterial injury, aortic or arterial dissection.
    2. **Venous insufficiency.** Compartment syndrome, DVT, SVC syndrome, tumor compression.
  B. **Neurologic**
    1. **Acute**
      a. **Traumatic.** Spinal cord injury, head injury with epidural or subdural hematoma, peripheral nerve laceration or crush.
      b. **Cerebrovascular insufficiency.** Stroke, TIA, or subarachnoid hemorrhage.
      c. **Acute transverse myelitis**
      d. **Nerve compression.** Disc herniation, Saturday night palsy.
      e. **Hyperventilation**
    2. **Subacute or chronic**
      a. **Nerve compression.** Tumor, carpal tunnel syndrome.
      b. **Demyelinating disease.** Multiple sclerosis.
      c. **Migraines.**
      d. **Bell's palsy.**
      e. **Peripheral neuropathy** due to alcoholism, diabetes, metabolic derangements.
      f. **Drug- or toxin-induced** isoniazid, antiretroviral, cholesterol-lowering agents, lead, arsenic.

IV. **Database**
  A. **Physical Exam Key Points**
    1. **Vascular exam.** Carefully document presence and quality of peripheral pulses and perfusion in all extremities.

    2. Check for carotid bruit.

    3. Neurologic exam. Map out distribution of numbness using pin prick, check motor strength and reflexes, carefully search for any other neurologic deficits.

B. Laboratory Data

    1. Consider checking renal panel.

    2. Consider D-dimer if concerned about low to moderate probability of DVT.

C. Radiographic and Other Studies

    1. In setting of trauma or other spinal cord injuries or, consider plain radiographs of the spine, CT, or MRI.

    2. In the setting of suspicion of metastatic cord compression, MRI.

    3. In setting of suspicion of cerebrovascular cause, head CT and carotid US or MRI/MRA.

V. Plan

    A. Overall Plan. Suspicion of acute arterial insufficiency, compartment syndrome, or cerebral bleed requires emergent surgical consultation. Suspicion of spinal cord compression requires emergent MRI and consultation with neurosurgery and oncology. Other causes must be managed according to their individual etiologies.

    B. Specific Plans

        1. Acute arterial insufficiency. High-flow O_2, vascular access, prompt reduction of dislocations or fractures, emergent vascular surgery consultation, and admission.

        a. Compartment syndrome. High-flow O_2, vascular access, emergent orthopedic surgery consultation, and admission.

        b. DVT. Anticoagulation and admission or outpatient enoxaparin.

        c. Stroke. High-flow O_2, vascular access neurology consultation, aspirin, consider anticoagulation and thrombolytics. Admit.

        d. Spinal cord injury or spinal nerve compression. Neurosurgical consultation and admit where appropriate.

        e. Metabolic or drug-induced. Treat accordingly.

        All others require further work-up and treatment as outpatients.

VI. ICD-9 Diagnoses: Paresthesia; Electrolyte imbalance; Hyperventilation; Peripheral neuropathy (due to drug, dietary deficiency, diabetes mellitus).

VII. Problem Case Diagnosis: Metastatic breast cancer to L4 directly compressing the L4 nerve root.

VIII. Teaching Pearl Question: What percentage of patients with known metastatic cancer develop spinal cord compression? What are the most common neoplastic causes?

IX. Teaching Pearl Answer: 5%. Lung, breast, and prostate cancer and multiple myeloma.

REFERENCES

Johansen K, Watson J. Compartment syndrome: New insights. *Semin Vasc Surg* 1998;11(4):294–301.

Pascuzzi RM, Fleck JD. Acute peripheral neuropathy in adults. Guillain-Barré syndrome and related disorders. *Neurol Clin* 1997;15(3):529–547.

Quinn JA, De Angelis LM. Neurologic emergencies in the cancer patient. *Semin Oncol* 2000;27(3):311–321.

55. PENILE PROBLEMS

I. **Problem:** A 19-year-old male approaches the triage nurse and asks to see a male doctor for a problem "down there."

II. **Immediate Questions**
   A. **Are the vital signs stable?**
   B. **Please explain more clearly what the problem "down there" is.** Don't assume anything. A very serious injury or problem may still be too embarrassing for a young person to admit readily.

III. **Differential Diagnosis, Database, and Specific Plans by Lesion Type**
   A. **Sexually Transmitted Lesions**
      1. **Genital herpes**
         a. **Symptoms.** Grouped painful, tingling, superficial vesicles/pustules on red base that ulcerate in 1–7 days; can get inguinal lymphadenopathy and constitutional symptoms.
         b. **Etiology.** Herpes simplex type II (90%) and type I (10%).
         c. **Incubation.** 2–21 days.
         d. **Complications.** HIV transmission, herpetic sacral radiculomyelitis, erythema multiforme.
         e. **Diagnosis.** Herpes culture of vesicular fluid or debrided ulcer.
         f. **Treatment.** Acyclovir or valacyclovir.
      2. **Condylomata acuminata** (genital warts)
         a. **Symptoms.** Numerous, pale pink, projections that can coalesce to form a cauliflower-like mass; can be pruritic or painful.
         b. **Etiology.** Human papillomavirus.
         c. **Risk factor.** Immunocompromised.
         d. **Complication.** Penile squamous cell carcinoma.
         e. **Treatment.** *Topical:* Liquid nitrogen, podophyllum 20%, podofilox (Condylox) 0.5 %, trichloracetic acid 35% up to 85%. *Excision:* Surgery or CO_2 laser.
      3. **Primary syphilis**
         a. **Symptoms.** Begins as a firm papule, then painless ulcer (chancre) with indurated raised borders that lasts 2–6 weeks; usually only single papule but multiple ones can be present; inguinal lymphadenopathy possible.
         b. **Etiology.** *Treponema pallidum.*
         c. **Incubation.** 10–90 days.

      d. Complications. Cutaneous syphilis; neurosyphilis.
      e. Diagnosis. Darkfield microscopy of smear from lesion; serum VDRL or RPR.
      f. Treatment. Bicillin LA 2.4 million units IM or doxycycline 100 mg PO bid × 14 days.

4. Molluscum contagiosum
    a. Symptoms. Benign epidermal tumors that are small, waxy, smooth, dome-shaped, pink or flesh-colored, firm, papules with umbilicated centers; can be mildly pruritic or painful; not always an STD (high incidence in kids).
    b. Etiology. Molluscum contagiosum virus.
    c. Risk factor. HIV disease.
    d. Incubation. 2–8 weeks.
    e. Complications. Secondary bacterial infections.
    f. Treatment. Usually resolves spontaneously in 6–9 months; may use curettage, liquid nitrogen, silver nitrate, trichloracetic acid 35%, salicylic acid, cantharidin 0.7%.

5. Chancroid
    a. Symptoms. Begins as red papule, then pustule, then painful ulcer with irregular borders, moist malodorous base, and gray exudate; usually only single papule but multiple ones can be present; 50% have inguinal lymphadenopathy, which can ulcerate.
    b. Etiology. *Hemophilus ducreyi.*
    c. Incidence. Rare in U.S., but more common than syphilis worldwide.
    d. Incubation. 2–14 days.
    e. Complication. HIV transmission.
    f. Treatment. Single dose of ceftriaxone 250 mg IM or azithromycin 1 gm PO.

6. Lymphogranuloma venereum (LGV)
    a. Symptoms. Begins as small papule or vesicle, then painless ulcer (25%), then tender inguinal lymphadenopathy (100%); urethritis and constitutional symptoms possible.
    b. Etiology. *Chlamydia trachomatis.*
    c. Incidence. 20 times more common in males.
    d. Incubation. 1–12 weeks.
    e. Complications. Inguinal fistulas, genital lymphedema/elephantiasis.
    f. Diagnosis. *Chlamydia* culture of urethra, ulcer, or lymph node.
    g. Treatment. Azithromycin or doxycycline.

7. Granuloma inguinale
    a. Symptoms. Begins as a subcutaneous nodule, then painless beefy elevated granuloma, then painful necrotic ulcer on penis, inguinal regions, and/or anus.
    b. Etiology. *Calymmatobacterium granulomatis.*
    c. Incidence. 100 cases annually in U.S.

      d. Incubation. 1–12 weeks.

      e. Complication. Penile squamous cell carcinoma.

      f. Diagnosis. Intracellular Donovan bodies by Wright's or Giesma's stain.

      g. Treatment. 3 weeks of tetracycline 500 mg PO qid or TMP-SMX DS PO bid.

B. Sexually transmitted urethritis

1. Gonorrhea

      a. Symptoms. Yellow purulent urethral discharge, dysuria, urethral pruritus.

      b. Etiology. *Neisseria gonorrhea.*

      c. Incubation. 2–7 days.

      d. Complications. Urethral stricture, epididymitis, prostatitis, disseminated gonococcal infection, *Chlamydia* coinfection.

      e. Diagnosis. Intracellular gram-negative diplococci on Gram's stain; gonorrhea urethral culture.

      f. Treatment. Single dose of ceftriaxone 125 mg IM, cefixime (Suprax) 400 mg PO, cefuroxime (Ceftin) 1 g PO, ciprofloxacin 500 mg PO, ofloxacin (Floxin) 400 mg PO, spectinomycin 2 g IM, or azithromycin 2 g PO (has high incidence of GI side effects); and antichlamydial antibiotic.

2. Nongonococcal urethritis

      a. Symptoms. Yellow mucopurulent urethral discharge, dysuria, urethral pruritus; 50% are asymptomatic.

      b. Etiology. *Ureaplasma urealyticum* (50%), *Chlamydia trachomatis* (35%), *Mycoplasma hominis* (10%), *Trichomonas vaginalis* (5%).

      c. Incubation. 1–5 weeks.

      d. Complications. Epididymitis, prostatitis, gonorrhea coinfection.

      e. Diagnosis. *Chlamydia* urethral culture, DNA probe, or enzyme immunoassay.

      f. Treatment. Azithromycin 1 g PO × 1, doxycycline 100 mg PO bid × 7 days, ofloxacin (Floxin) 300 mg PO bid × 7 days, or erythromycin 500 mg PO qid × 7 days; and antigonorrhea antibiotic.

C. Acquired Phimosis

1. Symptoms. Foreskin becomes stuck over the glans like a muzzle and can't be retracted.

2. Risk factors. Balanoposthitis, poor hygiene, scarring due to prior foreskin injury, penile cancer, balanitis xerotica obliterans.

3. Complications. Urinary retention, balanitis.

4. Treatment

      a. Temporary. Hemostatic dilation of foreskin ostium to relieve urinary retention.

      b. Definitive. Dorsal slit incision or circumcision.

D. Paraphimosis

1. **Symptoms.** Edematous foreskin is stuck proximal to the corona and can't be reduced over the glans.
2. **Risk factor.** Vigorous sexual activity, balanoposthitis, poor hygiene, frequent catheters.
3. **Complications.** Glans ischemia or gangrene, urinary retention.
4. **Treatment.** Manual reduction or dorsal slit incision of constricting fibrotic band.

E. Foreign Body Constriction (Incarceration)

1. **Symptoms.** Swollen glans and penile shaft distal to circumferential foreign body.
2. **Etiology.** Hair, sex toy, string, or other object around penile shaft.
3. **Complications.** Ischemia, urethral trauma, urinary retention.
4. **Treatment.** Remove or cut away the object, then consider obtaining Doppler US of the penis to evaluate blood flow and/or retrograde urethrogram to evaluate urethra.

F. Zipper Entrapment

Can involve penile shaft, foreskin, or glans.

1. **Treatment**
   a. Cut median bar (diamond or bridge) of zipper slider with bone cutter or wire clippers, which causes the zipper's interlocking teeth to fall apart.
   b. Anesthetizing the skin and forcing the zipper open without cutting its median bar may increase the amount of tissue caught in the zipper and/or lacerate the skin.

G. Infectious Balanitis

1. **Symptoms.** Infectious inflammation of the glans (balanoposthitis also involves the foreskin).
2. **Etiology.** *Candida,* group B streptococci, *Gardnerella vaginalis.*
3. **Risk factors.** Uncircumcised, diabetes, poor hygiene, sex partner has vaginal candidiasis, morbid obesity, penile squamous cell carcinoma.
4. **Complications.** Secondary bacterial infection, phimosis, balanitis xerotica obliterans.
5. **Treatment**
   a. Daily mild soap cleansings of glans.
   b. **Candidal balanitis**
      i. **Topical powder.** Clotrimazole (Lotrimin), miconazole (Micatin), nystatin (Mycostatin), or tolnaftate (Tinactin) bid till resolved.
      ii. **Oral pill.** Fluconazole (Diflucan) 150 mg PO once.
   c. **Secondary bacterial infections.** Bacitracin and/or cephalexin (Keflex) or dicloxacillin.
   d. Circumcision if recurrent.

H. Balanitis Xerotica Obliterans

Also known as lichen sclerosus et atrophicus of the penis.

1. **Symptoms.** 1. Smooth, white, atrophic glans; foreskin erosions; narrow meatus; and urethral stricture.
2. **Complications.** Phimosis, urinary retention, penile squamous cell carcinoma.
3. **Treatment.** Topical steroids, dilations, surgical excision.

I. **Balanitis Circinata**
Papulosquamous (psoriasiform) plaques called keratoderma blennorrhagica on glans.
   1. **Symptoms.** Due to Reiter's syndrome (also have urethritis, peripheral arthritis, conjunctivitis, and plaques on feet and toes due to reactive immune response to *Yersinia* or other infection).

J. **Zoon's (Plasma Cell) Balanitis**
   1. **Symptoms.** Benign, idiopathic, red, smooth, glistening erosion on glans from plasma cell infiltration.
   2. **Risk factors.** Only in uncircumcised males.
   3. **Treatment.** Topical steroids, CO_2 laser, circumcision.

K. **Priapism**
   1. **Symptoms.** Painful prolonged pathologic erection (no detumescence). Glans isn't involved.
   2. **Complications.** Penile ischemia, cavernosal arterial thrombosis, penile fibrosis, impotence, urinary retention.
   3. **Etiology**
      a. **Drug**
         i. **Cardiac.** β-Blockers, calcium channel blockers, prazosin, hydralazine.
         ii. **Psychotropic.** Phenothiazines, trazodone (Desyrel), citalopram (Celexa).
         iii. **Illicit.** Ecstasy, cocaine, marijuana.
         iv. **Other.** Metoclopramide (Reglan), omeprazole (Prilosec), hydroxyzine (Atarax).
      b. **Intracavernosal injection for impotence.** Phentolamine, papaverine, prostaglandin E_1.
      c. **Hematologic.** Sickle cell anemia, thalassemias, leukemia, multiple myeloma.
      d. **Other.** Idiopathic, spinal cord lesion, amyloidosis, tumor infiltration.
   4. **Treatment**
      Ice and/or ejaculation are not helpful.
      a. **Of all etiologies.** Terbutaline 0.25–0.5 mg SQ (or 5 mg PO); repeat in 15 min prn.
      b. **Of impotence injections.** 30–90 mL lateral corporal aspiration; if persists then instill 30–90 mL of 10 mg of phenylephrine (Neo-Synephrine) mixed in 500 mL of NS; repeat 10–20 mL q 5–10 min prn up to 10 doses.
      c. **Of drug.** Corporal aspiration, pseudoephedrine instillation, heparin irrigation of corporal bodies, corpus cavernosum-spongiosum shunt surgery.

L. Penile Fracture
1. **Symptoms.** Blunt trauma to or abrupt lateral bending of erect penis causes sudden pain, swelling, hematoma, palpable tunical defect, deformity, and angulation of penile shaft.
2. **Etiology.** Due to rupture of the tunica albuginea of the corpus cavernosum.
3. **Risk factor.** Female dominant position during sexual intercourse.
4. **Complications.** Meatal blood, hematuria, and dysuria due to urethral injury (10–38%); perineal, scrotal, and/or lower abdominal wall ecchymosis to due Buck's fascia injury; urinary retention due to periurethral hematoma; erectile dysfunction.
5. **Diagnosis.** Cavernosography or MRI; and retrograde urethrogram.
6. **Treatment.** Ice compress, pressure dressing, analgesia, and surgery.

M. Penile Traumatic Lymphangitis
1. **Symptoms**
   a. Self-limiting nontender, translucent, firm, nodular penile tissue beginning at the corona.
   b. Can be diffuse or unilateral cord-like.
2. **Etiology.** Vigorous/prolonged intercourse or masturbation; external penile pumps.
3. **Treatment.** Resolves in 1–2 months with sexual abstinence.

N. Peyronie's Disease
1. **Symptoms.** Painful abnormally curved erections due to fibrosis in corpora cavernosum.
2. **Risk factors.** Age 40–60 years old, mild penile trauma, Dupuytren's hand contractures, HLA-B7.
3. **Treatment.** Urology referral.

O. Pearly Penile Papules
1. **Symptoms.** Dome-shaped or hair-like angiofibromas on corona.
2. **Treatment.** None needed.

P. Penile squamous cell carcinoma
1. **Symptoms.** Painless mass or persistent lesion/ulcer on glans or foreskin (shaft < 2%).
2. **Risk factors.** Age 40–60 years old, uncircumcised, third world countries, smegma, genital warts, balanitis xerotica obliterans, granuloma inguinale, leukoplakia.

VI. ICD-9 Diagnoses: Acute prostatitis; Balanitis; Balanoposthitis; Paraphimosis; Phimosis; Priapism; Urethritis (state organism if known).

VII. Problem Case Diagnosis: Genital herpes.

VIII. Teaching Pearl Question: What is a reason for the high incidence of AIDS disease in Africa?

IX. Teaching Pearl Answer: Due to the high incidence of genital ulcers, which promote the transmission of the human immunodeficiency virus.

REFERENCES

Adimora AA, Hamilton H, Holmes KK, Sparling PF. *Sexually Transmitted Diseases: Companion Handbook.* McGraw-Hill, 1994.

Centers for Disease Control and Prevention. 1998 Guidelines for treatment of sexually transmitted diseases. *MMWR* 1998;47:RR.

56. PREGNANCY PROBLEMS

I. **Problem:** A 19-year-old female presents with severe sudden pelvic pain.

II. **Immediate Questions**

A. **What are the vital signs?** Manage appropriately. Endotracheal intubation (RSI) if hypoxic or unresponsive. Large-bore IV access. IV hydration if tachycardic, hypotensive, or orthostatic with normal pulse Ox.

B. **Date of last menstrual period or gestational age?** What trimester? Multiple gestations (eg, twins)? Previous US? If so, at what gestational age, and what were the findings? Stat urine pregnancy test if not known to be pregnant.

C. **Vaginal bleeding** or rupture of membranes? Any passed tissue? If tissue, send to pathology for POC analysis.

D. **Contractions?** If greater than 20 weeks gestation, contact on-call or patient's OB/GYN for STAT evaluation or admission. If delivery seems imminent, do not attempt to transfer the patient!

E. **Previous obstetrical history?** Number of pregnancies, number of live births (term?), spontaneous abortions, therapeutic abortions, complications during/after pregnancy (premature labor, high blood pressure, preeclampsia or "toxemia," diabetes, hyperemesis gravidarum, prenatal care, blood type).

F. **Other medical problems?** Hypertension, diabetes, seizure disorder, cardiac problems, asthma, or pulmonary problems. Medications and allergies.

G. **Review of systems.** Any recent abdominal trauma or domestic violence, headache, seizure or altered mentation, visual changes, facial or lower extremity swelling (symmetric or asymmetric?), fever, cough, shortness of breath, chest pain, flank pain, back pain, abdominal pain, nausea/vomiting, vaginal bleeding or discharge, dysuria, increased urinary frequency, fetal movement.

III. **Differential Diagnosis**

A. **Pelvic Pain or Vaginal Bleeding**

1. **Ectopic pregnancy.** During first trimester, ANY pelvic pain is "ectopic until proven otherwise." Risk factors: prior ectopic, Hx STDs, PID, IUD, tubal ligation, recent elective abortion, infertility.

2. **Spontaneous abortion.** Consider during first or second trimester. Pain usually resolves after passage of tissue or fetus. If in doubt about the diagnosis, confirm with US.

3. **Threatened abortion.** Consider during first or second trimester. Pelvic pain or vaginal bleeding with IUP and no evidence of ectopic attachment.
4. **Placental abruption.** Consider during second or third trimester. Pelvic/abdominal pain with/without vaginal bleeding. Trauma? Confirm by US.
5. **Placenta previa.** Consider during second or third trimester. Painless vaginal bleeding. Confirm by US.

B. **Neurologic Signs or Symptoms**
   1. **Preeclampsia.** Hypertension (140/90 mm Hg, but may be less), proteinuria, pathologic edema.
   2. **Eclampsia.** Preeclampsia + seizure or coma. Most frequent > 20 weeks gestation, 20–25% occur postpartum (98% on first postpartum day).
   3. **Intracranial hemorrhage.** Headache, syncope, visual or other neurologic complaints. Frequent cause of death in severe preeclampsia/eclampsia.
   4. **Seizure.** During first trimester, NOT related to preeclampsia. Work-up as seizure in nonpregnant patient.

C. **Chest Pain, Hypoxia, or Dyspnea**
   1. **Pneumonia.** Cough, fever, dyspnea, chest/back pain.
   2. **Pulmonary embolus.** Dyspnea, chest/back pain. DVT and PE are common during all trimesters of pregnancy and for 6–12 weeks after delivery.
   3. **Noncardiac pulmonary edema.** Common complication of pneumonia, pyelonephritis, and other infections, due to low oncotic pressure state during pregnancy.
   4. **Peripartum cardiomyopathy.** Occurs during last month of pregnancy to within 5 months postpartum. Rule out other causes of pulmonary edema/heart failure.

D. **Abdominal Pain or Contractions, Flank Pain, Fever, or Vomiting**
   1. **Hyperemesis gravidarum.** Check urine for ketones, infection. Rule out other causes of vomiting.
   2. **UTI/pyelonephritis.** May be asymptomatic. Dysuria, frequency, flank/back pain.
   3. **HELLP syndrome.** Right upper quadrant pain or epigastric pain accompanied with nausea, vomiting, and malaise.
   4. **Appendicitis.** Pain/tenderness often displaced superiorly and laterally, may cause RUQ pain in late pregnancy. Peritoneal signs may be absent due to elevation of abdominal wall by gravid uterus.
   5. **Cholecystitis.** Incidence may be increased in pregnancy, especially in teens. Differentiate from HELLP syndrome.
   6. **Preterm labor.** Evaluate for precipitating factors—UTI, DKA, trauma, others.
   7. **Pregnancy-induced diabetes.** Consider first-onset DKA, rule out precipitating infections.

E. Other (should not be missed!)

1. **Pregnancy-induced hypertension.** Rule out preeclampsia—no proteinuria or edema!
2. **DVT.** Asymmetric leg pain/swelling.
3. **Fetal demise.** 20+-week gestation, no fetal activity.

IV. Database

A. Physical Exam Key Points

1. **Mental status.** Glasgow Coma Scale; postictal?
2. **Vital signs.** Check carefully and repeat during evaluation.
3. **HEENT.** Check for facial swelling (preeclampsia) or dry mucous membranes (volume depletion). Check pupils for reactivity (CVA), fundi for hemorrhages (CVA).
4. **Lungs.** Check for crackles (cardiogenic or noncardiogenic pulmonary edema) or wheezes (asthma, CHF).
5. **Abdomen.** Gravid? RUQ or RLQ tenderness (cholecystitis, hepatitis, HELLP, preeclampsia, appendicitis), approximate fundal height (estimate gestational age). Are there fetal heart tones (IUP vs early pregnancy, threatened abortion, fetal demise), and what is the fetal rate (fetal distress).
6. **Back.** Flank tenderness (pyelonephritis, pneumonia).
7. **Pelvic.** (Avoid if greater than 20 weeks AND vaginal bleeding (r/o placenta previa first!) Identify source of vaginal bleeding (from the os, or from a laceration/trauma). Is the cervical os open or closed? Is tissue present? (If so, send for POC) Is there adnexal tenderness or a mass (ectopic or appendicitis)? Are there fetal parts presenting? What is the fetal presentation (breech, etc)?
8. **Extremities.** Check for edema, tenderness, asymmetry (preeclampsia, DVT, heart failure).
9. **Neurologic.** Are there global or focal deficits, or is there seizure activity? (Seizure, eclampsia, subarachnoid hemorrhage).

B. Laboratory Data.
In general, depends on clinical suspicion, gestational age, history, and physical exam. Consider type and Rh or T&C, CBC, LFTs, coagulation rates, UA and culture, quantitative β-HCG, Lytes, cardiac enzymes, and D-dimer.

C. Radiographic and Other Studies

1. **Pelvic US** if first trimester pelvic pain or bleeding, to evaluate for ectopic (mass, free fluid in the pelvis), threatened/completed abortion, retained POC.
2. **Abdominal US** if second or third trimester pregnancy with significant abdominal pain, vaginal bleeding, or absent fetal heart tones to evaluate for placental abruption, placenta previa, uterine rupture or fetal demise. Any trimester for cholecystitis, appendicitis, HELLP.
3. **Head CT** (no contrast) if coma, altered mentation, seizure, or abnormal neurologic exam, to evaluate for intracranial hemorrhage.
4. **ECG** if considering PE, eclampsia, cardiogenic pulmonary edema.

5. **Doppler** ("duplex") US of the lower extremities to evaluate for DVT.
6. **CXR** (with abdominal shielding) for PE (cardiogenic vs non-cardiogenic) or crackles or wheezing (pneumonia).
7. **V/Q scan** (or spiral CT scan of chest) if considering PE. Often not necessary if positive DVT study (similar treatment).

V. Plan

A. **Overall Plan.** Fetal well-being depends on adequate maternal diagnosis and treatment. Gestations of less than 20 weeks are considered nonviable outside the uterus, thus gestational age greater or less than 20 weeks often determines specific management. In trauma, work-up and treat as nonpregnant first, with radiographic studies as needed. Obtain a concurrent OB consult if greater than 20 weeks, and consider admission for fetal monitoring even if no maternal injury is apparent.

B. **Specific Plans**
1. **Ectopic pregnancy.** T&C, good IV access, stat OB/GYN consult.
2. **Threatened abortion.** May discharge home, threatened abortion instructions, follow-up within 48 h.
3. **Spontaneous abortion.** Tissue to pathology for POC, may discharge home, OB follow-up 48–72 h.
4. **Molar pregnancy.** OB consult.
5. **Placental abruption.** Stat OB consult.
6. **Placenta previa.** Stat OB consult.
7. **Preeclampsia.** Control BP, stat OB consult.
8. **Eclampsia.** Load with magnesium (4 g IV) to terminate seizures, add benzodiazepines as needed, control BP, intubate if indicated, rule out intracranial hemorrhage, admit. May need emergent delivery.
9. **Intracranial hemorrhage.** Control BP, intubate if indicated, admit.
10. **Seizure.** During first trimester, work up and treat as seizure in nonpregnant patient. Consult OB. second–third trimester, treat as eclampsia.
11. **Pneumonia.** Oxygen, blood cultures, IV antibiotics, consult OB. If discharged home, requires close follow-up.
12. **PE.** IV heparin, pain medication, oxygen, admit.
13. **Noncardiac PE.** Treat underlying cause, intubate if indicated, admit.
14. **Peripartum cardiomyopathy.** Treat as in nonpregnant heart failure. Stat OB and cardiology consults, admit.
15. **Hyperemesis gravidarum.** IV hydration, antiemetics, may discharge home with close OB follow-up if symptoms resolve and urine is cleared of ketones.
16. **UTI/pyelonephritis.** Treat even asymptomatic bacteriuria (untreated increases the risk of spontaneous abortion/preterm labor). Consider admission if pyelonephritis.

17. **HELLP syndrome.** OB consult, antiemetics, pain medication, admit.
18. **Appendicitis.** Surgical/OB consults, antibiotics, admit.
19. **Cholecystitis.** Surgical/OB consults, antibiotics, admit.
20. **Preterm labor.** OB consult.
21. **Pregnancy-induced diabetes.** OB consult.
22. **Pregnancy-induced HTN.** OB consult.
23. **DVT.** Treat like PE.
24. **Fetal demise.** OB consult. May discharge home with OB follow-up within 72 h for induction/delivery.

VI. **ICD-9 Diagnoses:** Ectopic pregnancy (state site if known); Pregnancy complicated by \\ (list disease state, ie, diabetes); Hyperemesis gravidarum; Placental abruption; Placenta previa; Preeclampsia; Pyelonephritis; Threatened abortion.

VII. **Problem Case Diagnosis:** Ectopic pregnancy.

VIII. **Teaching Pearl Question:** What is the most common cause of death from eclampsia?

IX. **Teaching Pearl Answer:** Intracranial hemorrhage.

REFERENCES

Duley L, Henderson-Smart D. Magnesium sulphate versus diazepam for eclampsia. *Cochrane Database Syst Rev* 2000;(2):CD000127.

Duley L, Henderson-Smart D. Magnesium sulphate versus phenytoin for eclampsia. *Cochrane Database Syst Rev* 2000;(2):CD000128.

McGregor JA, French JI, Richter R, Franco-Buff A, Johnson A, Hillier S, et al. Antenatal microbiologic and maternal risk factors associated with prematurity. *Am J Obstet Gynecol* 1990;163(5 Pt 1):1465–1473.

Munro PT. Management of eclampsia in the accident and emergency department. *J Accid Emerg Med* 2000;17(1):7–11.

Ros HS, Lichtenstein P, Bellocco R, Petersson G, Cnattingius S. Pulmonary embolism and stroke in relation to pregnancy: How can high-risk women be identified? *Am J Obstet Gynecol* 2002;186(2):198–203.

57. PSYCHIATRIC PROBLEMS

I. **Problem:** A 20-year-old male is brought to the ED by police after being called to residence because the man was "acting weird" and talking to himself

II. **Immediate Questions**
   A. **Primary survey?** Hypoxia, trauma, exposure, environment found in.
   B. **Vital signs?** Hypothermia/hyperthermia, hypotension/HTN.
   C. **Timing of symptoms?** If acute onset, age < 12 or > 40, decreased LOC, postexposure to toxin, think of medical illness vs functional illness.

    D. Any past medical history? Previous psychiatric diagnosis? New meds (esp. anticholinergic/benzodiazepines)? Alcohol/drugs? DM? STD? Seizures?

III. Differential Diagnosis
    A. Infectious. Meningitis, encephalitis, neurosyphilis, hepatitis.
    B. Metabolic. Electrolyte abnormalities (hypoglycemia/hyperglycemia, hyponatremia, uremia), hypothyroidism/hyperthyroidism.
    C. Neurologic. Seizure (prolonged postictal, complex partial), trauma (bleeds [SDH, EDH, SAH], concussive syndrome), CVA, HTN, encephalopathy.
    D. Toxicologic. Illicit drugs (phencyclidine, mescaline, amphetamines), anticholinergics (diphenhydramine), alcohol withdrawal.
    E. Psychiatric. Psychosis, delirium, mood disorder.

IV. Database
    A. Physical Exam Key Points
        1. Vital signs. Address any abnormalities carefully.
        2. Mental status. Mini-mental status exam (See Table A-4, page 656.).
        3. General appearance. Personal hygiene, response to environment (agitation, confusion), rash (syphilis, meningococcemia).
        4. Neurologic exam. Pupil reactivity (CVA, drugs, SDH, EDH), focal deficits (CVA), meningismus, hallucinations (tactile/visual/olfactory = medical, auditory = psych).
    B. Laboratory Data
        1. If previous psych history, negative ROS, normal PE and vital signs, no ancillary testing necessary. Psych consult for stabilization of disorder.
        2. If new onset of symptoms, negative ROS, NL PE/VS, negative PMH: UDS, ABG, CBC, BMP, alcohol, LFTs, and CT+/-LP.
    C. Radiographic and Other Studies. Other studies indicated by H&P, TFTs, PT/PTT, RPR, HIV, ammonia.

V. Plan
    A. Overall Plan. Correct all abnormal vital signs and lab abnormalities. Maintain patient in a safe environment.
    B. Specific Plans
        1. Infectious. Appropriate antibiotics and admit.
        2. Metabolic. Treat accordingly to normalize.
        3. Neurologic. If known seizure disorder and mental status clears may discharge. CVA, trauma with altered mental status, HTN encephalopathy should be admitted.
        4. Toxicologic. Observation for agents that clear. Benzodiazepines for sedation, antidotes for specific ingestions. DT admit.
        5. Psychiatric. Consultation and joint decision for inpatient vs outpatient management.

VI. **ICD-9 Diagnoses:** Acute psychosis; Anorexia nervosa; Bipolar disorder; Generalized anxiety disorder; Panic disorder; Schizophrenia (chronic, acute exacerbation, remission); Somatization disorder; Suicidal risk.

VII. **Problem Case Diagnosis:** Acute psychosis secondary to new-onset schizophrenia

VIII. **Teaching Pearl Question:** Describe the typical presentation of anticholinergic delirium.

IX. **Teaching Pearl Answer:** Mad as a hatter (delirium/hallucinations), hot as a hare (hyperpyrexia), dry as a bone (dry mouth/anhydrosis), blind as a bat (blurred vision), plugged as a pig (urinary retention/constipation), and fast as a fibrillation (tachycardia) (Lagomasino, et al).

REFERENCES

Korn CS, Currier GW, Henderson SO. "Medical clearance" of psychiatric patients without medical complaints in the emergency department. *J Emerg Med* 2000;18(2):173–176.

Lagomasino I, Daly R, Stoudemire A. Medical assessment of patients presenting with psychiatric symptoms in the emergency setting. *Psych Clin North Am* 1999;22(4):819–850.

Olshaker JS, Browne B, Jerrard DA, Prendergast H, Stair TO. Medical clearance and screening of psychiatric patients in the emergency department. *Acad Emerg Med* 1997;4(2):124–128.

Reeves RR, Pendarvis EJ, Kimble R. Unrecognized medical emergencies admitted to psychiatric units. *Am J Emerg Med* 2000;18(4):390–393.

58. RESPIRATORY DISTRESS

I. **Problem:** One day after having her hip surgically repaired, an elderly female *suddenly* feels short of breath.

II. **Immediate Questions**
   A. **How sudden is sudden?** Hours? Minutes? (key to estimating prior probabilities of the diagnostic alternatives).
   B. **Is the airway intact?** Clear, establish, and maintain (See Section VIII, 15. Rapid Sequence Endotracheal Intubation, page 470.).
   C. **What are the vitals and mental status?** Is the patient normocardic, normotensive, normocapnic, afebrile, and alert? Initiate cardiac and oximetry monitoring; Intravenous line, and oxygen. Is the patient hypotensive, confused, or cyanotic? Is the cardiac rhythm abnormal?

III. **Differential Diagnosis**
   A. **Obstructive.** Consider foreign body, anaphylaxis, infectious causes (consular/submandibular/retropharyngeal abscess, epiglottis, glossitis), expanding hematoma, angioedema, burn, vocal cord paralysis.
   B. **Pulmonary.** PE, fat or air embolus, pneumothorax (esp. tension), hemothorax, COPD, asthma, flail chest, diaphragmatic rupture.

    C. Cardiac. Atypical presentation AMI, acute cardiac failure, dysrhythmias, acute cardiac tamponade, myocarditis, valvular disorder.

    D. Abdominal. Hemoperitoneum, ascites, mass.

    E. Other. Neuromuscular, anxiety, toxicity, hiccups, increased intracranial pressure.

IV. Database

  A. Physical Exam Key Points. Quickly assess for use of secondary respiratory muscles, retractions, nasal flaring, and cyanosis.

    1. Mental status. Is the patient able to speak sentences, phrases, words, or not at all? If patient becomes unconscious, GCS < 8, no longer able to protect airway, or fatiguing—consider intubation. (See Section VIII, 15. Rapid Sequence Endotracheal Intubation, page 470.)

    2. Vital signs. Reevaluate at regular intervals.

    3. HEENT. Is the patient able to clear secretions? Deviated uvula or asymmetry (abscess), perioral or lingual swelling (angioedema), tracheal deviation (mass effect vs tension pneumothorax), presence of JVD (tension pneumothorax, PE, or cardiac tamponade). Examine for singed nasal hairs or carbonaceous sputum (burns).

    4. Chest wall. Look for flail chest segment and penetrating trauma. (Examine *front and back!*)

    5. Lungs. Do both sides of the chest expand and contract symmetrically? Are breath sounds present and equal? Bilateral absence suggests complete upper airway obstruction, whereas unilateral breath sounds suggests pneumothorax. Quality? If too shallow, may suggest fatigue. Dull to percussion (hemothorax or empyema). Listen for bowel sounds in chest (ruptured diaphragm).

    6. Heart sounds. Distant heart sounds suggest cardiac tamponade or pericarditis. **Beck's triad:** JVD, distant heart sounds, hypotension.

  B. Laboratory Data. ABG will identify hypoxemia and hyperventilation/hypoventilation, underlying acid–base disorder. Consider D-dimer.

  C. Radiographic and Other Studies. CXR is essential. ECG to look for diffuse ST segment elevation (pericarditis). The most common finding on ECG for PE is tachycardia and < 15% have the classic $S_1Q_3T_3$. Chest CT, V/Q scan, angiography, MRI, Doppler US of lower extremities are selected based on results of the initial evaluation, CXR, and ABG results.

V. Plan

  A. Overall Plan. Supplemental oxygen, maintain airway, identify underlying cause.

  B. Specific Plans

    1. Oropharyngeal abscess. Avoid laryngospasm by minimizing airway manipulation. Begin IV antibiotics (no steroids.) Incision and drainage if cooperative patient and necessary equipment available.

    2. Foreign body. No blind finger sweeps. Bronchoscopy.

3. **PE.** If no contraindications begin anticoagulation with heparin (80 U/kg bolus followed by 18 U/kg/h). Goal aPTT of 50–90 s. Emergency thrombolytics are considered in the patient with proven diagnosis and acute shock or in high suspicion when signs of right-heart failure (as diagnosed by CVP, echo, ECG) are present. Benefit of thrombolysis achieved up to 2 weeks in stable patients. If anticoagulation contraindicated consider inferior vena cava filter.

4. **Pneumothorax/hemothorax.** Place chest tube. Tension pneumothorax may be temporarily decompressed with 18 G needle.

5. **Cardiac tamponade.** Needle decompression followed by surgical consult for pericardial window.

6. **Burns.** Have a low threshold for intubation because swelling will progress.

VI. **ICD-9 Diagnoses:** Acute myocardial infarction (state which wall); Acute pulmonary edema; Acute respiratory distress; Anaphylaxis; Asthma exacerbation; Hypoxia; Pneumonia; Pneumothorax; Pulmonary embolus.

VII. **Problem Case Diagnosis:** Pulmonary embolism.

VIII. **Teaching Pearl Question:** What is the typical presentation for PE?

IX. **Teaching Pearl Answer:** There is no typical presentation for PE. The classic triad of dyspnea, hemoptysis, and pleuritic chest pain occurs in less than 20 % of patients.

REFERENCES

Goldhaber SZ. Pulmonary embolism. *N Engl J Med* 1998;339(2):93–104.

Valenzuela T, Croghan M. Pulmonary embolism. In: Harwood-Nuss A, Luten R, Shepherd S, Wolfson A, eds. *The Clinical Practice of Emergency Medicine.* 2nd ed. Lippincott-Raven Publishers, 1996:148–165.

Shoenfeld CN. Pulmonary embolism. In: Tintinalli JE, Kelen GD, Stapczynski JS, eds. *Emergency Medicine: A Comprehensive Study Guide.* 5th ed. McGraw-Hill, 2000: 396–401.

59. SCROTAL PROBLEMS

I. **Problem:** A 35-year-old man presents with a swollen scrotum, which was first noticed 6 h ago.

II. **Immediate Questions**
   A. **Does he have scrotal pain?**
   B. **Recent trauma?**
   C. **Fever?**
   D. **Urinary symptoms, urethral discharge?**
   E. **Genital lesions?**
   F. **History of similar symptoms? STD, anal intercourse?**
   G. **Testicular emergency probable?** Yes. Consult a urologist **immediately,** even before a scrotal US is done.

III. Differential Diagnosis: (85–90% of acute scrotal pain is due to the first 3 diagnoses)

A. Testicular Torsion. Testis twists on the spermatic cord within the tunica vaginalis. Risks include trauma, exercise, sexual activity, cryptorchidism, age 12–16 years old, a redundant cord resulting in a dangling testis (bell-clapper deformity) in a horizontal lie, a history of similar pain that resolved spontaneously (41%), and right testis (71%). Complications include testicular infarction, necrosis, and infertility. Testis salvage rate drops to < 70% at 6 h.

B. Intrascrotal Appendageal Torsion. A piece of tissue protruding from the testis (92%) or epididymis (8%) twists on itself. Primary cause of scrotal pain in patients 3–13 years old.

C. Epididymitis. Bacterial (from STDs, prostatitis, or stool) or noninfectious (amiodarone, systemic diseases, or retrograde reflux of sterile urine) inflammation of the epididymis. Complications include orchitis, intrascrotal abscess, infertility, testicular infarction, and chronic pain.

D. Orchitis. Infection of the testis due to bacterial epididymitis, mumps, other viruses, TB, fungi, and syphilis. Complications include infertility.

E. Scrotal Abscess. Superficial (benign) or intrascrotal (emergent).

F. Varicocele. Painless dilated pampiniform plexus veins of the spermatic cord due to retrograde renal venous blood flow. 90% in the left scrotum. Causes 40% of infertility.

G. Spermatocele. Painless sperm-containing retention cyst of the epididymis or rete testis.

H. Testicular Tumor. Most common cancer in males 20–34 years old. Risk factors include right testis and cryptorchidism.

I. Inguinal Hernia. Complications include incarceration resulting in bowel obstruction; strangulation resulting in ischemia, necrosis; and perforation resulting in peritonitis, abscess, and/or sepsis.

J. Testicular Trauma. Can cause contusion (intact parietal tunica vaginalis) or disruption of the parietal tunica vaginalis, causing a laceration, fracture (incomplete rupture), complete rupture, amputation, or dislocation (testis displaced outside of scrotum, 80% into the abdomen). Complications include hematocele (blood in tunica vaginalis) and loss of testis.

K. Fournier's Gangrene. Bacterial perineal necrotic infection. Risks include perineal trauma, age 20–50 years old, and immunocompromised. 5–10% mortality rate.

L. Urethral Phlegmon. Urethral extravasation of infected urine due to urethral stricture or trauma, causing skin necrosis, scrotal infection, and cephalad extension.

IV. Database

A. Physical Exam Key Points

1. **Thorough exam.** Scrotum, testicles (normally align vertically), epididymis, spermatic cords, penile shaft, glans, meatus, prostate, and inguinal regions.

2. **Transillumination.** Place a bright light near the scrotum in a dark room. Tumors don't pass light and are dark. Hydroceles transmit light, appear red, and are due to an imbalance in the secretory and absorptive capacities of the parietal and visceral layers of the tunica vaginalis.
3. **Cremasteric reflex.** The testicle rises > 0.5 cm when stroking the ipsilateral inner thigh.
4. **Prehn's sign.** Elevating the testicle improves the pain. Is unreliable.
5. **Dresner's sign.** Scrotal blue dot due to intrascrotal appendageal torsion.
6. **Specific exam findings**
   a. **Testicular torsion.** Scrotal tenderness, edema and erythema; high-riding testis in horizontal lie; fever (20%); hydrocele; absent cremasteric reflex; and/or negative Prehn's sign.
   b. **Intrascrotal appendageal torsion.** Scrotal erythema and edema; tender pea-sized nodule of anterosuperior testis; Dresner's sign; and/or hydrocele.
   c. **Epididymitis.** Epididymal tenderness, swelling, and induration of posterosuperior testis; fever (95%); urethral discharge; positive cremasteric reflex; and/or positive Prehn's sign.
   d. **Orchitis.** Testicular swelling and tenderness; usually with fever.
   e. **Scrotal abscess.** Superficial or intrascrotal fluctuance, tenderness, erythema, and swelling.
   f. **Varicocele.** Soft mass or swelling (collapsible "bag of worms") superior to testis that fluctuates in size (increases when standing or straining, and decreases when supine).
   g. **Spermatocele.** Mobile, small (< 1 cm), transilluminable mass that doesn't fluctuate in size.
   h. **Testicular tumor.** Firm distinct mass.
   i. **Inguinal hernia.** Mass in inguinal ring, which can fluctuate in size, transilluminates minimally, and usually is reducible.
   j. **Testicular trauma.** Scrotal tenderness, ecchymosis, and swelling; and/or hematocele.
   k. **Fournier's gangrene.** Perineal swelling, edema, necrosis, gangrene, crepitus, and/or subcutaneous emphysema.
   l. **Urethral phlegmon.** Scrotal swelling/edema; urinary retention; and/or overflow incontinence.
B. **Laboratory Data.** *Urethral culture:* For GC/*Chlamydia* (before UA obtained). UA and culture. Sterile pyuria is present in 24% of testicular torsions. Bacteriuria is frequently seen in epididymitis. *Wound culture:* For Fournier's gangrene and intrascrotal abscess.
C. **Radiographic and Other Studies.** *Scrotal Doppler US:* Decreased pulsatile blood flow in testicular torsion, and increased pulsatile blood flow in epididymitis. Don't permit studies to delay time to surgery if testicular torsion is clinically obvious ("avoid castration by procrastination"). If diagnosis of epididymitis isn't definitive clinically, get US to rule out testicular torsion.

V. Plan

    A. Overall Plan. Do NOT miss or delay referring a testicular torsion!

    B. Specific Plans

        1. **Testicular torsion.** Immediate urologic consultation, IV analgesics, scrotum ice packing to increase salvage rate, emergent manual (via external rotation) or surgical detorsion, and emergent bilateral orchiopexy.

        2. **Intrascrotal appendageal torsion.** Bed rest, scrotal elevation, analgesics, anticipate calcification or degeneration in 10–14 days, and rarely surgery.

        3. **Epididymitis.** Antibiotics, bed rest, scrotal elevation, ice packs, analgesics, sitz baths, stool softeners, athletic supporter when ambulating, and STD education/testing.

        4. **Orchitis.** Antibiotics and other measures used in epididymitis.

        5. **Scrotal abscess.** I&D if superficial; emergent surgical debridement if intrascrotal.

        6. **Varicocele.** Surgical removal if severe, low sperm count, or testicular atrophy.

        7. **Spermatocele.** Usually no treatment needed.

        8. **Inguinal hernia.** Manual reduction and elective herniorrhaphy if not incarcerated or strangulated; otherwise emergent herniorrhaphy.

        9. **Testicular trauma.** Emergent surgery if the parietal tunica vaginalis is disrupted.

      10. **Fournier's gangrene.** Emergent surgical debridement, suprapubic catheter, IV antibiotics, aggressive IV fluid, and hyperbaric oxygen.

      11. **Urethral phlegmon.** Antibiotics, surgical debridement, and suprapubic catheter.

      12. **Tumors.** Urologic referral.

VI. ICD-9 Diagnoses. Acute epididymitis; Cryptorchidism; Fournier's gangrene; Hydrocele; Inguinal hernia; Neoplasm; Orchitis; Torsion of appendix epididymis or testicle; Varicocele.

VII. Problem Case Diagnosis: Epididymitis.

VIII. Teaching Pearl Question: What role does a serum WBC have in distinguishing testicular torsion from epididymitis?

IX. Teaching Pearl Answer: Not much help, as up to 50–60% of patients with testicular torsion will have leukocytosis.

REFERENCES

Lindsey D, Stanisic TH. Diagnosis and management of testicular torsion: Pitfalls and perils. *Am J Emerg Med* 1988;6:42–46.

Paltiel HJ, Connolly LP, Atala A, Paltiel AD, Zurakowski D, Treves ST. Acute scrotal symptoms in boys with an indeterminate clinical presentation: Comparison of color Doppler sonography and scintigraphy. *Radiology* 1998;207:223–231.

60. SEIZURE

I. **Problem:** A 50-year-old man was observed to have a grand mal seizure while waiting in line to purchase a bottle of wine at the local liquor store.

II. **Immediate Questions**
   A. **Is the airway intact?**
   B. **What are the vital signs and mental status?** Initiate IV, place on pulse ox, cardiac monitor, and oxygen. Cardiac arrhythmias, hypoxemia, and focal neurologic deficits offer a clue as to cause.
   C. **Is there a cervical spine injury as a result of the seizure?**
   D. **What was he doing before, during, and after seizure?** Is there a possible traumatic injury? Was there an aura, loss of consciousness, tongue biting or incontinence? Was there a post-ictal phase?
   E. **What type of seizure was it?** Focal versus generalized?
   F. **Previous history of seizures?** Antiseizure medication.
   G. **Recent traumatic head injury?**
   H. **History of illicit drug or alcohol use?**
   I. **Recent headaches, vomiting, or febrile illness?** May indicate underlying undiagnosed CNS neoplasm, meningitis, and encephalitis.
   J. **Is this status epilepticus?** Defined as persistent seizures for at least 30 min or recurrent seizures without return to baseline mental status in between episodes.

III. **Differential Diagnosis**
   A. **Hypoxia.** Consider causes for respiratory failure including fire and suicide attempt because when the carboxyhemoglobin concentration is greater than 50%, seizures are likely to occur.
   B. **Hypoglycemia.** Hypoglycemia is the most common metabolic cause of seizure.
   C. **Cardiac Dysrhythmias.** Ventricular fibrillation causes hypoxic encephalopathy leading to seizures.
   D. **Intracranial Hemorrhage.** Seizures occur in 16% of patients within cerebrovascular events.
   E. **Tumor.** Approximately 30% of brain tumors present as a first-time seizure.
   F. **Trauma.** Traumatic head injuries.
   G. **Infection.** Meningitis, cerebral abscesses, and viral meningitis are all associated with seizures. In the southwestern United States as well as in developing countries, consider neurocysticercosis. In patients with HIV, consider toxoplasmosis as well as cryptococcal meningitis.
   H. **Metabolic.** Hypoglycemia, hyponatremia or hypernatremia, hypocalcemia or hypercalcemia should be considered. Hypomagnesemia causes seizures especially in alcoholics. Uremia causes seizures occurring 2–3 days after the patient becomes anuric.
   I. **Drugs/Toxins.** Consider cyanide, TCAs, meperidine, penicillin, theophylline, methanol, isoniazid, and ethylene glycol. Lead poisoning should be considered in children and mercury poisoning in adults.

Also consider cocaine, amphetamines, heroin, and methylenedioxy-methamphetamine (MDMA - "ecstasy"). (See Section V, 12. Designer Drug Overdose, page 348.)

J. Alcohol. Alcohol withdrawal seizures occur between 6 h and 7 days after the cessation of alcohol ingestion.

K. Fever. Lowers the seizure threshold in children.
1. Simple febrile seizures: less than 15 min.
2. Complex febrile seizures: longer than 15 min.

L. Pregnancy. Eclampsia

M. Epilepsy

N. Pseudoseizures. Injuries, incontinence, tongue biting, and postictal period rare.

IV. **Database**
   A. **Physical Exam Key Points.** Don't forget to consider associated injuries from possible fall.
      1. **Vital signs.** Vital signs including temperature and pulse ox.
      2. **HEENT.** Check for signs of trauma, eg, possible contusions, lacerations, "raccoon eyes," or Battle's sign. Check for hemotympanum as well as for otitis media. Extraocular motions, reactive pupils, and optic discs. Tongue lacerations should be documented, and gingival hyperplasia may suggest that the patient is taking phenytoin.
      3. **Neck.** The cervical spine should be palpated for possible injury, including tenderness, crepitus or stepoffs. Also assess the neck for signs of meningismus and carotid bruits.
      4. **Chest.** Look for signs of trauma, including subcutaneous emphysema. Also, auscultation may yield evidence of rales, rhonchi, or other evidence of pulmonary disease.
      5. **Cardiovascular.** Check for AF, murmurs, or rubs.
      6. **Spine.** The patient should be rolled, maintaining cervical, thoracic, and lumbar spine precautions, because vertebral compression fractures are associated with seizure.
      7. **Extremities.** Examine the extremities for any evidence of trauma. Seizure is the most common cause of posterior shoulder dislocation.
      8. **Neurologic examination.** Needs to be repeated several times as the patient recovers from their postictal period. Check for focal deficit that may indicate a structural lesion in the brain. A reliable neurologic exam cannot be obtained in a patient younger than 18 months of age. Also note that some patients with epilepsy experience a Todd's paralysis during the postictal phase, which is a temporary focal deficit usually consisting of a hemiparesis, aphasia, or a facial droop. This typically resolves in less than 24 h but occasionally lasts several days.
         a. **Mental status examination.**
         b. **Cranial nerve function.**
         c. **Motor strength in all four extremities.**

      d. **Reflexes.**

      e. **Sensory examination.**

      f. **Cerebellar function.**

      g. **Gait and stance.**

B. Laboratory Data. Consider hypoglycemia and hypoxemia immediately. Bedside glucose, Lytes, magnesium, and calcium. Based on the history consider CBC, toxicology screen, anticonvulsant levels, and urine pregnancy. Consider prolactin level if pseudoseizures likely. In children younger than 18 months of age, an adequate neurologic assessment is difficult and a more thorough evaluation is required including LP.

C. Radiographic and Other Studies. Based on physical exam, consider CT of head, cervical, thoracic, lumbar spine series if indicated, possible shoulder series to evaluate for dislocation, ECG and LP. Consider possible MRI or EEG.

V. Plan

A. Overall Plan

1. **Admit**

    a. Status epilepticus.

    b. Seizures secondary to infectious cause.

    c. New-onset seizures in patients older than 50 years.

    d. Eclampsia.

    e. Seizures due to intracranial hemorrhage or tumor.

    f. Seizures due to hypoxia, hyponatremia, hypoglycemia, cardiac dysrhythmias, or drug toxicity.

2. **Discharge.** Patients with a known seizure disorder and subtherapeutic drug levels.

3. **Neurology consult**

    a. All admitted patients.

    b. Patients with new-onset seizures.

    c. Breakthrough seizures in a patient with therapeutic anticonvulsant drug levels.

B. Specific Plan

1. **Airway control.** IV, oxygen, glucose.

2. **Seizure control.** Benzodiazepines are first-line drugs of choice.

    a. **Benzodiazepines.** Lorazepam (2–10 mg IV) or diazepam (5–20 mg IV). Midazolam can be used and is rapidly absorbed IM, PR, as well as IV.

    b. **Fosphenytoin.** Loading dose is 18 mg/kg and can be given at 150 mg/min. Watch for hypotension. Can be given IM.

    c. **Phenytoin.** Loading dose is 10–20 mg/kg IV no faster than 50 mg/min. *Adult oral load suggestion:* 400 mg initially, then 300 mg at 2 h and then 4 h post (1000 mg total).

    d. **Phenobarbital.** Loading dose is 20 mg/kg and can be given at 100 mg/min. Watch for sedation, respiratory depression, and hypotension, which may require endotracheal intubation.

      e. Pentobarbital. Usually reserved for refractory cases of status epilepticus. Endotracheal intubation is usually required as the amount of respiratory depression is quite significant. In addition, all motor activity is suppressed so continuous EEG monitoring is required to determine when the seizure activity is halted. The loading dose is 5 mg/kg at 50 mg/min followed by a continuous infusion of 0.5–3 mg/kg/h. Hypotension is common and may require vasopressors.

VI. ICD-9 Diagnosis: Seizure; Drug/narcotic withdrawal; Dysrhythmia; Epilepsy; Focal/partial seizure; Pseudoseizure; Status epilepticus; Syncope; Todd's paralysis; Intoxication (state substance).

VII. Problem Case Diagnosis: Alcohol withdrawal seizure.

VIII. Teaching Pearl Question: What percent of the general population will have a seizure in their lifetime?

IX. Teaching Pearl Answer: 10%.

REFERENCES

American College of Emergency Physicians: Clinical policy for the initial approach to patients with a chief complaint of seizure that are not in status epilepticus. *Ann Emerg Med* 1997;29.706–724.

American College of Emergency Physicians: Practice Parameter: Neuroimaging in the emergency patient presenting with seizure (summary statement). *Ann Emerg Med* 1996;28:114–118.

Bradford JC, Kyriakedes CG. Evidence based emergency medicine evaluation and diagnostic testing: Evaluation of the patient with seizures: An evidence based approach. *Emerg Med Clin North Am* 1999;17(1):1–20.

Roth HL, Drislane FW. Neurologic emergencies: Seizures. *Neurol Clin* 1998;16(2):1–33.

61. SEPSIS

I. Problem: Elderly male presents with fever, confusion, tachycardia, hypotension.

II. Immediate Questions

    A. Primary survey. Check ABCs. Are there diminished pulses or other signs of poor peripheral perfusion?

    B. What are the vitals and mental status? Is the patient stable and alert? Apply monitors (cardiac and pulse ox), start IV, apply oxygen.

    C. Generalized signs and symptoms. Hyperthermia or hypothermia, tachycardia, tachypnea, initially warm, hyperperfused periphery (warm sepsis) then as hypotension develops, signs of poor peripheral perfusion develop such as cool extremities, poor capillary refill, confusion, decreased urine output (cold sepsis).

D. **Was their any history of specific localizing complaints?**
Clues that can lead to identifying the source of the septic infection include:
1. **Pulmonary.** Cough, dyspnea, tachypnea, pleuritic chest pain, sputum production, or hemoptysis.
2. **Genitourinary.** Dysuria, frequency, urgency, hematuria, abdominal pain, flank pain, vomiting. History of urinary catheterization. History of prostate disease. Recent pregnancy or abortion. Testicular/vulvar or perineal pain and swelling.
3. **CNS.** Headache, meningismus, confusion, coma, recent adjacent infection such as otitis media or sinusitis.
4. **GI/Intra-abdominal.** Abdominal pain, vomiting, anorexia, stool changes, jaundice.
5. **Skin.** Recent trauma or burns, cellulitis, abscesses, decubitus ulcers, rashes such as petechiae. History of IV drug use.
6. **Cardiovascular.** Chest pain, CHF complaints, peripheral embolization signs such as Osler's nodes, splinter hemorrhages. History of known congenital or acquired cardiac defects, prosthetic valves, IV drug use.
7. **Musculoskeletal.** Localized swelling, pain, and warmth over affected joints, muscles, or bones. History of recent penetrating trauma, especially open fractures. History of surgery or prosthetic joints.
E. **Any past medical history?** Besides the preceding specific conditions, any disorders that cause immunosuppression, eg, HIV, diabetes, autoimmune disorders, malignancies.
F. **Medications?** Immunosuppressive medications, eg, corticosteroids, methotrexate, antirejection medications, chemotherapy.

III. **Differential Diagnosis**
A. **Sepsis**
B. **Thyrotoxicosis**
C. **Addison's Disease**

IV. **Database**
A. **Physical Exam Key Points**
1. **Mental status.** Mini mental status exam. (See Table A-4, page 656.)
2. **Vital signs.** Check carefully and repeat during evaluation.
3. **Skin.** Check for rashes, petechiae, wound infections, cellulitis, or lymphangitis. Line sites.
4. **HEENT.** Often the initial infection will be present here, eg, otitis media, sinusitis, dental sources.
5. **Neck.** Examine for nuchal rigidity, lymphadenopathy
6. **Lung sounds.** Acute respiratory distress, localized wheezing, rhonchi or rales, tachypnea, cough
7. **Heart sounds.** Tachycardia, new or changed murmurs indicative of endocarditis

8. **Abdomen.** Abdominal tenderness that may localize source, eg, RLQ pain suggestive of appendicitis, LLQ pain characteristic for diverticulitis, etc.

9. **Genitourinary.** Suprapubic or flank tenderness. Vaginal discharge or bleeding. Testicular/vulvar and peritoneal pain with subcutaneous air.

10. **Musculoskeletal.** Examine for focal redness, swelling, tenderness, crepitance, or joint swelling.

11. **Neurologic exam.** Mental status changes with confusion, delirium. or coma.

B. **Laboratory Data**

1. **Blood.** CBC with Diff, focused chemistry tests based on exam, blood cultures from two separate sites, Lactate, ABG.

2. **Urine.** UA with culture.

3. **CSF.** *Tube 1:* Cell count and Diff; *Tube 2:* Protein and glucose; *Tube 3:* Culture and Gram's stain; *Tube 4:* Repeat cell count, viral, and fungal studies.

4. **Sputum.** Culture and Gram's stain.

5. **Wound drainage.** Culture and Gram's stain.

C. **Radiographic and Other Studies.** CXR, US of abdomen/pelvis, CT scan of abdomen/pelvis or localized area or concern.

V. **Plan**

A. **Overall Plan.** Identify source of sepsis, collect cultures expeditiously, and immediately start supportive measures, eg, airway protection, ventilatory support, and BP support. Start antibiotics as soon as appropriate.

B. **Specific Plans**

1. **Airway.** Indications include need for ventilatory support or airway compromise. Keep O_2 sats > 95% to maximize O_2 delivery to tissues.

2. **Breathing.** Sepsis is the most common cause of ARDS. Initial therapy for ARDS is mechanical ventilation with high-flow oxygen and PEEP with optimal levels in the 10–15 cm H_2O range. This may decrease cardiac output and can cause barotrauma.

3. **IV Fluids**

   a. Initially these patients will require large amounts of isotonic crystalloids, eg, NS or RL. Fluid resuscitation should be guided by vital signs, repeat exams, and clinical course. If the patient is to be spending significant time in the ED, invasive monitoring may be necessary, eg, CVP or right-heart catheterization.

4. **Transfusion** may be necessary in some patients. Maintain hemoglobin at 10–12 g/dL.

5. **Pressors.** If volume resuscitation does not seem to be sufficient to maintain perfusion, then vasoactive pressors may be indicated. Clinical indications include very low initial MAP or a persistently low MAP (< 60–65 mm Hg) after adequate fluid resuscitation.

6. **Dopamine.** Conventional teaching is for progressive levels of dopamine dosing, starting from 1–5 μg/kg/min dopaminergic receptors predominate (renal dose); 5–10 μg/kg/min β-adrenergic effects; 10–20 α/β-adrenergic effects; > 20 predominantly α-adrenergic effects. New data indicate little conclusive evidence for renal dosing of dopamine.

7. **Norepinephrine.** Recent evidence indicates that norepinephrine is superior to other vasopressors in maintaining splanchnic blood flow and improving refractory hypotension and oliguria. Dosing range is 5–20 μg/min.

8. **Phenylephrine.** This is a selective α_1-adrenergic agonist that provides specific vasoconstriction without inotropic effect or increasing heart rate. It may be a good choice when tachyarrhythmias limit use of other vasopressors. Dosing range is 5–20 μg/min.

9. **Surgical intervention.** Abscesses, intraabdominal causes, septic joints, necrotizing fasciitis all will need to be addressed surgically after initial stabilization.

10. **ICU admission.** All nonsurgical cases of sepsis will need ICU admission.

VI. **ICD-9 Diagnosis:** Adrenal insufficiency; Anaphylaxis; Circulatory/hypovolemic shock (state due to surgery or trauma if applicable); Sepsis/septicemia; Septic shock; Toxic shock syndrome.

VII. **Problem Case Diagnosis:** Sepsis.

VIII. **Teaching Pearls Question:** True or False: Antibiotics are the most important initial therapy for a patient who presents acutely septic.

IX. **Teaching Pearls Answer:** False. Antibiotic effects often are not seen for 24–48 h. Supportive therapy and establishing a diagnosis are the most important initial interventions.

REFERENCES

Balk RA. Sepsis and septic shock. *Crit Care Clin* 2000;16:179–192.

Dellinger RP. Current therapy for sepsis. and septic shock. *Infect Dis Clin North Am* 1999;13(2.):495–509.

Ferguson KL, Brown L. Bacteremia and sepsis. *Emerg Med Clin North Am* 1996;14: 185–195.

Meier-Hellerman A, Bredle DL, Reinhart K. Letter to the Editor. Treating patients with severe sepsis. *New Engl J Med* 1999;341:56.

Wheeler AP, Bernard GR. Treating patients with severe sepsis. *New Engl J Med* 1999; 340:207–214.

62. SEXUAL ASSAULT

I. **Problem:** A 25-year-old female states she was attacked by a man she met at a bar earlier tonight.

II. Immediate Questions

A. Are vitals stable? (See Problems 47. Hypotension, page 142, 40. Hemorrhagic Shock page 122.)

B. Does the patient want the police involved? Depending on the state law, physicians may not be required to report this crime, but the patient must provide informed consent for an evidentiary exam.

C. History

1. **Who?** Stranger, acquaintance, family, significant other.
2. **What happened?** Oral, anal, or vaginal penetration? Brief sequence of events (too many details may conflict with police report). Use of objects? Physical force? Weapons? Number of assailants?
3. **When/where?** How long ago did this occur? Location? Sperm or acid phosphatase can be detected up to 72 h out
4. **Activities since assault?** Bathing/showering? Douching? Change of clothing? Use of tampons? Dental hygiene? Wiping/bathroom use?

D. Medical

1. **Last menstrual period?** At high risk for pregnancy?
2. **Last consensual intercourse?** Important for laboratory analysis to separate body fluids/typing from consensual partner and assailant
3. **Other medical problems?** Any other medical issues to address at this visit?
4. **Allergies?** Important to obtain prior to prescribing antibiotics or pregnancy prophylaxis.

III. Differential Diagnosis

A. Domestic Violence. 38% of females who reported sexual assault were assaulted by someone with whom they had a relationship. (Riggs et al) Depending on state law, injuries from domestic violence may also need to be reported to the police. Involve social work early in the course.

B. Child Abuse. Should remain in the differential for juvenile sexual assault victims. Without the parent in the room, ask the child questions about the assault. Involve social work early in the course.

C. Sexual Assault. Lifetime prevalence of sexual assault in women is 39% (Feldhaus et al); only 43% will seek medical care after the assault, and only 46% will report the assault to the police. Involve social work and contact your local rape crisis team during the patient's ED course.

IV. Database

A. Physical Exam Key Points

1. **Vital signs.** Check for any abnormalities.
2. **General.** Check for bruises, lacerations, or other signs of trauma. Use a body map or photographs when applicable.
3. **Genital.** Check for discharge, abrasions, or lacerations. Toluidine blue can also be used to look for lacerations. Colposcopy can also be useful for identifying injuries in the posterior fourchette. Both

toluidine blue and colposcopy are not mandatory for the evidentiary exam and may not be available in the ED. Examine penis and testicles for signs of trauma if the victim is male.

4. **Rectal.** Anoscopy or rectal exam for anal assault. Check for tears, blood, or other signs of trauma.

5. **Evidentiary.** Informed consent required. Use rape kit required by the jurisdiction in which the assault occurred. Body fluid samples should be obtained from each orifice that was penetrated. Some hospitals have sexual assault nurse examiners (SANE) who perform this exam.

B. **Laboratory Data**

1. **Pregnancy test.** Important to obtain prior to initiating pregnancy prophylaxis.

2. **Blood typing.** For forensics lab; used to compare victim and assailant's blood types.

3. **STD tests.** The incidence of STDs in sexual assault victims is comparable to the general population, thus prophylactic treatment with antibiotics is recommended over testing for STDs.

4. **HIV test.** If this was a known high-risk assailant or the patient wishes to be tested for HIV, appropriate referrals should be given and prophylaxis can be offered to the patient.

5. **Drug screen.** Should be done only if the patient requests a tox screen or if specifically looking for a substance. All drug use will be detected so the patient should be warned of this prior to initiating the test. If suspicious for GHB, send urine to lab for analysis.

6. **Forensic tests.** Sperm can be detected up to 24 h after assault. Acid phosphatase can be detected up to 72 h assault. Crime laboratories can detect sperm or semen in up to 48% of samples (compared with 13% in the ED). All evidence collected should be labeled with victim's name and source of evidence; chain of custody should be upheld.

C. **Radiographic and Other Studies.** Unnecessary if a normal physical exam. Order appropriate tests based on physical exam findings.

V. **Plan**

A. **Overall Plan.** Contact local social worker or rape counselor to arrange follow-up for patient or provide this information to patient. Ensure patient's safety. Involve police with patient's permission. Very few patients will sustain injuries severe enough to require hospitalization.

B. **Specific Plans**

1. **Pregnancy prophylaxis.** *Plan A:* Ovral 2 tabs bid × 1 day; *Plan B:* 1 tab PO bid × 1 day; Premarin 25 mg PO qd × 5 days.

2. **STD prophylaxis.** Ciprofloxacin 500 mg PO, cefixime 400 mg PO, or ceftriaxone 125 mg IM for gonorrhea; azithromycin 1 g PO or doxycycline 100 mg PO bid × 7 days for *chlamydia;* 2 g PO metronidazole for bacterial vaginosis and trichomoniasis.

VI. ICD-9 Diagnoses: Adult physical abuse; Adult sexual abuse; Child physical abuse; Child sexual abuse; Rape-alleged (observe for or examine for).

VII. Problem Case Diagnosis: Lifetime prevalence of sexual assault in women is 39% (Feldhaus et al); assailant is a first-time acquaintance in 24% of cases (Riggs et al).

VIII. Teaching Pearls Question. What percentage of patients will have signs of trauma?

IX. Teaching Pearls Answer: 67% will have general body trauma; 53% will have genital trauma (Riggs et al).

REFERENCES

Feldhaus KM, Houry D, Kaminsky R. Lifetime sexual assault prevalence rates and reporting practices in an emergency department setting. *Ann Emerg Med* 2000;36:23–27.
Hampton HL. Care of the woman who has been raped. *N Engl J Med* 1995;332:234–237.
Riggs N, Houry D, Long G, Markovchick V, Feldhaus KM. Analysis of 1,076 cases of sexual assault. *Ann Emerg Med* 2000;35:358–362.

63. SKIN INFECTIONS

I. Problem: A "skin popping" heroin user presents with fever, tachycardia, BP 86/50, RR 32, a painful, rapidly advancing area of erythema, and marked edema from his left arm.

II. Immediate Questions

    A. Is the patient toxic? If so, begin initial resuscitation: Start IV, O_2, and monitors.

    B. Are the ABCDs intact? Does the disease process threaten to invade the soft tissues of the neck and airway? Is the patient able to ventilate and oxygenate adequately? Manage appropriately. (See Section VIII, 15. Rapid Sequence Endotracheal Intubation, p 470.) Hypotensive, tachycardic? Assume septic shock, start fluid resuscitation and, if necessary, a vasoactive agent with α and β-adrenergic activity (dopamine). Mental status/level of consciousness? Monitor closely.

    C. Distribution, character, and temporal aspects of skin findings? Generalized, facial, extremity, mucosal? Crepitus, edema, sandpaper-like, easy separation of outer portion of the epidermis from the basal layer on exertion of pressure (Nikolsky's sign). Bulla? Red, blue, purple? Is there evidence of deep space infection, compartment syndrome (pain, paresthesia, paralysis, pallor, pulselessness), or osteomyelitis? Smoldering for a week or rapid evolution over 24 h?

    D. Evidence of other organ system dysfunction? Vomiting or diarrhea? Oliguria or anuria? Myalgias? Spontaneous petechiae, purpura, or hemorrhage?

   E. Inciting events? Vaginal tampon user? IV or subcutaneous drug
      user? Trauma? Recent surgery?
   F. Immunocompromised patient? Diabetes, cancer/chemotherapy,
      alcoholic, asplenic?

III. Differential Diagnosis
A. Emergent
   1. **Systemic**
      a. **Toxic shock syndrome (TSS).** Staph or Strep. Blanching,
         macular, sandpaper-like rash with desquamation 1–2 weeks
         after resolution, fever > 38.9°C, hypotensive, and three of
         seven organ systems involved (renal, hepatic, hematologic,
         gastrointestinal, musculoskeletal, mucosal, CNS). Associ-
         ated soft-tissue pain and/or swelling? Risk factors include
         use of superabsorbent vaginal tampons and nasal packing.
      b. **Necrotizing fasciitis.** Quickly advancing area of erythema,
         marked edema, crepitus, and possibly gangrenous (purple/
         blue discoloration). Pain is intense then may resolve as sen-
         sory pathways are destroyed. Septic shock common and DIC
         possible. Hypocalcemia from tissue necrosis. Predisposing
         factors include trauma, surgery, diabetes, and cellulitis. Mor-
         tality > 30%.
      c. **Myositis/Myonecrosis.** Variable skin findings from minimal
         to gangrenous. Massive edema and crepitus; brawny skin
         with purplish blebs; thin, brown, foul-smelling exudate. Pain
         extreme and out of proportion with physical findings. Septic
         shock. Predisposing factors include trauma, surgery, and
         contaminated wounds. Mortality > 30%.
   2. **Superficial**
      a. **Cellulitis.** Poorly defined erythematous area; edema; warmth;
         mildly tender; located in extremities, face, or perineum. Mild
         systemic toxicity, fever uncommon. Predisposing factors
         include trauma, preexisting skin lesions, and vascular or
         immune compromise.
      b. **Erysipelas.** Tender, indurated, warm area of sharply demar-
         cated erythema (fiery red) over face or extremities. Toxicity
         variable. Extremes of age.
B. Nonemergent
   1. **Bacterial**
      a. **Abscess.** Tender, erythematous area of swelling and fluc-
         tuance.
      b. **Impetigo.** Bullous or nonbullous areas that ruptures, leaving
         a honey crust.
      c. **Folliculitis.** Pustules around hair follicles that can result
         in furuncles (superficial abscesses) or carbuncles (deep
         abscesses).

2. **Viral**
   a. **Herpes simplex.** Painful, vesicular eruption on lips or mucous membranes (type I) or perineum (type II). Recurrence is the hallmark.
   b. **Herpes zoster.** Painful, vesicular eruption occurring in a dermatomal distribution. Common in patients older than 50 years.
   c. **Molluscum.** Discrete, umbilicated papules with a pearly-pink color found on face, neck, and trunk.
3. **Fungal**
   a. **Candidiasis.** White plaques adhere to mucous membranes in the mouth and vagina and to intertriginous areas.
   b. **Dermatophytes.** Annular plaques with scaling and erythema at the edges and central clearing. Pustules and vesicles may also be seen. Locations include trunk and limbs, groin, scalp, and feet.

IV. **Database**
A. **Physical Exam Key Points**
1. **Vital signs.** Check BP, pulse, temp, RR and oxygen saturation
2. **Mental status and overall toxicity.** Level of responsiveness and gestalt.
3. **Skin.** Head to toe examination! Note the areas involved, extent, and character of lesions. Is it limited to one small area like the face or generalized? Sharply demarcated or poorly defined. Red/pink, fiery red, purple, blue or brawny. Macular, papular, vesicular, bullous, petechial, or sandpaper-like. Is there easy separation of the outer portion of the epidermis from the basal layer on exertion of pressure (Nikolsky's sign)? Can you feel or hear a crackle with palpation of involved skin (crepitus)? Check for discharge from area of concern.
4. **Mucous membranes.** Examine the oral mucosa for vesicles, bullae, petechiae.
B. **Laboratory Data.** The majority of diagnoses are **clinical!** In patients with shock or toxic appearance obtain an ABG, CBC, with Diff, Lytes, calcium, magnesium, phosphorus, renal panel, liver panel, CPK, PT/INR/PTT, fibrinogen, and blood cultures.
C. **Radiographic and Other Studies.** Plain radiographs may be obtained to visualize gas (poor sensitivity). CT defines the extent of fasciitis and myonecrosis in planning for wide debridement and excision. MRI helps differentiate between acute cellulitis and necrotizing fasciitis.

V. **Plan**
A. **Overall Plan.** Patients in shock require resuscitation with IV fluids, pressors, antibiotics, and ICU admission. Toxic appearing patients or those at the extremes of age or immunocompromised with erysipelas, or cellulitis can be admitted to a step-down unit or ward bed for IV

antibiotic treatment. Only nontoxic, afebrile, immunocompetent patients with close follow-up may be discharged.

B. Specific Plans

    1. Cellulitis. Elevation, cool compresses, analgesia and an anti-Staph antibiotic (cefazolin/cephalexin or dicloxacillin, or clindamycin). Facial cellulitis requires coverage for anaerobes (clindamycin or amoxicillin clavulanate, or erythromycin).

    2. Toxic shock syndromes. IV fluids (often > 5 L), pressors, antibiotics (nafcillin or oxacillin or clindamycin or vancomycin).

    3. Necrotizing fasciitis. IV fluids, pressors, blood products if DIC occurs, antibiotics to cover gram-positive, -negative, and anaerobes (penicillin or first-generation cephalosporin **and** aminoglycoside **and** clindamycin or metronidazole), surgical debridement (obligatory).

    4. Myositis/myonecrosis. IV fluids, pressors, antibiotic coverage (same as for necrotizing fasciitis). Surgical debridement/excision is a must.

    5. Erysipelas. In clear cases of erysipelas, Pen G or Pen VK is effective. If there's a question of underlying cellulitis, use an antipenicillinase antibiotic (cephalexin/cefazolin or dicloxacillin). Children need coverage for *Haemophilus influenzae,* so cefuroxime is appropriate.

VI. ICD-9 Diagnoses: Abscess (state site); Cellulitis (specify site); Erysipelas; Folliculitis; Herpes simplex; Herpes zoster; Impetigo; Necrotizing fasciitis; Tinea (corpora, cruris, capitis); Varicella.

VII. Problem Case Diagnosis: Necrotizing fasciitis.

VIII. Teaching Pearl Question: Name the three most common organisms found to cause cellulitis?

IX. Teaching Pearl Answer: *Staphylococcus aureus, Streptococcus pyogenes, H. influenzae.*

REFERENCES

Bobrow BJ, Pollack CV Jr, Gamble S, Seligson RA. Incision and drainage of cutaneous abscesses is not associated with bacteremia in afebrile adults. *Ann Emerg Med* 1997;29:404–408.

Folstad SG. Soft tissue infections. In: Tintinalli JE. J *Emergency Medicine: A Comprehensive Study Guide.* 5th ed., McGraw-Hill, 2000:1001–1008.

Meislin HW, Guisto JA. Soft tissue infections. In: Marx J. *Rosen's. Emergency Medicine: Concepts and Clinical Practice.* 5th ed. Mosby Inc, 2002:1944–1957.

64. SORE THROAT

    I. Problem: A 29-year-old male with sore throat, no fever or cough; pharynx is red, no exudates, and tender lymph nodes.

II. Immediate Questions

A. Are there any signs of airway compromise?
1. Stridor.
2. Labored respirations.
3. Inability to swallow secretions.
4. Change in voice (hoarseness, "hot potato" voice).

B. How sick does the patient look?

C. What are the vital signs?

D. Is the patient dehydrated from fever and/or decreased fluid intake? Antipyretic and IV fluids.

E. Does the patient have valvular heart disease?

F. Is the patient immunocompromised or HIV-positive?

G. Oral sex? Multiple partners? STD?

H. What noninfectious causes should be promptly considered? In older patients, consider referred pain from cardiac ischemia. History of burns or trauma? Malignancy? Foreign body (esp. fish/chicken bones)?

III. Differential Diagnosis

A. Infectious
1. **Simple pharyngitis.** Group A strep, gonorrhea, or viral.
2. **Tonsillitis.** Exudative, purulent patches, enlarged, "kissing."
3. **Epiglottitis.** Major concern in unvaccinated (H. flu) sick looking children. Adults, dysphagia out of proportion to exam, may not look sick.
4. **Retropharyngeal abscess.** Rare in adults. 96% younger than 6 years. Dysphagia, odynophagia, drooling, fever, dysphonia, neck extended, prefer the supine position. High fever, edema, and erythema of the post pharynx, nodes, occasional trismus.
5. **Ludwig's angina.** Progressive cellulitis of the floor of the mouth, can rapidly obstruct the airway. 70–98% of cases have lower molar disease. Dysphagia, neck swelling, odynophagia, dysarthria, drooling, tongue swelling, bilateral submandibular swelling, and elevation of the tongue.
6. **Peritonsillar abscess.** Tonsil and soft palate displaced downward, may have uvular deviation. Bilateral in 5%. "Hot potato" voice.
7. **Diphtheria.** Grey "membrane". In lost or no immunity.
8. **Candida esophagitis.** Only in immunocompromised.

B. Noninfectious
1. **Referred pain from an AMI**
2. **Burn, chemical exposure, or trauma**
3. **Neoplastic disease**
4. **Thyroiditis**

IV. Database

A. Physical Exam Key Points
1. **General appearance.** Ill-appearing, dehydrated, drooling, hoarse or "hot potato" voice, trismus.

    2. Are there signs or symptoms predictive of group A strep?
      a. Fever.
      b. Tender cervical lymphadenopathy.
      c. No cough or rhinorrhea.
      d. Tonsillar exudate.
    3. If benign exam, check for causes of referred neck pain.
      a. Thyroid masses or tenderness, ear exam.
  B. Laboratory Data. Rapid antigen tests for group A strep (65–91% sensitivity, specificities 62–97%) may be useful. WBC not helpful. Throat culture takes too long.
  C. Radiographic and Other Studies. Soft-tissue lateral of the neck if epiglottitis or retropharyngeal abscess is suspected.
    1. Epiglottitis. Width > 50% of the C3 body or > 60% of the height of the epiglottis.
    2. Retropharyngeal abscess. Inspect film with neck extended. Retropharyngeal space < 7 mm at the anteroinferior aspect of C2, or 14 mm (children), 22 mm (adults) at C6. Nasopharyngo-scope, in adults, to directly view epiglottis, cords (and valleculae if foreign body is suspected).

V. Plan
  A. Overall Plan. Identify life-threatening infections, monitor airway, IV antibiotics and ENT/oral surgery consult.
  B. Specific Plans
    1. Simple pharyngitis. Penicillin or erythromycin if three or four group A strep risk factors or positive rapid strep antigen test.
    2. Epiglottitis. ENT consult and IV cefotaxime or ceftriaxone. Steroids controversial. Admit to ICU.
    3. Retropharyngeal abscess. ENT consult, IV antibiotics, and likely surgery. Admit to a monitored setting or the OR.
    4. Ludwig's angina. Monitor airway closely. Keep patient sitting up and suction secretions. Intubation best in OR. Consult ENT for I&D. IV antibiotics (clindamycin, high-dose penicillin, ticarcillin-clavulanate, piperacillin-tazobactam or ampicillin-sulbactam).
    5. Peritonsillar abscess. Drain (needle aspiration vs I&D). Admit if toxic appearance or can't take PO fluids. Antibiotics and analgesics. Many patients have already been on penicillin. Clindamycin is a good choice.

VI. ICD-9 Diagnoses: Acute pharyngitis; Aphthous pharyngitis; Peritonsillar abscess; Peritonsillar cellulitis; Pharyngotonsillitis; Pharyngolaryngitis; Retropharyngeal abscess; Streptococcal pharyngitis.

VII. Problem Case Diagnosis: Our patient has two of four predictors of group A strep (no cough and tender lymphadenopathy). A rapid antigen test was negative. The patient was prescribed analgesics for viral pharyngitis.

VIII. Teaching Pearl Question: What is the prevalence of group A strep in adults with sore throat?

IX. Teaching Pearl Answer: 10% (1).

REFERENCES

Cooper RJ, Hoffman JR, Bartlett JG, Besser RE, Gonzales R, Hickner JM et al. Principles of appropriate antibiotic use for acute pharyngitis in adults: Background. *Ann Emerg Med* 2001;37:711–719.

Melio FR, Holmes DK. Upper respiratory tract infections. In: Rosen P, Barkin R. *Emergency Medicine: Concepts and Clinical Practice.* 5th ed. Mosby, 2001.

Pfaff JA, Moore GP. Eye, ear, nose, and throat. In Pearls, Pitfalls, and Updates. *Emerg Med Clin North Am* 1997;15(2):327–341.

65. STROKE/TIA

I. **Problem:** An elderly male presents to the ED with difficulty talking and weakness of his right arm and leg.

II. **Immediate Questions**

  A. **Is the airway intact?** Manage appropriately (See Section VIII, 15. Rapid Sequence Endotracheal Intubation, page 470.).

  B. **What are the vital signs and mental status?** Apply O_2, place the patient on a monitor, measure O_2 saturation and blood glucose, start an IV and obtain a 12-lead ECG. (See Problems 45. Hypertension, page 136, and 47. Hypotension, page 142.).

  C. **Determine the onset of symptoms and the cadence of events.** Were symptoms maximal at onset? Are they getting worse or better since they started? The risk/benefit of thrombolysis is directly proportional to the time from initiation of symptoms to start of therapy.

  D. **Were there any associated events or other complaints?** Trauma? Headache, neck pain, chest pain, shortness of breadth, palpitations?

  E. **Any past medical history?** Previous CVA? Hypertension? Diabetes? Heart disease? History of AF? Previous episodes of similar symptoms?

  F. **Medication use?** Antihypertensive agents, oral hypoglycemic drugs, insulin, anticoagulants or antiplatelet drugs, illicit drug use—cocaine or amphetamines.

III. **Differential Diagnosis**

  A. **Stroke**

  1. **Ischemic**

    a. **Thrombotic.** Occlusion of blood vessel, ie, clot formation at an ulcerated atherosclerotic plaque.

    b. **Embolic.** Acute blockage of a cerebral artery by a piece of foreign material from outside the brain, ie, a cardiac mural thrombus secondary to MI, cardiomyopathy, or AF, or material from an ulcerated atheromatous plaque of an internal carotid artery.

    c. **Carotid dissection.** Temporary complete or partial occlusion of carotid lumen with formation and subsequent embolization of clot.

  2. **Hemorrhagic.** Intracranial or subarachnoid hemorrhage.

B. Transient Ischemic Attack (TIA). Focal neurologic deficits that completely resolve in < 24 h.

C. Seizure. (See Problem 60. Seizure, page 180.) Consider Todd's paralysis.

D. Head Trauma. Resulting in subdural or epidural hematoma, cerebral contusion.

E. Meningitis. Consider if fever, immunosuppression, headache, stiff neck, or rash is evident.

F. Atypical Migraine. Consider if history of migraine with focal neurologic symptoms, or if typical migraine headache is present.

G. Metabolic. Consider hypoglycemia, electrolyte abnormality (hyponatremia/hypernatremia, hypocalcemia/hypercalcemia), drug or alcohol ingestion, infection particularly in the elderly, and carbon monoxide poisoning.

H. Neoplasm. Consider if history of malignancy, symptoms more chronic in nature, preceding or persistent headache, significant weight loss, progressive neurologic symptoms.

I. Vasculitis. Consider if history or autoimmune disorder such as SLE, Behçet's syndrome.

J. Psychiatric. Consider as diagnosis of exclusion—even with known psychiatric patient.

L. Miscellaneous. Hyperviscosity state, Thrombotic thrombocytopenic purpura.

IV. Database

A. Physical Exam Key Points

1. **Mental status.** Mini-mental status exam (See Table A-4, page 656.).

2. **Vital signs.** Closely monitor BP throughout evaluation.

3. **Head/neck.** Facial musculature asymmetry, tongue injury, carotid or vertebral bruits, meningismus.

4. **Heart.** Rate and rhythm; S_3; S_4 gallops indicative of CHF, MI, or cardiomyopathy; murmurs (bacterial endocarditis).

5. **Rectal exam.** Needed if considering thrombolysis.

6. **Skin:** Look for rashes, signs of drug use, embolic manifestations.

7. **Neurologic exam.** Pupils for asymmetry, fundi for papilledema or hemorrhages, focal deficits, strength/sensation, coordination, speech, deep tendon reflexes and Babinski's reflex, National Institute of Neurological Disorders and Stroke stroke score.

B. Laboratory Data

1. **Blood/serum tests.** CBC, Lytes, BUN, creatinine, PT, PTT, INR, consider CPK/troponin.

2. **UA.** Hematuria may be seen in SBE.

3. **ESR.** Elevated in SBE, vasculitis, or hyperviscosity syndromes.

4. **ECG.** To assess rhythm, presence of silent infarct.

C. Radiographic and Other Studies

1. **Emergent noncontrast head CT scan.** To determine if a hemorrhagic event has occurred. Although a CT scan will often be normal within 48 h of a nonhemorrhagic CVA, it may reveal the presence of an acute stroke (middle cerebral artery sign) or prior CVA.

    2. Carotid US. When symptoms are in the distribution of carotid circulation. Subsequent endarterectomy in those patients found to have moderate or severe stenosis reduces the risk of major stroke and death.

    3. Echocardiography. If considering mural thrombus or SBE. MRI can detect ischemic changes within 2 h of onset of event. Can also detect carotid or vertebral artery dissection.

V. Plan
  A. Overall Plan. Stabilize airway and blood pressure.
  B. Specific Plans. Manage and refer specific type of stroke/TIA.
    1. Stroke
      a. Early involvement of neurologic specialist if patient is within treatment window for thrombolytic therapy and has no contraindications. Studies have shown benefit with treatment within 6 h; however, an increase benefit to risk ratio is seen with patients treated within 3 h.
      b. If patient determined ineligible for thrombolytic therapy admission to a neurologic specialized unit has been found to decrease morbidity and mortality.
      c. There is no evidence to suggest BP reduction is of benefit in people with acute ischemic stroke.
      d. No short- or long-term benefit in acute ischemic stroke with immediate systemic anticoagulants.
    2. TIA
      a. Prolonged antiplatelet treatment is beneficial for people with a prior (presumed ischemic) stroke or TIA.
      b. Consider admission to the hospital for facilitating above-mentioned tests and or differentiating other possible causes of symptoms.

VI. ICD-9 Diagnoses: Acute cerebrovascular accident; Late effects of cerebrovascular disease with (aphasia, cognitive defects, hemiplegia, etc); Transient ischemic attack; Transient paralysis arm/leg.

VII. Problem Case Diagnosis: Left ICA ischemic stroke

VIII. Teaching Pearls Question: What percentage of patients who present with TIA, if untreated will eventually have a stroke.

IX. Teaching Pearls Answer: 10.5 % (Johnston et al.)

REFERENCES

Kothari R, Barsan WG. Stroke. In Marx J. *Rosen's Emergency Medicine: Concepts and Clinical Practice.* 5th ed. Mosby, 2002:1433–1445.

Johnston SC, Gress DR, Browner WS, Sidner S. Short-term prognosis after emergency department diagnosis of TIA. *JAMA* 2000;284(22):2901–2906.

NINDS rt-PA Stroke Study Group. Tissue plasminogen activator for acute ischemic stroke. *N Engl J Med* 1995;333:1581–1587.

North American Symptomatic Carotid Endarterectomy Trial Collaborators. Beneficial effect of carotid endarterectomy in symptomatic patients with high-grade carotid stenosis. *N Engl J Med* 1991;325:445–453.

66. SWOLLEN, WARM, OR COLD EXTREMITY

I. **Problem:** An elderly woman presents with a swollen arm 2 days after a fall.

II. **Immediate Questions**
   A. **Is the extremity neurovascularly intact?** Able to move, feel extremity? Painful?
   B. **Mechanism of injury?** Fall? Compression? Burn? Cold exposure? Submersion injury?
   C. **Has the patient ever injured the extremity before?** Any prior surgery to extremity?
   D. **Is the extremity warm or cold?** Ischemia versus perfused limb. Necrosis?
   E. **What are the patient's vital signs?** Febrile? Tachycardic? Hypoxic?
   F. **Is the extremity painful?** To touch? Full range of motion? Pain out of proportion to exam? Paresthesias? Pain with movement? Deformity?
   G. **Any comorbid conditions?** Diabetes? Vascular disease? Trauma? Heart disease? Sedentary? Renal disease? Smoker?
   H. **Duration of symptoms?** Hours? Days (rhabdomyolysis)?

III. **Differential Diagnosis**
   A. **Cardiovascular.** PVD, venous stasis, DVT, peripheral valvular incompetence, thromboembolism, Raynaud's phenomenon.
   B. **Musculoskeletal.** Fracture, dislocation, compartment syndrome, fasciitis, arthritis, synovitis, tenosynovitis, IV infiltrate, rhabdomyolysis, myositis, osteomyelitis.
   C. **Dermatologic.** Cellulitis, bites, burns, frost bite.
   D. **Lymphatic.** Lymphedema, lymphangitis.
   E. **Renal.** Nephrotic syndrome.
   F. **Neurologic.** Neuropraxia.

IV. **Database**
   A. **Physical Exam Key Points**
      1. **Vital signs.** Tachycardic, febrile, hypotensive, hypoxic?
      2. **Neurologic exam.** Careful motor and sensory exam (including light touch and two point discrimination) of extremity
      3. **Musculoskeletal exam.** Strength, joint versus compartment, range of motion (passive and active), pain with passive movement, point tenderness, deformity, circumference of swollen extremity compared with normal extremity
      4. **Vascular exam.** Distal pulses, capillary refill, bruits, arterial versus venous cause.
      5. **Dermatologic exam.** Color of skin (hyperemic vs pale), overlying rash/erythema, skin intact; temperature of skin compared with "normal" extremity, necrosis, crepitance, edema (pitting?), malodorous, signs of lymphangitis.
      6. **Pressures.** Compartment pressures (wick catheter).

    B. Laboratory Data. WBC, D-dimer, albumin, arthrocentesis (WBC count with Diff, cultures, Gram's stain, crystals, glucose, protein), CPK, blood cultures, CRP, ESR.

    C. Radiographic and Other Studies. Plain films, Doppler/duplex US, arteriogram, venogram, lymphogram, Doppler pulses.

V. Plan

    A. Overall Plan. Consult *early* for threatened limb (ie, orthopedic or vascular surgery). Consider admission if comorbidities.

    B. Specific Plans

        1. **Vascular compromise needs immediate vascular surgical evaluation.**

        2. **DVT.** Anticoagulate (heparin vs LMWH); consider admission.

        3. **Compartment syndrome.** Remove splint or cast if patient has one on, measure compartment pressure, place extremity in neutral position, immediate orthopedic evaluation.

        4. **Infectious.** Cultures, IV antibiotics, Gram's stain, cell count.

        5. **Fracture.** Immobilize, splint/cast, ice, elevate, orthopedic evaluation, pain control.

VI. ICD-9 Diagnoses: Arthritis; Cellulitis; Compartment syndrome; Deep venous thrombosis; Fasciitis; Fracture; Lymphangitis (state if associated with cellulitis); Nephrotic syndrome; Neuropraxia osteomyelitis; Peripheral vascular disease; Synovitis; Tenosynovitis; Thromboembolus; Thrombophlebitis; Venous stasis.

VII. Problem Case Diagnosis: Fractured radius—nondisplaced. Apply splint, medications for pain control, and follow up with orthopedics if neurovascularly intact.

VIII. Teaching Pearl Question: What is the first symptom of compartment syndrome?

IX. Teaching Pearl Answer: Pain. Persistent pain out of proportion to original injury is a symptom of compartment syndrome. The "5 p's" of compartment syndrome are pain, pallor, paresthesias, pulselessness, paralysis.

REFERENCES

Cohen SR, Payne DK, Tunkel RS. Lymphedema: Strategies for management. *Cancer* 2001;92(4):980–987.

Harwood-Nuss A. *The Clinical Practice of Emergency Medicine.* 3rd ed. Lippincott Williams (Wilkins, 2001:612–616.

Kroger K, Rudofsky G. Duplex sonography of venous stasis. *Angiology* 1997;48(6):523–527.

Moore III RE, Friedman RJ. Current concepts in pathophysiology and diagnosis of compartment syndromes. *J Emerg Med* 1989;7:657–662.

Simonart T, Simonart JM, Derdelinckx I, De Dobbeleer G, Verleysen A, Verraes S, et al. Value of standard laboratory tests for the early recognition of group A beta-hemolytic streptococcal necrotizing fasciitis. *Clin Infect Dis* 2001;32(1):E9–12.

Somjen GM, Donlan J, Hurse J, Bartholomew J, Weir E, Johnston AH, et al. Duplex ultrasound of the acutely painful and swollen leg. *Dermatol Surg* 1996;22(4):383–387.

Witte CL, Witte MH. Disorders of lymph flow. *Acad Radiol* 1995;2(4):324–334.

67. SYNCOPE

I. **Problem:** An elderly male "passes out" after finishing water aerobics.

II. **Immediate Questions**
   A. **Is the airway intact?** Manage appropriately. (See Section VIII, 15. Rapid Sequence Intubation, page 470.)
   B. **What are the vitals and mental status?** Is the patient stable and alert? Apply monitors (ECG and pulse ox), start IV, apply oxygen. Confusion? Orthostatic changes? Heart rate and rhythm, and BP discrepancy between arms may offer clues to cause.
   C. **Did pt have a witnessed loss of consciousness? If so, what did it look like? Seizure activity?** Interview any witness after stability ensured for description of syncopal event, evidence of seizure activity, injury?
   D. **What was he doing when it happened?** Exertion or other stress?
   E. **Status immediately before?** Precipitating events (stress, postural change, micturition, defecation, shaving, severe headache, CP)? Prodrome (nausea, visual changes, aura)? *Note:* If no prodrome think **cardiac!**
   F. **Status immediately after?** Postictal phase? Confusion? Aphasia?
   G. **Any past medical history? Heart disease? Diabetes? Seizure disorder? Medications?** Previous syncope, MI, valvular disease, known aneurysm, DVT or PE, diabetes, seizure disorder, malignancy, new medications or QT interval drugs (class IA, IC antiarrhythmics, antihistamines, phenothiazines, cyclic antidepressants)?

III. **Differential Diagnosis**
   A. **Cardiovascular.** Sudden onset without prodrome.
      1. **Tachydysrhythmia.** (See Problems 53. Palpitations, page 157, and 68. Tachycardia, page 202.) Consider VT (old or new MI), PAT (dig toxicity), AF, A-flutter, PSVT, WPW (short PR with delta wave), long QT interval (acquired or congenital).
      2. **Bradydysrhythmia.** (See Problem 11. Bradycardia, page 36) Consider heart blocks (old or new MI), sick sinus syndrome, pacer malfunction, AF with slow response, vagal.
      3. **Outflow obstruction.** Consider aortic stenosis in elderly, HCM (IHSS) in young adult, atrial myxoma.
      4. **Pump failure.** Consider AMI with cardiogenic shock, aortic dissection, pulmonary hypertension, cardiac tamponade, PE, massive blood loss.
   B. **Noncardiovascular**
      1. **Vasovagal or reflex-mediated.** History of precipitating event (upright thorax and stressful event), prodrome (lightheadedness, diaphoresis, nausea, visual changes), previous history of same. Most common cause of syncope. May be precipitated by cough, micturition, defecation, swallowing, pain, shaving or head-turning (carotid sinus hypersensitivity).

2. **Seizure.** Witness? Preceding aura, postictal phase, prior history, metastatic malignancy? Diabetic?
3. **Metabolic.** Consider hypoglycemia, hyperventilation, intoxication, overdose, electrolyte abnormality, carbon monoxide poisoning, hypoxemia.
4. **TIA or CVA.** Consider sudden "drop attack" in elderly with vertebral basilar insufficiency sometimes when looking upward, SAH, CVA.
5. **Orthostatic hypotension.** Blood loss, dehydration, new medication, autonomic dysfunction (diabetes, Parkinson's).
6. **Psychiatric.** Consider all other causes first—even in known psychiatric patient.

IV. **Database**
   A. **Physical Exam Key Points.** Don't forget to consider injuries from fall.
      1. **Mental status.** Mini mental status exam (See Table A-4, page 656.).
      2. **Vital signs.** Check carefully and repeat during evaluation.
      3. **Mouth and neck.** Check the mouth for bitten tongue. Check the carotids for bruits, neck for tenderness from possible fall.
      4. **Heart sounds.** Systolic murmur (aortic stenosis in elderly or HCM in young adult). S_3 or S_4 (MI, CHF).
      5. **Abdomen, rectal and pelvic.** Check for pulsatile abdominal mass (AAA). Check vagina and stool for blood. Pelvic exam for pregnancy or asymmetric tenderness (ectopic).
      6. **Neurologic exam.** Check pupils for reactivity (CVA), fundi for hemorrhages (SAH), focal deficits (CVA), cerebellar deficits (VBI), persistent confusion (metabolic).
   B. **Laboratory Data.** *Normal H&P:* Bedside glucose (fingerstick) and pregnancy test **only** with the following studies. Other studies if risk factors uncovered in history and physical.
   C. **Radiographic and Other Studies.** *Normal H&P:* Cardiac monitor, ECG, and orthostatic BP **only.** Consider maneuvers to reproduce the event (orthostasis, hyperventilation, cough) with care not to harm or injure patient. *If risk factors uncovered in H&P:* Cardiac enzymes, CXR, CBC, Lytes, echo, Holter monitor, head CT, EEG, Tilt-table.

V. **Plan**
   A. **Overall Plan.** Patients with cardiac or suspected cardiac causes should be admitted. Elderly with functional decline should be considered for admission as well. Other conditions must be managed according to their individual causes.
   B. **Specific Plans**
      1. **Vasovagal or reflex-mediated.** Avoid precipitating events (stressful environments, quick postural changes with or without micturition, defecation, prolonged standing, carotid sinus stimulation. Stay hydrated. Primary care follow-up.
      2. **Cardiovascular.** Treat dysrhythmias accordingly (See Problems 68. Tachycardia, page 202, and 11. Bradycardia, page 36, 15.

Chest Pain, page 51, 16. CHF, page 54, 38. Heart Murmur, page 118, 52. Pacemaker Problems, page 154.). All should be admitted until problem clarified and resolved.
3. **Seizure.** Treat seizure (see Problem 60. Seizure, page 180.). If known seizure disorder and uncomplicated may discharge home with follow-up. If first seizure and uncomplicated and ED work-up negative may discharge home with further outpatient work-up (EEG, MRI) and follow-up. If complicated seizure, admit and treat accordingly.
4. **TIA.** (See Problem 65. Stroke/TIA, page 195.)
5. **Metabolic.** Treat accordingly.

VI. **ICD-9 Diagnoses:** Syncope/collapse; Alteration of consciousness, transient; Arrhythmia/dysrhythmia; Cardiac arrest; Coma; Dehydration; Dizziness/vertigo; Epilepsy; Heart block complete; Heart block third degree; Heart murmur; Hyperventilation; Hypoglycemia; Orthostatic hypotension; Palpitation; Paroxysmal ventricular tachycardia; Critical care time.

VII. **Problem Case Diagnosis:** Aortic stenosis.

VIII. **Teaching Pearl Question.** What percent of patients diagnosed with PE have an initial syncopal episode?

IX. **Teaching Pearl Answer.** Up to 13% (Thames et al)

REFERENCES

Kapoor WN. Evaluation and management of the patient with syncope. *JAMA* 1992; 268(18):2553–2560.

Martin TP, Hanusa BH, Kapoor WN. Risk stratification of patients with syncope. *Ann Emerg Med* 1997;29:459–466.

Thames MD, Alpert JS, Dalen JE. Syncope in patients with pulmonary embolism. *JAMA* 1977;238:2509–2511.

68. TACHYCARDIA

I. **Problem:** A 24-year-old woman complains that her "heart is racing." Her mouth is dry and her lips and fingertips are numb. She states that she "has been under a lot of stress lately." On cardiac auscultation, she has a distinct midsystolic click.

II. **Immediate Questions**
   A. **Is she stable?** Are there signs of respiratory distress or vascular instability?
   B. **Does she have symptoms** or a history of chest pain, dyspnea, near-syncope, syncope, or mental confusion?
   C. **How fast is the heart rate?**
   D. **Are P waves present?**
   E. **Is the rhythm regular or irregular?**

F. **Is the QRS complex wide** (greater than 120 ms)?

G. **Is the tachycardia a primary arrhythmia** or the result of an underlying condition (see Differential Diagnosis)?

H. **Could any medications,** herbs, or illicit drugs be causing the tachycardia

III. Differential Diagnosis

A. **Primary Tachyarrhythmias.** (See Problem 53. Palpitations, page 157.)

   1. **Wide complex with regular rhythm.**

      a. VT.

      b. SVT with WPW, BBBs or other aberrant conduction pathway.

      c. Wide complex with irregular rhythm.

      d. AF with WPW, BBB or other aberrant conduction pathway.

      e. Torsades de pointes.

   2. **Narrow complex with a regular rhythm.**

      a. Sinus tachycardia.

      b. Reentrant SVT.

      c. Atrial flutter.

      d. Accelerated junctional rhythm.

   3. **Narrow complex with irregular rhythm.**

      a. AF.

      b. Multifocal atrial tachycardia.

      c. Atrial flutter with variable blocks.

B. **Secondary Causes**

   1. **Intravascular volume.**

      a. Hypovolemia from dehydration or anemia.

   2. **Cardiovascular**

      a. Myocardial ischemia or infarction.

      b. Mitral valve prolapse and valvular disease.

      c. Cardiomyopathies with or without heart failure.

      d. Endocarditis, myocarditis, pericarditis, and pericardial tamponade.

   3. **Respiratory**

      a. PE, pneumonia, and pneumothorax.

      b. Exacerbations of COPD, asthma, and restrictive lung disease.

   4. **CNS**

      a. Cerebral vascular events.

   5. **Metabolic**

      a. Hyperthyroidism from an endogenous overproduction or excess exogenous use of levothyroxine.

   6. Medications, illicit drugs, and herbs.

      a. Sympathomimetic effects of cocaine, amphetamines, caffeine, albuterol, and aminophylline.

      b. Anticholinergic effects of atropine, diphenhydramine, and TCA.

      c. Withdrawal of alcohol, opiates, and benzodiazepines.

    7. Miscellaneous.
       a. Sepsis with or without evidence of shock.
       b. Hyperthermia—infectious and noninfectious.
       c. Anxiety and pain.
       d. Carbon monoxide toxicity.
       e. Methemoglobinemia.

IV. Database
A. Physical Exam Key Points
  1. General
    a. Assess the patient's general appearance and hemodynamic stability. Review all vital signs. Look for pallor, diaphoresis, and apprehension.
  2. HEENT
    a. Dilated pupils suggest sympathomimetic or anticholinergic effects. JVD suggests CHF or cardiac tamponade.
  3. Heart
    a. Irregular rate and rhythm is seen in AF and multiple atrial tachycardia. Rubs can be heard in pericarditis and muffled heart sounds with cardiac tamponade. A midsystolic click suggests MVP and murmurs valvular disease.
  4. Lungs
    a. Listen for rhonchi, rales, and decreased breath sounds.
B. Laboratory Data
  1. Hemoglobin, BUN-creatinine, qualitative drug assays ("tox screen"), quantitative drug levels (eg, digoxin), Lytes, cardiac enzymes (eg, CPK, troponin)
C. Radiographic and Other Studies
  1. Monitor the rhythm.
  2. ECG to determine the rate, rhythm, PR interval, and QRS width.
  3. CXR if pneumonia or CHF is suspected.
  4. Spiral CT or V/Q scan if PE is suspected.

V. Plan
A. Overall Plan
  1. Address any obvious life-threatening abnormalities regarding the ABCs.
  2. Immediately focus on identifying an underlying cause before treating tachycardias as a primary tachyarrhythmia.
  3. Immediate IV access and oxygen.
  4. Converted reentrant tachycardias may be discharged if there is no sign of ischemia or instability.
  5. In AF focus on rate control in the ED, rather than conversion.
  6. Poor cardiac function increases the risk of stroke during electrical cardioversion of supraventricular tachycardias.
  7. Place defibrillator at the bedside and consider immediate electrical cardioversion in unstable patients.

       8. Cardioversion is seldom needed for heart rates slower than 150 bpm.

B. Specific Plan

  1. PRBC for anemia and NS if dehydrated.

  2. Benzodiazepines are used to treat sympathomimetic effects, drug withdrawal, and anxiety.

  3. Bicarbonate is the first-line drug therapy for wide complex tachycardias caused by most toxin overdoses.

  4. Use antipyretics for fever and core cooling in environmental hyperthermia.

  5. Analgesics for pain-induced tachycardia.

  6. Arrhythmia treatment

    a. Wide complex with regular rhythm.

      i. VT—amiodarone, lidocaine, procainamide, and sotalol.

      ii. SVT with WPW, BBBs or other aberrant conductions.

    b. Wide complex with irregular rhythm.

      i. AF with WPW—Amiodarone or procainamide, avoid AV nodal blockade (calcium channel blockade, β-blockers, digoxin, and adenosine).

      ii. Torsades de pointe—Magnesium, phenytoin, lidocaine overdrive pacing, isoproterenol, electrolyte correction.

    c. Narrow complex with a regular rhythm.

      i. Sinus tachycardia—Treat the underlying cause.

      ii. Reentrant SVT—Vasovagal maneuvers followed by pharmacologic AV nodal blockade (eg, adenosine, diltiazem, or esmolol).

      iii. Atrial flutter—Diltiazem or esmolol.

    d. Narrow complex with irregular rhythm.

      i. AF with normal cardiac function—Diltiazem or esmolol.

      ii. AF with impaired cardiac function—Diltiazem with caution or use other alternatives such as amiodarone or digoxin.

      iii. Multiple atrial tachycardia—Treat the underlying cause, may use diltiazem if no obvious cause.

VI. ICD-9 Diagnoses: Arrhythmia/dysrhythmia; Hyperventilation; Palpitation; Paroxysmal ventricular tachycardia; Ventricular tachycardia; Pulmonary embolism; Dehydration; Anemia; Hypoxemia; Exacerbation chronic obstructed lung disease; Exacerbation of asthma; Sepsis; Atrial fibrillation; Atrial flutter; Multiple atrial tachycardia.

VII. Problem Case Diagnosis: Tachycardia associated with mitral valve prolapse and a panic (anxiety) attack.

VIII. Teaching Pearl Question: What is holiday heart?

IX. Teaching Pearl Answer: Atrial fibrillation from excess ethanol ingestion.

REFERENCES

Bolton E. Disturbances of cardiac conduction. In Tintinalli JE, Kelen GD, Stapczynski JS. *Emergency Medicine. A Comprehensive Study Guide.* 5th ed. McGraw-Hill, 2000: 169–177, 180–182, 187–191.

Shah CP, Thakur RK, Xie B, Hoon VH. Clinical differentiation of narrow QRS complex tachycardias. *Emerg Med Clin North Am* 1998;16:331–360.

Xie B, Thakur RK, Shah CP, Hoon VH. Clinical differentiation of narrow QRS complex tachycardias. *Emerg Med Clin North Am* 1998;16:295–330.

Yealy DM, Delbridge TR. Dysrhythmias. In: Marx JA. *Rosen's Emergency Medicine. Concepts and Clinical Practice.* 5th ed. Mosby, 2002:1079–1096.

69. TRANSFUSION REACTION

I. **Problem:** An elderly man has fevers, chills, hypotension while receiving transfusion in outpatient treatment facility.

II. **Immediate Questions**

A. **Is the airway intact?** Manage appropriately.

B. **What are the vitals?** Is the patient alert? Obtain IV access, apply oxygen, and apply monitors (pulse ox and ECG).

C. **Is the transfusion stopped?** Immediately stop infusion, save donor bag, tubing.

D. **What other medicines** did the patient receive? Premedications, steroids, Tylenol.

E. **Any prior history of allergies or transfusion reactions?** Including family history.

F. **Past medical history.** Important information, precipitants of hypotension or fever, anticipate secondary complications.

III. **Differential Diagnosis**

A. **Anaphylaxis.** (See Problem 5. Anaphylaxis, page 18.). History of allergies, IgA-deficient patients. Respiratory distress, shock, angioedema. Immediate and systemic reaction. Usually occurs very early in transfusion. Death from upper airway obstruction and severe cardiovascular collapse.

B. **Acute Hemolytic Reaction.** Fever, chills, tachycardia, hypotension, joint pain, shock. Feeling of impending doom. Typically dramatic sudden change clinically. Anxiety, chest/back pain, flushing. If under anesthesia, severe hypotension, evidence of oozing, hemoglobinuria only clues.

C. **Febrile Nonhemolytic Reaction** (FNHTR). Fever, chills, diaphoresis, rigors, headache usually within 1–2 h. More common in multiply and heavily transfused patients. Diagnosis of exclusion.

D. **Delayed Transfusion Reaction.** Transfusion 3–10 d prior. Fatigue, jaundice, dark urine.

E. **Urticarial Reaction.** Pruritus, urticaria (hives).

F. **Transfusion Related Acute Lung Injury.** Dyspnea, hypoxemia, cyanosis developing within 2–8 h after transfusion.

IV. Database
A. Physical Exam Key Points
1. **Vital signs.** Especially BP (hypotension).
2. **Skin.** Urticaria, erythema, pain at infusion site, oozing, cyanosis, flushing, jaundice.
3. **Pulmonary.** Check for wheeze, diminished lung sounds.

B. Laboratory Data
1. Send samples of pretransfusion, posttransfusion serum or plasma for smear, check for hemolysis, direct Coombs's test, direct antiglobulin test.
2. Repeat type and screen, repeat cross match.
3. UA, esp. for hemoglobin. LFTs.
4. Send donor blood for culture.

C. Radiographic and Other Studies.
If pulmonary issues, consider CXR for pulmonary edema/ARDS pattern.

V. Plan
A. Overall Plan.
Stop transfusion, start vigorous fluid therapy, consider diuretic. Maintain adequate ventilation. Obtain blood, urine specimens and notify blood bank. Most commonly should be admitted for observation and further testing.

B. Specific Plans
1. **Anaphylaxis.** (See Problem 5. Anaphylaxis, page 5.). ABCs, epinephrine 1:1000 0.3 mL SQ, airway and cardiovascular support, antihistamines.
2. **Acute hemolytic reaction.** Usually admit ICU. IV fluids to keep urine output 100 mL/h, also diuresis, to prevent renal failure. Can consider dopamine, mannitol. In massive reactions, can consider exchange transfusion.
3. **Delayed transfusion reaction.** Most times, no specific therapy. Adequate hydration. Check antibody screens for future transfusions.
4. **Febrile nonhemolytic transfusion reactions.** Supportive therapy, rule out hemolysis. Observation.
5. **Transfusion related acute lung injury.** Supportive measures for pulmonary edema, hypoxia. Ventilatory support as needed (O_2, CPAP, or intubation with PEEP).
6. **Urticaria.** (See 22. Dermatologic Problems, p 73.) Antihistamines. Monitor airway, hemodynamics.

VI. ICD-9 Diagnoses:
Anaphylactic shock due to serum; Complication blood transfusion; Incompatibility reaction (ABO or Rh); Hemolysis; Infection.

VII. Problem Case Diagnosis:
Acute hemolytic transfusion reaction.

VIII. Teaching Pearls Question:
Do transfusion reactions occur more frequently in men or women?

IX. Teaching Pearls Answer:
Women, because of prior red cell immunization during pregnancy.

REFERENCES

Jeter EK, Spivey MA. Noninfectious complications of blood transfusion. *Hematol Oncol Clin North Am* 1995;9(1):187–204.

Manno CS. What's new in transfusion medicine? *Ped Clinic North Am* 1996;43(3):793–808.

Sloop GD, Friedberg RC. Complications of blood transfusion. How to recognize and respond to noninfectious reactions. *Postgrad Med* 1995;98(1):159–62, 166, 169–172.

70. URINARY TRACT PROBLEMS

I. **Problem:** A young female complains of low back pain and burning with urination.

II. **Immediate Questions**
   A. **What are the symptoms?** Check for urinary frequency, dysuria, hematuria, fever, flank pain, abdominal pain, vomiting.
   B. **Is the patient pregnant** (no fluoroquinolones!), **elderly or neonate, diabetic, or do they have multiple medical problems?** If so, consider need for admission.
   C. **What are the vitals?** Febrile? Orthostatic?
   D. **Any past medical history?** Check history for recent UTI, pyelonephritis, kidney stones, prostatitis or epididymitis, antibiotic failures or allergies.
   E. **Sexually active?** Any history of STDs, new sexual partners, vaginal or urethral discharge?
   F. **Time since last void?** History of urinary retention? Recent instrumentation or surgery?

III. **Differential Diagnosis**
   A. **UTI.** Dysuria, increased frequency, low back pain. Vaginal discharge/itching are negatively associated with UTI.
   B. **Pyelonephritis.** As with UTI, plus flank pain, fever, or vomiting.
   C. **Perinephric Abscess.** Consider if recent antibiotics and persistent flank pain.
   D. **Pregnancy.** Often increases urinary frequency.
   E. **Urethritis.** Consider if dysuria or urethral discharge, especially in males.
   F. **Prostatitis.** Consider if urethritis, especially if rectal/scrotal pain or tenesmus.
   G. **Benign Prostatic Hypertrophy.** Consider in older males if urinary hesitancy or retention.
   G. **Prostate Cancer.** Consider with low back pain, urinary hesitancy or retention.
   H. **Kidney or Ureteral Stone.** Consider if severe flank pain, often with radiation to suprapubic area. Pain usually not positional, sudden onset, nothing makes better/worse. Often with nausea or vomiting.

    I. Urinary Retention. Consider if recent catheterization or surgery, decreased urine output, suprapubic distension, or history of prostate enlargement or cancer.

    J. Urosepsis. Consider in neonates and elderly if UTI plus change in mentation or lethargy.

IV. Database

A. Physical Exam Key Points

1. **Mental status.** Confused? (Consider sepsis).
2. **Vital signs.** Check orthostatics if toxic appearing or tachycardic.
3. **Flank (CVA) tenderness to percussion** (pyelonephritis).
4. **Abdomen.** Check for RLQ tenderness (appendicitis) and RUQ tenderness (cholecystitis), suprapubic distension (urinary retention).
5. **Rectal and genitourinary.** External lesions (eg, herpes)? Vaginal or urethral discharge (STDs)? Check prostate for bogginess/tenderness (prostatitis), and nodules (prostate cancer). Bimanual pelvic exam for asymmetric tenderness (ectopic), pregnancy.

B. Laboratory Data.
If otherwise healthy with normal exam and history, UA and pregnancy test **only**; if multiple medical problems, diabetes, elderly, or toxic appearing, add CBC and Lytes (chem 8) and urine culture. In girls younger than 2 years and boys younger than 6 months old, **always** get a catheterized urine specimen (**not** a "bag" specimen) **and** a urine culture! If possible STD, do *Chlamydia*/GC cultures, VDRL, wet prep, and Gram's stain.

C. Radiographic and Other Studies.
Noncontrast spiral CT of the abdomen and pelvis (or IVP) if suspected kidney/ureteral stone. Contrasted CT if apparent treatment failure after recent pyelonephritis (r/o perinephric abscess).

V. Plan

A. Overall Plan.
Septic, elderly, pregnant, immunocompromised, or pediatric patients with pyelonephritis should be admitted—initiate the first dose of antibiotics in the ED. Give fluids if dehydrated, pain medication if needed, and antiemetics if nauseated or vomiting.

B. Specific Plans

1. **Urinary retention.** Foley catheter. Stat urology consult if not able to pass a Foley catheter. Follow-up with primary care physician, surgical (post-op), or urology (suspected BPH or prostate cancer).
2. **Kidney or ureteral stone.** Early pain management. Antibiotics/close follow-up if infected urine, with primary care physician or urologist.
3. **Simple UTI in adult.** Pyridium for 2 days, antibiotic for 3 days. Follow-up with primary care physician if symptoms do not resolve. Consider a first-generation cephalosporin or fluoroquinolone if high community resistance to sulfa.
4. **Complicated UTI, pyelonephritis, pediatric UTI, prostatitis, urethritis (> 35 years old).** Antibiotics for 10–14 days. Pain

medication as needed. IV hydration as needed. If planning to discharge home, consider starting therapy with IV/IM dose of antibiotic. Sulfa not recommended for *empiric* therapy in adults with pyelonephritis due to frequent microbial resistance.

5. **Pregnant with UTI/pyelonephritis**. IV fluids and pain medication as needed. Antibiotics for 7–14 days. Avoid fluoroquinolones (fetal arthropathy), sulfamethoxazole (third trimester—kernicterus), and tetra/doxycycline (stain teeth and bones). Needs **close follow-up** with obstetrician, or admission. Treat asymptomatic bacteriuria to decrease risk of spontaneous abortion and preterm labor.

6. **STD or urethritis (< 35 years old).** Follow CDC guidelines.

VI. **ICD-9 Diagnoses:** Acute pyelonephritis; Acute urinary retention; Hematuria; Nephrolithiasis; Renal colic; Urinary tract infection.

VII. **Problem Case Diagnosis:** Simple UTI.

VIII. **Teaching Pearl Question.** What diagnoses should be considered with sterile pyuria (urine with an elevated number of WBCs and no bacteria)?

IX. **Teaching Pearl Answer:** *Chlamydia* infection and tuberculosis.

REFERENCES

Bent S, Nallamothu BK, Simel DL, Fihn SD, Saint S. Does this woman have an acute uncomplicated urinary tract infection? *JAMA* 2002;287(20):2701–2710.

Gupta K, Scholes D, Stamm WE. Increasing prevalence of antimicrobial resistance among uropathogens causing acute uncomplicated cystitis in women. *JAMA* 1999;281(8): 736–738.

McGregor JA, French JI, Richter R, Franco-Buff A, Johnson A, Hillier S, Judson FN, Todd JK. Antenatal microbiologic and maternal risk factors associated with prematurity. *Am J Obstet Gynecol* 1990;163(5 Pt 1):1465–1473.

71. VAGINAL BLEEDING/DISCHARGE

I. **Problem:** A 19-year-old woman complains of vaginal bleeding, abdominal cramps, and lightheadedness upon standing.

II. **Immediate Questions**

A. **What are the vital signs?** Is she tachycardic, hypotensive, or orthostatic? Associated symptoms of syncope, dizziness, or weakness may also imply significant blood loss. Start an IV(s) and place patient on a cardiac monitor if vitals concerning. Include fetal heart tones and fetal monitoring if patient is in second half of pregnancy.

B. **Is the patient having any vaginal bleeding?** When did it start, is there any tissue, clots, or associated abdominal pain/cramping. Quantify blood loss (pads/h). What was she doing when bleeding started?

C. **Is the patient pregnant?** Assume all patients of childbearing age are pregnant until proven otherwise. When was her last menstrual period and was it normal? How far along is the pregnancy? Are there any contractions? Has she had any prenatal care, OB US, or complications with past or present pregnancy?

D. Is there any vaginal discharge? How long have symptoms and discharge been present? Is she sexually active? Is there a history of previous STD or other vaginal infections? Ask about fever, pruritus, dyspareunia, and dysuria.

E. Any past medical history? Specifically ectopic pregnancies, fertility drugs, tubal ligation, IUD, STD, diabetes, cancer, or bleeding disorders? **Medications?** Coumadin, oral contraceptives or Depo-Provera?

III. Differential Diagnosis

A. Vaginal Bleeding

1. **Pregnant**
   a. **Ectopic pregnancy.** The first consideration in any patient, regardless of history of birth control, including tubal ligation, or sexual abstinence.
   b. **Threatened, inevitable, incomplete or complete spontaneous abortions**
   c. **Placenta previa or abruption**
   d. **Labor**
   e. **Postpartum hemorrhage**
2. **Nonpregnant**
   a. **Menses**
   b. **Dysfunctional uterine bleeding**
   c. **Tumors or fibroids**
   d. **Vaginal or cervical lacerations or trauma**
   e. **Postpartum endometritis**

B. Vaginal Discharge

1. **Candidal vaginitis.** Diabetic patients, patients taking antibiotics.
2. **Bacterial vaginosis.** Copious or "fishy" smelling discharge.
3. *Trichomonas vaginitis.*
4. *Neisseria gonorrhea.*
5. *Chlamydia trachomatis.*
6. **Vaginal foreign body.** Insertion of objects most common by children. *Adults:* Forgotten tampons, retained diaphragms, or condoms.

IV. Database

A. Physical Exam Key Points

1. **Vital signs.** Always check and recheck if there is a change in symptoms or concern of significant blood loss.
2. **Mental status.** Awake and alert? Postural changes?
3. **Abdomen.** Check for a gravid abdomen and tenderness. *Pregnant patients:* Check for fetal heart tones and uterine tenderness and estimate dates by fundal height.
4. **Pelvic exam.** Check for vaginal trauma or lacerations. Note the color and odor of the vaginal fluid or blood. Note any POC. Evaluate the inner cervical os to see if it is open or closed (to a ring

forceps tip). Check for cervical motion tenderness, adnexal tenderness, adnexal masses, and estimate the uterine size. **Note: Pelvic examination should NOT be done in patents in the second half of pregnancy until an US is performed to rule out placenta previa.**

B. **Laboratory Data. A pregnancy test (qualitative β-HCG) should be checked in all patients of childbearing age.**
   1. **Vaginal bleeding.** Hct. If pregnant check Rh status, if Rh-negative treat patient with RhoGAM (300 μg, IM, if > 13 weeks gestation; 50 μg, IM, if < 13 weeks gestation).
   2. **Vaginal discharge.** Saline for *Trichomonas* and bacterial vaginosis (clue cells), KOH wet mount for *Candida,* and cultures for *Chlamydia* and gonorrhea.

C. **Radiographic and Other Studies.** If pregnancy test is positive evaluate for ectopic by US. In late pregnancy US is needed to evaluate for placenta previa. Quantitative β-HCG is useful if US is nondiagnostic. Other ED studies depending on the H&P could include CBC, T&C, PT, PTT, TSH, and pelvic US for the nonpregnant patient.

V. **Plan**
A. **Overall Plan.** Pregnant patients with vaginal bleeding need US for evaluation regardless of the history or physical exam findings. Most non-pregnant vaginal bleeding and discharge can be managed and discharged with appropriate follow up. Any patient with significant blood loss or toxicity should be aggressively resuscitated and admitted.

B. **Specific Plans.** (See also Problem 56. Pregnancy Problems, page 168.)
   1. **Early pregnancy.** US to evaluate for ectopic position. If ectopic, resuscitate appropriately, T&C blood, and consult OB for definitive management. If the transvaginal US is nondiagnostic for IUP or ectopic and quantitative β-HCG less than discriminative zone (usually ~ 1500) and patient stable and thought to be low risk and reliable may be discharged with precautions and follow-up in 48 h for repeat quantitative β-HCG. All others should be admitted until pregnancy location clarified.
   2. **Abortions.** Threatened abortion (bleeding, closed os): If US demonstrates IUP and negative ED work-up, may discharge patient with precautions. Others generally require OB consultation for definitive management (Possible D&C vs expectant management). All fetal tissue should be sent to pathology.
   3. **Late pregnancy and postpartum bleeding.** Monitor and stabilize patient and fetus. T&C for blood and consult OB for admission and definitive management. Oxytocin (10 U in 500 mL of NS at 120–240 mL/h) may be used to treat postpartum hemorrhage.
   4. **Nonpregnant vaginal bleeding.** Unless unstable or with significant blood loss, most require only phone consultation and good follow-up. Hormone manipulation, US, and D&C may be required depending on the cause and severity of the bleeding.

5. **Vaginal discharge.** *Trichomonas, Candida,* bacterial specimens. Treat accordingly (antifungals or antibiotics). Gonorrhea and *Chlamydia* infections may be treated on the basis of H&P or positive cultures. Both should be treated if diagnosis is considered. Sexual partners need treatment for gonorrhea and *Chlamydia* and *Trichomonas* infections.

VI. ICD-9 Diagnoses: Abortion (spontaneous, threatened, complete/incomplete); Dysfunctional uterine bleeding; Ectopic pregnancy; Foreign body-vagina; Hemorrhage (antepartum, postpartum, ectopic/postabortion); Menorrhagia, Menstruation disorder, Vaginitis (specify type).

VII. Problem Case Diagnosis: Ectopic pregnancy.

VIII. Teaching Pearls Question: True or false? A patient with vaginal bleeding and open cervical os cannot have an ectopic pregnancy.

IX. Teaching Pearls Answer: False; up to 7% of women with an ectopic pregnancy will present with vaginal bleeding and open cervical os. (Dart et al)

REFERENCES

American College of Emerg Physicians. Clinical policy for the initial approach to patients presenting with a chief complaint of vaginal bleed. *Ann Emerg Med* 1997;29:435–458.
Dart RG, Kaplan B, Varaklis K. Predictive value of history and physical examination in patients with suspected ectopic pregnancy. *Ann Emerg Med* 1999;33:283–290.
Egan ME, Lipsky MS. Diagnosis of vaginitis. *Am Fam Physician* 2000;62:1095–1104.

72. WEAKNESS

I. Problem: A young adult with severe weakness following a mild cold.

II. Immediate Questions
   A. Is the airway intact? Is the patient maintaining adequate tidal volume? Manage appropriately. (See Section VIII, 15. Rapid Sequence Endotracheal Intubation, p 470.)
   B. Altered mental status? Central causes need to be considered rapidly. Remember to check the glucose and pulse ox.
   C. What are the vital signs? Place on monitor (ECG and pulse ox), consider oxygen and IV.
   D. Is there bowel or bladder involvement? Incontinence or retention implies cord pathology.
   E. Is there pain? Think cord compression or muscle inflammation.
   F. Location, progression, and time course of symptoms? Proximal versus distal involvement, ascending or descending, and rapidity of onset will help determine cause.
   G. Past medical history? Diabetes? Alcoholism? Medications? Prior episodes? (MS, myasthenia gravis, familial periodic paralysis, myositis.) Diabetic and alcoholic neuropathy in susceptible patients. Look

for new medications that may cause weakness (diuretics, β-blockers, sedatives). Ask about ingestions: honey, insecticides, fish.

III. Differential Diagnosis

A. Neurologic Causes.
Present with acute to subacute onset (minutes to hours to days) of moderate to severe focal muscle weakness. Determine location of lesion based on H&P (see Database) and then consider diagnoses based on location.

1. **Brain.** Infarction/hemorrhage (See Problem 65. Stroke/TIA, page 195.), mass, demyelination.
2. **Cord.** Pain indicates compression (tumor, abscess, herniated disc). Cord infarction and transverse myelitis are painless.
3. **Peripheral nerve.** Guillain-Barré (most common), tick paralysis, diabetic/toxic neuropathy, porphyria, diphtheria, ciguatoxin (fish).
4. **Motor end plate.** Myasthenic crisis, botulism (canned food/ wounds in adults, honey in infants), organophosphate poisoning (insecticide exposure).
5. **Muscle.** Myositis, alcoholic myopathy, polymyalgia rheumatica, familial periodic paralysis.

B. Nonneurologic Causes.
Occasionally present acutely (MI, hypokalemia) but more commonly with subacute to chronic onset (days to weeks to months) of mild to moderate generalized weakness.

1. **Infection.** Especially in very young/old: UTI, pneumonia, sepsis.
2. **Cardiac.** MI in older patients.
3. **Lytes/Toxic.** Abnormal potassium, calcium, phosphate, magnesium. Medications which sedate or make orthostatic. Street drugs.
4. **Constitutional.** Dehydration, malnutrition. Also anemia, hypothyroidism, adrenal insufficiency.
5. **Psychiatric.** Diagnosis of exclusion. Consider depression and suicide risk.

IV. Database

A. Physical Exam Key Points

1. **Airway/breathing.** Monitor closely for compromise (inability to maintain airway, hypoventilation, hypoxemia).
2. **Vital signs.** Fever (infection), bradycardia (organophosphates or severe CNS event), orthostasis (cardiac meds, dehydration).
3. **Head and neck.** Pharyngeal exudates (diphtheria), dry mucous membranes (dehydration), conjunctival pallor (anemia).
4. **Neurologic exam.** (If a lesion exists, locate it.)
   a. **Cord.** Diminished reflexes, sensation, and rectal tone (the latter two are only seen with cord pathology). *Distribution:* Progressive at fixed level.
   b. **Peripheral nerve.** Diminished reflexes, normal sensation or paresthesias, normal rectal tone. *Distribution:* Distal and ascends.

      c. Motor end plate. Variable reflexes, normal sensation, normal rectal tone. *Distribution:* Head/neck and descends. Fatigability in myasthenia gravis.

      d. Muscle. Variable reflexes, normal sensation (possible tenderness), normal rectal tone. *Distribution:* Proximal.

    5. Skin. Look for tick (tick paralysis), wound (botulism), rash (dermatomyositis), profuse sweating (organophosphates).

  B. Laboratory Data. If H&P does not make diagnosis clear: CBC, Lytes, UA (infection). For muscle, evaluate for rhabdomyolysis: CK, BUN/Cr, potassium, urine myoglobin. Other studies if indicated (eg, ESR for polymyositis).

  C. Radiographic and Other Studies. In older patients, ECG and CXR. Head CT if suspect CVA. MRI for cord lesion. Vital capacity or inspiratory force to evaluate respiratory compromise (especially in peripheral nerve and motor end plate disorders). Tensilon test for myasthenia gravis. Other studies as appropriate to differential.

V. Plan

  A. Overall Plan. Secure airway if compromised or borderline. Almost all patients with acute weakness are admitted. Ominous (place in monitored setting) if weakness is severe, ascending, or bulbar.

  B. Specific Plans

    1. Cord. Observe for paralysis (complications determined by level of lesion). Admit for treatment (based on MRI).

    2. Peripheral nerve. Airway management. Remove ticks if found. Admit if acute or progressive or potentially life-threatening.

    3. Motor end plate. Airway management. Consider Tensilon test. Treat organophosphate poisoning (see Section V. Organophosphate Poisoning, page 353.). Treat botulism and diphtheria if indicated (obtain antitoxin).

    4. Muscle. Treat rhabdomyolysis if present. Correct electrolyte abnormalities. Possible biopsy and/or steroids.

    5. Nonneurologic. As indicated: Rehydrate, correct Lytes, blood transfusion if significantly anemic, treat infection, cardiac care for MI, steroids for adrenal insufficiency, psychiatric evaluation for severe depression.

VI. ICD-9 Diagnoses: Adverse effect of medication; Anemia; Arrhythmia; Congestive heart failure; CVA-acute; Electrolyte imbalance; Generalized weakness; Guillain-Barré disease; Hypothyroidism; Myasthenia gravis; Myelitis; Neoplasm (specify site).

VII. Problem Case Diagnosis: Guillain-Barré syndrome.

VIII. Teaching Pearls Question: What percent of myasthenia gravis patients have ocular involvement only?

IX. Teaching Pearls Answer: Twenty percent. (LoVecchio et al)

REFERENCES

Chew WM, Birnbaumer DM. Evaluation of the elderly patient with weakness: An evidence based approach. *Emerg Med Clin North Am* 1999;17(1):265–278.

Jacobson RD. Approach to the child with weakness or clumsiness. *Pediatr Clin North Am* 1998;45(1):145–168.

LoVecchio F, Jacobson S. Approach to generalized weakness and peripheral neuromuscular disease. *Emerg Med Clin North Am* 1997;15(3):605–623.

73. WHEEZING

I. **Problem:** A young adult female returns from a hike with worsening dyspnea and wheezing.

II. **Immediate Questions**
   A. **Is the airway intact?** Manage appropriately.
   B. **What are the vitals and mental status?** Is the patient stable and alert? Apply monitors including pulse ox and apply oxygen. Observe respiratory effort—does patient have labored respirations or signs of fatigue?
   C. **What were circumstances of current symptoms?** Exposed to any allergens such as pollens, molds, animals, new medications? Symptoms of URI? Any chest pain? Any associated symptoms such as fever, orthopnea, edema?
   D. **What is the progression of current attack?** Sudden onset or have symptoms continued for a period of time? Has the patient used any medications such as inhalers or nebulizers? Have treatments helped?
   E. **Any past medical history? Medications? Allergies?** Does patient have known history of asthma, COPD, allergic reactions? Determine pulmonary history including extent of previous exacerbations and history of hospital or ICU admissions, intubations, need for home oxygen or chronic steroids.

III. **Differential Diagnosis**
   A. **Pulmonary.** Asthma exacerbation, COPD/emphysema, pneumonia, bronchitis, bronchiolitis, croup, pneumonitis, pulmonary embolus, smoke inhalation injury, foreign body aspiration.
   B. **Cardiovascular.** CHF, myocardial ischemia, cor pulmonale.
   C. **Other.** Anaphylaxis, acute allergic reaction, angioedema.

IV. **Database**
   A. **Physical Exam Key Points**
      1. **Mental status.** Confusion is likely secondary to hypoxia or CO_2 retention and necessitates immediate intervention.
      2. **Vital signs.** Pulse ox is considered a fifth vital sign in pulmonary patients. Pulse ox less the 90% indicates severe respiratory distress.

3. **Respiratory.** Note respiratory rate, depth, effort, breath sounds. Signs of respiratory distress include use of accessory muscles, retractions, poor air movement, inability to speak in full sentences.
4. **Cardiac.** Note tachycardia, new murmurs, gallops. Evidence of JVD.
5. **Other.** Sitting upright or leaning forward and diaphoresis are other signs of respiratory distress. Look for rashes or signs of edema.

B. **Laboratory Data.** Few blood tests indicated with clear asthma or COPD exacerbation. ABG is useful only in patients with severe, prolonged attacks or with altered mental status. Obtain other labs if diagnosis is unclear, such as cardiac enzymes in suspected myocardial ischemia.

C. **Radiographic and Other Studies.** Peak flow is very useful in patients trained in the use and determining progression of illness or effectiveness of treatment. CXR should be obtained in patients with pneumothorax, fever or if CHF suspected. ECG in patients with possible cardiac cause.

V. **Plan**

A. **Overall Plan.** Recognize and treat underlying cause of respiratory symptoms. Perform necessary interventions to prevent or treat respiratory failure.

B. **Specific Plans**

1. **Mild to moderate asthma exacerbation.** Pre- and posttreatment peak flow to predict initial extent of illness and progression. O_2 to keep pulse ox greater than 90%. Inhaled β-agonists (albuterol 2.5 mg) every 20 min with reassessment after each treatment. Include inhaled ipratropium bromide (0.5 mg) in moderate to severe exacerbations (evidence supports using in **all** treatments) can be repeated 20 min for 3 doses. Steroids—either prednisone (40–60 mg PO adult; 1–2 mg/kg pediatric) or methylprednisolone (60–125 mg IV adult; 1–2 mg/kg IV/PO q6h × 24 h pediatric).

   a. **Discharge criteria.** Subjective improvement, essentially clear breath sounds with good air movement, peak flow greater than 70% predicted, or greater than 300 (adults), access to adequate follow-up.

   b. **Discharge medications/instructions.** $β_2$-Agonist MDI with instructions, consider spacer if unfamiliar with use; systemic steroids: 5–10 day prednisone burst (adults 30–50 mg/day, children 1 mg/kg/day), no taper indicated. Inhaled steroids for prevention of further attacks and daily management, although not proven effective in initial management of acute exacerbations. Start inhaled steroids at end of PO steroid burst. Ensure adequate follow-up care.

2. **Severe asthma exacerbation.** O_2 to keep saturation > 90%, initiate continuous $β_2$-agonist nebulized treatments with ipratropium bromide. Consider subcutaneous terbutaline (10 μg/kg)

or epinephrine (0.01 mg/kg). Systemic corticosteroids (see item b., give IV/IM with significant respiratory distress), consider magnesium (2 g IV), consider BiPAP ventilation. Be alert for pneumothorax (sudden decompensation).

    a. Indications for intubation. Worsening peak flow despite therapy (< 50% predicted), worsening hypoxia, increasing P_{CO_2} (> 42 mm Hg), increasing respiratory acidosis, declining mental status, increasing agitation.

    b. Rapid sequence intubation. Use Ketamine (1–1.5 mg/kg IV) or etomidate (0.3 mg/kg IV) as induction agent; ketamine provides additional bronchodilation. (See Section VIII, 15. Rapid Sequence Endotracheal Intubation, p 470.)

  3. COPD exacerbation. Supplemental O_2, increase as indicated (suppression of ventilatory drive is rare), systemic corticosteroids, initiate bronchodilator therapy with β_2-agonists and ipratropium bromide (See item 2.). Consider terbutaline (0.25 mg SQ, can repeat × 1). Use ABG to monitor worsening CO_2 retention or hypoxia.

VI. ICD-9 Diagnoses: Wheezing; Acute asthma exacerbation; Allergic reaction; Asphyxia-food or foreign body; Acute bronchitis; Congestive heart failure; Neoplasm.

VII. Problem Case Diagnosis: Asthma exacerbation stimulated by environmental allergens.

VIII. Teaching Pearl Question: What is the approximate peak flow in a normal adult male and female?

IX. Teaching Pearl Answer: Male: about 550 L/min; female: 450–500 L/min, will vary depending on patient's size.

REFERENCES

American Thoracic Society. Standards for the diagnosis and care of patients with chronic obstructive pulmonary disease. *Am J Respir Crit Care Med* 1995;152:S77–121.

Jagoda A, Shephard SM, Spevitz A, Joseph MM. Refractory asthma, part 1: Epidemiology, pathophysiology, pharmacologic interventions. *Ann Emerg Med* 1997;29:262–274.

Manthous CA. Management of severe exacerbations of asthma. *Am J Med* 1995;99: 298–308.

II. Pediatric Emergency On-Call Problems

1. GENERAL PEDIATRIC ASSESSMENT

I. Problem: A 9-month-old afebrile infant is "not acting right" according to his parents—he seems alert but is not feeding well, and is less active than usual.

II. Immediate Questions

A. Airway intact? Reposition patient, remove from car seat.

B. Breathing adequate? Crying means yes.

C. Circulation adequate? Mottling is common in infants who are cold, delayed capillary refill less common.

D. Vital signs? Fever indicates infection. Heart rate may indicate arrhythmias, especially if rapid and unvarying. Respiratory rate and BP often depend on degree of emotional distress.

E. Mental status? Terminology counts. "Lethargic" indicates abnormal mental status, eg, an intoxicated patient. "Fatigued" should be used to describe most children who appear ill at first glance. Children who cry throughout the exam but were calm before it are not "irritable," they are acting appropriately for age.

F. How is patient different from normal? Regardless of the examiner's medical expertise, parents are the experts about their children. Try to draw out as much information as possible about how the child seems different from normal.

III. Differential Diagnosis of an Infant Who Is "Not Acting Right." By definition this term is quite broad—some of the most serious conditions are:

A. Cardiovascular

1. **SVT.** Consider when a rapid unvarying heart rate > 200 bpm is present; cause may be RSV, congenital problems (WPW), idiopathic.

2. **CHF.** May be due to congenital lesions, cardiomyopathy.

B. Neurologic

1. **Intoxication.** Exposure to a variety of toxins affecting the CNS.

2. **Mass lesions.** Tumor (usually posterior fossa in the young), bleeding or swelling (from head trauma, which may be nonaccidental), hydrocephalus (congenital, but can present many months after birth).

3. **Seizures.** Their presentation may be subtle among the young and neurologically immature.

C. Hematologic

1. **Malignancies, anemia.** Leukemia is the most common childhood malignancy.

D. Metabolic

1. **Hypoglycemia.** May be a primary cause but can occur secondarily with many problems.

E. Gastrointestinal

1. **Intussusception.** Profound lethargy (out of proportion to dehydration) may occur between episodes of vomiting.
2. **Infant botulism.** These infants are alert but weak.
3. **Improper feeding.** Excessive free water intake leading to hyponatremia, improper formula reconstitution leading to hyponatremia/hypernatremia.
4. **Surgical conditions.** Appendicitis can occur in infants and young children and produces crankiness, vomiting, and fever. Localized tenderness is absent because perforation almost always occurs.

IV. Database

A. Physical Exam Key Points

1. What is the child's general appearance **before** you start examining him (pre-exam baseline)? Is he consolable by his parents? Is he eating, smiling, and interacting?
2. Minimize patient fear (and crying) by staying low, keeping the child on a parental lap, and talking to him during your exam. Common useful distraction techniques include the use of penlights, small toys.
3. The abdomen exam is most affected by crying, followed by heart and lungs. Do these first. Save ears for next to last and the mouth/throat for last.
4. Patient position may need to vary during exam. Typically young patients are examined while sitting on a caregiver's lap facing the examiner. Adequate inspection of ears and throat may require repositioning child so that he is face to face with caregiver, then lower him down to lie on both the caregiver and examiner's laps, looking upward at the ceiling, with his head on the examiner's lap. This allows the caregiver to hold the patient's arms, while the examiner controls the patient's head movement.

B. Laboratory Data.
Lytes reveal improper feeding (abnormal sodium), dehydration (bicarbonate), and metabolic abnormalities (glucose, calcium, ammonia). CBCs are often obtained but rarely useful unless a hematologic condition present.

C. Radiographic and Other Studies.
If suspect cardiac or respiratory problem, CXR indicated (with ECG if cardiac). Neurologic abnormalities should lead to noncontrast head CT. Concerns of intussusception are addressed with an air contrast or barium enema.

V. Plan

A. Overall Plan.
Cardiac or other important causes of abnormal overall appearance should be ruled out. Infants and young children who have persistently abnormal overall state, or who are not feeding well, are admitted for observation at the least.

B. Specific Plans

1. **SVT.** Place IV in antecubital location, rapidly administer 0.1 mg/kg of adenosine, increase to 0.2 then 0.3 mg/kg if not successful.
2. **CHF.** Admit to cardiology, perform echocardiogram, consider use of diuretics and/or pressors.
3. **Intoxication.** Consider screens for drug of abuse, consider meds taken by breastfeeding mothers, consider CO poisoning.
4. **CNS mass lesions.** Includes tumors, bleeding, swelling, hydrocephalus, consider increased ICP as cause of patient's abnormal state. Pretreat with sedation, intubation, paralysis, head elevation, mild hyperventilation. Neurosurgical consultation mandatory.
5. **Seizures.** Obtain EEG, load with anticonvulsants if needed.
6. **Intussusception.** Perform contrast enema to diagnose and (usually) cure.
7. **Infant botulism.** Admit to monitor for worsening respiratory compromise.

VI. ICD-9 Diagnoses

VII. Problem Case Diagnosis: SVT

VIII. Teaching Pearl Question: How does the pathophysiology of infant botulism differ from the adult form of the disease?

IX. Teaching Pearl Answer: Infants become colonized by *Clostridium botulinum,* the organism that produced the neurotoxin causing botulism, adults ingest preformed toxin, not the live organisms that produce it.

REFERENCES

Bonadio WA. The history and physical assessments of the febrile infant. *Pediatr Clin North Am* 1998;45(1):65–77.
Barkin RM. Pediatrics. A potpourri of clinical pearls. *Emerg Med Clin North Am* 1997; 15(2):381–388.

2. ABDOMINAL PAIN IN CHILDREN

I. **Problem:** A 6 month-old infant presents with 1 day of intermittent abdominal pain and vomiting.

II. **Immediate Questions**

A. **Is the patient clinically stable?** Assess and address ABCs; oxygen, IV access for isotonic (NS or LR 20 mL/kg boluses) fluid, NG suction

B. **What is the nature of the abdominal pain?** Constant (appendicitis) vs intermittent or colicky (intussusception)? Worsening? Awakens from sleep? Duration? Improved by eating (gastritis) or position (gastroesophageal reflux)? Worsened by drinking (renal obstruction) or eating (cholelithiasis, pancreatitis)?

C. **Vomiting?** Bilious (bowel obstruction until proven otherwise) or bloody? How frequent and for how long?

D. Stools? Any blood? Diarrhea or constipation? How often, and when?

E. Eating or drinking? How much? Dehydration (last urine, number of diapers?) Anorexia?

F. Other symptoms? Fever? Respiratory difficulty? Lethargy (sepsis, dehydration, or intussusception) or altered mental status? Sore throat? Last menstruation? Vaginal bleeding or discharge? Scrotal pain or swelling? Dysuria? Umbilical redness (omphalitis) or discharge (urachal anomalies)? Evidence of injury or abuse?

G. Past medical history? Congenital or chromosomal anomalies associated with GI tract abnormalities? (ie, Down syndrome with duodenal atresia). Prior abdominal surgery (10% lifetime risk of obstruction from adhesions) or prior episodes of pain? Chronic constipation (Hirschsprung's disease) or malabsorption (cystic fibrosis, chronic volvulus)?

III. Differential Diagnosis

A. Surgical

1. **Appendicitis.** Early perforation in younger patients, 4% of pediatric abdominal pain.
2. **Bowel obstruction.** Intussusception, volvulus, pyloric stenosis (nonbilious, < 2 months of age).
3. **Abdominal mass.** Renal, neuroblastoma, Wilms's tumor, lymphoma.
4. **Other.** Nephrolithiasis, cholecystitis, ovarian torsion, testicular torsion, ectopic pregnancy.

B. Medical

1. Ten diagnoses account for 85% of pediatric abdominal pain, from most to least common, they are:
   a. "Nonspecific" abdominal pain (diagnosis of exclusion, *next day follow-up mandatory!*).
   b. Gastroenteritis.
   c. Appendicitis.
   d. Constipation.
   e. UTI.
   f. Viral URI.
   g. Streptococcal pharyngitis.
   h. Viral pharyngitis/stomatitis.
   i. Pneumonia (lower lobes).
   j. Otitis media.
2. *Always* consider pregnancy or pelvic inflammatory disease in sexually active adolescents.
3. If no acute surgical or medical cause is identified, arrange *next day* outpatient follow-up for further evaluation.

IV. Database

A. Physical Exam Key Points

1. **Address ABCs.**
2. **HEENT exam.** Pharyngitis, otitis media.

      3. **Pulmonary exam.** Pneumonia, grunting respiration.
      4. **Abdominal exam.**
         a. Serial abdominal exams (persistent RLQ tenderness is 90% sensitive for appendicitis).
         b. Bowel sounds (diminished with ileus, surgical conditions).
         c. Peritonitis (involuntary guarding with gentle percussion).
         d. Hepatosplenomegaly.
         e. Distention (obstruction, constipation, mass).
         f. Mass.
      5. **Rectal exam.** Mass, blood, RLQ tenderness.
      6. **Genitourinary exam.** Testicular tenderness or mass, vaginal discharge or bleeding, pelvic exam for adolescent female.
   B. **Laboratory Data.** CBC and UA/culture. Consider basic Lytes and glucose with dehydration, serum pregnancy test in adolescent females. Other studies if risk factors uncovered in history and physical exam.
   C. **Radiographic and Other Studies**
      1. **Abdominal flat/upright radiograph.** Indicated for peritonitis, distention, prior surgery, mass.
      2. **Abdominal CT scan.** Indicated for suspected appendicitis, mass.
      3. **Ultrasound.** Indicated for suspected biliary tract disease, pregnancy, mass, appendicitis (less sensitive than CT scan).
      4. **Air-contrast enema.** Diagnosis and treatment (95% effective) for intussusception.

V. Plan
   A. **Overall Plan.** Admit patients with acute surgical conditions and those with acute medical conditions who require further stabilization or evaluation. Consider admission for patients with an unclear cause who have significant pain or vomiting.
   B. **Specific Plans**
      1. **Acute surgical conditions.** Address ABCs, IV fluid resuscitate, place NG tube, keep patient NPO. Consider IV pain relief. Notify surgical service.
      2. **Acute medical conditions.** Address ABCs, IV fluid resuscitate as needed. Treatment as appropriate for diagnosis. Consider admission as in Overall plan.
      3. **Nonacute conditions.** Treatment as appropriate for diagnosis. Arrange next day outpatient follow-up.

VI. ICD-9 Diagnoses: Abdominal pain (state which quadrant); Acute appendicitis; Constipation; Henoch-Schönlein purpura; Infantile colic; Intussusception; Urinary tract infection.

VII. Problem Case Diagnosis: Intussusception.

VIII. Teaching Pearls Question: What percent of pediatric intussusception patients have a normal exam? A normal abdominal ray?

IX. Teaching Pearls Answer: Fifty percent of intussusception patients have a normal exam, 25% have normal radiographs.

REFERENCE

Schafermeyer RW. Pediatric abdominal emergencies. In: Tintinalli J. Emergency Medicine—A Comprehensive Guide. McGraw-Hill, 2000:844–852.

3. ACUTE LIFE-THREATENING EVENT (ALTE)

I. **Problem:** A 2-month-old infant with a runny nose and cough was found limp and pale at home; he did not seem to be breathing. Stimulated by family member and brought to the ED, he is awake on his mother's lap.

II. **Immediate Questions**

A. **Is the airway open and is child breathing?** Manage according to BLS and PALS guidelines.

B. **What are the child's vital signs, oxygenation, cardiac rhythm, and mental status?** In most evaluations for ALTE these are normal; persistent abnormalities require further investigation.

C. **Duration of episode?** Abnormalities lasting a few seconds are less worrisome than those lasting minutes. Pauses in respiration up to 20 s may be normal.

D. **Skin color abnormal?** Blue or purple may suggest significant respiratory or cardiac problems; red occurs for other reasons, usually a choking or gagging episode. Paleness in a limp infant suggests a CNS event or abnormal perfusion to the brain.

E. **Was there abnormal body tone or movements?** May suggest a seizure disorder, primary neurologic problem, inadequate brain perfusion, or inadequate metabolic supply (eg, low glucose).

F. **Were the patient's eyes open during event?** Apnea usually occurs during sleep; babies who are choking generally have their eyes open.

G. **Underlying conditions or maternal infections?** Especially history of prematurity with past apnea and bradycardia, or intracranial complications such as intraventricular hemorrhage. Seek history of congenital anomalies (eg, congenital heart disease) or maternal infections (eg, herpes).

H. **History of infant death in a sibling?** Family history of infant deaths may suggest underlying metabolic disease, inherited cardiac problem, SIDS, or abuse.

I. **History of trauma?** Always ask early in evaluation. Even when knowledge of nonaccidental trauma is withheld from the physician, a plausible history for trauma may be offered. Phrase questions in a nonjudgmental manner such as "Do you have any concerns that someone may have injured your child?"

J. **When was the child most recently feed? When did he have anything in his mouth prior to the episode?** Choking is the most common cause of ALTE.

III. Differential Diagnosis

An apparent life-threatening event occurs when an infant is believed to be seriously ill (not breathing) because he exhibits some combination of apnea, color change, change in muscle tone, choking, or gagging.

A. Central Nervous System

1. **Central apnea.** Not common, can be associated with sepsis, acute CNS event (nonaccidental head trauma), seizure, intraventricular hemorrhage, CNS congenital anomaly (eg, hydrocephalus), and respiratory infections (RSV, pertussis).

B. Respiratory

1. **Obstructive apnea** from a foreign body, or congenital anomalies.
2. **Laryngospasm (choking)** from liquids in airway such as phlegm, mucus, formula, breast milk, or stomach contents (emesis, GER). Most common reason for ALTE work-up.
3. **LRIs** or congenital anomalies.

C. Gastrointestinal

1. **GER** (with or without aspiration) as may induce laryngospasm (choking).

D. Other

1. **Deception.** True histories are not always provided. Infants may be subjected to smothering, shaking, or given medications inappropriately.
2. **Cardiovascular.** Uncommon causes include SVT and myocarditis.
3. **Breath-holding episode.** Usually over 6 months with precipitating frustration or minor injury history. Presents with cry, cessation of breathing, loss of tone and rapid color change to blue or pale, and altered level of consciousness with spontaneous resolution.
4. **Near SIDS.** Some SIDS episodes, caught at the onset, successfully aborted.
5. **Toxins.** CO, opiates, OTC cough/cold medicines.

IV. Database

A. Physical Exam Key Points

1. **Vital signs.** Check cardiac rhythm; recheck for fever or hypothermia, and hypotension.
2. **Mental status.** Appropriate responses for developmental age of the child.
3. **Head.** Signs of injury? Consider dilating pupils to check for retinal hemorrhages. Nasal congestion, patency of airway.
4. **Respiratory.** Wheezes, rapid breathing, or respiratory distress.
5. **Neurologic exam.** Especially level of alertness, appropriate interaction for age, symmetric movements, and tone.

B. Laboratory Data. Screening chemistry for electrolyte levels and glucose, and anion gap. Fever and ALTE (and not clearly a simple febrile seizure) then complete "sepsis" evaluation to include CBC and blood culture, UA and urine culture, CSF studies to include cell count, protein, glucose, and culture. Consider drug screen when unclear cause present. Check HCT if first breath-holding episode (anemia makes these worse).

C. Other studies. CT scan in any case with clearly altered level of consciousness, any seizure activity, or any suspicion of inflicted injury. ECG if any abnormalities in rhythm or past cardiac history.

V. Plan
A. Admit infants that
1. Required resuscitation with rescue breaths or chest compressions.
2. Had color change to blue or purple.
3. Have fever.
4. Have any abnormality on neurologic exam.
5. Have a history clearly suggesting seizure.
6. Had siblings die of SIDS.
7. Present with excessively stressed families.
8. Have a history, physical exam, or caregivers that make you concerned about nonaccidental trauma.

B. Specific Plans
1. **GER.** UGI or pH study to confirm. Start antacid and motility agent.
2. **Possible seizure.** Outpatient evaluation with CNS imaging and EEG if stable and family not stressed; admit infant with many "episodes" for observation.
3. **Lower respiratory infection.** Admit and monitor if apnea, hypoxia, or respiratory distress is clearly present. Intubate if episodes recur or child requires stimulation to resolve.
4. **Toxin identified.** Supportive care.
5. **Near SIDS.** Admit, BLS training, follow-up MD to consider home monitoring.
6. **CNS infections.** IV antibiotics until infecting agent identified.
7. **Breath holding episode.** Reassurance, education, treat Fe deficiency.

VI. ICD-9 Diagnoses:
Apnea/apneic spells; Asphyxia—food or foreign body; Bronchiolitis; Gastroesophageal reflux; Laryngospasm; Newborn apnea; Newborn hypoxia; Pneumonia; Seizure; Sudden infant death syndrome.

VII. Problem Case Diagnosis:
RSV bronchiolitis, a cause of apnea in young infants.

VIII. Teaching Pearls Question:
What is a leading cause of death in infants after SIDS, and death related to congenital defects?

IX. Teaching Pearls Answer:
Infant homicide.

REFERENCES

Gray C, Davies F, Molyneux E. Apparent life-threatening events presenting to a pediatric emergency department. *Pediatr Emerg Care* 1999;15(3):195–199.

Torrey SB. Apnea. In: Fleisher GR, Ludwig S, Henretig FM, Ruddy RM, Silverman BK, eds. *Pediatric Emergency Medicine.* 4th ed. Lippincott Williams & Wilkins, 2000:147–152.

4. COUGH IN CHILDREN

I. **Problem:** A 1-year-old is being seen for a chronic cough, not improving after multiple courses of antibiotics.

II. **Immediate Questions**

A. **Is the patient in respiratory distress or impending respiratory failure?** Administer oxygen, place patient on monitors, secure the airway.

B. **Does the patient look toxic or appear ill?** Establish IV access, send labs, administer fluids.

C. **Is the cough acute or chronic?** Does the family remember any triggering event (choking episode, viral URI, fever)?

D. **What makes it better or worse?** Has the family tried any treatment modalities (albuterol, cool air, water or saline mist, antibiotics, cough suppressants)?

E. **Other associated symptoms?** Fever, nasal congestion, vomiting, sore throat, facial pain, abdominal pain? How has the cough affected the patient's activity level?

F. **Quality of the cough?** Barking, "seal like," wheezy, paroxysmal?

G. **When it is worse?** Night vs day, during rest, feeding or activity?

H. **Medical and family/social history**—Heart disease, immunocompromise, GERD, family history of asthma, social history of day care, multiple ill contacts, pets.

III. **Differential Diagnosis**

A. **Reactive airway disease/asthma.** Lower airway wheezing.

B. **Croup.** Inspiratory stridor, barking or "seal like" cough.

C. **Bronchiolitis.** Winter onset, lower airway wheezing. Severe cases may lead to respiratory failure or apnea, especially in young infants or those born prematurely.

D. **Foreign body.** May not get history of acute coughing or choking episode. Unilateral wheezing on physical exam.

E. **Pneumonia.** Usually acute associated with a fever and increased respiratory rate. In the younger child, auscultatory findings often absent.

F. **Pertussis.** Paroxysms of coughing associated with cyanosis, inspiratory "whoop" and posttussive emesis.

G. **CHF.** Check for heart murmur, enlarged liver, poor perfusion, absent femoral pulses.

H. **Bacterial tracheitis.** Patient appears toxic with inspiratory stridor, fever. Often confused with severe croup.

I. **Epiglottitis.** Patient appears toxic with fever and inspiratory stridor, often leaning forward in "tripod" position.

J. **URI,** influenza syndrome.

K. **GERD.**

L. **Sinusitis.** Postnasal drip.

IV. **Database**

A. **Physical Exam Key Points**

1. **Severe respiratory distress or impending respiratory failure.** Proceed with ABCs and PALS protocols.
2. **Vital signs.** Does the patient have a fever, tachycardia, tachypnea, hypotension, or hypoxia?
3. **Nose, Ears, and Mouth.** Rhinorrhea, otitis media, postnasal secretions, sinus tenderness, pharyngitis, pharyngeal foreign body.
4. **Neck.** Masses, unilateral swelling, and retractions.
5. **Chest.** Retractions, breathing depth.
6. **Lungs.** Stridor (upper tract disease), wheezing (lower tract disease), rhonchi, rales, or unequal breath sounds.
7. **Cardiovascular.** Murmur, abnormal heart sounds.
8. **Abdomen.** Hepatosplenomegaly, use of abdominal muscles in breathing.
9. **Musculoskeletal.** Fingernail cyanosis or clubbing.

B. Laboratory Data
1. ABG if severe respiratory distress or impending respiratory failure. Capillary gas adequate to check approximate pH and presence of CO_2 retention.
2. Pertussis DFA and/or culture if history and exam concerning for pertussis.

C. Radiographic and Other Studies
1. CXR if bacterial pneumonia, foreign body, or congestive heart failure suspected.
2. Lateral neck if bacterial tracheitis, epiglottitis, or foreign body is suspected. Bacterial tracheitis may sometimes be visible as "shaggy" tracheal shadow.
3. Inspiratory/expiratory CXR or fluoroscopy if foreign body is suspected. Bronchoscopy is the gold standard for ruling out foreign body.
4. UGI or pH probe study to evaluate for GERD.
5. CT of the sinuses if sinusitis unresponsive to antibiotic treatment suspected.

V. Plan
  A. Overall Plan. Any patient with severe respiratory or impending respiratory failure should be treated per the Pediatric Advanced Life Support protocol and if the etiology is known, treatment initiated immediately.
  B. Specific Plans
1. **Viral upper respiratory infection.** Supportive care only, antibiotics not indicated. This may include
    a. Increasing room humidity (humidifier, vaporizer).
    b. OTC cough suppressants (dextromethorphan).
    c. Sleeping in more upright position (pillows, in car seat).
    d. Suction of nasal secretions.
    e. Avoidance of exposure to cigarette smoke.
2. **Bronchiolitis.** May try nebulized racemic epinephrine or an albuterol treatment, though majority of patients do not respond. Anti-

biotics not indicated. Recent studies indicate large doses of dex-amethasone may be helpful.

3. **Reactive airway disease/asthma.** Nebulized albuterol and ipra-tropium treatments supplemented with oral steroid therapy.

4. **Pneumonia.** Antibiotics for most common pathogens. Consider if patient could have an atypical organism (*Mycoplasma*).

5. **Croup.** Dexamethasone (0.6 mg/kg given PO, IM, IV equally effec-tive) and cool mist. Nebulized racemic epinephrine for patients in moderate to severe respiratory distress, especially at rest.

6. **Epiglottitis.** Keep patient comfortable. Patient should be taken immediately to the operating room for direct visualization of the epiglottis and securing of airway. Radiographs or IV placement are not indicated in a patient with suspected epiglottitis.

7. **Bacterial tracheitis.** IV antibiotics with admission to the hospi-tal for careful airway observation and monitoring.

8. **Foreign body.** Surgical consultation and bronchoscopy.

9. **Pertussis.** Admission to isolation room for observation of any potential life-threatening events (apnea). Treat patient and all exposed contacts with erythromycin.

10. **GERD.** Place patient on an H_2-blocker and/or a GI motility drug.

VI. ICD-9 Diagnoses: Allergy; Allergic rhinitis; Asthma exacerbation; Bron-chiolitis; Foreign body; Pneumonia; Sinusitis: Upper respiratory infection.

VII. Problem Case Diagnosis: Foreign body aspiration.

VIII. Teaching Pearl Question: How often do you get a history of choking or aspiration of an object in a patient with a potential foreign body aspiration?

IX. Teaching Pearl Answer: In only half to two thirds of the time.

REFERENCES

Bachur R. Cough. In: Fleisher GR, Ludwig S, eds. *Textbook of Pediatric Emergency Med-icine.* 4th ed. Lippincott, Williams & Williams, 2000:183–186.

Cheng W, Tam. Foreign body ingestion in children: Experience with 1265 cases. *J Pediatr Surg* 1999;(10):1472–1476.

5. EAR PAIN IN CHILDREN

I. **Problem:** A 2-year-old male presents with 2-day history of fever and pulling at left ear.

II. **Immediate Questions**

A. **Are the vital signs and mental status normal for age?** If not, treat these first.

B. **When did the pain and associated symptoms start?** How long has the child been pulling at the ear? Duration and quantification of fever? Does the child have nausea, vomiting, diarrhea, sore throat, oral pain, otorrhea? Does the child have decreased hearing, tinnitus, vertigo? Is there a history of trauma, recent air travel, diving or swimming?

C. **Past medical history.** Is the patient immunocompromised? Does the patient have a history of recurrent ear infections, tympanostomy tubes, mastoiditis? Is the patient on any medication (antibiotics, antipyretics, analgesics)? Is the analgesic working? Why is the patient on antibiotics and which antibiotic? Does the patient have a syndrome that predisposes him to ear infections?

D. **Social history and immunizations.** Are there smokers in the house, does the child attend daycare? Are the patient's immunizations up to date?

III. **Differential Diagnosis**

A. **Otogenic.** Arising from ear.

1. **Acute otitis media.** Most common cause. Common bacterial causes *Streptococcus pneumonia, Haemophilus influenza, Moraxella catarrhalis. Otoscopic findings:* TM hyperemia, dullness, bulging, pus behind TM, decreased TM motility with pneumatic otoscopy. Classify as suppurative if drainage.

2. **Otitis externa.** AKA swimmer's ear. Pinna tender to movement. *Causes: Staphylococcus aureus, Pseudomonas,* uncommonly *Aspergillus* and *Candida.*

3. **Foreign body.** Insects, beads, vegetable matter common. Remove button batteries immediately.

4. **Otitis media with effusion.** Collection of serous (noninfected) fluid behind TM. Common after resolution of otitis media and URIs.

5. **Ear piercing.** Pain caused by infection with skin flora or allergic reaction to earring metals such as nickel.

6. **Tympanic membrane perforation.** Can be caused by otitis media, external trauma.

7. **Perichondritis or perichondral hematoma.** Require antibiotics and drainage, respectively.

8. **Thermal injury.** Burns or frostbite.

9. **Herpes zoster oticus.** Ramsay-Hunt syndrome. Vesicles.

10. **Furunculosis.** Infection of hair follicle at the external auditory meatus.

B. **Nonotogenic**

1. **Dental.** Cavities, trauma dental abscess, or impaction.

2. **Pharyngitis.** Retropharyngeal abscess, peritonsillar abscess.

3. **Temporomandibular joint dysfunction.** Bruxism.

4. **Sinusitis.**

5. **Lymphadenitis.** Cervical, preauricular.

C. **Life-threatening causes of otalgia**

1. **Hemotympanum.** Secondary to basilar skull fracture, may be nonaccidental.

2. **Intracranial.** Meningitis, subdural empyema (altered mental status, meningismus, seizures, headache).

      3. Mastoiditis. Tender protruding auricle, swelling and tenderness along mastoid area.

IV. Database
A. Physical Exam Key Points. Ear exam often done last.
    1. General. Overall appearance of child, mental and hydration status.
    2. HEENT.
        a. Head. Full or bulging fontanelle, signs of trauma. *Eyes:* Drainage, conjunctival injection.
        b. Ears. External: bruises, lacerations, tenderness, erythema, rashes, excoriations, vesicles, preauricular LAD, mastoid swelling or tenderness, displacement of pinna.
        c. Otoscopy. Foreign bodies, erythema of canal, blood or drainage in canal.
        d. TM. Landmarks, light reflex, erythema, bulging, retraction, perforations, quality of fluid behind TM (blood, pus, serous).
        e. Nose. Nasal septal hematoma, bleeding. *Throat:* Erythema, exudate, tonsillitis, petechiae.
    3. Mouth and face. Dental caries, abscesses, loose teeth, facial swelling, tenderness, erythema, TMJ clicking/grinding/tenderness.
    4. Neck. Meningismus, lymphadenopathy, tenderness.
    5. Neurologic. GCS, focal deficits, age-appropriate behavior.
B. Laboratory Data. Consider culturing purulent drainage from OM with perforation. Tympanocentesis if chronic nonperforated OM or risk of resistant organism is high (patient failing first- and second-line therapy or if patient is immunocompromised and at risk for uncommon pathogen).
C. Radiographic and Other Studies. Focal neurologic deficits, hemotympanum, or mastoiditis usually requires CT to confirm diagnosis and direct therapy.

V. Plan
A. Overall Plan. Otogenic causes of otalgia can generally be treated on an outpatient basis. Other causes can be handled based on infection source.
B. Specific Plans
    1. Otitis media, nonperforated. *Antibiotics:* Amoxicillin PO 80–90 mg/kg/day (max 2.0 g/day) ÷ q8h. This is the high dose recommended for intermediate and some highly resistant *S. pneumonia* seen in certain geographic areas, in children exposed to antibiotics in previous 3 months, those younger than 2 years old, and for those who attend daycare. Otherwise, amoxicillin 40–45 mg/kg/day ÷ q8h provides the standard dose. *Alternatives:* Amoxicillin-clavulanate, cefuroxime axetil, intramuscular ceftriaxone 50 mg/kg/day × 3 days. *Analgesics:* Acetaminophen, ibuprofen. *Topical anesthetic:* Antipyrine and benzocaine (contraindication TM perforation). Use for only 3 days.

    2. **Otitis media with perforation.** Consider adding the use of ophthalmic (won't harm middle ear) antibiotic drops such as to-bramycin or ciprofloxacin to oral antibiotics.

    3. **Otitis externa.** *Antibiotics:* Ciprofloxacin otic. *Antibiotic and hydrocortisone:* Ciprofloxacin otic and Cortisporin suspension.

    4. **Mastoiditis.** Admission, IV antibiotics, ENT consultation.

VI. ICD-9 Diagnoses: Acute otitis media; Acute otitis externa; Chronic otitis media with effusion; Foreign body; Pharyngitis; Ruptured tympanic membrana.

VII. Problem Case Diagnosis: Left otitis media.

VIII. Teaching Pearl Question: What percentage of acute OM caused by *H. influenzae* and *M. catarrhalis* resolves spontaneously?

IX. Teaching Pearl Answer: Fifty percent of *H. influenzae* and 80% of *M. catarrhalis* infections (Hoberman, et al).

REFERENCES

Dowell SF, Butler JC, Giebink GS, Jacobs MR, Jernigan D, Musher DM, et al. Acute otitis media: Management and surveillance in an era of pneumococcal resistance—A report from the Drug-resistance Streptococcus pneumoniae Therapeutic Working Group. *Pediatr Infect Dis J* 1999;18(1):1–9.

Hoberman A, Paradise J. Acute otitis media: Diagnosis and management in the year 2000. *Pediatr Ann* 2000;29(10):609–620.

6. FEBRILE INFANT

    I. Problem: A 9-year-old child with sickle cell disease presents with a fever.

    II. Immediate Questions

        A. Is the child stable? ABCs come before evaluation of fever.

        B. Are there other features of concern? Signs of sepsis, toxicity, meningitis, or shock may warrant resuscitation (plus immediate antibiotics after a stat blood culture).

        C. What is the child's age? The approach to fever varies markedly by age.

        D. Is the child immune-deficient, high-risk, or carrying medical devices? *Examples:* Sickle cell, cancer, transplant, central line, CSF shunt; cardiac patients and many others need special caution or consultation.

        E. How high is the temperature? A relatively weak predictor of illness severity. Ill appearance more important. No single "cutoff" for fever in young infants (0–3 mon) but 38.0°C (rectal) used most frequently.

    III. Differential Diagnosis

        A. Infection

1. **Viral**
   a. **Common or benign** (eg, chickenpox, roseola, gastroenteritis)
   b. **Serious.** Viral meningitis, encephalitis, myocarditis—signs often subtle.
2. **Bacterial**
   a. **Focal, identifiable.** Otitis, symptomatic UTI, pneumonia, cellulitis, etc.
   b. **Occult.** May include bacteremia, UTI, pneumonia, meningitis, bone, joint, or muscle infections.
3. **Other.** Parasites, fungi (rare).
B. **Infection-like.** Kawasaki disease, serum sickness, toxic-shock syndrome, appendicitis, etc.
C. **Metabolic.** Hyperthyroidism.
D. **Neoplastic.** Rare cause of acute fever.
E. **Toxic.** Drug fevers and salicylism or phencyclidine use.
F. **Factitious.** Due to erroneous or intentional mismeasurement.
G. **Miscellaneous.** Heat illness, trauma, CNS dysfunction.

IV. **Database**
A. **Physical Exam Key Points.** After 3–6 mon of age in the well-appearing child, a detectable focus of infection may be a diagnostic endpoint.
   1. **General appearance.** Most important. Document, when present, simple, clear descriptors of "optimal observation": Alert, interactive, cheerful, comfortable, calm, curious, responsive, consolable, smiles, plays, etc.
   2. **Vital signs.** Increases in HR, RR due to fever usually moderate.
   3. **ENT.** Red TMs, tender sinuses; erythematous papules in pharynx or at base of uvula most common sign of viral infection.
   4. **Neck** (and fontanelle). Document neck supple to chest, anterior fontanelle slack or scaphoid?
   5. **Chest and respiratory.** Bronchiolitis or pneumonia may be signaled more by breathing pattern than auscultation.
   6. **Cardiac.** Murmur (endocarditis risk?), rub, PMI, pulse quality, pulse pressure, perfusion.
   7. **Abdomen.** Bladder or CVA tenderness? Hepatomegaly or splenomegaly?
   8. **Skin.** Know the rashes associated with dangerous or bacterial disease (Rocky Mountain spotted fever, meningococcemia, toxic shock); most of the rest will be viral.
B. **Laboratory Data**
   1. **CBC.** Most useful if part of evidence-based screening process for sicker or younger children; consider getting with blood culture.
   2. **UA and urine culture.** Helpful in younger children (< 2 or 3), especially newborns, girls, uncircumcised boys if ill appearance but no obvious source, as UTIs often occult. Catheterized samples (or suprapubic in infants) are indicated if child is too young to give clean-catch.

3. **Blood culture.** If concerned about possible sepsis, immune deficiency, or occult bacteremia (T > 39–40°C without source in child < age 3).
4. **Throat culture** (± rapid test). May be useful after age 2 if no source for fever and no clear signs against Strep (eg, runny nose, cough). Recall most cases of Strep lack classic signs, and fever with headache, vomiting, or abdominal pain may predominate. A positive Strep test does not rule out the presence of another disease.

C. **Radiographic and Other Studies.** CXR may be helpful if tachypnea and ill appearance present in younger child in whom pneumonia may be occult.

V. **Plan**

A. **Overall Plan.** *Septic, toxic, or meningitic:* Patients should be evaluated emergently and admitted for IV antibiotics. Immune-deficient patients may also require admission. In the remaining patients plans depend on age and specific diagnosis.

B. **Specific Plans**
1. **Younger than 29 d of age.** Most experts perform full sepsis evaluation (checking blood, urine, CSF) and admit for IV antibiotics.
2. **From 29 to 90 d.** Complete evaluation usually indicated; management may vary if well-appearing, but usually admit if ill.
3. **From 3 mon to 3 y.** Caution mixes with judgment. If child passes "optimal observation," may treat specific infections as indicated. If fails "optimal observation," perform lumbar puncture.
4. **From 3 to 12 y.** Approach is similar to adults, but with consideration of pediatric diseases and precautions.

VI. **ICD-9 Diagnoses:** Bacteremia; Fever; Fever unknown origin; Newborn bacteremia; Septicemia.

VII. **Problem Case Diagnosis:** The child develops acute chest syndrome (bacterial pneumonia with sickle crisis) over 12 h and requires admission to the PICU.

VIII. **Teaching Pearls Question:** List three reasons children are at increased risk due to serious bacterial infections in the first 1–2 mon of life.

IX. **Teaching Pearls Answer:** (1) Bacterial infection is more common (occurring in approximately 6–15% of patients with fever). (2) The immune system is immature and relatively incompetent. (3) The appearance of serious illness, useful in older infants, is often absent (Baker 1999).

REFERENCES

Baker MD. Evaluation and management of infants with fever. *Pediatr Clin North Am* 1999;46:1061–1072.

Baraff LJ. Management of fever without source in infants and children. *Ann Emerg Med* 2000;36:602–614.

Baskin MN, O'Rourke EJ, Fleisher GR. Outpatient treatment of febrile infants 28 to 89 days of age with intramuscular administration of ceftriaxone [see comments]. *J Pediatr* 1992;120:22–27.

7. IRRITABLE CHILD

I. **Problem:** Four-month-old male brought to ED for episodic crying for 8 h; he is afebrile and intermittently listless.

II. **Immediate Questions**
   A. **Vital signs stable?** ABCs come before evaluation of neurologic status.
   B. **Mental status normal?** Is infant "toxic" or "lethargic"? Consolable, or "paradoxically" more irritable when held or moved? Visually interact, want to eat, responsively smile? How long has infant been crying? Is it acute or chronic, constant or paroxysmal? Appearance of baby between crying spells?
   C. **Associated symptoms?** Fever, vomiting, diarrhea? Cough, rhinitis, respiratory distress? Poor feeding? Pain with limb movement? Apnea or seizure-like episodes?
   D. **Past medical or family history?** Current or recent medications, history of trauma, previous ED visits, immunization history, past illnesses or diagnoses, ill contacts, daycare exposures.

III. **Differential Diagnosis**
   A. **Infectious**
      1. **Meningitis.** Nuchal rigidity inconsistent in infants; fever may be lacking. A full fontanelle and/or vomiting may be seen. Antibiotic pretreatment should lower threshold for LP.
      2. **UTI.** One third of young children are afebrile. Infants with culture-proven UTIs frequently have normal UA.
      3. **Septic arthritis/osteomyelitis.** Lower extremity involvement most common; toxicity and fever may be absent. The infant may exhibit pseudoparalysis and pain on passive movement.
      4. **Otitis media.** Often overcalled in young infants. Be wary of treating infants < 3 mon without additional laboratory evaluation.
      5. **Viral gastroenteritis, URI.** Crying should not be persistent; systemic toxicity is lacking.
   B. **Traumatic**
      1. **Nonaccidental trauma.** Highest risk in children < 2. May present as a crying, irritable infant, although many have a chief complaint of listlessness or lethargy. Most infants with shaken baby syndrome do not have external signs of trauma. Any facial bruising in infancy is suggestive of physical abuse.
      2. **Corneal abrasion.** Common, use fluorescein to check. Conjunctivitis, fever absent.
   C. **Gastrointestinal**
      1. **Intussusception.** Peak incidence, 2 mon–2 years. Paroxysms of crying from abdominal pain usually an early symptom. Between

episodes child initially appears well, later is lethargic. Presence of "currant jelly stool" a late finding—if absent, do rectal exam. Misdiagnosed as sepsis, shaken baby syndrome, or drug ingestion. Upper quadrant mass may be palpable.

2. **GERD/esophagitis.** History of frequent nonforceful, nonbilious regurgitation following feedings. Infant may take sips from breast or bottle then cry.
3. **Constipation.** Defined by consistency of stool (hard is not normal) rather than frequency (soft stools every few days are fine).
4. **Incarcerated inguinal hernia.** Always open the diaper.
5. **Appendicitis.** Unusual, presents without focal RLQ pain because perforation rate in young children approaches 100%.

D. **Integument**
  1. **Hair tourniquet syndrome.** An encircling hair may lead to strangulation of a toe, finger, penis, clitoris, or uvula.

E. **Cardiovascular**
  1. **SVT.** The cause of "unexplained intractable crying" in 4% of afebrile infants.

F. **Miscellaneous**
  1. **Infant colic syndrome.** Characterized by recurrent paroxysms of usually nocturnal crying beginning at 1–4 wk of age, peaking at 6 wk of age, diminishing by 4 mon. Vomiting, diarrhea, or fever are not features of infant colic syndrome.
  2. **Teething.** Onset no earlier than 4 mon, associated with a swollen, tender gum, does not account for fever.
  3. **Foreign body.** Infants too young to do this by themselves often "helped" by older siblings.

IV. **Database**
  A. **Physical Exam Key Points.** A brief period of nonthreatening observation while child sits on parent's lap yields vital information regarding interaction, playfulness, willingness to smile, ability to be comforted, respiratory rate and pattern, and extremity movement. Distraction is the essence of a successful pediatric examination. The most annoying aspects of the examination (tympanic membranes, pharynx, rectum) should be deferred until last.
    1. **Vital signs.** Fever indicates infection.
    2. **General appearance.** Most important part of exam.
    3. **HEENT.** Fontanelle, facial bruising, oropharyngeal lesions, corneal abrasions, foreign body.
    4. **Neck.** Nuchal rigidity.
    5. **Cardiac.** Tachyarrhythmia.
    6. **Abdomen.** Tenderness, guarding, masses.
    7. **Skin.** Bruising, hair tourniquet.
    8. **Musculoskeletal.** Point tenderness, extremity pain with passive range of motion.
    9. **Genital/Rectal.** Hernia, scrotal redness, testicular swelling or tenderness, anal fissures, bloody or hard stool.

B. Laboratory Data

1. **Routine screening tests.** Of little value. If a careful physical exam does not reveal abnormalities, try fluorescein staining of cornea and catheterized UA with urine culture.
2. **CBC with Diff, blood culture, and LP.** Should be done as clinically indicated. More extensive evaluation generally warranted in young infants (particularly if fever present).

C. Radiographic and Other Studies

1. **CXR,** other plain films. Done as clinically indicated.
2. **Air or barium enema.** If intussusception suspected.
3. **Head CT.** If abuse suspected.

V. Plan

A. Overall Plan.
Persistent crying or toxicity after initial ED evaluation warrants additional investigation, and/or admission. Arrangement and documentation of appropriate follow-up important, especially if cause of crying obscure at discharge.

B. Specific Plans

1. **Infectious.** Obtain cultures and start therapy. Young children are admitted for treatment more often than older children and adults.
2. **Traumatic.** If nonaccidental, comprehensive evaluation indicated.
3. **Hair tourniquet syndrome.** Cut hair or use depilatory cream.
4. **Esophagitis.** An empiric trial of flavored antacid, 2.5 mL 5 min before each feeding for several days is reasonable. Ranitidine and metoclopramide may be considered in highly suggestive cases with follow-up.
5. **Infant colic syndrome.** Counseling regarding natural history of colic should be done for all cases. Chamomile tea may be helpful. Simethicone is a high-grade placebo. Avoid paregoric dicyclomine, hyoscyamine sulfate, and empiric formula changes. Arrange follow-up.

VI. ICD-9 Diagnoses:
Child abuse, unspecified; Constipation; Corneal abrasion; Gastroesophageal reflux; Hernia—obstructed; Infantile colic; Intussusception; Meningitis; Supraventricular tachycardia; Teething; Urinary tract infection.

VII. Problem Case Diagnosis:
Intussusception.

VIII. Teaching Pearls Question:
How often is abusive head trauma in children missed?

IX. Teaching Pearls Answer:
Thirty-one percent of children with an acute episode of abusive head trauma were initially "missed" by physician; 28% of these children were reinjured during period of diagnostic delay. Most frequent misdiagnoses were viral gastroenteritis, accidental head trauma, rule-out sepsis, and colic (Jenny, 1999).

REFERENCES

Bolte RG. Intractable crying in infancy and early childhood. In: Aghababian RV, ed. *Emergency Medicine: The Core Curriculum.* Lippincott-Raven, 1998:622–630.

Jenny C, Hymel KP, Ritzen A, Reinert SE, Hay TC. Analysis of missed cases of abusive head trauma. *JAMA* 1999;281:621–626.

Poole SR. The infant with acute, unexplained, excessive crying. *Pediatrics* 1991;88: 450–455.

8. MUSCULOSKELETAL PROBLEMS IN CHILDREN

I. **Problem:** A 3-year-old male is brought by his parents for evaluation of a limp.

II. **Immediate Questions**

   A. **What are the vitals and mental status?** Is the patient stable and alert? Signs of toxicity, ill appearance, or obvious trauma may provide immediate clues.

   B. **Was there a history of trauma preceding onset of symptom?** May be relatively minor or absent in young children. Consider nonaccidental trauma if obvious injury without consistent history. Consider possible associated injuries.

   C. **Is there a fever?** Duration and intensity? Presence indicates infectious or inflammatory condition, but absence does not rule out.

   D. **How long has he been limping?** Acute or insidious onset? Recurrent? Worsening over time?

   E. **Any associated symptoms?** Pain, swelling, morning stiffness, night sweats, or weight loss? Remember knee pain may be referred from the hip in children.

   F. **Is there related past medical history?** Include birth and developmental history. Recent viral or strep infection? Recent medication use? Joint pain or swelling? Unexplained injuries? Family history of autoimmune or bleeding disorders?

III. **Differential Diagnosis**

   A. **Traumatic.** Sudden onset without systemic symptoms.

      1. **Fracture.** Torus, greenstick, and physeal fractures are unique to immature skeleton and may be subtle on radiographs. Consider toddler's fracture in 1–3-year-olds with minor mechanism. Pelvic avulsion fractures and slipped capital femoral epiphysis occur in adolescents.

      2. **Sprain/strain.** Less likely than fractures in skeletally immature patient.

      3. **Contusion.** Consider compartment syndrome in severe crush injury.

      4. **Hemarthrosis.** Consider bleeding disorder or ligament disruption.

   B. **Infectious/inflammatory.** Fever often present.

1. **Septic arthritis.** Most serious infectious cause and true surgical emergency. Usually due to hematogenous spread. Joint often warm and swollen with severe pain on movement. May be toxic appearing.
2. **Transient synovitis.** History of recent viral infection common. Usually milder course but may mimic early septic arthritis.
3. **Osteomyelitis.** Presentation is more chronic than septic arthritis. Usually due to hematogenous spread.
4. **Rheumatic.** Lyme disease, Henoch-Schönlein purpura, acute rheumatic fever, JRA, SLE.
5. **Discitis.** Back pain and local tenderness may not be present.

C. **Neurologic.** Consider central (transverse myelitis, MS), peripheral (Guillain-Barré, reflex sympathetic dystrophy), muscular (muscular dystrophy, myositis) etiologies.

D. **Neoplastic.** Bone pain from systemic (ALL, AML) and localized (osteosarcoma, Ewing's sarcoma, spinal cord tumor) malignancies.

E. **Metabolic.** Consider rickets.

F. **Other.** Consider Legg-Calvé-Perthes disease, Osgood-Schlatter disease, foreign body in the foot, testicular torsion, appendicitis, inguinal hernia.

IV. **Database**

A. **Physical Exam Key Points**
1. **Vital signs.** Check for fever, and repeat during evaluation. Check for signs of systemic illness or toxicity.
2. **Head and neck.** Check for associated head or neck trauma. Check for cervical lymphadenopathy.
3. **Abdomen.** Check for hepatosplenomegaly or mass. Check for RLQ tenderness that may indicate appendicitis. Check for inguinal hernia and testicular torsion.
4. **Back.** Check for CVA or focal spinal column tenderness.
5. **Extremities.** Observe position child holds extremity (flexion with external rotation of thigh indicates intraarticular hip pathology). Check for localized redness, swelling, deformity, or tenderness. Check for effusion or limited ROM of joints. Check feet for foreign bodies. Check for regional or diffuse lymphadenopathy.
6. **Neurologic.** Check strength, sensation, and reflexes.
7. **Gait.** Watch patient walk without shoes on and with legs exposed. Check stride length, time spent in stance phase, joint flexibility.

B. **Laboratory Data.** If fever present, check CBC, ESR, CRP. Consider also in afebrile child with normal radiographs. If history or physical is suggestive of malignancy consider CBC, LDH, uric acid. Consider Lyme titer in child with arthritis living in endemic area.

C. **Radiographic and Other Studies.** If history of trauma or focal findings on PE, obtain radiographs of involved area. Comparison views may be helpful. For limp in toddler without obvious source on PE, obtain AP and frog-leg lateral radiograph of both hips; consider femur and lower leg films. Obtain hip US to look for effusion in children with increased joint space on hip films or history and PE highly suggestive of septic arthritis. Consider bone scan if work-up does not indicate cause and symptoms persist.

V. Plan
    A. Overall Plan. Evaluate for traumatic injuries and systemic illness and stabilize as necessary. Evaluate for serious bacterial infections. Treat injuries as indicated.

    B. Specific Plans
        1. Fractures. Provide appropriate definitive care (splint, cast, or orthopedic evaluation for reduction/surgery) depending on fracture location and type.

        2. Septic arthritis or osteomyelitis. Admit for IV antibiotics and possible surgical debridement. Orthopedics consult recommended.

        3. Transient synovitis. Rest, NSAIDs, reevaluate the following day. Consider further work-up for worsening symptoms.

        4. Neoplastic. May require admission after consultation with oncologist.

VI. ICD-9 Diagnoses:
Abnormality of gait; Juvenile rheumatoid arthritis; Osgood–Schlatter's disease; Osteogenesis imperfecta; Scoliosis; Septic arthritis; Slipped capital femoral epiphysis.

VII. Problem Case Diagnosis:
Transient synovitis.

VIII. Teaching Pearl Question:
What is the most common pathogen in both septic arthritis and osteomyelitis in children?

IX. Teaching Pearl Answer:
Staphylococcus aureus.

REFERENCES

Clark MC. The limping child: Meeting the challenges of an accurate assessment and diagnosis. *Pediatr Emerg Med Reports* 1997;2:123–134.

Del Beccaro MA, Champoux AN, Bockers T, Mendelman PM. Septic arthritis versus transient synovitis of the hip: The value of screening laboratory tests. *Ann Emerg Med* 1992;21:1418–1422.

Myers MT, Thompson GH. Imaging the child with a limp. *Pediatr Clin North Am* 1997;44: 637–658.

9. NONACCIDENTAL TRAUMA IN CHILDREN

I. Problem:
Ambulance brings in 3-month-old male found unresponsive by his father. Child has bruising. Father states child "rolled off the bed."

II. Immediate Questions
    A. Is airway patent and child breathing adequately? Airway management according to BLS and PALS guidelines.

  B. **Vital signs and mental status?** Is patient still unresponsive? If so, proceed with PALS/ATLS guidelines. Check pupils for retinal hemorrhages and reactivity.

  C. **Trauma history?** History of minor trauma (fall off couch or bed) with subsequent major head trauma indicates nonaccidental trauma/abusive head injury.

  D. **How was child acting before he became unresponsive?** Any seizure activity? If "acting well" immediately prior to episode, unlikely to be sepsis, CNS infection, meningoencephalitis.

  E. **Any history of sudden or infant death in a sibling?** Raises concern of metabolic disease or dysrhythmia (prolonged QT syndrome). Family history of previous or multiple SIDS victim should raise concern for nonaccidental trauma. Extensive history of trauma in siblings may indicate poor care at the least, abuse at worst.

  F. **Significant past medical history?** Cardiac dysrhythmias, seizures, major infections, fractures.

  G. **Could this be an ingestion?** What medications are in the home? More common in children 1–5 years old, unlikely in infants younger than 12 months unless older sibling or caretaker gave child medication.

III. Differential Diagnosis

  A. **Nonaccidental Trauma.** Suspect when the severity of injury/injuries is not explained by the history provided by the caretaker. Bruising is *quite* rare in nonambulatory infants (Sugar et al, 1999).

  B. **Accidental Trauma.** Minor falls cause minor (head) injuries. May rarely (1–3%) cause skull fracture.

  C. **Metabolic.** Rarely presents with sudden onset of abnormal mental status. May have family history or previous developmental concerns. Osteogenesis imperfecta is rare, abuse is common. Patients with osteogenesis imperfecta often have positive family histories, blue sclera, abnormal teeth, hearing impairment, osteoporosis, abnormal fracture healing, short stature, and other features that allow them to be distinguished by those with experience in this field.

  D. **CNS Infection.** Meningoencephalitis should have symptoms. Herpes simplex encephalitis can have associated intracranial hemorrhage.

  E. **Intracranial Hemorrhage.** From vitamin K deficiency (usually occurs within first 4–8 weeks after birth) or ruptured A-V malformation.

  F. **ALTE.** See Problem 3. Apparent Life-Threatening Event.

  G. **Hematologic.** New-onset bruising may represent thrombocytopenia (from leukemia or ITP) or clotting factor disorder (hemophilia).

IV. Database

  A. **Physical Exam Key Points.** Evidence of external injury may be subtle or absent. Look for any external evidence of trauma such as facial bruising or abrasions (seen in over a third of missed cases of abusive head injury [Jenny et al, 1999]); bruising elsewhere; scalp swelling. Feel for a bulging fontanel.

    B. Laboratory Data. CBC and PT/PTT looking for evidence of bleeding disorder. LFTs, amylase, lipase looking for associated occult abdominal injury.

    C. Radiographic and Other Studies. Head CT looking for evidence of abusive head injury may reveal acute or chronic subdural hemorrhage, skull fracture, cerebral edema, or other intracranial processes. MRI may facilitate the dating of hemorrhages.

V. Plan

    A. Overall Plan. Contact child protective services for *any* child with an injury suggestive of nonaccidental trauma. This is a legal mandate. Admit any child with suggestive injuries until a safe environment is found for the child.

    B. Specific Plans

        1. Nonaccidental trauma. If ED evaluation showed classic constellation of findings of abusive head injury/shaken baby syndrome (SDH, retinal hemorrhages, cerebral edema), obtain a skeletal survey. Look for associated skeletal injuries (seen in up to half of cases of abusive head injury) such as (posterior) rib fractures or classic metaphyseal lesions ("bucket handle," "corner" fractures) of the long bones. Document any bruising seen with photographs. Obtain ophthalmology consult for a dilated retinal exam. Consult the child protection team/child abuse evaluation team.

        2. Accidental trauma. Corroborate history provided.

        3. Metabolic. Obtain basic metabolic profile, looking for acidosis, hypoglycemia. . .

        4. Sepsis/CNS infection. Treat with intravenous antibiotics if any evidence of possible infection.

        5. Seizure. EEG.

        6. Ingestion. Toxicologic screen or specialized testing for substances often missed on standard screening tests (hair samples for methamphetamine exposure).

VI. ICD-9 Diagnoses: Child abuse, unspecified; Child emotional/psychologic abuse; Child sexual abuse; Child physical abuse; Shaken infant syndrome.

VII. Problem Case Diagnosis: Nonaccidental trauma, child abuse, shaken baby syndrome, abusive head injury.

VIII. Teaching Pearls Question: What percentage of healthy 3-month-old/nonambulatory infants will have bruises?

IX. Teaching Pearls Answer: Less than 1% (Sugar et al, 1999).

REFERENCES

Jenny C, Hymel KP, Ritzen A, Reinert SE, Hay TC. Analysis of missed cases of abusive head trauma. *JAMA* 1999;281:621–626.

Levin A. Retinal hemorrhages and child abuse. *Rec Adv Paediatr* 2000;18:151–219.

Sugar N, Taylor J, Feldman K. Those that don't cruise rarely bruise. *Arch Pediatr Adolesc Med* 1999;153:399–403.

10. SWALLOWED FOREIGN BODY

I. **Problem:** A child presents with drooling and chest pain after swallowing a penny.

II. **Immediate Questions**
   A. **Respiratory distress present?** If child is unable to phonate and is in extreme distress, perform foreign body removal technique (usually Heimlich maneuver) appropriate for age. If the child is in respiratory distress or failure, suspect tracheal location.
   B. **Any blue spells or significant choking spell related to the ingestion?** When did ingestion occur? Just because parents did not see ingestion does not mean one did not occur. Suspect foreign body in cases of stridor, poor feeding, chest pain of hours to weeks duration.
   C. **Has the child been able to eat or drink after the ingestion?** Chest pain, foreign body sensation, drooling present? Time of last PO intake?
   D. **Any past medical history?** Esophageal stenosis? History of pica or previous foreign body removals?

III. **Differential Diagnosis**
   A. **Airway Foreign Body**
      1. History of significant choking episode usually present, often associated with blue spell.
      2. Degree of respiratory distress may range from mild to severe, depending on size, shape, and location of foreign body.
   B. **Esophageal Foreign Body**
      1. History may also include gagging/choking spell, foreign body sensation.
      2. Physical exam may reveal drooling.
      3. Minimal or no respiratory distress should be present.
   C. **GI Foreign Body**
      1. History of ingestion usually present.
      2. Foreign body sensation often present due to mucosal trauma.
      3. Physical findings (abdominal pain) rarely present.

IV. **Database**
   A. **Physical Exam Key Points**
      1. **Presence of respiratory distress.** Differential breath sounds, wheezing, or diminished air movement suggests an airway foreign body.
      2. **Oropharynx.** Inspect for retained foreign body. Inspect for drooling.
   B. **Metal Detector.** Helpful for the location and presence of coins. Unreliable for other metallic foreign bodies.
   C. **Radiographic and Other Studies**
      1. **CXR.** Will detect radiopaque foreign body in thorax
      2. **Abdominal film.** Often done in conjunction with a CXR for GI foreign body.

3. **Barium swallow.** Recommended for nonradiopaque objects in symptomatic child (drooling, chest pain, vomiting) when esophageal foreign body a concern.

V. **Plan**
   A. **Overall Plan.** All esophageal foreign bodies and aspirated foreign bodies warrant removal.
   B. **Specific Plans**
      1. **Disc button batteries.** Warrant prompt removal if esophageal in location. Disc batteries in GI tract rarely require removal, unless not moving within several days.
      2. **Esophageal coins.** Patients with asymptomatic esophageal coins may be observed at home for 24 h to attempt spontaneous passage. Esophageal coins with duration of 24 h are frequently removed by radiologists under fluoroscopy using a Foley catheter. Other options include rigid endoscopic surgical removal.
      3. **Other esophageal foreign bodies.** Warrant prompt removal endoscopically.
      4. **Foreign bodies distal to the esophagus.** Rarely require removal unless the object is 2 in. in length or is a long sewing needle.

VI. **ICD-9 Diagnoses:** Foreign body—swallowed.

VII. **Problem Case Diagnosis:** Penny in the esophagus.

VIII. **Teaching Pearls Question:** How many hours after ingestion of a button battery can esophageal rupture occur?

IX. **Teaching Pearls Answer:** Six hours after ingestion (Litovitz et al).

REFERENCES

Bassett KE, Schunk JE, Logan L. Localizing ingested coins with a metal detector. *Am J Emerg Med* 1999;(17):338–341.

Litovitz TL, Schmitz BF. Ingestion of cylindrical and button batteries: An analysis of 2382 cases. *Pediatrics* 1992;89:747–757.

Schunk JE, Harrison AM, Corneli HM, Nixon GW. Fluoroscopic Foley catheter removal of esophageal foreign bodies in children: Experience with 415 episodes. *Pediatrics* 1994;(94):709–714.

Soprano JV, Fleisher GR, Mandl KD. The spontaneous passage of esophageal coins in children. *Arch Pediatr Adolesc Med* 1999;(153):1073–1076.

11. VOMITING AND DIARRHEA IN CHILDREN

I. **Problem:** A child presents with nonbilious, nonbloody vomiting and watery diarrhea with a normal activity level, but slightly sunken eyes and dry mucous membranes.

II. **Immediate Questions**
   A. **Is the patient clinically stable?** Are airway, breathing, circulation adequate, are vital signs within normal limits for age?

B. **Are any of the following risk factors for more serious illness present?**
  1. Abdominal pain with tenderness, with or without guarding?
  2. Bilious or bloody emesis?
  3. Pallor, jaundice, oliguria/anuria, bloody diarrhea?
  4. Systemically unwell, out of proportion to level of dehydration?
C. **Is the child clinically dehydrated?**
  1. Decreased skin turgor, peripheral perfusion?
  2. Kussmaul breathing?
  3. Dry oral mucosa, sunken eyes?
  4. Listlessness, inconsolability?
D. **Pertinent History**
  1. How long has the child been ill? Consider bacterial or parasitic causes for problems that persist, especially if longer than a week.
  2. How much is the child drinking, urinating?
  3. Is the vomiting projectile?
  4. Volume and frequency of diarrhea?
  5. Is the child in daycare? Are there known ill contacts? Have others who have eaten the same food as the affected child developed similar symptoms?
  6. Travel outside of the country, pets, well water?
E. **Medications**
  Prolonged antibiotic use? Makes Clostridium difficile infection more likely. Antimotility agents used?
F. **Past medical history.** Is the child immunocompromised? History of UTI?

III. **Differential Diagnosis**
  A. **Acute Life-Threatening Causes**
    1. **Intussusception**/surgical abdomen/obstruction.
        a. Abdominal pain with tenderness, with or without guarding.
        b. Bilious or bloody emesis, bloody diarrhea.
        c. Systemically unwell, out of proportion to the level of dehydration.
        d. Shock.
    2. **Nonaccidental trauma.**
        a. Ecchymosis, facial and/or scalp injuries.
        b. Inconsolability, irritability.
        c. Altered mental status, seizure.
    3. **HUS.**
        a. Pallor, jaundice.
        b. Oliguria/anuria.
        c. Bloody diarrhea.
        d. Shock.
    4. **Pseudomembranous colitis.**
        a. History of antibiotic use.
        b. Ill-appearing child with bloody diarrhea.

5. *Salmonella* gastroenteritis in a neonate.
   a. Can lead to bacteremia and meningitis.
6. **Toxic megacolon.**
   a. Seen in Hirschsprung's disease or inflammatory bowel disease.
7. **Appendicitis.**
   a. Gastroenteritis most frequent misdiagnosis.
   b. Children perforate at far higher rate than adults.
   c. Pediatric exam more difficult, less focal.
8. **Head trauma** (nonaccidental).
   a. Vomiting may be accompanied by diarrhea.
   b. True history may not be revealed.
   c. Consider in the ill-appearing, vomiting infant.
9. **Hydrocephalus.**
   a. Often presents with vomiting.

B. **Common Causes**
   1. Viral gastroenteritis.
   2. Food poisoning.
   3. Hepatitis.
   4. Pyelonephritis (complicated UTI).
   5. GERD.
   6. Pyloric stenosis (young infant only).
   7. Guardianships.

IV. **Database**
   A. **Physical Exam Key Points**
      1. **General**
         a. Listlessness, fatigue, irritability.
      2. **HEENT.**
         a. Dry oral mucosa, sunken eyes.
         b. Fontanelle sunken (dehydration), or full (increased ICP).
      3. **Cardiorespiratory.**
         a. Shock, decreased peripheral perfusion.
         b. Deep acidotic breathing, grunting.
      4. **Abdominal exam.**
         a. Presence, location, quality of pain, guarding, rebound, or distention.
      5. **Skin exam.**
         a. Pallor, jaundice, petechiae, or purpura.
         b. Decreased skin turgor, check on abdominal wall.
         c. Ecchymosis, facial and/or scalp injuries.
   B. **Laboratory Data**
      1. **Stool for guaiac, culture, ova & parasites** if:
         a. Bloody diarrhea, associated high fever.
         b. Chronic diarrhea.
      2. **Lytes, BUN, creatinine,** if:
         a. Severe dehydration with circulatory compromise.
         b. Moderate dehydration—"doughy" skin may indicate hypernatremia.

   c. Moderately dehydrated children whose histories or physical findings are inconsistent with straightforward diarrheal episodes.

  3. UA and urine culture if
   a. Vomiting and fever are the primary components of the illness in girls < 3 years or uncircumcised boys < 6 months.

  4. CBC, Lytes, coagulation studies, stool for *Escherichia coli* 0157:H7 and UA if diarrhea bloody, concerns for HUS.

 C. Radiographic and Other Studies
  1. Abdominal film to rule out obstruction if emesis bilious.
  2. Air contrast enema if concerns for intussusception.
  3. Head CT for concerns of nonaccidental trauma.

V. Plan
 A. Overall Plan. Rule out life-threatening causes of vomiting and diarrhea. Treat dehydration, and regularly assess success of rehydration.

 B. Specific Plans
  1. Mild to moderate dehydration (3–8% body wt).
   a. Oral rehydration solution (ORS) 30–80 mL/kg given little and often (5 mL every 1–2 min) over 3–4 h.
   b. If PO ORS not tolerated or large ongoing losses present, consider use of ORS via NG tube, or IV NS or LR 20 mL/kg repeated once.

  2. Severe dehydration (9–10% body wt).
   a. NS or LR IV 20 mL/kg repeated up to twice.

  3. Refeeding following rehydration.
   a. Breast-feeding children should continue to breast-feed.
   b. In the dehydrated child with gastroenteritis who is normally formula-fed, feeds may be stopped during rehydration but should be restarted when possible.

  4. Disposition.
   a. Admit children with severe dehydration.
   b. Those with mild-moderate dehydration should be observed in a for a period of at least 6 h.
   c. Those at high risk of dehydration (< 6 mon, high frequency of watery stools or vomiting) should be closely monitored.

  5. Treatment recommendations.
   a. Infants and children with gastroenteritis are not treated with antidiarrheal agents.
   b. Most bacterial gastroenteritis does not require or benefit from antibiotic treatment. *Exceptions: Salmonella* gastroenteritis in infants, immunocompromised patients, and those systemically ill, or shigellosis in any patient.

VI. ICD-9 Diagnoses: Diarrhea; Infectious diarrhea; Presumed infectious diarrhea; Dehydration; Newborn dehydration; Gastroenteritis; Viral gastroenteritis; Vomiting; Newborn vomiting; Uncontrollable vomiting.

VII. **Problem Case Diagnosis:** Viral gastroenteritis with moderate dehydration.

VII. **Teaching Pearl Question:** Should antimotility agents be given in the setting of high frequency diarrhea?

VIII. **Teaching Pearl Answer:** Antimotility agents should be avoided as these may increase the risk of HUS.

REFERENCES

Armon K, Stephenson T, MacFaul R, Eccleston P, Werneke U. An evidence and consensus based guideline for acute diarrhea management. *Arch Dis Child* 2001;85:132–142.

Bell BP, Griffin PM, Lozano P, Christie DL, Kobayashi JM, Tarr PI. Predictors of hemolytic uremic syndrome in children during a large outbreak of Escherichia coli 0157:H7 infections. *Pediatrics* 1997;100(1):E12.

Liebelt EL. Clinical and laboratory evaluation and management of children with vomiting, diarrhea, and dehydration. *Curr Opin Pediatr* 1998;10(5):461–469.

Murphy MS. "Guidelines for managing acute gastroenteritis based on a systemic review of published research." *Arch Dis Child* 1998;79:279–284.

12. WHEEZING IN CHILDREN

I. **Problem:** A 16-month-old female presents during winter with new-onset cough and difficulty breathing, worsening progressively over 2 days. She "felt warm" last night. Diffuse wheezing is noted bilaterally on auscultation.

II. **Immediate Questions**
   A. **Is the patient in severe respiratory distress or impending respiratory failure?** Observe breathing difficulties (stridor, retractions, nasal flaring, tachypnea, grunting, coughing, hoarseness, agitation). Marked respiratory distress and/or a blood gas showing significant respiratory acidosis can indicate respiratory failure. Administer oxygen, place patient on monitors, establish IV access, secure airway as needed.
   B. **Previous episodes of respiratory distress?** Wheezing, pneumonia, "bronchitis," RSV infection.
   C. **Risk factors for respiratory problems?** History of prematurity, cardiac conditions, failure to thrive, exposure to smoke or allergens, winter season, family history of asthma, allergy, atopy.
   D. **Possibility of aspiration or foreign body?** Did distress start when child was eating or had something in her mouth?

III. **Differential Diagnosis**
   A. **Asthma.** Viral URI most common trigger for children.
   B. **Bronchiolitis.** Infant age group, winter onset, community outbreaks.
   C. **Pneumonia** (may be viral, bacterial, atypical). CXR helps distinguish type.
   D. **GERD.** May have history of severe "spitting up," fussiness with feeds, twisting and arching with feeds (Sandifer's syndrome).
   E. **Foreign Body.** Always consider, even with history of asthma.

    F. **CHF.** Due to myocarditis, congenital heart defects, severe anemia. Recognition difficult in young child; high index of suspicion is needed to cull these patients from children with wheezing and cough due to viral infections. Physical exam may reveal other congenital defects, an enlarged liver, hypotension, absent or abnormal pulses.

    G. **Complications of Prematurity.** Bronchopulmonary dysplasia, tracheomalacia.

    H. **Anaphylaxis.** Usually accompanied by skin findings and historical clues.

    I. **Genetic Disorders.** CF, vascular rings, tracheoesophageal fistula.

    J. **Tumors** (eg, lymphoma). Often visible on CXR as "retrocardiac pneumonia."

IV. Database

  A. **Physical Exam Key Points**

    1. **Vital signs.** RR (often high at triage due to excitement or fear, measure again when calm), fever (affects RR, remeasure after antipyresis), HR (tachycardia may be a measure of respiratory distress), pulse ox (the "fifth vital sign").

    2. **General appearance.** Ill vs well, cyanosis, evidence of atopy, tripod positioning.

    3. **Respiratory status.** Shortness of breath, fatigue; presence and location of wheezing; diminished breath sounds; measured FEV_1 using peak flow meter (in older, cooperative children).

    4. **Cardiac.** Cyanosis; clubbing; heart murmur.

  B. **Laboratory Data.** Consider blood gas, CBC, blood culture, chemistry panel, ECG.

  C. **Radiographic and Other Studies.** Consider CXR (AP and lateral); inspiratory/expiratory films or lateral decubitus films in smaller infants for possible foreign bodies.

V. Plan

  A. **Overall Plan.** May require some or all of the following: Oxygen, pulse ox, cardiac monitor, portable CXR, blood gas, intubation.

  B. **Specific Plans**

    1. **Asthma.** If no previous management, give several nebulized β_2-agonist (albuterol) treatments. Consider adding nebulized ipratropium bromide (an anticholinergic) in patients with moderate to severe distress. Consider steroid use (orally or parenterally) immediately for severe exacerbation, and in mild to moderate exacerbation if no immediate response to inhaled therapy. Parenteral magnesium sulfate (40 mg/kg IV) may help a subset of severely ill patients. Consider CXR to rule out other causes of wheezing/hypoxia/fever. Recommend transfer to an ICU for progressive respiratory distress despite management with steroids and nebulized medications. Theophylline is no longer used in the acute management of asthma.

2. **Pneumonia.** Administer oxygen. Often accompanied by dehydration, consider IV fluid administration. If without respiratory distress and nonhypoxic, consider outpatient management with antibiotics. If hypoxic, in respiratory distress, or with significant infiltrate/effusion on CXR, consider CBC, blood culture, and admission for parenteral antibiotics. In older children, consider atypical pneumonia (eg, *Mycoplasma*) when choosing treatment.

3. **Foreign body.** Portable radiographs if child in distress. Consultants from general surgery, ENT, and gastroenterology may remove foreign bodies, depending on institution.

4. **CHF.** CXR may show cardiomegaly and/or increased pulmonary vascular markings (pulmonary edema). Child may be wheezing with respiratory distress and be hypotensive due to heart failure. Recommend supplemental oxygen, ECG if heart failure suspected, inotropic support PRN, cardiology consultation, admission.

VI. **ICD-9 Diagnoses:** Wheezing; Asphyxia—food or foreign body; Bronchiolitis; Pneumonia; Vascular ring—congenital.

VII. **Problem Case Diagnosis:** New-onset reactive airways disease triggered by winter respiratory viral infection.

VIII. **Teaching Pearls Question:** In a child with asymmetry on auscultation with the suspected history of a foreign body aspiration, what might an inspiratory/expiratory CXR reveal?

IX. **Teaching Pearls Answer:** Unilateral obstructive hyperinflation or atelectasis. Pneumonia may be present if presentation delayed. If history and physical exam are strongly suggestive of pneumonic foreign body, a normal CXR does not rule out this possibility.

REFERENCES

Rosenthal B. Wheezing. In: Fleisher GR, Ludwig S, Henretig FM, Ruddy RM, Silverman BK, eds. *Textbook of Pediatric Emergency Medicine.* 4th ed. Lippincott Williams & Wilkins, 2000:643–649.

Scarfone RJ. Bronchiolitis—Or Is It? *Pediatr Ann* 2000;29:89–92.

III. Trauma Emergency On-Call Problems

1. TRAUMA ASSESSMENT AND RESUSCITATION

I. **Problem:** An 18-year-old unhelmeted woman is unconscious and hypotensive (BP 80/50 mm Hg) with multiple injuries after a motorcycle crash (MCC).

II. **Immediate Questions**
- **A. Is airway intact?** Manage appropriately (see Section VIII, 15. Rapid Sequence Endotracheal Intubation, page 470). Commence/maintain C-spine immobilization.
- **B. Breathing?** High-flow O_2, relieve tension pneumothorax, ventilate if needed. ICC for hemothorax or pneumothorax.
- **C. Circulation.** Check for tamponade bleeding, immobilize fractures, establish 2 IV access points ≥ #16. 1–2 L crystalloid (LR) stat if shocked (SBP < 90 mm Hg or pulse > 100).
- **D. Disability.** Record pupil size and reaction, response to voice, pain, and nil stimuli, reflexes, plantars. (See 3. Blunt Head Trauma, page 256, and 11. Neck and Spinal Cord Trauma, page 282)
- **E. Exposure.** Remove all clothing, examine whole body (and back), cover to keep warm.

III. **Differential Diagnosis**
- **A. Hypoxia or Airway Obstruction.** Most important to identify and treat.
- **B. Hypotension.** External and internal blood loss, fractures long bones.
- **C. Head Injury.**
- **D. Hypoglycemia.** May have caused crash. Check medic alerts, SQ injection marks. Bedside glucose.
- **E. Drugs/Alcohol.** May have caused crash. Check medic alerts, SQ injection marks.
- **F. Seizure.** Cause or complication.

IV. **Database**
- **A. Physical Exam Key Points**
  1. Identify and treat each life-threatening condition in order (A., B., C., D., E.) **before** moving on. Restart ABCDE if patient deteriorates.
  2. Check distal pulses before and after reducing fractures and dislocations.
  3. Don't forget back (log roll), ears (hemotympanum), rectum, and vagina in systematic head-to-toe exam. "Fingers and tubes in every orifice."
  4. Beware of possible spinal injury in unconscious patients. Patients with spinal cord injury are typically hypotensive and bradycardic.
  5. Consider pregnancy.

B. **Laboratory Data.** CBC, coagulation studies, chemistries, alcohol and drug screen, T&C, blood gas. Beta-HCG in female of childbearing age. Repeat H/H at least every 15 min in severely injured patients. Consider RL and repeat ABG to assess adequacy of resuscitation.

C. **Radiographic and Other Studies.** Lateral C-spine, CXR, pelvic radiograph as initial studies. Trauma US (if available). Limb radiographs, head CT, and other imaging only when patient stable.

V. Plan

A. Overall Plan

1. Activate trauma team early.
2. Identify and treat immediate life threats as they are found. Team members to be assigned to A. B. and C. Designated team leader to coordinate.
3. Sequence of further studies/surgery to be decided by relevant specialties in discussion.

B. Specific Plans

1. **Airway.** Clearing and protection highest priority.
2. **Breathing.** O_2 and adequate ventilation vital. Tension pneumothorax to be vented before CXR.
3. **Circulation** must be stabilized before patient leaves trauma room. Tamponade bleeding and splint fractures can be source of major blood loss. Commence blood after 2 L crystalloid. Use O-negative if no time for type-specific. Abdominal exam unreliable—patient may have 3 L of blood loss before distension. Suspect intra-abdominal bleeding if shock not explained by external loss, hemothorax, or limb fractures or if patient not responding to fluids. If not responsive to fluids or ICC drainage > 1.5 L initially or > 300 mL/h, will require immediate operation. Foley catheter to monitor urine output—suprapubic if blood present at urethral meatus or if prostate is mobile or high riding on rectal exam. Use gastric tube to decompress stomach—oral if midfacial injuries or suspect injuries at base of skull.
4. **Disability.** No unstable patient should go for CT. Neurosurgery, orthopedics, etc may review patient in OR or after patient is stabilized.
5. **Exposure.** Perform systematic head-to-toe exam once stabilized. Cover with blankets or external warming to prevent hypothermia. Suspect spinal injury in all major trauma patients. Spinal precautions and log roll at all times. Judicious use of IV analgesia once patient assessed fully—titrate to effect.
6. **History if possible** (Family/friends). Minimum necessary details: AMPLE = *a*llergies, *m*edications, *p*ast history/illnesses, *l*ast ate/drank, *e*vent details (mechanism of injury).
7. **Reassess frequently.** If patient deteriorates, recommence from A. Examine specifically for major life threats—ATOMIC = *a*irway obstruction, *t*ension pneumothorax, *o*pen pneumothorax, *m*assive hemothorax, *i*ncomplete (flail) chest, *c*ardiac tamponade.

VI. ICD-9 Diagnoses: As appropriate

VII. Problem Case Diagnosis: Hemopneumothorax, Liver laceration, Splenic hematoma, Left parietal cerebral contusion, Fractures of right wrist, left femur, left ankle.

VIII. Teaching Pearls Question: How much blood must be lost acutely before the systolic blood pressure falls?

IX. Teaching Pearls Answer: 30–40% of blood volume (1.5–2 L in a 70-kg adult) = class III shock.

REFERENCE

American College of Surgeons. *Advanced Trauma Life Support Student Manual.* 6th ed. American College of Surgeons Committee on Trauma, 1997:17–37.

2. BLUNT ABDOMINAL TRAUMA

I. Problem: A 35-year-old male, unrestrained driver in highway speed MVA, hypotensive, with severe abdominal pain, presents to the ED.

II. Immediate Questions/Primary Survey

A. Airway? Manage appropriately (See Section VIII, 15. Rapid Sequence Endotracheal Intubation, page 470, and Section III, 1. Trauma Assessment and Resuscitation, page 251).

B. Breathing? Signs of chest or abdominal injury? Note character of respiratory effort, rate, and breathing pattern. Are lung sounds equal? Abnormal breath sounds? Crepitance with palpation? Flail chest? High-flow O_2, pulse oximetry, assisted ventilations as indicated, needle or tube thoracostomy.

C. Circulation? Heart tones normal? Equal peripheral pulses? Obtain blood pressure, pulse, start two large-bore IVs, administer LR boluses.

D. Disability? AVPU? Pupils? Moving all extremities? Abdominal wall sensation intact? Consider blood glucose measurement.

E. Exposure? Remove all clothing from the patient. Check for abrasions, contusions, lacerations, deformities, bleeding. Note patterns of injuries. Remember to then cover patient to prevent hypothermia.

III. Differential Diagnosis

A. Solid visceral injuries
1. **Spleen.** Most commonly injured organ.
2. **Liver.** Second most commonly injured organ.

B. Hollow visceral injuries
1. **Small bowel**
2. **Stomach**
3. **Colon**
4. **Bladder**

    C. **Retroperitoneal injuries**
       1. **Kidney**
       2. **Duodenal rupture**
       3. **Pancreas**
       4. **Neurovascular structures**
    D. **Diaphragmatic injury**

IV. **Database/Secondary Survey.** (This will focus on the abdominal exam. For other aspects of trauma care, see the appropriate chapter).
    A. **Physical Exam Key Points**
       1. **Lungs.** Chest wall contusion, wounds, crepitance? Flail chest? Breath sounds equal or abnormal sounds?
       2. **Heart.** Rate, extra sounds (gallop, friction rub, murmur).
       3. **Abdomen.** Inspect (signs of injury, abdominal breathing, distension?). Auscultate (bowel sounds, bruits). Percuss (pain, hyperresonance). Palpate (rigid, doughy). Consider NG/OG tube as indicated.
       4. **Pelvis.** Stable? Equal pulses? Perineum? Blood at urethral meatus or introitus? Scrotal hematoma?
       5. **Back.** Midline tenderness? Ecchymosis? Other signs of injury?
       6. **Rectal.** Gross blood? Prostate position? Sphincter tone? Insert Foley catheter after normal rectal exam.
       7. **Neurologic.** Sensory exam of abdomen, pelvis should be performed; any loss of sensation is worrisome for spinal cord injury and interferes with abdominal exam.
    B. **History key points.** Do not delay primary survey and correction of life-threatening conditions to take the history.
       1. **Mechanism.** Shearing and compression forces are most common in blunt trauma. Speed of car? Seat belts? Ejection? Vehicle damage (interior and exterior)?
       2. **AMPLE history. A**llergies, **m**edications, **p**ast medical history, **l**ast meal, **e**vents leading to presentation.
    C. **Laboratory studies**
       1. **Hct.** (May be normal initially—Do not delay transfusion if normal Hct but patient shows signs of shock and is unresponsive to bolus fluid therapy).
       2. **Platelets.** Transfuse platelets for platelet count < 50,000 and signs of shock.
       3. **T&S or T&C.** All patients should have T&S. T&C—For clear evidence of injury, shock, T&C 4–6 units. Transfuse O-negative blood initially if patient unresponsive to fluid boluses or shock is profound.
       4. **Chemistries.** Rapid bedside glucose. CO_2 levels. Consider CO-oximetry if patient was exposed to fire or toxic substances. Other chemistry values should be based on patient's condition, medications, and comorbidities.
       5. **ABG.** Will give hemoglobin determination more rapidly than CBC. Important acid–base information. Base deficit > 5 mmol/L in-

dicates need for continued aggressive resuscitation. Base deficit > 15 mmol/L may indicate 25% mortality rate (Rutherford et al)

6. **LFTs.** AST or ALT > 130 correlates with serious hepatic injury.
7. **Amylase.** More accurate 3–6 h after injury.
8. **UA.** Indicated for gross hematuria or if mechanism of injury is a deceleration. Urine pregnancy test (women).
9. **Coagulation profiles.** Perform if patient takes anticoagulation medication, has liver disease, or blood dyscrasias, or profound shock is present anticipating DIC development.
10. **Drug and alcohol screens.**
11. **Lactate.** Inability to clear serum lactate may predict nonsurvivors. Some find this helpful along with ABG in determining severity of perfusion–resuscitation deficit. Target: < 2 mmol/L deficit.

D. **Radiographic and Other Studies**
   1. **C-spine, chest, pelvis radiographs**. Standard for almost every trauma patient.
   2. **Focused abdominal ultrasound for trauma (FAST exam).** Sensitivity and specificity approaches 85–95% for **free** fluid in hemodynamically unstable patient, which suggests emergent laparotomy.
      a. **Drawbacks.** Operator- and machine-dependent.
      b. **Advantages.** Rapid, relatively inexpensive, can be performed in the resuscitation room. (See Section VIII, 4. Bedside Ultrasound, page 424)
   3. **CT scan.** Higher specificity and detail than US or DPL.
      a. **Drawbacks.** Time-consuming, patient must be taken out of resuscitation area, expensive. May miss GI perforation, diaphragmatic rupture, and pancreatic injuries.
      b. **Advantages.** Provides, by far, the most detailed images of traumatic pathology.
   4. **Diagnostic peritoneal lavage (DPL).** Rapidly determines the presence of intraperitoneal blood.
      a. **Absolute contraindication.** Patient will undergo laparotomy regardless of results.
      b. **Exploration indicated.** > 10 mL blood aspirated on catheter insertion, > 100,000 RBC/mm^3 or 50,000 WBC/mm^3 after infusion of LR, presence of bile, or elevated amylase in fluid.
      c. **Complications.** Bleeding, infection, damage to intraperitoneal structures.

V. **Plan**
   A. **Overall Plan.** Laparotomy is the definitive therapy for intraabdominal injuries. Nonoperative management of injury should only be made by surgeon who will follow the patient.
   B. **Specific Plans**
      1. **Suspected intraabdominal injury.** Consult trauma surgeon as soon as possible. If no surgeon is available, transfer the patient

to nearest trauma center after patient is stabilized. Do not delay transfer for labs or imaging studies.

2. **Doubt intraabdominal injury.** Patients with minimal tenderness may still have injuries. Elderly, children, patients with distracting injuries and those who are intoxicated are at higher risk for missed injuries. Safest plan is to admit for 24-h observation with serial exams and repeat of Hct. Discharge only those patients with negative work-up, very low suspicion of injury. and good follow-up (recommend 24-h recheck).

VI. ICD-9 Diagnoses: Bladder and urethra injury; Kidney injury (unspecified); Liver contusion; Liver laceration; Nonspecified intraabdominal injury; Pancreatic injury (unspecified); Splenic injury (unspecified); Unspecified liver injury; Uterus injury (unspecified).

VII. Problem Case Diagnosis: Intraperitoneal hemorrhage.

VIII. Teaching Pearls Question: What areas are imaged for a FAST exam?

IX. Teaching Pearls Answer: Pericardium, hepatorenal recess (Morison's pouch), splenorenal recess, right and left paracolic gutters, urinary bladder and pelvic recess.

REFERENCES

Boulanger BR, McLellan BA: Blunt abdominal trauma. *Emerg Med Clin North Am* 1996; 14(1):151–171.

Rutherford EJ, Morris JA, Reed GW, Hall KS: Base deficit stratifies mortality and determines therapy. *J Trauma* 1992;33:417–423.

Salomone JA, Salomone JP: Abdominal trauma, blunt. *eMed J* 2001;2:5.

3. BLUNT HEAD TRAUMA

I. Problem: a 21-year-old male struck the windshield head on in an MVA. On arrival of paramedics, patient is unresponsive to verbal or painful stimuli without obvious focal neurologic Deficit.

II. Immediate Questions

A. Is the airway intact? Manage appropriately.

B. Is breathing adequate? Assist with BVM and manage airway.

C. Is spine immobilized? Place C-collar and backboard.

D. Is there an immediate threat to life? Perform a quick (primary) survey. Check for and manage massive thoracic injury, exsanguinating hemorrhage. Order IV, 100% O_2, monitors (ECG and pulse ox).

E. What are the vitals and neurologic exam? Use IV fluid and blood to normalize vitals. Do not withhold fluid because of concern about brain swelling. Check mental status, pupils, and motor response. Establish score on GCS (GCS, see Table A-29, p 680). If GCS ≤ 8 or deteriorating, intubate—use neuromuscular blockers to decrease ICP response to intubation. If signs of herniation syndrome—depressed mental status with anisocoria, posturing, or worsening level of consciousness—give mannitol and hyperventilate until herniation syndrome resolves. Goal P_{CO_2} is 30–35 mm Hg; further hyperventilation may dangerously decrease cerebral perfusion. Obtain noncontrast head CT in stable patient with serious head trauma, unless other injuries (chest, abdomen) require immediate treatment. Need C-spine radiographs in all patients with altered sensorium, posterior midline cervical tenderness, distracting injury, or neurologic deficit.

III. Differential Diagnosis
Head trauma is usually straightforward; however, consider other causes of LOC in patients with suspected head trauma. (See Section I, 3. Altered Mental Status, p II) Conversely, consider head trauma in all patients with LOC, even without history or exam findings suggestive of trauma.
  A. Scalp laceration. Can lead to significant blood loss. Close promptly.
  B. Skull fracture. Complicated: open, depressed, involve sinus or cause pneumocephalus. Basilar skull Fx can lead to traumatic meningitis. Consider prophylactic antibiotics in consult with neurosurgeon.
  C. Cerebral contusion/intracerebral hemorrhage. Contusion is most frequent blunt brain injury. May be contrecoup. Bleeding into contused parenchyma may be delayed and require neurosurgical intervention.
  D. Subarachnoid hemorrhage. Most common CT scan abnormality in patients with moderate and severe blunt brain injury. The amount of blood inversely related to presenting GCS.
  E. Epidural hematoma. Eighty percent lead to uncal herniation if untreated. Early recognition and intervention crucial.
  F. Subdural hematoma. Caused by sudden acceleration–deceleration of brain. Elderly and other atrophied brains are at high risk. More associated parenchymal injury than from epidurals. Treatment depends on type and associated brain injuries.
  G. Diffuse axonal injury. Disruption of axonal fibers in white matter and brainstem. Shearing forces of sudden deceleration are the cause. Injury occurs immediately and is irreversible.

IV. Database
  ### A. Physical Exam Key Points
    1. Carefully assess for other injuries (chest, abdomen, pelvis, extremities).
    2. Examine for scalp wounds, which can cause major blood loss.
    3. Baseline neurologic exam—at a minimum, examine level of consciousness, pupils, and motor response at both hands and feet. Assign GCS.
    4. Shock? Manage aggressively with NS, LR, or blood to maintain normal vital signs for optimal brain perfusion.
    5. Seizure activity? Manage with benzodiazepines and phenytoin. Monitor for hypotension caused by these medications.

      6. Are there comorbidities contributing to patient's status or ability to respond to stress?

         a. PMH, meds.

      7. Reassess frequently.

         a. Neurologic deterioration is caused by intracranial bleeding until proven otherwise.

B. Laboratory Data

    1. T&S, Hct, platelets, and coagulopathies (head trauma can cause DIC) if severe head trauma or multisystem trauma. Alcohol and toxicology screen may be useful.

    2. Other tests guided by comorbidities.

C. Radiographic and Other Studies

    1. Noncontrast head CT if suspect traumatic cause of altered mental status or abnormal neurologic exam.

      a. Head CT after traumatic LOC not needed if all of the following are met: between 3 and 60 years old, normal mental status, GCS 15, normal neurologic exam, no coagulopathy, no headache (local or diffuse), no vomiting, no drug or alcohol intoxication, no deficits in short-term memory, no seizure, and presentation less than 24 h after the event.

    2. C-spine imaging in patients with altered sensorium, posterior midline cervical tenderness, abnormal neurologic exam, or distracting injury.

    3. Other imaging studies as guided by suspicion of other injuries or comorbidities.

    4. Repeat CT if deterioration or if initial CT equivocal.

V. Plan

A. Overall Plan

    1. Admit all with abnormal CT or altered mental status, even with negative head CT.

    2. If discharged home, provide aftercare instructions.

      a. Standard head sheet.

      b. Be sure to address other injuries, real or potential.

B. Specific Plans

    1. Assume C-spine fracture until ruled out—immobilize spine.

    2. Manage airway early.

    3. Aggressively treat shock and hypoxia.

    4. Search for other injuries.

    5. Consider other causes of LOC.

    6. Obtain pulse ox, bedside glucose.

    7. Reassess frequently and at short intervals.

    8. Obtain a noncontrast head CT in stable patients with serious head trauma. Definitive management of life-threatening thoracoabdominal injuries takes precedence over head injury, unless hemodynamic stability can be maintained.

9. Prompt neurosurgical consultation in patients with abnormal neurologic exam, especially with intracranial hemorrhage. May need evacuation of hematoma or monitoring and treatment of ICP.

VI. **ICD-9 Diagnoses:** Cerebral contusion; Concussion—with loss of consciousness, mental confusion, without loss of consciousness; Intracranial injury (specify no, brief, moderate, prolonged loss of consciousness); Intracranial hemorrhage (extradural, subdural, subarachnoid).

VII. **Problem Case Diagnosis:** Diffuse axonal injury.

VIII. **Teaching Pearls Question:** Name the two most important modifiable extracranial parameters that influence the outcome of traumatic brain injury.

IX. **Teaching Pearls Answer:** Hypotension and hypoxia. A single episode of hypotension (SBP < 90 mm Hg in adults) can double mortality rate. Early endotracheal intubation and correction of hypotension are associated with improved outcomes.

REFERENCES

Ghajar J. Traumatic brain injury. *Lancet* 2000;9;923–929.
Haydel MJ, Preston CA, Mills TJ, Luber S, Blaudeau E, DeBlieux PM. Indications for computed tomography in patients with minor head injury. *N Engl J Med* 2000;343(2):100–105.

4. BURNS

I. **Problem:** Victim of house fire has stridor and singed nasal hairs.

II. **Immediate Questions**
   A. **Is the airway intact?** Is breathing labored or restricted? Manage per ATLS guidelines (See 1. Trauma Assessment and Resuscitation, pages 251, and Section VIII, 15. Rapid Sequence Endotracheal Intubation, page 470). Early intubation if suspect inhalation injury. Perform chest escharotomy if breathing restricted. Administer oxygen.
   B. **What are vital signs and mental status?** If in shock consider other causes (trauma, MI, spinal shock). If patient has altered mental status, consider carbon monoxide (CO) toxicity and give high-flow oxygen (decrease half-life carboxyhemoglobin). Pulse ox may be normal but patient hypoxic if CO-toxic.
   C. **What caused the burn and how long was contact?** Flash burns and splashed substances (less severe burns). Direct flame or prolonged contact with hot substance or chemical (more severe burns). Was lightning or high-voltage electricity involved? (severe burns, internal injury and arrhythmias).
   D. **Was fire in confined space?** Increased risk of CO toxicity and inhalational injury.
   E. **Is there potential for coexisting trauma?** MVA. Fall from height. Blunt injury from blast or lightning strike.

    F. Past medical history? Age of patient? Increased morbidity and mortality in very young and elderly. Diabetes, heart disease, immune suppression increase risk.

    G. Any suspicion for child or elder abuse? Is history consistent with injuries? Are caregivers reliable? Look for suspicious patterns of burns (immersion).

III. Differential Diagnosis

    A. Estimate Depth of Burn.

        1. **Superficial partial thickness.** Red, painful, no blisters.

        2. **Deep partial thickness.** Red, painful, weeping, blisters.

        3. **Full thickness.** White, charred, nonpainful (insensate).

    B. Calculate % BSA Burned.

        1. **Rule of nines.** Assign 9% to head, each upper extremity, and half of each lower extremity. Front and back torso are 18% each, and genitalia 1% (Figure III–1).

        2. **Palm rule.** Palm of patient's hand approximately 1% BSA.

    C. Classify Severity of Burn. (American Burn Association Grading System).

        1. **Minor burn injury.**

            a. Partial thickness < 15% BSA adults, 10% kids and elderly.

            b. Full thickness < 2% BSA not involving face, ears, eyes, hands, feet, or genitalia.

        2. **Moderate burn injury.**

            a. Partial thickness. 15–25% BSA adults, 10–20% BSA kids/elderly

            b. Full thickness burns. 2–10% BSA not involving face, ears, eyes, hands, feet or genitalia

        3. **Major burn injury**

            a. Partial thickness. > 25% BSA adults, > 20% BSA kids/elderly

            b. Full thickness. > 10% BSA or involving face, ears, eyes, hands, feet or genitalia

            c. All high-voltage electrical injuries.

            d. All burns complicated by inhalational injury or major trauma.

    D. Inhalational Injury.

        1. **Thermal injury.** Stridor, respiratory distress, hypoxia, carbonaceous sputum, or singed nasal hairs.

        2. **Carbon monoxide toxicity.** History of fire in confined space and decreased mental status, focal neurologic symptoms or cardiac arrhythmia or ischemia.

    E. Restrictive Injury.

        1. **Respiratory.** Mechanical restriction of chest wall or neck from eschar.

        2. **Extremity.** Circumferential burns cause vascular compromise. Distal pain, paresthesias, or cyanosis. Loss of pulses late finding.

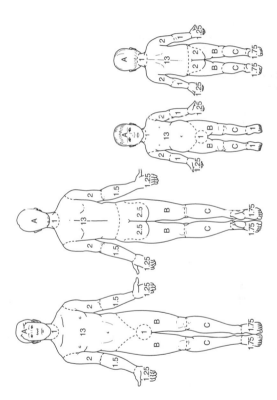

Figure III–1. Tables of estimating the extent of burns in adults and children. In adults a reasonable system for calculating the percentage of body burned is the "Rule of nines": Each arm equals 9%; the head equals 9%; the anterior and posterior trunk each equal 18%; each leg equals 18%; and the perineum equals 1%. (Reproduced, with permission, from Demling RH, Way LW: Burns and other thermal injuries. In : Way WL, ed. Current Surgical Treatment & Diagnosis, 10th ed. Originally published by Appleton & Lange. Copyright © 1994 by the McGraw-Hill Companies, Inc.)

IV. **Database**
   A. **Physical Exam Key Points.** Continuously reassess airway and breathing.
      1. **Mental status.** Confusion, obtundation.
      2. **Vital signs.** Reassess often for signs of hypovolemia or hypoxia.
      3. **HEENT.** Signs of head trauma, burns to cornea (singed eyebrows), facial burns, singed nasal hairs, stridor, hoarse voice, carbon stained sputum.
      4. **Pulmonary.** Full expansion of chest with ventilation, presence of large, deep burn to anterior chest or neck.
      5. **Cardiac.** Presence of cardiac arrhythmia (CO toxicity).
      6. **Abdomen/pelvis.** Tenderness suggests coexisting trauma.
      7. **Genitalia.** Look for burns and "immersion burns" in toddlers.
      8. **Extremities.** Look for burns on hands and feet. Look for circumferential burns and assess neurovascular status.
   B. **Laboratory Data.** ABG and carboxyhemoglobin level. CPK, BUN, creatinine, and UA to monitor myoglobinemia. Hct and coagulation studies. Pregnancy test.
   C. **Radiographic and Other Studies.** CXR. Other radiographs as indicated to detect trauma. ECG if suspect CO toxicity.

V. **Plan**
   A. **Overall Plan.** Determine depth of burns, total % BSA burned, and classify severity of burn. Evaluate for trauma and other burn-related injuries while initiating resuscitation. Classification of burn will determine disposition.
   B. **Specific Plans**
      1. **Airway.** Intubate if suspect inhalational injury. Bronchoscopy if suspect thermal injury. High-flow oxygen if suspect CO toxicity.
      2. **Resuscitation.** Establish IVs through unburned skin.
         a. Administer crystalloid:
         b. 4 mL LR/kg/% BSA burn half in first 8 h.
            i. Monitor urine output.
            ii. 0.5–1.0 mL/kg/h
      3. **Carbon monoxide toxicity.** Carboxyhemoglobin levels do not correlate with severity. Obtain toxicology consult if elevated level and symptomatic.
      4. **Pain.** Anticipate severe pain in partial-thickness burns. Treat with morphine after fluids started. Provide adequate outpatient pain meds.
      5. **Wound care.** Infection risk substantial. Clean with mild soap solution and cover with cool, sterile compresses if transfer or consultation imminent. If discharging, cover with antibiotic ointment or silver sulfadiazine (Silvadene) cream before sterile dressing. May aseptically aspirate blister fluid but leave intact blisters in place.
      6. **Severity of burn determines disposition.**
         a. **Minor burns.** Treat as outpatient. Follow up in 24–48 h.

   b. **Moderate burns.** Treat as inpatient with general or plastic
      surgery consult.
   c. **Major burns.** Treat as for moderate burns and transfer to
      burn center.
 VI. ICD-9 Diagnoses: Burn (specify location and degree); Burn of internal
      organs (specify site).

 VII. Problem Case Diagnosis: Inhalational/thermal injury requires intubation.

 VIII. Teaching Pearls Question: Calculate 24-h fluid requirement for adult
       male (70 kg) with 20% BSA burn.

 IX. Teaching Pearls Answer: 5600 mL (2800 mL in first 8 h).

REFERENCES

Baxter CR, Waeckerle JF. Emergency treatment of burn injury. *Ann Emerg Med* 1988;
   17:1305–1315.
Monaco WW. Initial management of burns. *N Engl J Med* 1996;335:1581–15.
Nguyen TT. Current treatment of severely burned patients. *Am Surgeon* 1996;223(1):14–25.

5. CHEST TRAUMA

 I. Problem: An elderly male presents after an MVA. He was a restrained
    driver and his airbag deployed. He complains of chest pain and worsen-
    ing shortness of breath.

 II: Immediate Questions
   A. Is the airway intact? Manage appropriately; some indications for
       trauma intubation: GCS < 9, respiratory distress, need for PPV (flail
       chest, open pneumothorax), combative patient (remember that pneu-
       mothorax may become a tension pneumothorax under positive pres-
       sure). (See Section VIII, 15. Rapid Sequence Endotracheal Intubation,
       page 470).
   B. Breathing assessment? Evaluation of respiratory pattern, appropri-
       ate rate/depth, evidence of splinting, paradoxical movement. Assess
       breath sounds, pulse ox. Intervene appropriately with supplemental O_2,
       selective intubation, PPV, chest tube, needle thoracostomy.
   C. Circulation assessment? Assess pulses in all extremities, BP, men-
       tal status. IV fluid resuscitation as indicated. (See this section, Prob-
       lem 1. Trauma Assessment and Resuscitation, page 251).
   D. What are the vitals and mental status?
      1. Is patient awake/alert, intubate if GCS < 9.
      2. Any signs of shock: tachycardia before hypotension, think spinal
         shock if not tachycardic. Initiate IV fluid resuscitation.
      3. Evaluate gross neurologic function: moving all extremities, does
         it require verbal or painful stimuli? Any gross sensory or motor
         deficits?

E. **What was the mechanism of injury?** Blunt vs penetrating trauma, or combination.

F. **What is the patient's medical history? Any medications or known allergies?** Assess for any other possible explanation for dyspnea, hypoxia, hypotension, altered mental status.

III. **Differential Diagnosis**
   A. **Blunt Trauma.** Pneumothorax, tension pneumothorax, open pneumothorax, hemothorax, rib fractures, flail chest, pulmonary contusion, cardiac contusion, cardiac laceration/rupture, cardiac tamponade, traumatic aortic injury, large vessel injury, esophageal injury, tracheobronchial injury, diaphragmatic injury.
   B. **Penetrating Trauma.** Consider all of previously mentioned possibilities, include associated risk of intraabdominal injury, spinal cord injury; increased risk of lung parenchymal injury, cardiac and vessel injury.

IV. **Database**
   A. **Physical Exam Key Points.** Follow American College of Surgeons ATLS protocols. Resuscitation measures take place concurrently with primary and secondary survey.
      1. **Airway.** GCS, associated facial trauma, potential for airway obstruction. Does patient have gag reflex? Intubate when indicated.
      2. **Breathing.** Rate and depth of respirations? Any signs of respiratory distress? Paradoxical movement? Feel chest wall for tenderness, deformities, subcutaneous air, and crepitus. Assess breath sounds and check for symmetry.
      3. **Circulation.** Assess for pulses in all extremities: radial, femoral, dorsalis pedis. Check capillary refill. Initiate immediate fluid resuscitation in tachycardic or hypotensive patients. Apply pressure dressings to any significant bleeding.
      4. **Disability.** Brief neurologic evaluation. What is GCS? Does patient respond to verbal or painful stimuli, or unresponsive? Are there any gross motor or sensory deficits? What is rectal tone?
      5. **Secondary survey.** Head-to-toe evaluation after initial primary survey and appropriate interventions initiated.
   B. **Laboratory Data.** Obtain baseline CBC, T&S, cross-match blood if patient hypotensive, ABG or VBG to assess for possible base deficit—may suggest early shock state. UA for hematuria. Consider blood alcohol and tox screens if patient has altered mental status. Order appropriate labs for specific patients: pregnancy tests in women, blood glucose in diabetics, TSH in persistent unexplained tachycardia or patients with goiter, etc.
   C. **Radiographic and Other Studies.** Significant blunt trauma will require at least CXR, C-spine, and pelvic radiographs. Consider helical CT chest in stable patients with suspicious mediastinal widening (> 8 cm in supine AP film) or in patients with mechanism suggestive of aortic injury. TEE is alternative to helical CT if available. Other extremity views and CT head as indicated. CT abdominal/pelvis if indicated and patient

hemodynamically stable (See this section, 2. Blunt Abdominal Trauma, page 253). Monitor pulse ox for signs of hypoxia. ECG to evaluate blunt myocardial injury. Bedside ultrasound (FAST) in experienced hands can be useful screening study for hemothorax and pericardial tamponade (see Section VIII, 4. Bedside Ultrasound, page 424).

V. Plan

A. Overall Plan.
Anticipate injuries by presentation and mechanism of injury; recognize and diagnose theses injuries and perform therapeutic interventions when indicated. Refer to trauma surgeon early if admission likely.

B. Specific Plans

1. **Pneumothorax.** Treat with 100% oxygen. Most require tube thoracostomy (chest tube—See Section VIII, 17. Thoracostomy Tube Placement, page 473) to decompress. Small pneumothorax (< 25%) can sometimes be closely observed by experienced trauma surgeon.

2. **Tension pneumothorax.** Should be clinical diagnoses made by absent breath sounds, JVD, and hemodynamic instability. Other signs include tracheal deviation and cyanosis. Immediate decompression indicated with needle thoracostomy (See Section VIII, 17. Thoracostomy Tube Placement, page 473), followed with chest tube, unless chest tube readily available.

3. **Open pneumothorax.** EMS workers should cover wound with three-sided occlusive dressing. ED management includes placement of chest tube thoracostomy, not into or through injury, and PPV. Consider intubation and mechanical ventilation.

4. **Hemothorax.** Placement of large-bore (36 Fr) chest tube. Indications for thoracotomy by CT surgeon or trauma surgeon include immediate output of > 1500 mL blood or continuous output of > 200 mL/h.

5. **Rib fractures.** Most can be managed conservatively with adequate pain control. Consider incentive spirometer use with patient to decrease risk of pneumonia. Superior rib fractures may be associated with significant vascular trauma.

6. **Flail chest.** Three or more consecutive rib fractures results in loss of chest wall integrity and ability to generate adequate negative intrathoracic pressure for inspiration. Adequate pain control and PPV most important, consider mechanical ventilation. Strapping or sand bags to area may help stabilize chest wall. May benefit from epidural block (consult anesthesia consult)

7. **Pulmonary contusion.** Noted by worsening hypoxia, dyspnea, tachypnea, and tachycardia. ABG will show widening A-a gradient and CXR will demonstrate a developing consolidation. Provide supplemental O_2, consider intubation if hypoxia worsens.

8. **Blunt myocardial injury including myocardial contusion.** Initial diagnosis typically made on ECG with evidence of conduction

blocks, frequent ectopy, or ischemic changes. Enzymes not typically helpful in making diagnosis. Admit for close monitoring.

9. **Cardiac tamponade.** Suspect tamponade in patients with worsening hypotension and distended neck veins, but with equal breath sounds. Additional evidence: bedside US (See Section VIII, 4. Bedside Ultrasound, page 424) or increasing CVP (> 15 cm H_2O) and muffled heart tones. Treatment includes pericardiocentesis or placement of a pericardial window.

10. **Traumatic aortic injury.** Suspect aortic injury in patients with rapid deceleration injury and blunt chest trauma (MVA, falls). Physical exam suggestions include harsh systolic murmur, pulse deficits, extremity hypertension, or differing blood pressures in upper and lower extremities. CXR findings include superior mediastinal widening (> 8 cm in supine AP film), deviation of esophagus or trachea (at T4), deviation of NG or ET tube, obscured aortic knob, apical cap, left pleural effusion, left mainstem bronchus displaced > 40 degrees below horizontal. If aortic injury suspected and patient stable, aortography or helical chest CT to confirm. Bedside TEE or immediate thoracotomy if patient unstable.

11. **Esophageal injury.** Typically occurs with other significant chest injuries and can be initially overlooked. Common signs and symptoms include pain, pneumomediastinum or pneumothorax, dyspnea, subcutaneous air, or hematemesis. Do not occur often but require surgical evaluation when suspected.

12. **Diaphragmatic injury.** Presentation depends on size of defect and amount of viscous fluid herniated. May complain of cough or dyspnea, or abdominal pain radiating to shoulder. Patient may have decreased breath sounds or audible bowel sounds in chest if significant herniation. Evaluate CXR for elevated or obscured hemidiaphragm, elevation of NG tube. Simple diaphragmatic tears without herniation are often asymptomatic.

13. **Tracheobronchial injury.** Will present with dyspnea, chest pain, hemoptysis, subcutaneous air, pneumothorax, or pneumomediastinum. Often will require chest tube and possibly ventilatory support. Bronchoscopy for definitive diagnosis.

VI. **ICD-9 Diagnoses:** Cardiac contusion; Flail chest; Pulmonary contusion; Rib fracture(s); Tamponade cardiac; Traumatic aortic rupture; Traumatic diaphragm rupture; Traumatic pneumothorax (with or without hemothorax);Traumatic tension pneumothorax.

VII. **Problem Case Diagnosis:** Pulmonary contusion.

VIII. **Teaching Pearls Question:** How much pleural fluid needs to collect to be evident on upright CXR?

IX. **Teaching Pearls Answer:** 200–300 mL.

REFERENCES

Calhoon JH, Grover FL, Trinkle JK. Chest trauma: Approach and management. *Clin Chest Med* 1992;13:55–67.

Feliciano DV. The diagnostic and therapeutic approach to chest trauma. *Semin Thorac Cardiovasc Surg* 1992;4:156–162.

Mansour KA. Trauma of the diaphragm. *Chest Surg Clin North Am* 1997;7:373–383.

6. ELECTRICAL INJURY

I. **Problem:** A 36-year-old utility worker is brought to the ED after being electrocuted.

II. **Immediate Questions**

A. **Is the airway intact?** Manage appropriately (See Section VIII, 15. Rapid Sequence Endotracheal Intubation, page 470).

B. **What are the vital signs and mental status?** Is the patient stable, awake, and alert? In all but the most trivial injuries apply monitors (ECG, pulse ox, BP), initiate oxygen therapy, IV access. Electrical injuries are often associated with burns and traumatic injuries secondary to falls or explosions.

C. **What type of current was the patient exposed to?**

1. **Alternating current (AC)** exists in both high voltage (> 600 V) and low voltage. Typical U.S. household electricity is stepped down to 220 V for major appliances and 110 V for general household service. Injuries may range from trivial to fatal. Immersion in water increases morbidity and mortality.

2. **Direct current (DC)** is used in medical devices such as defibrillators and pacemakers.

3. **Lightning** is a massive short-lived impulse of current. Although the initial phase of a lightning strike may course through the body, it quickly flashes over to transit over the outside of the body. The severity of injury is difficult to predict. Injuries range from trivial to fatal.

D. **How long was the patient exposed to the source of electricity?** Injury is worsened with prolonged exposure. Chest wall tetany may cause prolonged apnea.

E. **Did a flash or an arc occur?** Flash and arc burns differ in severity and implications.

1. **Flash burns** are thermal burn and alone do not imply internal injury.

2. **Electrical arcs** are high-voltage currents that pass through the air and may transmit through a person. Extensive internal injury may occur.

F. **What body parts were in the path of the current?**

1. Head-to-toe and arm-to-foot are more dangerous than arm-to-arm, or foot-to-foot.

2. Children who bite electrical cords may sustain severe oral and facial burns. Delayed lingual artery hemorrhage may occur.

G. Does the patient have any preexisting medical problems?

H. What resuscitative measures were taken in the prehospital setting?

III. Differential Diagnosis

A. Neurologic

1. **Syncope** (See Section I, 67. Syncope, page 200). Sudden collapse preceded by scream might be a clue to an electrical cause. Transient LOC is common.

2. **Seizure.** Electrocution may mimic or cause seizure activity. Evaluate for postictal state; may require intervention (See Section I, 60. Seizure, page 180).

3. **Head trauma.** Consider trauma secondary to falls. Intracranial hemorrhage may result from cranial electrical contact.

B. Cardiac

1. **Sudden cardiac death.** An ECG should be performed on anyone with a suspected electrical injury. Asystole and ventricular fibrillation are common in AC electrical injury. (See Section I, 13. Cardiac Arrest, page 41).

2. **Tachyarrhythmia.** Other cardiac electrical abnormalities include ST segment elevations, prolonged QT, PVCs PACs, AF, and BBB. Treat arrhythmias as indicated (See Section I, 68. Tachycardia, page 202) Prolonged asystole might respond to CPR in electrical injury victims.

3. **MI.** Elevated CK, CK-MB, myoglobin, and the troponin cardiac markers may be elevated due to MI but also may be elevated secondary to massive myonecrosis. CK-MB relative index may be less specific in electrical injury. (See Section I, 15. Chest Pain, page 51)

C. Thermal Burns

1. **Arc burns** have a central area of desiccation surrounded by erythema. Arc burns should prompt evaluation for internal burns and muscle injury (See this section, 4. Burns, page 259).

2. **Flash burns** resemble thermal burns and do not imply internal injury. Treat as thermal injury.

3. **Contact burns** resemble the object that was touched. Source and ground contact burns may be useful for predicting current path through patient. Treat burns as indicated, size of burn underestimates potential internal injury.

D. Trauma

1. **Head trauma.** Many patients are thrown or fall in association with the electrical injury. Altered mental status may indicate serious head trauma (See this section, Blunt Head Trauma, page 256).

2. **Thoracic and abdominal trauma.** Evaluate and treat as indicated (See this section, 2. Blunt Abdominal Trauma, page 253, and 5. Chest Trauma, page 263).

   3. Orthopedic injury may result from falls or secondary to severe muscle contractions (See this section, 7. Extremity Fractures and Dislocations, page 271).

IV. Database
A. Physical Exam Key Points
   1. **ABCs.** Manage the airway as indicated. Assess circulation, paying particular attention to pulses in limbs with contact burns because muscle necrosis, vascular thrombosis, and hemorrhage may cause compartment syndrome.
   2. **Vital signs.** Check carefully and repeat during evaluation.
   3. **Mental status and neurologic exam.** Mental status and neurologic exams should be performed to detect any alterations in consciousness or disability. Neurologic deficits may be immediate or delayed and may include intracranial hemorrhage, brain injury, spinal cord injury, or peripheral nerve deficits.
   4. **Head.** Evaluate ears for hemotympanum or membrane perforation. May be present in lightning injury and head trauma. Evaluate the mouth, lips, and tongue in children suspected of biting extension cords.
   5. **Chest and abdomen.** Inspect and palpate for signs of trauma and burns.
   6. **Extremities.** Inspect, palpate, and test each limb for signs of neurologic, vascular, or orthopedic compromise. Treat burns as indicated.

B. Laboratory Data
   1. In patients with all but trivial electrical contact obtain CBC, Lytes (sodium, potassium, chloride, bicarbonate), BUN, creatinine, and UA (specific gravity, pH, color, glucose, and hemoglobin).
   2. In patients with suspected internal electrical injury obtain CPK, total and fractionated. Obtain urine, serum myoglobin if UA is positive for hemoglobin.
   3. Suspected abdominal injury should prompt evaluation of LFT and coagulation tests.
   4. In cases of hemorrhage or extensive burns that may require grafting, blood should be typed and cross-matched.
   5. Obtain ABG if ventilatory assistance is required or prolonged ventilatory arrest is suspected.

C. Radiographic and Other Studies
   1. **ECG.** Electrocardiography should be obtained on all victims of electrical injury. Findings of abnormal rhythms should prompt further monitoring and evaluation.
   2. **Plain films** should be obtained on all deformed limbs or joints. A standard trauma series of lateral C-spine, AP chest, and AP pelvis should be obtained in case of suspected trauma. Obtain CXR in cases of prolonged arrest or respiratory complaints. Abdominal plain films can be used to evaluate for electrical and burn ileus.

3. **CAT** of the head should be obtained in situations of altered mental status or suspected head trauma.
4. **MRI** should be obtained to evaluate any lasting neurologic deficits not explained by CT or plain radiography.

V. Plan

A. Overall Plan

Rapidly evaluate and treat any patient suspected of electrical injury. Treat any findings appropriately. Be suspicious that apparent injuries may underrepresent the total extent of injuries. Admission or transfer to a burn center is recommended for any patient with significant injuries. Admission for observation and cardiac monitoring is recommended for all patients with high-voltage exposure (> 600 V) regardless of injuries. Adults with low-voltage injury may be discharged home if an ECG shows no abnormalities, the physical exam is normal, and they have no symptoms. Children rarely suffer delayed cardiac arrhythmias. They may be discharged home if their injuries are limited, the ECG is normal, follow-up is ensured, and parents are reliable.

B. Specific Plans

1. **Initial resuscitation should be aggressive.** Airway management and prolonged CPR may prevent death.
2. **Continuous ECG and pulse oximetry** should be provided.
3. **Spinal immobilization** should be ensured in patients with suspected injuries.
4. **Cardiac arrhythmias** should be treated as recommended by the ACLS guidelines. Cardiac monitoring should be instituted in all cases of high-voltage exposure, high-risk low-voltage exposure, those with an abnormal ECG, and those with cardiac or respiratory symptoms.
5. **Fluid resuscitation** should be instituted early using LR or NS through two large-bore IVs. Fluid requirements in severe electrical injury will be underestimated using traditional methods.
6. **Treat rhabdomyolysis** as needed. Consider bicarbonate to alkalinize urine (pH > 6.5) to prevent acute renal failure.
7. **Muscle injury and vascular thrombosis** and spasm lead to both **compartment syndromes** and delayed hemorrhage. Fasciotomy or amputation may be required.
8. **Wound and burn care.** Early consultation with plastic or burn surgical specialists or transfer to a certified burn center is recommended for all significant electrical burn patients.
9. **Delayed complications** include ophthalmic and neurologic problems. Ensure that follow-up is available.

VI. ICD-9 Diagnoses:
Burn (specify location and degree—includes electrical burns); Effect of lightening (ie, lightening strike); Electrocution and nonfatal effect of electric current (ie, electrical shock); Rhabdomyolysis.

VII. Problem Case Diagnosis:
High-voltage AC electrical injury.

VIII. Teaching Pearl Question: What delayed complication should be considered in a child who sustains an oral burn from biting an electrical cord?

IX. Teaching Pearl Answer: Delayed hemorrhage from the lingual artery.

REFERENCES

Bailey B, Gauderault P, Thivierge RL, Turgeon JP. Cardiac monitoring in children with household electrical injuries. *Ann Emerg Med* 1995;25:612–617.
Canady JW, Thompson SA, Bardach J. Oral commissure burns in children. *Plast Reconstr Surg* 1996;97:738–744.
Fish R. Electric shock: I, II, III, *J Emerg Med* 1993;11:309, 457, and 599.
Lee C. Injury by electrical forces: Pathophysiology, manifestations, and therapy. *Curr Probl Surg* 1997;34:677–764.

7. EXTREMITY FRACTURES AND DISLOCATIONS

I. **Problem:** A 25-year-old male presents following an MVA with a deformed left thigh with an anterior laceration through which bone shards are protruding.

II. **Immediate Questions**
   A. **What is the overall status of the patient?** Patients who sustain orthopedic injuries often are victims of polytrauma, and no matter how impressive fractures appear attention should always focus on resuscitation and the ABCs.
   B. **Is an "orthopedic emergency" present?** These include open fractures (delays in treatment increase risk of osteomyelitis), neurovascular deficit (immediate reduction indicated), compartment syndrome (compartmental pressures greater than 30 mm Hg require emergent fasciotomy), associated dislocations (delay in reduction makes reduction more difficult and, in the case of the hip, may lead to avascular necrosis).
   C. **What is the PMH?** Any allergies to antibiotics? When was the last meal (in case of surgery)? Is there a history of cancer or other disease to suggest a pathologic fracture? Are there significant comorbid diseases that may complicate surgery?
   D. **How are you going to describe the fracture to the orthopedist?**
      1. Anatomic location (eg, distal radius).
      2. Type (eg, simple, comminuted).
      3. Angulation (describe angle between the longitudinal axes of the two fracture fragments).
      4. Displacement (measure the percentage of the width of the bone that the cortices are separated from each other).
      5. Fracture line (eg, transverse, oblique, spiral, impacted).
      6. Associated injuries (open vs closed, neurovascular complications).

III. Differential Diagnosis: Fracture Patterns

A. **Clavicle.** Typically treated with sling and rest except for displaced distal fractures, which may require surgery. May be associated with subclavian artery and brachial plexus injuries.

B. **Scapula.** Greater than 80% are associated with injury to the ipsilateral lung, thoracic cage, and shoulder girdle. Majority are treated with sling and early ROM exercises. Fractures involving the glenoid and neck should be evaluated by CT scan and may require surgery.

C. **Humerus.** Humeral head fractures are classified by how many parts they result in (Neer system). May be associated with axillary nerve and artery injuries. Two-part fractures may generally be treated with a sling. Three- and four-part fractures may require open fixation. Humeral shaft fractures are usually treated with sling and swath. Indications for surgery include neurovascular injury, segmental fracture, floating elbow, open fractures, and bilateral fractures. May be associated with injuries to the brachial artery and median, ulnar, or radial (most common) nerves.

D. **Elbow.** Supracondylar fracture is the most common pediatric elbow fracture. The only sign may be a posterior fat pad (always indicative of blood in the joint), an anterior fat pad that is superiorly displaced (sailed), or an anterior humeral line that does not intersect the posterior two thirds of the capitellum as it should. Displaced fractures have a high incidence of neurovascular injury and usually require surgery to prevent compartment syndrome and an ischemic (Volkmann's) contracture.

E. **Forearm.** *Nightstick fracture:* Isolated midshaft ulna fracture. Treatment with splint unless more than 50% displaced or 10 degrees angulated. *Monteggia fracture:* Proximal ulna fracture with associated radial head dislocation. *Galeazzi fracture:* Fracture of distal third of radius with associated distal radioulnar dislocation. Always assess proximal and distal joints for pain in cases of fractures.

F. **Wrist.** *Colles's fracture:* Dorsally angulated fracture of the distal radius. *Smith's fracture:* Distal radius fracture with volar angulation. *Chauffeur fracture*: Radial styloid avulsion—frequently associated with unstable ligamentous injury. *Occult fractures of the scaphoid* and other carpals are common; significant pain or tenderness is indication for splinting and orthopedic referral because of the high incidence of morbidity with untreated fractures.

G. **Hand.** *Game keeper's (skier's) thumb:* Caused by radial stress of MCP joint resulting in damage to ulnar collateral ligament with or without associated fracture; surgery frequently required—splint in thumb spica and obtain urgent orthopedic consultation. *Distal phalanx fractures:* Place in protective splint leaving other joints free. *Metacarpal neck fractures:* Fractures of fourth and fifth metacarpals (boxer's fracture) can tolerate up to 30 degrees of angulation without needing reduction. *Metacarpal shaft fractures:* Assess rotational deformity clinically—should be reduced then splinted.

H. Hip. Femoral neck and intertrochanteric fractures will typically present with shortening and external rotation of the affected leg. Surgical fixation leads to earlier mobilization and lower mortality. Be highly suspicious of fracture in elderly patients with groin, hip, or thigh pain who have hip range of motion. Nondisplaced fractures may not be apparent on plain films and MRI may be required; if missed, displacement may occur, increasing morbidity and mortality.

I. Femur. Associated complications include hemorrhage (≤ 1.5 L of blood may be lost into the thigh), fat emboli syndrome, and ARDS. High incidence of injury to the ipsilateral limb and pelvic girdle requires diligent assessment of entire patient.

J. Knee. *Ottawa knee rules:* Obtain radiographs for patients who are over 55, have tenderness over the fibular head or patella, cannot flex to 90 degrees, or cannot bear weight for four steps (97% sensitivity, 27% specificity). *Pittsburgh knee rules:* Obtain radiographs for patients who are younger than 12 or older than 55, and patients between these ages with a history of fall or direct blow to the knee who cannot bear weight for four steps (99% sensitivity, 60% specificity). Patella fractures will require surgery if displaced by more than 3 mm or if extensor mechanism is disrupted (test patient's ability to extend leg against gravity).

K. Tibia/Fibula. Because of scant soft-tissue coverage, there is a high incidence of open fractures and compartment syndrome with tib/fib fractures. Nondisplaced fractures of the fibula may be treated with elastic bandage wrapping. Fibular head fractures may be associated with damage to the common peroneal nerve (Check for weakness of dorsiflexion).

L. Ankle. *Weber classification:* Type A—fibula fracture below joint line; usually stable and treated conservatively; Type B—fibula fracture at joint line extending proximally; may require surgery if there is clinical or radiographic evidence of medial injury; Type C—fibular fracture above the joint line; indicates syndesmotic injury and requires surgery. Always assess the proximal fibula in ankle injuries for a Maisonneuve's fracture. *Maisonneuve's fracture:* Lateral displacement of lateral malleolus with or without fracture of the medial malleolus in association with a proximal fibula fracture—indicates unstable syndesmosis injury and requires surgery.

M. Foot. *Calcaneous fracture:* 10% are associated with spinal injuries; typically require CT evaluation for surgery planning. *Lisfranc fracture/dislocation:* Usually involves fracture of the base of the second MT (pathognomonic) with disruption of the Lisfranc joint (attachment of the metatarsals with the cuneiforms and cuboid)—requires emergent consultation. *Fifth metatarsal fractures:* Avulsion fracture (within the proximal 1.5 cm of the metatarsal)—may be treated with only hard-soled shoe. *Jones fracture*: Fracture line is 1.5–2 cm distal to proximal end of MT—high rate of nonunion requires splinting and urgent orthopedic referral.

N. **Pediatric.** Four unique fracture types result from the more porous and pliable nature of pediatric bone: Plastic deformity (appears on radiograph as excessive bowing); torus (buckle); greenstick (only one side of the cortex is disrupted); fractures involving the physes. Physeal fractures are classified using the Salter-Harris system: Type I (fracture through the physis only—radiographs appear normal—clinical diagnosis); type II (through the physis and metaphysis—most common type); type III (fracture line begins intraarticularly and extends through the epiphysis into the physis); type IV (begins intraarticularly and extends through the epiphysis, physis and metaphysis); type V (physis is crushed without any other injury). The higher the Salter-Harris type, the worse the prognosis for normal growth.

O. **Fractures of Abuse.** Suspicion should be raised if the injury is not consistent with the proposed mechanism of injury or child's developmental stage. Fractures that are particularly suggestive of abuse include: healing fractures of different ages; "bucket-handle" or metaphyseal corner fracture (typically caused by torsional stress rather than falling); humeral fractures in children younger than 3 years old; complex skull fractures; posterior rib fractures, vertebral body and spinous process fractures; spiral or oblique long bone fractures (with the exception of the "toddler's fracture"—nondisplaced spiral fracture of the distal tibia that is not associated with abuse).

IV. **Database**
   A. **Physical Exam Key Points**
      1. **ABCs.**
      2. **Distal vascular and neurologic function.** Repeat exam and document findings before **and** after joint or fracture reduction.
      3. **Distal and proximal joints.** Always assess the joints adjacent to long bone fractures.
      4. **Skin.** Any associated laceration should suggest an open fracture.
      5. **Associated injuries.** Certain fractures are commonly associated with other injuries (eg, calcaneous fractures and lumbar vertebrae fractures).
   B. **Laboratory Data.** Consider preoperative CBC, coagulation studies, and T&C, especially for surgeries with a potential for large blood loss (eg, hip).
   C. **Radiographic and Other Studies.** Generally AP and lateral films are adequate. Some anatomic regions require specialized views, and the consulting orthopedist may have further requests.

V. **Plan**
   A. **Overall Plan.** ABCs! Address potentially life-threatening injuries before all else. Provide adequate analgesia.
   B. **Specific Plans.** Fracture stabilization. Apply ice and elevate limb to reduce swelling. Remove all distal rings and other constrictions. All extremity deformities should be immediately splinted to improve patient comfort and decrease chance of neurovascular and skin injuries. Trac-

tion splints (Hare or Sager) are used for femur fractures to reduce hemorrhage, promote length restoration, and decrease discomfort.

C. **Antibiotics.** Make sure tetanus immunization is up to date. Administer antibiotics for open fractures. A first-generation cephalosporin (eg, cefazolin) is adequate for clean lacerations of less than 1 cm. Lacerations greater than 1 cm extensively damaged soft tissues, and grossly contaminated wounds should be treated with an aminoglycoside (eg, gentamicin) as well. Dirty fractures, especially those sustained in agricultural settings should receive coverage for *Clostridia* (eg, penicillin).

D. **Analgesia.** If hemodynamic status permits, be sure to supply adequate analgesia. (See Section VIII. 13. Procedural Sedation in Adults, page 464 and 14. Procedural Sedation in Children, page 467)

E. **Consultation.** Most nondisplaced, closed fractures of the hand, wrist, foot, and ankle can be splinted and referred for outpatient orthopedic consultation. Most other fractures will require emergent consultation.

VI. **ICD-9 Diagnoses:** For all fractures specify location/bone and open vs closed, also specify part of bone fractured, ie, metacarpal head. For all dislocations specify joint, open vs closed, and direction of dislocation, ie, anterior elbow dislocation.

VII. **Problem Case Diagnosis:** Open transverse fracture of the midshaft of the left femur. There is 50% displacement and 30 degrees of angulation with the apex anterior.

VIII. **Teaching Pearls Question:** An 18-year-old presents with a severe sprain of the medial aspect of the ankle. What associated injury must never be missed?

IX. **Teaching Pearls Answer:** Maisonneuve's fracture. Always assess the proximal fibula in ankle injuries. Missed fractures carry a high rate of morbidity and liability.

REFERENCES

Beaty JH. Orthopedic aspects of child abuse. *Curr Opin Pediatr* 1997;9:100–103.

Blake R, Hoffman J. Emergency department evaluation and treatment of the shoulder and humerus. Emerg Med Clin North Am 1999;17(4):859–876.

Della-Giustina K, Della-Giustina DA. Emergency department evaluation and treatment of pediatric orthopedic injuries. Emerg Med Clin North Am 1999;17(4):895–922.

Harrison BP, Hilliard MW. Emergency department evaluation and treatment of hand injuries. *Emerg Med Clin North Am* 1999;17(4):793–822.

Ritchie JV, Munter DW. Emergency department evaluation and treatment of wrist injuries. *Emerg Med Clin North Am* 1999;17(4):823–842.

Roberts DM, Stallard TC: Emergency department evaluation and treatment of knee and leg injuries. *Emerg Med Clin North Am* 2000;18(1):67–84.

Rudman N, McIlmail D. Emergency department evaluation and treatment of hip and thigh injuries. *Emerg Med Clin North Am* 2000;18(1):29–66.

Skaggs D, Pershad J: Pediatric elbow trauma. Pediatr Emerg Care 1997;13(6):425–434.

Wedmore IS, Charette J. Emergency department evaluation and treatment of ankle and foot injuries. Emerg Med Clin North Am 2000;18(1):85–113.

8. EYE TRAUMA

I. **Problem:** A young male was assaulted in a fist and knife fight one hour ago and is complaining of a change in vision in his right eye.

II. **Immediate Questions**
   A. **ABCs?** Are there signs of blunt/penetrating trauma to neck? The patient should be completely undressed and examined for additional trauma.
   B. **Are there signs/symptoms of intracranial injury?** Mental status normal? Any focal neurologic findings?
   C. **What are the patient's vital signs?**
   D. **What is the patient's visual acuity in each eye?** Measure each eye independently with glasses if appropriate.
   E. **What obvious signs are present on initial ocular observation?** Any periorbital or orbital lacerations? Swelling, chemosis, or proptosis?

III. **Differential Diagnosis**
   A. **Blunt Trauma.**
      1. Periorbital contusion.
      2. Orbital wall fractures.
      3. Retrobulbar hemorrhage.
      4. Corneal abrasion.
      5. Foreign body.
      6. Subconjunctival hemorrhage.
      7. Hyphema.
      8. Traumatic mydriasis or miosis.
      9. Iridodialysis.
      10. Traumatic cataract.
      11. Lens subluxation/dislocation.
      12. Scleral rupture.
      13. Vitreous hemorrhage.
      14. Retinal hemorrhage, tear/detachment.
      15. Optic nerve injury.
   B. **Penetrating Trauma.**
      1. Eyelid lacerations.
      2. Conjunctival lacerations.
      3. Corneal lacerations.
      4. Scleral lacerations.
      5. Intraocular foreign body.

IV. **Database**
   A. **Complete Eye Exam.**
      1. **Visual acuity.**
      2. **Gross inspection** of periorbital tissues, lids, sclera, cornea, iris, conjunctiva.
      3. **Palpation** of orbital rim to diagnose fractures.
      4. **Extra-ocular muscle movement.**

   5. **Pupillary exam** including testing for an afferent pupillary defect.
   6. **Visual field testing.**
   7. **Funduscopic** examination with direct ophthalmoscope.
   8. **Slit lamp** examination to examine cornea and anterior chamber.
   9. **Intraocular pressure measurement.**
B. **Physical Exam Key Points**
   1. **Visual acuity** is a vital sign of the eye. Each eye should be tested independently and with glasses if patient wears them. Use the pinhole method to correct for any uncorrected refractive errors.
   2. **Periorbital lacerations** should be evaluated for possible intracranial involvement. Fat coming out of an eyelid laceration indicates orbital involvement because the eyelids have little to no fat.
   3. **Significant bloody chemosis** or a "bag of blood" subconjunctival hemorrhage is suggestive of eye rupture or penetration.
   4. **Proptosis, limitation of extraocular muscles, and elevated intraocular pressure** are indicative of retrobulbar hematoma.
   5. **Enophthalmos** indicates potential orbital floor blowout fracture.
   6. **A teardrop-shaped pupil,** or any pigmented material prolapsing through the sclera indicates corneal and scleral rupture or penetration, respectively.
   7. **Afferent pupillary defect** is not usually caused by hyphema or vitreous hemorrhage. Afferent pupillary defects are generally caused by large retinal injuries involving the macula, or optic nerve injury.
   8. **Iridodialysis,** a secondary pupil, is a tearing of the iris root from the ciliary body.
   9. **Iridodonesis,** a shimmering of the iris with rapid eye movement, is a helpful sign of lens subluxation/dislocation.
   10. **Diminished red eye reflex** and the inability to visualize the fundus well with a direct ophthalmoscope are signs of vitreous hemorrhage.
   11. **Large retinal tears** may be seen with the direct ophthalmoscope as a billowing forward of the membrane, but many tears are smaller and peripherally located and will be missed with plain direct ophthalmoscopic exam. Visual acuity will be normal except if the macula is involved.
   12. **Mydriasis,** especially when associated with ptosis, should be concerning for a third nerve compression process.
   13. **Loss of vision with normal visual acuity testing** should be carefully examined for a visual field cut.
B. **Laboratory Data.** Rarely needed.
C. **Radiographic and Other Studies**
   1. **Slit lamp examination.** Performed to look at the anterior structures of the eye. Corneal abrasion, foreign body, microscopic or small hyphema may be discovered.
   2. **Seidel test.** If aqueous humor is leaking through a corneal wound, streaming fluorescent dye surrounded by an orange pool of solution will be seen.

3. **Intraocular pressure measurement.** Can be helpful but should not be undertaken by a nonophthalmologist when signs of ocular rupture/penetration are present.
4. **Plain orbital radiographs.** Useful for diagnosing orbital rim or floor fractures, and metallic foreign bodies.
5. **CT and MRI scans.** Useful for diagnosis of foreign body, intra-cranial involvement, detailed examination of fractures, and determining globe penetration or rupture. MRI scans should not be used if a metallic foreign body is suspected.
6. **Formal visual field testing.**

V. **Plan**
   A. **Overall Plan.** Immediate ophthalmologic consultation is needed for retrobulbar hematoma, intraocular foreign body, hyphema, traumatic cataract, lens dislocation, scleral rupture, vitreous hemorrhage, retinal hemorrhage/tear/detachment, optic nerve injury, corneal/scleral lacerations or rupture, and complex lid lacerations.
   B. **Specific Plans**
      1. **Periorbital contusion.** Symptomatic treatment.
      2. **Orbital wall fractures.** Symptomatic treatment. Antibiotics if fracture involves an infected sinus, and avoid nose blowing/Valsalva's maneuver. Some ophthalmologists will treat with steroids for ocular entrapment.
      3. **Retrobulbar hematoma.** Confirm diagnosis with CT imaging. Lateral canthotomy as temporizing measure, and medications for reducing elevated intraocular pressure.
      4. **Corneal abrasions.** Symptomatic treatment, cycloplegia, topical nonsteroidal medication, and topical antibiotics.
      5. **Superficial foreign body.** Removal of foreign body and treatment as corneal abrasion.
      6. **Subconjunctival hemorrhage.** Symptomatic treatment.
      7. **Hyphema.** Specific treatment left up to ophthalmologist.
      8. **Traumatic mydriasis/miosis.** Symptomatic treatment.
      9. **Iridodialysis.** If no hyphema present, symptomatic treatment.
     10. **Traumatic cataract.** Medications for acutely elevated intraocular pressure.
     11. **Lens subluxation/dislocation.** Ophthalmologic consultation.
     12. **Scleral/corneal rupture or laceration.** Avoid manipulation of orbit, place protective shield over eye. Keep patients NPO, anti-emetics as needed, and broad-spectrum antibiotics.
     13. **Intraocular foreign body.** Treatment as scleral or corneal laceration/rupture.
     14. **Retinal tear/detachment or vitreous hemorrhage.** Head of bed elevated, avoid platelet-inhibiting drugs, and ophthalmologic consultation.
     15. **Optic nerve injury.** Orbital CT scan to define injury, and ophthalmologic consultation. High-dose steroids or orbital decompression may be used for compressive syndromes.
     16. **Complex lid lacerations.** Ophthalmologic consultation.

   VI. ICD-9 Diagnoses: Contusion of eye and adnexa; Corneal abrasion; Corneal foreign body; Fracture of orbital bone; Hyphema; Iridodialysis; Lacerations of the eyelids; Lens subluxation/dislocation; Miosis; Mydriasis; Ocular lacerations; Optic nerve injury; Penetrating wound of the orbit with foreign Body; Penetrating wound of the orbit(with or without foreign body); Retinal detachments; Retinal hemorrhage; Retrobulbar hemorrhage; Rupture of eye; Subconjunctival hemorrhage; Traumatic cataract; Traumatic enucleation; Traumatic iritis; Vitreous hemorrhage.

 VII. Problem Case Diagnosis: Retrobulbar hematoma.

VIII. Teaching Pearl Question: An eye with an acute optic nerve laceration resulting in blindness will have a dilated pupil when examined by ambient light? True or False.

  IX. Teaching Pearl Answer: False. Optic nerve transection results in an afferent, not an efferent loss. There will be an afferent papillary defect, but efferent pupillary control of the bad eye is intact and responds to the afferent input from the good eye.

REFERENCES

Brunette DD. Ophthalmology. In: Marx JA, Hockberger RS, Walls RM eds. *Rosen's Emergency Medicine: Concepts and Clinical Practice.* 5th ed, Mosby, 2002:908–928.
Janda AM. Ocular trauma. Triage and treatment. *Postgrad Med* 1991;90:51–52, 55–60.
Linden JA, Renner GS. Trauma to the globe. *Emerg Med Clin North Am* 1995;13:581–605.

9. FACIAL TRAUMA

   I. Problem: A young female is punched in the face during an argument and complains of diplopia.

 II. Immediate Questions
   A. Is the airway intact? Manage appropriately (See Section VIII, 15. Rapid Sequence Endotracheal Intubation, page 470).
   B. Is significant active hemorrhage present? Control with direct pressure. Don't blindly clamp bleeding sites.
   C. Is neck tenderness present? Immobilize the cervical spine if C-spine injury is suspected.
   D. When did the injury occur?
   E. What was the mechanism of injury? (MVA, assault, sports injury, fall).
   F. Was there a LOC? If so, evaluate for possible closed head injury.
   G. Is the vision normal? If not, evaluate for ocular injury.
   H. Are there any areas of facial numbness? If so, evaluate for a fracture along the course of that specific nerve.
   I. Do the teeth fit together normally? If not, evaluate for mandibular fracture.

III. Differential Diagnosis
   A. Airway Failure. (See Section VIII, 15. Rapid Sequence Endotracheal Intubation, page 470) Consider obstruction from hemorrhage, debris, foreign body, tongue swelling, flail mandible.

B. **Facial Fractures.** Consider frontal, orbital/periorbital, nasal, ethmoid, zygomatic, Le Fort, mandibular, and open fractures.

C. **Eye Injuries.** (See this section, 8. Eye Trauma, page 276) Consider blowout fracture with extraocular muscle entrapment, third nerve injury, enophthalmos, penetrating globe, hyphema, corneal abrasion.

D. **Soft-Tissue Injuries.** (See Section VIII, 9. Laceration and Wound Care, page 455) Consider complex laceration, lacrimal duct injury, parotid duct laceration, nerve injury, intraoral laceration, lip laceration.

E. **Intracranial Injury.** (See this section, 3. Blunt Head Trauma, page 256) Consider intracranial hemorrhage, diffuse axonal injury, concussion syndrome, CSF leak.

F. **Domestic Violence.** Verify history with screening questions. Do you feel safe at home? Have you ever been a victim of physical abuse? Social services must evaluate patients with suspected domestic violence. Women with orbital fractures have a 30% likelihood of domestic violence or sexual assault.

IV. **Database**

A. **Physical Exam Key Points**

1. **Determine visual acuity and check extraocular movements.** Patients with altered visual acuity need a thorough eye exam. Patients with binocular diplopia should be evaluated for blowout fracture.

2. **Carefully inspect face** for deformity, asymmetry, ecchymosis lacerations, or hemorrhage. Inspect nose for deformity, epistaxis, septal hematoma, or CSF rhinorrhea. Inspect mouth for malocclusion, intraoral lacerations, or presence of a sublingual hematoma. Inspect ears for a tense ecchymosis of the pinnae, Battle's sign, hemotympanum, or CSF otorrhea.

3. **Carefully palpate facial bones** for tenderness, bony crepitus, and subcutaneous emphysema. Pay particular attention to the zygomaticofrontal suture (tripod fractures), zygomatic arch, nose, and infraorbital rim. Grasp the maxilla above the teeth between index finger and thumb and gently pull and push to assess midface stability (Le Fort fracture).

4. **Perform a thorough secondary survey** so that occult injuries are not overlooked.

B. **Laboratory Data.** Laboratory studies are not indicated for patients with isolated facial trauma.

C. **Radiographic and Other Studies.** Plain films are the initial screening study in most patients. Facial films should include a Waters's (infraorbital floor, orbital rims, maxillary sinuses) submentovertex or jug handle (zygomatic arch), PA or Caldwell (frontal bone and sinuses), and lateral. The mandible may be evaluated by a PA (body and symphysis) Towne's projection (condyles), and lateral obliques (rami). A Panorex view of the mandible visualizes all parts of the mandible except the symphysis. If a condylar fracture is suspected and plain films are negative, a coronal CT scan of the condyles should be obtained because plain films may miss these fractures. Nasal films are not indicated because they are neither sensitive nor specific and do not influence treatment. Frontal bone fractures require head CT because of the high forces required to cause these fractures. CT scan may be ordered in the ED or may be delayed until the time of outpatient follow-up. Some recommend CT as the initial study in patients who have a high likelihood of fracture based on clinical exam to save the cost of plain films, or in patients with suspected facial fractures who are already undergoing CT. CT scan is most useful for midface (tripod, Le Fort) and periorbital (blowout, orbital rim) fractures. Helical CT with 3D reconstruction can be helpful in evaluating difficult fractures in the midface and periorbital regions.

V. Plan

A. Overall Plan. Standard trauma resuscitation priorities remain in effect. If the airway is occluded perform a chin lift, or grab the tongue and pull it forward. Remove any foreign bodies. If active airway intervention is necessary, rapid sequence oral intubation should be performed (See Section VIII, 15, page 470). BVM ventilation may be difficult if facial instability is present. Control active hemorrhage with direct pressure. Do not clamp blindly. Although the face can bleed profusely, assume that hypotension is caused by nonfacial injuries.

D. Specific Plans

1. **Nondisplaced closed fractures** (blowout fracture, zygomatic arch, mandibular) can usually be treated on outpatient basis with maxillofacial surgery follow-up.
2. **Decreased visual acuity** should have immediate ophthalmology consultation.
3. **Nasal fractures** are treated with ice and elevation and patients are instructed not to blow their nose. If a septal hematoma is present, it should be drained. The patient is instructed to follow up in 5–7 days. If at that time the nose looks normal and is patent, no further treatment is necessary.
4. **Le Fort fractures** require admission due to the high-velocity nature of the injury.
5. **Open mandible fractures** should be admitted for IV antibiotics. Stable closed mandibular fractures are treated with a Barton's bandage (elastic wrapped around the head and mandible).
6. **Large pinna hematomas** should be drained to prevent cartilage necrosis and ear deformity.
7. **Frontal bone fractures** are caused by a high-impact force; these patients should undergo a cranial CT to rule out brain injury.
8. **Patients with CSF otorrhea**, rhinorrhea or other signs of basilar skull fracture should have neurosurgical consultation.

VI. ICD-9 Diagnoses: Multiple facial fractures; Epistaxis; Fracture of (specify bone); Orbital blowout fracture; "Le Fort fracture" coded as Maxilla fracture; Tooth avulsion; Tooth fracture.

VII. Problem Case Diagnosis: Orbital blowout fracture.

VIII. Teaching Pearls Question: What percentage of nasal fractures heal with a persistent fracture line?

IX. Teaching Pearls Answer: 50% (Ellis and Scott).

REFERENCES

Ellis E, Scott K. Assessment of patients with facial fractures. *Emerg Clin North Am* 2000;18(3):411–448.
Rhea JT, Rao PM, Novelline RA. Helical CT and three-dimensional CT of facial and orbital injury. *Radiol Clin North Am* 1999;37(3):489–513.

10. GENITOURINARY TRAUMA

I. Problem: A 37-year-old restrained driver in a moderate-speed MVA complains of abdominal pain and is found to have blood in the urine.

II. Immediate Questions
  A. Are there other, more serious injuries present? Head, chest, or abdominal injuries take precedence over the management of GU lesions in the multiply injured patient.
  B. Is it safe to pass a Foley catheter? If a partial disruption of the urethra is present, passage of a Foley catheter may convert it to a complete disruption. The integrity of the urethra must be ensured before passing a Foley.
  C. Is a pelvic fracture present? The presence of pelvic fractures significantly increases the probability of GU injuries.
  D. Is the lower GU tract or upper GU tract involved? It is important to localize the site of injury in the urinary system for definitive management.

III. Differential Diagnosis
  A. Lower Tract
    1. Urethral disruption. Urethral disruption is the significant injury that must be identified during the secondary survey.
    Pelvic fracture accounts for most posterior urethral disruptions (proximal to the urogenital diaphragm). Anterior urethral injuries are most frequently caused by straddle injuries, falls, gunshot wounds, and self-instrumentation.
    2. Bladder trauma
      a. Extraperitoneal bladder perforation is associated with pelvic fracture or direct trauma alone.
      b. Intraperitoneal bladder perforation may result from blunt forces causing increased intravesical pressure and bladder dome rupture.
  B. Upper Tract
    1. Renal trauma. Includes renal contusion (the most common form of GU trauma), renal laceration or rupture, and renal vascular pedi-

cle injury. It is important to identify which because without appropriate treatment the renal salvage rate may be very low, or renovascular hypertension may result.

2. **Ureteral disruption.** Rare, most often occurs in the setting of penetrating injury in the upper third of the ureter.

IV. **Database**
A. Physical Exam Key Points
1. **Compress the pelvis** or palpate over the pubic symphysis. Any elicited tenderness suggests pelvic fracture and increases the likelihood of GU trauma.
2. **Check for evidence of hematoma** or ecchymosis of the scrotum, perineum, or penis.
3. **Blood at the urethral meatus** suggests urethral injury. A Foley catheter should never be passed in this situation until the integrity of the urethra is evaluated.
4. **Rectal examination** must be performed to assess sphincter tone, bowel wall integrity, and **superior displacement (high riding) prostate.** Also evaluate if the prostate is boggy from hematoma.
5. **Pain in the abdomen,** palpable abdominal or flank mass may be present in cases of renal or ureteral injury.

B. Laboratory Data
1. **UA** to quantify the degree of hematoma. Gross hematuria or microhematuria ($\geq$3–5 RBC/hpf) with shock (BP < 90 mm Hg systolic) warrant further investigation of the GU tract. Patients who are not in shock, do not have other major traumatic injuries, and have < 50 RBC/hpf do not require imaging studies of the GU tract.
2. Other blood tests as indicated by patient condition.

C. Radiographic and Other Studies
1. **General strategy.** Radiologic work-up should proceed in a retrograde fashion if it is not immediately clear whether injuries are isolated to the lower or upper tract, with evaluation of the urethra first, bladder, and then upper tract.
2. **Retrograde urethrogram** is necessary for patients suspected of having urethral disruption (meatal blood, high-riding/boggy prostate, perineal/scrotal/penile hematoma).
3. **Retrograde cystogram** should be performed for patients with suspected bladder injury (pelvic fracture, hematuria).
4. **Contrast-enhanced helical CT for** suspected renal/ureteral injury (see UA section under Laboratory Data)

V. **Plan**
A. Overall Plan
Life-threatening injuries of the head, chest, and abdomen take precedence over GU injuries in the multiply injured patient. Follow the principles of trauma patient treatment.

B. Specific Plans
1. Place a Foley catheter once the integrity of the urethra has been ensured.

   2. Lower tract
   a. Urethra. If urethral trauma is identified, consult urology for definitive management. A suprapubic catheter may be necessary for urinary drainage.
   b. Bladder. Extraperitoneal bladder rupture may be treated expectantly with a Foley catheter for 7–14 days and allowed to spontaneously heal with close urology follow-up. Intraperitoneal bladder disruption requires operative repair.
   3. Upper tract
   a. Patients with < 50 RBC/hpf, stable vital signs, and no other major traumatic injuries may be safely treated as outpatients with appropriate follow-up.
   b. Patients with significant renal lacerations, disruptions, pedicle injuries, or ureteral disruption require prompt surgical intervention.
   c. Minor renal contusions or lacerations that do not extend into the collecting system or renal medulla can be managed nonsurgically with close urology monitoring.

VI. ICD-9 Diagnoses: Anterior and posterior urethral disruption/laceration; Extraperitoneal bladder rupture; Intraperitoneal bladder rupture; Pedicle disruption/laceration; Renal contusion; Renal laceration; Renal vascular ureteral disruption/laceration.

VII. Problem Case Diagnosis: Renal contusion.

VIII. Teaching Pearl Question: What is the kidney salvage rate when renal vascular injuries are identified and repaired promptly?

IX. Teaching Pearl Answer: Approximately 15–20%.

REFERENCES

Ahn JH, Morey AF, McAninch JW. Workup and management of traumatic hematuria. *Emerg Med Clin North Am* 1998;16(1):145–164.

Dreitlein DA, Suner S, Basler J. Genitourinary trauma. *Emerg Med Clin North Am* 2001; 19(3):569–590.

Uehara DT, Eisner RF. Indications for retrograde cystourethrography in trauma. *Ann Emerg Med* 1986;15(3):270–272.

11. NECK AND SPINAL CORD TRAUMA

   I. Problem: 65-year-old restrained male driver rear-ended, possible LOC, boarded and collared, BP 110/60, HR 68, RR 32. Patient C/O neck pain, left arm weakness, and tingling in his legs.

   II. Immediate Questions
   A. Does he have an adequate airway? Assess ABCs and treat as needed.

B. **What are the repeat vitals and GCS/AVPU?** Is patient responsive? IV, O_2, monitor, pulse ox, and temperature. Stable or unstable? Awake, alert, and oriented (person, place, and date) or confused?

C. **Chief complaint, what hurts?** Dyspnea, headache, neck or back pain, numbness or difficulty moving extremities. Patients who are intoxicated, have altered mental status, or have distracting injuries are unreliable

D. **AMPLE history.** Rate-controlling drugs, antihypertensives, illicit drugs, alcohol, hypertension, TIA, arrhythmia, osteoporosis, mechanism of injury, complete recall, before and after.

III. **Differential Diagnosis:** Assume injury to cord with significant falls, blunt trauma to head, neck, back or deceleration injuries.

A. **Spinal Cord Injury.** Incomplete or complete (may be from fracture fragment, dislocation, or disc compromising the canal), cord edema, or spinal shock.

B. **Cervical or Lumbar Spine Strain.** Pain with movement without neurologic deficit, fracture, or ligamentous instability on imaging studies.

C. **Ligamentous Injury.** Pain with movement disproportionate to clinical exam or radiographs. Flexion–extension radiographs or MRI.

D. **Multitrauma.** MVA with hypotension consider abdominal trauma (liver or spleen), vascular injury (aortic disruption or dissection), myocardial injury (contusion, MI, tamponade, valve rupture). Heart rate could be due to meds or arrhythmia.

IV. **Database**

A. **Physical Exam Key Points**

1. **Airway/breathing.** Evaluate patency and ability to maintain airway. Is there facial trauma or altered level of consciousness? Chest wall trauma or instability? Are breath sounds equal and symmetric? Monitor pulse oximetry.

2. **Vital signs.** Relative hypotension and paradoxical bradycardia suggest spinal shock; sudden loss of sympathetic tone below level of lesion, warm, dry skin, normal capillary refill. Hemorrhagic shock usually produces tachycardia, cool, clammy skin, and delayed capillary refill.

3. **Abdominal exam.** Check for ecchymosis, localized tenderness, distention or peritoneal signs; FAST exam.

4. **Neurologic exam**

a. **Mental status.** GCS, pupil reactivity and size.

b. **General.** Assess overall tone, motor strength (0–5 scale), and deep tendon and anogenital reflexes. Assess sensation, carefully map level of deficit. Posterior column dysfunction; loss of proprioception and vibratory sensation. Spinothalamic tract dysfunction; loss of pain and light touch, check for sacral sparing.

c. **Complete spinal cord transection.** (anatomic or physiologic): Flaccid paralysis and a sensory level. Priapism in males often present.

      d. **Anterior spinal cord syndrome.** Blunt trauma causing loss of motor and pain sensation bilaterally below level of lesion. Posterior cord function (proprioception, vibration) preserved.

      e. **Acute central cord syndrome.** Hyperextension injuries most common in the elderly after fall. Damage to the central cord fibers with motor loss greater in the upper extremities than lower. Variable sensory loss.

      f. **Brown–Séquard syndrome.** Penetrating injuries or unilateral facet dislocation. Hemicord injury with ipsilateral motor loss and contralateral sensory loss.

      g. **Cauda equina lesions.** L2 or lower, perineal (saddle) hypoesthesia with areflexic bowel, bladder, and lower extremities.

5. **CTL-spine exam.** Palpate C-spine supine, maintain neutral position, feel for stepoff, midline tenderness. Logroll, then palpate T and L spine. Assess rectal sphincter tone. If patient is unstable or unreliable, or if neurologic deficit is present, obtain screening radiographs, maintain immobilization.

6. **Extremity survey.** Look at and feel skin, check capillary refill, suspect injury to thoracolumbar spine with calcaneal fractures.

B. **Laboratory Data.** If multiple trauma or suspected head and/or spinal cord injury, then CBC, Chem 7, T&C, PT/PTT, Urine tox for drugs of abuse, and alcohol.

C. **Radiographic and Other Studies.** Clinically clear spine if no neurologic deficit, paresthesias, midline pain or tenderness, distracting injury, altered mental status, head injury, or intoxication present.

1. **Complete C-spine radiographs.** (AP, lateral, open-mouth) and obliques in pediatric patients. Must see from C1-T1. Check ABCs (alignment, bones, cartilage, soft tissue).

      a. **Lateral view of C-spine.** Assess atlantooccipital alignment, predental space ≤ 3 mm adult, < 5 mm child, prevertebral soft tissue < 5 mm anterior to C3, alignment and horizontal relationship of vertebral bodies, fanning of spinous processes, fractures.

      b. **Open-mouth/odontoid.** Assess dens for fractures, alignment, and spacing between C2 and lateral masses of C1.

      c. **AP.** Alignment of spinous processes and articular pillars, midline trachea.

      d. **Flexion–extension views.** Do when standard views normal, but pain is disproportionate to findings. Subluxation or flaring of spinous processes indicates ligamentous instability.

2. **Thoracolumbar radiographs.** Obtain lateral and AP views; can also get obliques.

3. **CT.** Subtle bony injuries, compromised canal, and some soft-tissue injuries.

4. **MRI.** Soft-tissue and ligamentous injuries.

V. Plan

A. Overall Plan. Immobilize until spinal cord injury excluded (normal radiographs and exam), keep warm, continuously monitor ABCD.

B. Specific Plans

1. **ABCs.** Intubate if necessary, maintain C-spine immobilization. Prepare to log roll and suction if vomiting.

2. **Shock.** Regardless of cause, initially resuscitate with isotonic crystalloid, use blood products when necessary. Use vasopressors if volume replacement unsuccessful and spinal shock suspected.

3. **Spinal cord injury.** Methylprednisolone 30 mg/kg bolus, followed by 5.4 mg/kg/h drip, start within 8 h of injury; consult orthopedics or neurosurgery for acute cord injuries, fractures, or subluxations. Transfer immobilized in collar and board if trauma service unavailable.

4. **Stable spinal column injuries.** Treat as outpatient.
   a. Acute cervical or lumbar strain.
   b. Isolated stable thoracolumbar fractures.

VI. ICD-9 Diagnoses:
Specify which vertebra is fractured/dislocated and if associated spinal cord injury present; Spinal cord contusion/injury.

VII. Problem Case Diagnosis:
Central cord syndrome.

VIII. Teaching Pearls Question:
What's the most commonly injured area of the TL spine?

IX. Teaching Pearls Answer:
Thoracolumbar junction because transition from fixed T-spine to mobile L-spine and from kyphosis to lordosis (Holmes et al).

REFERENCES

Hoffman JR, Mower WR, Wolfson AB, Todd KH, Zucker MI. Validity of a set of clinical criteria to rule out injury to the C-spine in patients with blunt trauma. National Emergency X-radiography Utilization Study Group. *N Engl J Med* 2000;343(2):94–99.

Holmes JF, Miller PQ, Panacek EA, Lin S, Horne NS, Mower WR. Epidemiology of thoracolumbar spine injury in blunt trauma. *Acad Emerg Med* 2001;8(9):866–872.

Shaw EV. Central cord syndrome presenting as unilateral weakness. *Am J Emerg Med* 1995;13(1):41–42.

12. NEEDLESTICK

I. Problem:
A 41-year-old surgeon presents after cutting his index finger with a scalpel in the OR.

II. Immediate Questions

A. Decontamination. Was the wound thoroughly cleaned and irrigated?

B. Disability. Is there any evidence of neurologic or vascular compromise?

C. **Delayed Disaster**
   1. **Type of exposure.** Splash, spill, stick, or slice? Body fluid: saliva, semen, blood? Blood in or on object?
   2. **Patient status.** Tetanus status? Hepatitis B immunization status (received immunization series **and** has titers demonstrating it worked)?
   3. **Source.** Hepatitis B (HBV)? Hepatitis C (HCV)? HIV? AIDS? Ill? Well? Unknown status? (See Section I, 43. HIV Problems, page 129)

III. **Differential Diagnosis**
   A. **HBV**
   B. **HCV**
   C. **HIV**
   D. **Tetanus**
   E. **Cellulites**

IV. **Database**
   A. **Physical Exam Key Points**
      1. **Neurologic exam.** Test each joint near injury for independent function against resistance. Also check each finger tip for two-point discrimination.
      2. **Vascular exam.** Make sure capillary refill is less then 2 s distal to injury.
      3. **Extent of injury.** Document evidence of cut, stab/stick, depth.
   B. **Laboratory Data**
      1. **Patient.** Baseline data for future reference: HIV, acute hepatitis panel (HAV IgM, HBsAg, HCV, HB core IgM), and for immunized patients HB surface antibody.
      2. **Source.** Obtain HBsAg, anti-HCV, and HIV antibody.
   C. **Radiographic and Other Studies**
      1. Radiograph only if high degree of suspicion for foreign body.

V. **Plan** (See Section I, 43. HIV Problems, page 129)
   A. **Overall Plan.** Minimize risk from exposure by thoroughly cleaning wound. Determine infectious state of source. Provide appropriate prophylaxis and treatment. Educate the patient so he can make informed consent about the choices of prophylaxis.
   B. **Specific Plans**
      1. **HBV.** Overall risk of infection from exposure 30%. Decrease risk of infection with hyperimmune globulin if source is infected and patient is not immunized, a nonresponder to immunization, or unknown response to immunization. Give vaccine if patient unvaccinated.
      2. **HCV.** Overall risk of infection from exposure 3%. No prophylaxis available. Wound care and close follow-up.
      3. **HIV.** Overall risk of infection from exposure 0.3%. Basically three levels of care, but refer to CDC recommendations (referenced)

and PEPline 888–448–4911 (See Section I, 43. HIV Problems, page 129)

   a. Do nothing.
      i. Source known to be HIV-negative.
      ii. Exposure was a splash to intact skin.
   b. Basic regimen. One month of two drugs (ZDV and 3TC; or 3TC and d4T; or d4T and ddl). (See Section I, 43. HIV Problems, page 129).
      i. Source unknown or HIV-positive without AIDS.
      ii. Exposure anything **but** penetrating hollow needle with source patient blood.
   c. Extended regimen. One month of three drugs (two basic drugs and a third as determined by expert consultation) (See Section I, 43. HIV Problems, page 129).
      i. Source has AIDS.
      ii. Exposure penetrating hollow needle with source patient blood in needle.
  4. Tetanus. A stick or cut is an open wound—update tetanus.
  5. Cellulites. Clean wound and monitor closely.

VI. ICD-9 Diagnoses: Needlestick (an E code only—relates mechanism); Prophylactic Immunotherapy (a V code); Puncture wound (specify site).

VII. Problem Case Diagnosis: Source patient not infected—no prophylaxis given.

VIII. Teaching Pearls Question: As of June 2000, occupational exposure to HIV has resulted in how many documented cases of HIV seroconversion among healthcare personnel in the United States.

IX. Teaching Pearls Answer: 56.

REFERENCES

Moran GJ. Emergency department management of blood and body fluid exposures. *Ann Emerg Med* 2000;35:47–62.
Preventing Occupational HIV Transmission to Healthcare Personnel
  http://www.cdc.gov/hiv/pubs/facts/hcwprev.htm

13. PELVIC AND HIP TRAUMA

I. Problem: Young man with hip pain and deformity after MVA.

II. Immediate Questions
  A. Is airway intact? Manage per ATLS guidelines (See this section 1. Trauma Assessment and Resuscitation, page 251, and Section VIII, 15. Rapid Sequence Endotracheal Intubation page 470).
  B. Is patient breathing adequately and hemodynamically stable? Consider pelvic fracture as source of hemorrhage. Recognize and

     treat other life-threatening injuries. Apply monitors, start IV, and evaluate per ATLS guidelines.

  C. What was mechanism of action? If MVA, was impact frontal or side, and how much intrusion into vehicle? If fall, from what height, and how did patient land?

  D. Does affected extremity have pulses? Can he move the limb and detect sensation? Loss of pulses may indicate arterial injury and need for immediate reduction. Nerve compromise requires early reduction as well and may indicate more serious injury (spinal cord).

  E. PMH? History of previous injury to extremity or artificial joint. Comorbid conditions may affect overall care.

  F. Last meal? Assess risk for intubation if emergent surgery indicated.

III. Differential Diagnosis

A. Pelvis Fracture

1. **Fracture stability**
   a. **Stable fracture.** Posterior sacroiliac joints intact, ring of pelvis intact (isolated ramus, iliac spine, or ischial tuberosity fracture), simple pubic diastasis, coccyx fracture.
   b. **Unstable fracture.** Posterior sacroiliac joint disruption, bilateral pubic ramus fractures.

2. **Mechanism**
   a. **Avulsion fracture.** Athletic injuries. Avulsion fracture off iliac spines or ischial tuberosity (stable).
   b. **Lateral compression.** MVA, pedestrian struck. Isolated pelvic wing and ramus fractures (stable). "Bucket handle" fracture (unstable).
   c. **AP compression.** MVA, pedestrian struck. Simple diastasis or ramus fracture (stable). "Open book" fracture with disruption sacroiliac joints and symphysis (unstable).
   d. **Straddle.** MCC. Bilateral rami fractures (unstable).
   e. **Vertical shear.** Fall. Malgaigne's fracture with rami fractures and diastasis and ipsilateral sacroiliac joint disruption (unstable).
   f. **Crush.** Combination of the previous.

B. Hip Dislocation

1. **Posterior dislocation.** Head-on MVA, knee hit dashboard. Leg adducted, internally rotated.
2. **Anterior dislocation.** Less common. Direct blow to abducted leg. Leg flexed, abducted, and externally rotated.

C. Hip Fracture

1. **Femoral head and neck.** Head fractures associated with dislocations. Neck fractures common in elderly with falls (may be ambulatory), younger patients in MVA. Leg shortened, abducted, and externally rotated.
2. **Intertrochanteric.** Most common. Fall in elderly. Leg shortened, externally rotated.

3. **Greater trochanteric.** Falls in elderly, MVA in younger patients. Leg flexed and externally rotated.
4. **Lesser trochanteric.** Iliopsoas muscle avulsion in athletes. Subtrochanteric. Majority are young patients in MVA. Leg flexed and externally rotated.
5. **Acetabular fracture.** Associated with hip dislocation and pelvic fractures.

IV. Database
A. Physical Exam Key Points
1. **Vital signs.** Consider pelvic fracture in unstable blunt trauma. Repeat during evaluation.
2. **Abdomen.** Tenderness, distention (hemoperitoneum). Grey Turner's sign (retroperitoneal hemorrhage).
3. **Pelvis.** Tender, unstable with compression.
4. **GU.** Blood at urethral meatus (urethral injury). Pelvic exam for vaginal bleeding or palpable open fracture. Scrotal exam for hematoma, ecchymosis.
5. **Rectal exam.** High-riding prostate (urethral injury). Palpate open fracture. Sphincter tone.
6. **Lower extremities.** Position (hip fracture, dislocation). Leg length discrepancy (hip fracture, vertical sheer pelvic fracture).
7. **Neurovascular exam.** Sensation and strength lower extremity. (Sciatic injury with posterior hip dislocation). Pulses (arterial injury with anterior dislocation).
B. Laboratory Data. Hct and coagulation studies. T&C for blood products. Renal function. Pregnancy test. UA.
C. Radiographic and Other Studies. AP pelvis and hip. Bedside abdominal US (hemoperitoneum). Urethrogram and cystogram (GU injury). CT scan (if patient stable). Pelvic angiogram (arterial bleeding in pelvic fracture). MRI hip (occult hip fracture).

V. Plan
A. Overall Plan. Anticipate and aggressively treat hemorrhage. Consider other causes of hypotension. Don't miss pelvic and hip trauma in obtunded patients. (See this section, 1. Trauma Assessment and Resuscitation, page 251, and Section I, 40. Hemorrhagic Shock, page 122, 47. Hypotension, page 142)
B. Specific Plans
1. **Pelvis trauma—unstable patient.** Treat hemorrhage aggressively and stabilize pelvis (lateral compression, early orthopedic consultation). Embolize arterial bleeding (early radiologic consultation). Recognize and treat GU trauma.
2. **Pelvis trauma—stable patient.** Anticipate hemorrhage. Unstable fractures admitted with orthopedic consult. Stable fractures discharged with weight bearing as tolerated if pain controlled.
3. **Hip fracture.** Orthopedic consultation and preoperative evaluation. Pain control and admission. Buck's traction for stability.

       4. Hip dislocation. Early reduction (prevent avascular necrosis). Orthopedic consultation and admission. Control pain.

       5. Acetabular fracture. Orthopedic consultation and admission.

VI. ICD-9 Diagnoses: Fracture or dislocation (state involved bone/joint, open vs closed, direction of dislocation).

VII. Problem Case Diagnosis: Posterior hip dislocation.

VIII. Teaching Pearls Question: What is the potential volume of blood loss into pelvis with open book pelvic fracture?

IX. Teaching Pearls Answer: Up to 6 L (Rubash and Mears).

REFERENCES

Coppola PT, Coppola M. Emergency department evaluation and treatment of pelvic fractures. *Emerg Med Clin North Am* 2000;18(1):1–27.

Rudman N, McIlmail D. Emergency department evaluation and treatment of hip and thigh injuries. *Emerg Med Clinics of North Am* 2000;18(1):29–66.

14. TRAUMA IN PREGNANCY

I. Problem: MVA victim is 34 weeks pregnant and has abdominal cramping and tachycardia.

II. Immediate Questions

    A. Is airway intact? Is patient oxygenating well? Manage per ATLS guidelines and administer high-flow oxygen. If intubation required, mother has lower oxygen reserves and increased risk of aspiration. (See this section, 1. Trauma Assessment and Resuscitation, page 251, and Section VIII, 15. Rapid Sequence Endotracheal Intubation, page 470)

    B. What are maternal vital signs? Is patient tachycardic or hypotensive? Maximize maternal hemodynamics. Vitals difficult to interpret because of physiologic changes in pregnancy (tachycardia, decreased blood pressure, and mild tachypnea).

    C. What is fetal heart rate? Recent fetal movement? Fetal tachycardia, bradycardia (normal 120–160 mm Hg), and decreased movement signal fetal distress.

    D. Is there abdominal pain/cramping? Vaginal bleeding or fluid? May signal placental abruption or the onset of labor.

    E. Mechanism of injury? Fetal and placental injury common even in minor trauma. Is there concern for physical abuse?

    F. Prenatal history? Last menstrual period, gestational age, complications of pregnancy, results of US.

III. Differential Diagnosis

    A. Maternal Injury. MVA, falls, abuse.

       1. Hypoxia. Limited oxygen reserves and decreased pulmonary function in pregnancy. Hypoxia and acidosis decrease uterine blood flow.

2. **Hemorrhage.** Solid organ injuries, pelvic fractures, and external blood loss. Increased lower extremity and pelvic blood flow increases blood loss.
3. **Coagulopathy.** Placental abruption, uterine injury, and fetal demise may lead to DIC.

B. **Fetal Injury.** Maternal death and shock, hypoxia, direct trauma.
1. **Hypoxia.** Maternal hypoxia or hypoperfusion results in fetal anoxia.
2. **Head injury and skull fractures.** Maternal pelvic fractures and lower abdominal blunt and penetrating trauma. Maternal injury may be minimal.

C. **Placental Injury.** Blunt and penetrating trauma.
1. **Abruption.** Placental separation leads to maternal hemorrhage, fetal distress, and death. Abdominal cramping, uterine tenderness, vaginal bleeding, maternal hypovolemia, enlarging uterus, and fetal distress may indicate abruption. Signs and symptoms may be minimal or absent.

D. **Uterine Injury.** Blunt and penetrating trauma.
1. **Contractions.** May indicate uterine irritability, uterine or placental injury.
2. **Rupture.** Rare but devastating event (fetal and maternal mortality high). Maternal shock, difficult to palpate fundus or easily palpable fetal parts may indicate rupture.

E. **Fetomaternal Hemorrhage.** Trauma may be minimal. After first trimester, fetomaternal hemorrhage should always be considered. Rh sensitization of mother against fetus may occur causing fetal hemolytic anemia. Affects this and future pregnancies.

F. **Amniotic Fluid Embolus.** Amniotic fluid enters maternal venous system and causes circulatory collapse. Sudden dyspnea, hypoxia, hypotension. Pulmonary edema and coagulopathy may ensue. Maternal and fetal mortality rate high.

G. **Supine Hypotension Syndrome.** Gravid uterus compresses inferior vena cava, causing decreased preload and hypotension. Maternal and placental hypoperfusion may result.

IV. **Database**
A. **Physical Exam Key Points.** Maternal well-being offers best chance of survival for fetus.
1. **Vital signs.** Second trimester heart rate 10–15 bpm above baseline and systolic blood pressure 5–10 mm Hg below. Returns to normal in third trimester. "Normal" vitals may be misleading. Auscultate or obtain Doppler fetal heart sounds. Fetal tachycardia or bradycardia indicate fetal distress.
2. **HEENT.** Continually reassess airway. Check for head trauma, cervical spine trauma.
3. **Cardiac.** Maternal flow murmurs common (high-flow state).
4. **Pulmonary.** Continually reassess respiratory performance (increased work of breathing and tachypnea) and oxygenation (pulse ox).

5. **Abdomen.** Palpate for size of uterus—should coincide with gestational age (umbilicus equals 20 weeks). Look for uterine tenderness, contractions, or increasing size. Abdominal tenderness (unreliable for hemoperitoneum in pregnancy).

6. **Genitourinary.** Check for vaginal bleeding. If no bleeding, perform sterile exam (assess cervical dilatation, presence of fetal parts in vagina, leakage of amniotic fluid: ferning on slide).

7. **Extremities.** Assess as in nonpregnant patient. Trauma to pelvis and lower extremities may exhibit large blood loss.

8. **Neurovascular exam.** As in nonpregnant patients.

B. **Laboratory Data.** Pregnancy test in all female trauma patients. Hct (32–34% normal in pregnancy), coagulation studies, blood type, and Rh. ABG or serum bicarbonate for occult maternal shock (21 mEq/L normal in pregnancy). Kleihauer–Betke (KB test) detects massive fetomaternal hemorrhage in Rh-negative mothers.

C. **Radiographic and Other Studies**

1. **Radiographs and CT** as needed to ensure maternal well-being (uterus shielded).

2. **Bedside US** to detect hemoperitoneum, placental abruption (sensitivity low).

3. **Cardiotocographic monitoring.** Abnormal fetal heart rate, decreased variability, and fetal decelerations after contractions indicate fetal distress. Fetal distress and uterine irritability sensitive indicator for placental abruption.

V. **Plan**

A. **Overall Plan.** Maternal resuscitation takes precedence over fetal evaluation. If mother is unstable, fetus is unstable. Initiate early cardiotocographic monitoring and obstetric consultation.

B. **Specific Plans**

1. **Maternal resuscitation.** Aggressive crystalloid infusion, high-flow oxygen, and left lateral decubitus positioning if > 20 weeks (avoid supine hypotension syndrome). Tilt backboard 15 degrees to left if immobilized. Avoid vasopressors (decreased uterine blood flow)

2. **Trauma care.** Laparotomy and surgical repair of fractures proceed as clinically indicated despite pregnancy.

3. **Placental abruption.** Emergency cesarean section indicated if fetal distress and abruption. Prepare for neonatal resuscitation. Expectant treatment if mother and fetus are stable or early gestational age (< 28 weeks). DIC common, monitor coagulation studies.

4. **Cardiopulmonary arrest.** Perimortem cesarean section if no response to ACLS within 5 min of ED arrival. Consider thoracotomy and open chest massage—do not cross-clamp aorta. Prepare for neonatal resuscitation.

5. **Monitor stable mother and fetus.** Admit all pregnant trauma patients (> 20 weeks) for 6–24 h for cardiotocographic monitoring. If discharged, patient needs close obstetrical follow-up and should

return for abdominal pain, bleeding. **Poor fetal outcome common** even with minimal trauma and no abnormal physical findings.
6. **Treat Rh-negative mothers.** Treat all traumatized Rh-negative mothers < 12 weeks with 50 µg RhIG. Treat >12 weeks with 300 µg dose. Use KB test to screen for massive fetomaternal hemorrhage that will require larger doses of RhIG.
7. **Tetanus booster.** Safe in pregnancy.
8. **Prevention.** Encourage three-point restraint in pregnant population, and screen patients for physical abuse.

VI. **ICD-9 Diagnoses:** Antepartum fetal-maternal hemorrhage; Antepartum fetal distress; Antepartum abnormality in fetal heart rate or rhythm; Placental abruption; Uterine rupture.

VII. **Problem Case Diagnosis:** Placental abruption.

VIII. **Teaching Pearls Question:** True or False: Mortality is higher in pregnant trauma patients than in nonpregnant patients.

IX. **Teaching Pearls Answer:** False.

REFERENCES

Shah KH, Simons RK. Trauma in pregnancy: Maternal and fetal outcomes. *J Trauma* 1998;45(1):83–86.
Smith EE, Cantrill SV. Clinical policy for the initial approach to patients presenting with acute blunt trauma. *Ann Emerg Med* 1998;31:422–454.

IV. Geriatric Emergency On-Call Problems

1. GENERAL GERIATRIC ASSESSMENT

I. **Problem:** Defining the chief complaint or the specific presenting problem in an elderly patient to accurately orient the emergency work-up may be challenging. Older patients frequently present to the ED with vague complaints such as weakness, decreased functional ability, dizziness, or falls. Emergency physicians must determine whether theses vague symptoms represent an important new disease processes such as sepsis, acute coronary syndromes, stroke, or acute metabolic abnormality.

II. **Immediate Questions**
Older patients have unique physiologic, emotional, and social needs that are often different from those of other adult patients. These needs must be taken into account as part of the ED evaluation, treatment, and disposition. Otherwise, the immediate questions should always include
   A. **Is the airway intact?** Manage appropriately.
   B. **What are the vitals and mental status?** Apply monitors, assess for changes in mental status.
   C. **Is a caregiver available or other person who knows the patient well?** If not present, locate to facilitate history taking.
   D. **What is the chief complaint?** This may be difficult to ascertain.

III. **Principles of Geriatric Emergency Medicine**
The following set of principles of geriatric emergency medicine has been defined by a multidisciplinary task force (See Sanders).
   A. **The older patient's presentation is frequently complex.** Older patients will often give vague and ambiguous symptoms for common medical conditions.
   B. **Common diseases present atypically in older patients.** Common diseases such as acute appendicitis and MI are often missed in older patients because they do not present with the typical symptoms such as right lower quadrant pain or chest pain.
   C. **The confounding effects of comorbid diseases must be considered.** Older patients often have comorbid diseases, and emergency physicians must consider whether the presenting complaint is an exacerbation of the existing condition or a new condition.
   D. **Polypharmacy is common.** Older patients also often take multiple medications. This may be a contributing factor for the cause of their presenting complaint. Medication interaction is also a problem when a new medication is added in the ED.
   E. **Recognition of the possibility for cognitive impairment is important.** Approximately 25–40% of older patients have cognitive impairment on presentation to the ED. This can affect the reliability of the

history as well as be indicative of specific conditions causing the chief complaint.

F. Some diagnostic tests may have different normal values. Some diagnostic tests change with age and others do not. Many laboratories do not provide age-adjusted normal values.

G. The likelihood of decreased functional reserve must be anticipated. Many physiologic parameters such as cardiac output decline with age. The lack of functional reserve may reflect how an older person responds to a common, treatable condition such as a UTI or multiple trauma.

H. Social support systems may not be adequate, and patients may need to rely on caregivers. A simple treatable condition such as an ankle sprain or fractured wrist may incapacitate an older patient who does not have adequate social support. This can then lead to other conditions such as malnutrition or functional decline.

I. Knowledge of baseline functional status is essential for evaluating new complaints. One method for assessing vague complaints is to determine whether the complaint represents functional decline. Functional decline can be assessed using standard activities of daily living scales. Acute functional decline can be a symptom of a serious medical condition (see this section, 6. Functional Decline).

J. Health problems must be evaluated for associated psychosocial adjustment. Emotional illness is common in older persons. The chief complaint must be evaluated in the context of the patient's emotional status.

K. The ED has an opportunity to assess important conditions in the patient's personal life. A number of conditions that may be important factors in evaluating the patient's chief complaint can be addressed in the ED visit. For example, the older patients suffering from domestic violence and elder abuse may present with a simple fall. Depression and alcoholism may be conditions that are readily assessed in an ED environment.

IV. Database

A. Mental Status. Older persons are screened for mental status abnormalities including delirium and cognitive decline. The initial screening can be done with orientation and three-item recall. Formal mental status testing can also be done for patients who fail the initial screening (see this section, 3. Altered Mental Status in the Older Patient).

B. Functional Assessment. A functional assessment of the patient's ability to function in his or her environment is done informally or formally (see this section, 6. Functional Decline).

C. Case Finding. Specific instruments to assess patients for elder abuse, depression, suicide risk, alcohol use, malnutrition, and incontinence can be applied in selected patients.

V. Differential Diagnosis

Key questions in the differential diagnosis include the following:

- **Does this patient's presentation represent sepsis?**

- **Does this patient's presentation represent an acute neurologic condition such as a CNS bleed or stroke?**
- **Does this patient's presentation represent an acute coronary syndrome or decompensated CHF?**
- **Does this patient's presentation represent an acute abdomen?**

VI. Plan

Between 30 and 40% of older patients seen in EDs are admitted to the hospital. Those patients who are discharged home are assessed to ensure, that (1) they have appropriate follow-up for the medical condition under evaluation and (2) their home environment is appropriate for their medical condition. Patients with relatively simple conditions such as rib fractures, bronchitis, pneumonia, contusions and sprains, etc may be at risk for complications if they do not have appropriate social support to care for their needs.

REFERENCES

Gerson LW, Schelble DT, Wilson JE. Using paramedics to identify at-risk elderly. *Ann Emerg Med* 1992;21:688–691.

Lachs MS, Williams CS, O'Brien S, Hurst L, Kossack A, Siegal A, Tinetti ME. ED use by older victims of family violence. *Ann Emerg Med* 1997;30:446–454.

Naughton BJ, Moran MB, Kadah H, Herman-Ackal Y, Longano J. Delirium and other cognitive impairment in older adults in and emergency department. *Ann Emerg Med* 1995; 25:751–755.

Sanders AB, ed. *Emergency Care of the Elder Person.* Beverly Craycom Publications, 1996.

Strange GR, Chen EH. Use of emergency departments by elder patients: A five-year follow-up study. *Acad Emerg Med* 1998;5:1157–1162.

2. ACUTE MYOCARDIAL INFARCTION IN THE OLDER PATIENT

I. **Problem:** 70-year-old female with history of CHF and arthritis, presents with a complaint of "just not feeling right." She reports symptoms of fatigue and mild shortness of breath and has had a vague sensation of pressure in her chest and upper abdomen for the last 12–24 h.

II. **Immediate Questions**

A. **Does the patient have risk factors for CAD?** Elderly patients are less likely to be diabetic, smoke tobacco, or have a history of prior revascularization procedures. CHF, CVA, and renal disease are more common in the elderly as are the precipitating factors of HTN and hyperlipidemia. Elderly females are at equal risk for MI as their male counterparts.

B. **Is there a history of similar episodes?** Elderly are more likely to have a prior history of angina or prior MI and to describe pain similar to previous MI.

C. **What is the location of the pain?** Is the pain pressure-like or crushing? Is there abdominal, back, or flank pain? Does the pain radiate?

Is it associated with any shortness of breath, diaphoresis, or nausea? Elderly patients with MI frequently present atypically without classic history or symptoms.

D. What is the time of onset? Elderly are more likely to delay seeking care, a large proportion present beyond the 6-h optimal therapy window for PTCA or thrombolytics.

III. Differential Diagnosis

A. CV. AMI, stable angina, AAA or thoracic dissection, pericarditis, myocarditis, mitral valve prolapse.

B. Pulmonary. PE, pneumothorax, pneumonia, asthma, COPD.

C. GI. GERD, esophageal spasm, peptic ulcer, pancreatitis, hepatitis, biliary colic, cholecystitis, colon or hepatobiliary malignancy, mesenteric ischemia, bowel obstruction, Boerhaave's syndrome.

D. Other. Herpes zoster, chest wall pain (costochondritis, muscle spasm), panic attack, anxiety disorder.

IV. Database

A. Physical Exam Key Points.

1. **General.** Evidence of trauma from fall.
2. **Pulmonary.** Check for signs of CHF—rales, jugular venous distention, and peripheral edema, wheezing, accessory muscle use.
3. **Cardiac.** Increased percentage of elderly have murmurs, rubs, and tachycardia, check BP in both upper extremities.
4. **GI.** Abdominal tenderness, masses, distention, melena, or hematochezia.
5. **Neurologic.** Lateralizing weakness, cranial nerve abnormalities, speech abnormalities.

B. Laboratory Data

1. **ECG.** Incidence of ST segment elevation with MI decreases with age. It is often difficult to interpret more frequent paced rhythms, LBBB, and AV blocks using ECG. Majority of elderly patients will have non-Q wave MI.
2. **Cardiac enzymes.** Lower total elevation in cardiac enzymes, particularly CK.
3. **Others.** Amylase, lactic acid (helpful in diagnosis of ischemic bowel), LFT, lipase.

C. Radiographic and Other Studies

1. **CXR.** Increased number with CHF findings and chronic lung disease. CXR must be obtained prior to anticoagulation/thrombolysis to rule out aortic dissection with wide mediastinum. Also may identify pneumonia and rib fracture.

V. Plan

A. Overall Plan. Suspected cardiac ischemia/infarction should be admitted. CHF exacerbation in the elderly should generally be admitted as well. Cardiac care should be initiated in the ED.

B. Specific Plans
   1. **Immediate**
      a. Evaluate for ABC issues.
      b. Oxygen, cardiac monitor, IV access.
      c. ECG.
      d. Aspirin (if no contraindications).
      e. Appropriate labs (cardiac enzymes, CBC, PT/PTT, Lytes, BUN, Cr, others as H&P warrant).
   2. **Symptomatic**
      a. 0.4 mg NTG, SL or IV (if SBP > 90 mm Hg) 5–200 µg/kg/min.
      b. Morphine for pain relief 1–2 mg IV, titrate to effect (*Caution:* Depressed CNS, respiratory drive).
      c. Avoid phenothiazines for nausea because sedative effects may be pronounced in the elderly.
   3. **Definitive.**
      a. **Thrombolytics.** Shown to decrease hospital deaths and increase long-term survival, underutilized compared with younger patients due to not meeting criteria (delayed presentation, large number of non-Q wave MI), and increased incidence of stroke. (*Caution:* Beyond age 75, risk/benefit ratio favors conservative therapy or PTCA)
      b. **PTCA/Angioplasty.** Shown to be effective but underutilized, slightly increases both short- and long-term survival over lytics. Beneficial in unstable patients but has higher overall complications including CHF, VT, CVA, distal embolization.
      c. **Beta-blockers.** Shown to increase survival in all AMI patients, including elderly. (*Caution:* Orthostatic hypotension.)

VI. ICD-9 Diagnoses: Acute myocardial infarction (state involved wall), Angina, Unstable angina, Acute pulmonary edema.

VII. Problem Case Diagnosis: The ECG showed ST depression with Q waves inferolaterally, the total CK was low but CK-MB and troponin were mildly elevated. CXR showed acute pulmonary edema. Patient was diagnosed with acute non-Q wave MI with associated pulmonary edema. She was started on aspirin, β-blockers, heparin, and NTG drip and transferred to the cardiac catheterization lab where she underwent PTCA with successful stenting of the right coronary artery.

VIII. Teaching Pearl Question: True or False? Elderly people will seek care for chest pain/MI sooner than younger people will.

IX. Teaching Pearl Answer: False. The proportion of elderly patients seeking care for chest pain/MI within 6 h of symptom onset actually declines significantly as patients age, and they present at significantly increased times from the onset of symptoms than younger patients.

REFERENCES

Berger AK, Schulman KA, Gersh BJ, Pirzada S, Breall JA, Johnson AE, et al. Primary coronary angioplasty vs. thrombolysis for the management of acute myocardial infarction in elderly patients. *JAMA* 1999;282:341–348.

Mehta RH, Rathore SS, Radford MJ, Wang Y, Wang Y, Krumholz HM. Acute myocardial infarction in the elderly: Differences by age. *J Am Coll Cardiol* 2001 38:736–741.

Solomon CG, Lee TH, Cook EF, Weisberg MC, Brand DA, Rouan GW, et al. Comparison of clinical presentation of acute myocardial infarction in patients older than 65 years of age to younger patients: The multicenter chest pain study experience. *Am J Cardiol* 1989;63:772–776.

Tresch DD, Brady WJ, Aufderheide TP, Lawrence SW, Williams KJ. Comparison of elderly and younger patients with out-of-hospital chest pain: clinical characteristics, acute myocardial infarction, therapy, and outcomes. *Arch Intern Med* 1996;156:1089–1093.

3. ALTERED MENTAL STATUS IN THE OLDER PATIENT

I. **Problem:** An elderly female is brought in by her daughter because "she is just not acting right."

II. **Immediate Questions**
   A. **Are the ABCs intact?** Manage appropriately
   B. **What are the vital signs and global mental status?** Is the patient stable and alert? Apply monitors (ECG and pulse ox), start IV, apply oxygen. **Check blood sugar level.** Consider naloxone and thiamine administration.
   C. **Advanced directives?**
   D. **Are caregivers or other sources available to aid in patient evaluation and treatment?**
   E. **When did the symptoms begin? Do the symptoms fluctuate?**
   F. **What is the patient's baseline mental status?** Preexisting dementia is common in elderly patients with altered mental status, and history of this should be specifically sought. Any history of psychiatric illness?
   G. **What is the patient's baseline functional status?** Ask about ADL and instrumental activities of daily living.
   H. **Is there evidence of delirium?** Delirium is frequently unrecognized in the elderly patient, and evidence for this should be specifically sought. Diagnose using the confusion assessment method (CAM): **acute** onset or **fluctuating** course **and** inattention (cardinal features) **and** either altered level of consciousness or disorganized thinking.
   I. **Specifically, how is the mental status altered?** Is there memory loss? Confusion? Disorientation? Hallucinations, and if so auditory or visual? Delusions? Alterations in affect? Behavior? Mood? Thought content? Alterations in level of consciousness, either agitated or stuporous/lethargic?
   J. **Any history of trauma?** May be recent or remote.
   K. **Any associated symptoms?** Is there fever? Chest pain? SOB? Symptoms indicating infection, urine, lung, skin, CNS? Remember in the elderly that presentations are frequently atypical.

L. **Is the patient taking medications or using recreational drugs or alcohol?** Polypharmacy, with resultant medication side effects and with drug-drug interactions, is a frequent problem in the elderly. Ask about alcohol, recreational drugs, complementary, and alternative medicines and food supplements.

M. **What is the PMH?** History of dementia, psychiatric illness, as mentioned earlier? Any metabolic or endocrine disorder, particularly diabetes? History of carcinoma?

III. **Differential Diagnosis**

In the elderly, alterations in mental status are more commonly due to toxic/metabolic rather than structural causes.

A. **CNS**
   1. **Meningitis/encephalitis/brain abscess.**
   2. **Dementia.**
   3. **Intracerebral bleeding, particularly subdural hematoma.**
   4. **Ischemia/infarct.**
   5. **Space-occupying lesion.**
   6. **Seizure/postictal state**

B. **Psychiatric.**
   1. **Depression.**
   2. **Schizophrenia/schizoaffective disorder.**

C. **Infectious.**
   1. **UTI.**
   2. **Pneumonia.**
   3. **Cellulitis/decubitus ulcer.**
   4. **Cholecystitis, diverticulitis, appendicitis.**

D. **Endocrine/Metabolic.**
   1. **Disorders of glucose, sodium, calcium, and magnesium metabolism.**
   2. **Disorders of thyroid function.**
   3. **Renal/hepatic failure.**
   4. **Wernicke/Korsakoff's syndrome or other vitamin-related deficiency.**
   5. **Volume depletion.**
   6. **Disorders of temperature regulation.**
   7. **Adrenal insufficiency.**

E. **Pharmacologic/Toxicologic.**
   1. **Polypharmacy/adverse drug reaction/drug-drug interaction.**
   2. **Alcohol or illicit drug intoxication or withdrawal.**
   3. **Complementary and alternative medicines.**
   4. **Carbon monoxide exposure.**

F. **Cardiovascular.**
   1. **MI/myocardial ischemia.**
   2. **Cardiac arrhythmia.**
   3. **CHF.**
   4. **Mesenteric ischemia.**
   5. **GI bleeding.**

G. **Pulmonary.**
  1. **Disorders of oxygenation and ventilation pneumonia, COPD, PE.**
H. **Neoplasm-Related.**
  1. **Primary or metastatic CNS lesion.**
  2. **Metabolic disorder, particularly hypercalcemia, SIADH.**
  3. **Anemia.**
  4. **Paraneoplastic syndrome.**

IV. **Database**
  A. **Physical Exam Key Points.**
    1. **Vital signs,** including pulse oximetry.
    2. **HEENT.** Head trauma/neck rigidity/hydration status?
    3. **Cardiopulmonary.** Signs of CHF/arrhythmia/pneumonia?
    4. **Abdominal/back.** Distension/peritoneal signs/hepatosplenomegaly/occult blood/CVA tenderness?
    5. **Skin.** Jaundice/cellulitis/decubitus ulcer?
    6. **Neurologic.** Including a detailed assessment of level of consciousness and mental status (see next item). Check pupils/fundi/EOMs. Check gait (if patient usually ambulatory).
    7. **Mental status.** As above, assess thought content, mood affect, judgment orientation, recall. Begin simply with orientation, three-item recall at 5 min. Use CAM to assess for evidence of delirium, Folstein Mini Mental Status Exam (See Table A-4, Mini Mental Status Exam, page 656) to assess dementia.
  B. **Laboratory Data.** Elderly patients frequently require more liberal use of diagnostic testing because presentations are frequently atypical and can be silent. CBC, basic metabolic screen (comprehensive or other if clinical presentation warrants eg, carcinoma, liver disease, thyroid disease, MI, etc); UA.
  C. **Radiographic and Other Studies.** CXR, ECG, ABG can be helpful. Body fluid cultures, including **spinal fluid,** as indicated. Consider CT scan or other neuroimaging, although remembering that only a small proportion of altered mental status presentations in the elderly are due to structural causes.

V. **Plan**
  A. **Overall Plan.** Disposition of the elderly patient requires a comprehensive assessment and plan, integrating the patient's highest level of function and independence with the needs of the patient, the patient's family, and the primary caregiver. If the patient is to be discharged, is a support system in place such that the management plan and follow-up can be ensured? In general, elderly patients with an acute alteration in mental status will require admission for further evaluation and treatment. This is especially the case for elderly patients with delirium.
  B. **Specific Plans**
    1. **Infectious.** Consider broader spectrum of pathogens, as well as increased morbidity and mortality, in the elderly. Refer to guidelines

for disposition that take into account age as a consideration for disposition, for example, the Infectious Disease Society of America and American Thoracic Society guidelines on community-acquired pneumonia.

2. **Thrombolysis.** Remember that thrombolysis may be of significant benefit in the elderly for treatment of both MI and stroke and should be considered in appropriately selected patients.

3. **Polypharmacy.** If prescribing medications, remember to take into account the possibility of altered drug effects, metabolism, and kinetics, as well as drug-drug interactions.

VI. ICD-9 Diagnoses: Acute cerebrovascular; Adverse drug effect; Alteration of consciousness; Cellulitis; Coma; Delirium; Dementia; Depression; Disease, Hematoma, subdural; Electrolyte imbalance; Neoplasm; Pneumonia; Psychosis; Septicemia; Stupor; Urinary tract infection.

VII. Problem Case Diagnosis: Delirium secondary to silent MI.

VIII. Teaching Pearls Question: True or false: Altered mental status in the elderly is most commonly due to subdural hematoma or other structural cause.

IX. Teaching Pearls Answer: False. Altered mental status in the elderly is more frequently due to toxic/metabolic, rather than structural causes (Kalbfleisch).

REFERENCES

Folstein SE, Folstein MF, McHugh PR. "Mini mental state": A practical method for grading the cognitive state of patients for the clinician. *J Psychiatr Res* 1975;12:189–198.

Inouye SK, van Dyck CH, Alessi CA, Balkin S, Siegal AP, Horwitz RI. Clarifying confusion: The confusion assessment method. *Ann Intern Med* 1990;113:941–948.

Kalbfleisch N. *Altered Mental Status in Emergency Care of the Elder Person.* Sanders AB, ed. Beverly Craycom Publications, St. Louis, Mo. 1996.

Lewis LM, Miller DK, Morley JE, Nork MJ, Lasater LC. Unrecognized delirium in ED geriatric patients. *Am J Emerg Med* 1995;13:142–145.

O'Keefe KP, Sanson TG. Elderly patients with altered mental status. *Emerg Med Clin North Am* 1998;16(4):701–715.

4. ELDER ABUSE

I. Problem: An elderly male presents with soiled clothing, lice, bruises in the shape of a belt buckle, confusion, and multiple rib fractures in various stages of healing.

II. Immediate Questions

A. **Is there evidence of physical abuse?**

1. **Bruises.** Unexplained, various stages of healing, regular patterns, shape of articles used, bite marks, unusual location.

    2. **Burns.** Immersion burns, patterned (eg, iron), rope burns, shape of cigarette/cigar, caustic burns.

    3. **Fractures.** Unexplained, various stages of healing, multiple, spiral.

    4. **Lacerations.** Unexplained, unusual location (eg, vulva).

    5. **Internal injuries.**

B. Is there evidence of physical neglect? Poor personal hygiene, inappropriate dress, consistent hunger, soiled clothing, weight loss, dehydration, urine burns, pressure sores, over/undermedication, lice, hypothermia, lack of functional aids such as glasses, dentures, hearing aids, and walking aids.

C. Is there evidence of sexual abuse? Bruised or bloody genitalia, bruises around breasts, vaginal bleeding or tears, anal tears or bruising, stained or bloody underwear, sexually transmitted diseases, and difficulty walking or sitting.

D. Is there evidence of emotional abuse? Antisocial, hypochondria, hysteria, compulsion, obsession, sleep disorder, habit disorder (eg, rocking, sucking, biting).

E. Is there evidence of financial abuse? Abrupt changes in a will, unexplained disappearance of money or other valuables, forging of an elder's signature, sudden appearance of previously uninvolved relatives claiming rights to an elder's possessions.

F. Any PMH? History of psychiatric illness, hospital visits, illicit drug use, alcohol abuse, and any current medications?

III. Differential Diagnosis

A. Coagulopathy. Consider if the patient is on warfarin (Coumadin), aspirin, or other blood thinners. May also see in sepsis or leukemia.

B. Ethanol or Other Substance Abuse. Consider acute intoxication or withdrawal.

C. Intracranial Hemorrhage. Consider subdural, epidural, or intracerebral bleed in a patient with acute mental status changes.

D. Metabolic Derangement.

E. Elder Abuse.

F. Drug Toxicity. Review patient's medication list and obtain appropriate drug levels.

G. Infection. Consider specific site of infection (eg, UTI) with or without sepsis.

H. Psychiatric Illness. Consider acute primary psychiatric cause (eg, acute psychosis).

IV. Database

A. Physical Exam Key Points. Don't forget to completely undress and examine the entire body, including the back.

    1. **General.** Check personal hygiene.

    2. **Mental status.** Mini mental status exam (See Tabe A-4, Mini Mental Status Exam, page 656).

    3. **Vital signs.** Check carefully and repeat during evaluation.

    4. **Mouth.** Check mouth for lacerations or dental fractures.

5. **Nose.** Check for epistaxis, septal hematoma.
6. **Neck and back.** Check for spinal tenderness.
7. **Chest.** Palpate for crepitance or rib irregularities.
8. **Abdomen.** Check for tenderness that may indicate intraabdominal organ injury.
9. **Rectal and pelvic.** Check external genitalia and anus for blood, bruising, or lacerations. Pelvic exam is necessary if there is vaginal bleeding.
10. **Skin.** Check for bruising, lacerations, burns, or imprints of objects.
11. **Extremities.** Check for deformities and joint effusions.
12. **Neurologic exam.** Check pupils for reactivity, fundi for hemorrhages, focal deficits, cerebellar deficits, and level of alertness.

B. **Laboratory Data.** If numerous bruises or unexplained bleeding are present, check a CBC with platelets, PT, INR, PTT, and bleeding time. Check Lytes and UA if weak, unexplained falls, or confused. Check a bedside glucose (fingerstick) if altered mentation. Check an alcohol level if inebriation suspected and obtain a drugs of abuse screen if other abused substances are suspected. Check specific drug levels if there is concern that patient may not be getting appropriate doses of medication.

C. **Radiographic and Other Studies.** Check appropriate radiographs for suspected fractures. Obtain old chart, and review previous visits for patterns of abuse. Head CT for patients with suspected head injury (skull fractures and subdural and epidural hemorrhages). Take photographs for appropriate documentation of injuries.

V. **Plan**
A. **Overall Plan.** Cases of suspected elder abuse should be referred to the medical social worker and adult protective services. If home situation is unsafe, then consider admission to the hospital. Specific problems due to the abuse (eg, fracture) should be addressed.

B. **Specific Plans.**
1. **Fractures.** Appropriate orthopedic involvement. Possibly splint or cast depending on the location.
2. **Bruises, lacerations, burns.** Appropriate repair (see Section VIII, Laceration and Wound Care, page 455) or dressings (see Section III, 4. Burns, page 259) with appropriate follow-up. Take pictures if possible.
3. **Dehydration, metabolic.** Treat accordingly.
4. **Hypothermia.** See Section I, 48. Hypothermia, page 144.
5. **Intracranial bleeds.** (See Subdural, Epidural bleeds).
6. **Social.** Medical social work evaluation and adult protective service involvement.

VI. **ICD-9 Diagnoses:** Adult emotional/psychologic abuse; Adult maltreatment, unspecified; Adult neglect; Adult physical abuse; Adult sexual abuse.

VII. **Problem Case Diagnosis:** Physical abuse and neglect.

VIII. **Teaching Pearls Question:** Which sex is disproportionately abused in the elderly population?

IX. **Teaching Pearls Answer:** Women (Jones, et al).

REFERENCES

Clarke ME, Pierson W. Management of elder abuse in the emergency department. *Emerg Med Clin North Am* 1999;17(3):631–644.

Jones JS, Holstege CP, Holstege H. Elder abuse and neglect: Understanding the causes and potential risk factors. *Am J Emerg Med* 1997;15:579–583.

Kleinschmidt KC. Elder abuse: A review. *Ann Emerg Med* 1997;30(4):463–472.

U.S. Administration on Aging. The National Elder Abuse Incidence Study; Final Report, 1998. http://www.aoa.dhhs.gov/abuse/report/default.htm

5. FALLS IN THE OLDER PATIENT

I. **Problem:** An elderly male is found awake on the living room floor by family.

II. **Immediate Questions**
   A. **Is the airway intact?** Manage appropriately (see Section VIII, 15. Rapid Sequence Endotracheal Intubation, page 470).
   B. **Is in-line stabilization in place?** C-collar and backboard.
   C. **What are the vitals and mental status?** Start IV, apply oxygen, apply monitors (ECG and pulse ox). Heart rate and rhythm, BP, Monitor orthostatic changes. Is fall from significant cardiovascular event? Confused? Change from baseline?
   D. **What was he doing when it happened?** Exertion or other stress?
   E. **Status immediately before?** Recent sitting to standing position? Prodromal symptoms (dizzy, giddy, light-headed, palpitations)?
   F. **Status immediately after?** Postictal phase? LOC (see Section I, 67. Syncope, page 200)? Circumstances following fall (assistance getting up, prolonged time on ground)? Aphasia?
   G. **Any PMH?** Heart disease? Diabetes? Medications (new or dose change, discontinued)? History of recurrent or increasing frequency of falls? History of recent illnesses?
   H. **Any obvious bony deformities?** Need for urgent reduction and splinting?

III. **Differential Diagnosis—Usually Multifactorial**
   A. **Intrinsic Cause**
      1. **Cardiac.** Sudden onset without prodrome.
         a. **Arrhythmia.** (See Section I, II. Bradycardia, page 36, 53 Palpitations, page 157, and 68. Tachycardia, page 202.) Consider VT, PAT, AF, A-flutter, PSVT, WPW, long QT interval, heart blocks, pacer malfunction.
         b. **Outflow obstruction.** Consider aortic stenosis.

        c. **Pump failure.** Consider AMI, aortic dissection, pulmonary HTN, cardiac tamponade, PE.
2. **Orthostatic hypotension.** Dehydration, blood loss, new medication, autonomic dysfunction (diabetes, Parkinson's disease).
3. **Vasovagal/vasomotor.** Stressful precipitating event? Prodrome of lightheadedness, diaphoresis, nausea, or visual changes? Consider carotid sinus hypersensitivity if associated with cough, micturition, postprandial state, defecation, head-turning, or emotional stress.
4. **Neurologic.** Consider stroke, TIA, vertebrobasilar insufficiency, SAH, subclavian steal syndrome, or seizure.
5. **Metabolic/respiratory.** Consider hypoxia (pneumonia, PE), hypoglycemia, electrolyte derangement (hypokalemia/hyperkalemia predisposing to arrhythmias), and hyperventilation.
6. **Musculoskeletal.** Consider arthritis pain and osteoporosis.
7. **Medications/polypharmacy.** Common agents include antihypertensives, diuretics, sedatives, hypnotics, antidepressants, corticosteroids, anticholinergics, and hypoglycemic agents. Consider discontinued, new, or dose changes as well.
8. **Acute Illness.** Sepsis, UTI, pneumonia.
9. **Normal physiologic aging.** Consider diminished visual acuity, hearing, balance, strength, gait, and reaction time.

B. **Extrinsic Cause** Consider environment, absent handrails, loose rugs, unstable furniture, slippery surfaces, inadequate lighting, and obstacles. Consider elder abuse.

IV. Database

A. **Physical Exam Key Points.** Identify injuries and clues to cause of fall.
1. **Vital signs.** Check carefully and repeat during evaluation. Orthostatic vitals.
2. **Mental status.** Mini mental status exam (See Table A-4, Mini Mental Status Exam, page 656).
3. **General.** Check for dry mucous membranes, sunken eyes, decreased skin turgor, and decreased axillary sweat.
4. **Head and neck.** Check for carotid bruits and neck tenderness from fall. Labyrinthine stimulation (inner ear problem).
5. **Chest.** Check for systolic murmur (aortic stenosis). S_3 or S_4 (MI, CHF). Loud bruit over left subclavian artery (subclavian steal syndrome).
6. **Abdomen, rectal and pelvis.** Check for pulsatile abdominal mass (AAA). Check stool for blood (source of blood loss). Check for pelvic instability and hematoma.
7. **Neurologic exam.** Check pupils for reactivity (CVA), fundi for hemorrhages (SAH), Focal deficits (CVA, intracranial bleed), cerebellar deficits (VBI), persistent confusion (metabolic). Balance and gait testing.

8. **Extremity and skin exam.** Check for obvious fractures, dislocations, lacerations, tenderness, hematomas, and contusions. Shortening and external rotation with hip fractures.

B. **Laboratory Data.** If complete history and PE are normal, bedside glucose, CBC, and BMP are sufficient to screen for most important conditions. Consider alcohol and tox screening. Other studies if risk factors uncovered in H&P.

C. **Radiographic and Other Studies.** *If complete H&P are normal:* Cardiac monitor, ECG, and orthostatic BP. Consider maneuvers to reproduce the event with care not to harm or injure patient. *Other studies if risk factors uncovered in H&P:* Cardiac enzymes, CXR, echocardiogram, Holter monitor, heat CT, extremity films.

V. **Plan**

A. **Overall Plan.** Rule out significant injury and life-threatening underlying conditions as cause of fall. Treat cause of fall to return patient to baseline functioning and reduce risk of recurrent falls. Elderly with functional decline should be considered for admission. Other causes must be managed according to their individual causes.

B. **Specific Plans.**

1. **Cardiac.** Treat dysrhythmias accordingly (See Section I, 11 Bradycardia, page 36, 15. Chest Pain, page 51, 16. CHF and Pulmonary Edema, page 54, 38. Heart Murmur, page 118, 52. Pacemaker Problems, page 154, and 68. Tachycardia, page 202). All should be admitted until problem clarified and resolved.

2. **Vasovagal.** Avoid precipitating events. Keep patient hydrated. Primary care follow-up.

3. **Elder considerations.** Wounds heal slower, sutures may need to stay in longer, immobilization advantage must be weighed against functional and balance status. Assess ADLs/IADLs for overall function. Consider behavioral modifications for postural hypotension, education on proper medication use, referral for conditioning and physical therapy, and arranging close follow-up with home safety visit.

4. **Analgesia.** Treat pain accordingly.

5. **Fractures.** Address need for urgent reduction and splinting.

VI. **ICD-9 Diagnoses:** Acute CVA; Adverse effect medication (specify med and reaction); Alteration of consciousness; Aortic stenosis; Arrhythmia/Dysrhythmia (specify type); Hypoglycemia; Hypotension-orthostatic; Pulmonary embolus; Ruptured aortic aneurysm; Syncope.

VII. **Problem Case Diagnosis:** Hypoglycemia.

VIII. **Teaching Pearl Questions.** What percent of elderly who need hospitalization after a fall die within 1 year? What percent of elder falls result in fracture, dislocation, or laceration requiring suturing?

IX. **Teaching Pearl Answers.** Up to 50% (Sanders); 10% (Sanders).

REFERENCES

Fuller G. Falls in the elderly. *Am Fam Physician* 2000;61(7):2159–2168, 2173–2174.
Przybelski RJ, Shea TA. Falls in the geriatric patient. *WMJ* 2001;100(2):53–56.
Sanders AB. Trauma and falls. In: Geriatric Emergency Medicine Task Force. *Emergency Care of the Elder Person.* Beverly Craycom Publications, 1996:153–170.

6. FUNCTIONAL DECLINE

I. **Problem:** Paramedics arrive with an elderly female whose family is concerned because she hasn't been doing well the past few days.

II. **Immediate Questions**
   A. **What is the code status of this elderly patient?** Would this patient desire aggressive airway management, CPR, or pharmacologic intervention if needed? Is there a durable power of attorney? Because these answers may not be immediately available, efforts should be made to obtain this information.
   B. **Is the airway intact?** Manage appropriately.
   C. **How is the patient's breathing?** Is it labored, shallow, fast, effective? Is central cyanosis present? Are the lips "pursed?" Is the patient using accessory muscles?
   D. **How is the patient's circulation?** Quickly assess skin color and temperature, capillary refill, and peripheral pulses.
   E. **What are the vital signs and mental status?** Is the patient stable and alert? Vital signs also include rhythm, temperature (rectal temperature may be necessary), oxygen saturation, and bedside glucose. When appropriate, consider visual and hearing acuity. Continuously monitor heart rate/rhythm, pulse ox, and BP.
   F. **Changes in functional status?** Which specific changes prompted this ED visit? Can patient no longer eat, cook, dress, bathe, go to the bathroom, or get out of bed? Is current living situation safe, including locking doors and turning off stove? Can patient pay bills, take medications, or take care of other needs?
   G. **Onset of changes in functional status?** Did changes occur rapidly or develop over several days/weeks? Any precipitating events (death of a spouse, family member, or friend, new medications, dose changes in current medications, new living situation, etc)? Any recent falls (head trauma or other internal injuries)?
   H. **Associated symptoms?** Chest pain; headache; difficulty breathing, speaking, or concentrating; insomnia; restlessness; nausea; vomiting; or change in urination, defecation, balance, coordination, or vision?
   I. **Sources of history?** Family members (living with patient or separately), caregivers, nursing home staff, friends, neighbors, paramedics?
   J. **Medical history?** Previous similar episodes? Heart or lung disease, diabetes, malignancies, seizures, medications (new medications, especially psychiatric, new doses, OTC, herbal supplements), urinary

tract problems, other infections? Review hospital records (inpatient/outpatient), nursing home notes, and prior lab/radiologic results.
- **K. Social history?** Does patient live alone? Do family members live close? Friends? When was patient's last known visitor? When (and what) was patient's last meal? Tobacco, alcohol, or drug use, previous (or present) occupation? How does patient spend the day? Does patient exercise (ambulation, cooking, cleaning, bathing are forms of exertion known as ADL).

III. Differential Diagnosis
A. Cardiovascular.
1. **Cardiac output-related.**
   - a. **Acute MI.**
   - b. **CHF.**
   - c. **Aortic stenosis and other valvulopathies.**
   - d. **Cardiac tamponade.**
   - e. **Atrial myxoma.**
2. **Rhythm disturbance.**
   - a. **Tachycardias.** SVT, VT, AF with fast ventricular response, atrial flutter, sinus rhythm, MAT, adverse drug response (especially β-agonists or NTG), pacemaker-mediated.
   - b. **Bradycardias.** Third-degree heart block, sick sinus syndrome, AF with slow ventricular response, digoxin toxicity, pacemaker malfunction.
   - c. **Irregular.** AF, PVC, bigeminy/trigeminy.
B. Pulmonary (with resultant hypoxia).
1. **Pneumonia/bronchitis.**
2. **COPD/asthma.**
3. **Pulmonary edema.**
4. **PE.**
5. **Pneumothorax.**
6. **Malignancy.** Primary or metastatic.
7. **Pleural effusion, empyema.**
8. **Primary lung problem.** Fibrosis, sarcoidosis, asbestosis.
9. **Infections.**
   - a. **Urinary tract.** Particularly common in elderly.
   - b. **Genitalia.** Consider Fournier's gangrene in elderly males (especially if Foley catheter is present), gynecologic infections (cervicitis, salpingitis), or malignancies.
   - c. **Lung.** Pneumonia, bronchitis, empyema.
   - d. **CNS.** Meningitis, encephalitis, brain abscess.
   - e. **HEENT.** Sinusitis, pharyngitis, otitis media/external (include malignant otitis externa).
   - f. **Abdominal.** Cholecystitis, cholangitis, appendicitis, gastroenteritis.
   - g. **Abscess/cellulitis.** Rectal area, skin, wounds.

C. **CNS.**
   1. **Stroke/TIA.**
   2. **Seizure, including postictal period.**
   3. **Subarachnoid, subdural, epidural, intracerebral hemorrhages.**
   4. **Dementia.**
D. **Metabolic.**
   1. **Sodium.** Hypernatremia, hyponatremia.
   2. **Glucose.** Hypoglycemia, hyperglycemia, DKA, hyperosmolar coma.
   3. **Adrenal insufficiency/crisis.**
   4. **Thyroid.** Hypothyroid, hyperthyroidism.
   5. **Calcium.** Hypercalcemia, hypocalcemia.
   6. **Magnesium.**
   7. **Acidemia.** Calculate anion gap, low bicarbonate?
   8. **Renal insufficiency/failure.**
   9. **Dehydration.**
   10. **Encephalopathy.**
E. **Medication-Related.**
   1. **Newly prescribed medications.** Especially β-blockers and β-blocker eye drops.
   2. **Changes in dosages of previous medications.**
   3. **Drug-drug interactions.**
   4. **Drug toxicity.** Including digoxin, lithium, anticonvulsants.
   5. **OTC meds.** Especially diphenhydramine or antihistamines.
   6. **Herbal supplements** (including vitamins).
F. **Psychiatric.**
   1. **Primary psychiatric diagnoses.** Occur in the elderly, but metabolic and organic causes must be considered first.
   2. **Suicidal gestures or attempts.** Including intentional drug ingestions.
   3. **Loneliness/depression.** Poor health habits, and potential functional decline.
G. **Vascular.**
   1. **Aortic dissection/aneurysm.**
   2. **Mesenteric ischemia.**
   3. **Blood loss.** GI bleed, trauma.
H. **Hematologic.**
   1. **Anemia.** Decreased production, increased consumption.
   2. **Malignancies** of the blood.
   3. **Problems of hemostasis,** including overanticoagulation.
I. **Malignancy-Related Complications.**
   1. **Hypercalcemia.**
   2. **Tumor** lysis syndrome.
   3. **Pain,** including its effect on vagal tone.
   4. **Malignant effusions.** Pericardium, lung.
   5. **Superior vena cava syndrome.**
   6. **Overmedication with narcotics.** Consider naloxone trial.

J. **Environmental.**
1. **Heat-related illness.** Exposure, drug reactions (malignant hyperthermia, neuroleptic malignant syndrome).
2. **Cold-related illness.** Exposure, sepsis (many elderly with overwhelming infections are hypothermic and do not mount a febrile response).
3. **Carbon monoxide.** From space heaters.
4. **Visual deficits.** May result in falls or inadvertent but incorrect medication doses—especially insulin.

K. **Nutritional.**
1. **Caloric deficiencies.**
2. **Vitamin deficiencies.** Especially if alcohol-dependent.

L. **Miscellaneous.**
1. **Elder abuse/neglect.** (See this section, 4. Elder Abuse, page 304)—physical, psychologic, financial.

IV. **Database**
A. **Physical Exam Key Points.**
1. **General appearance.** Does the patient appear ill, well-groomed, thin, obese, in apparent distress? What is the patient's position on the gurney?
2. **Mental status.** Briefly assess while speaking with the patient; Does he answer questions coherently? Assess memory (recent and remote) and perform a Mini Mental Status Exam (See this section, 1. General Geriatric Assessment, page 296, 3. Altered Mental Status in the Older Patient, page 301, and Table A-4, Mini Mental Status Exam, page 656).
3. **Vital signs.** Check carefully and repeat frequently. Include **rectal** temperature and oxygen saturation.
4. **Airway.** Patent and protected? Controlling secretions?
5. **Breathing.** Labored? Fast? Effective?
6. **Circulation.** Skin warm and dry? Peripheral pulses present, strong, regular, and symmetric?
7. **Head.** Evidence of trauma?
8. **Eyes.** Symmetric pupil response to light, conjugate gaze, clear corneas (cloudy corneas might suggest glaucoma), extraocular movements (include nystagmus)?
9. **Mouth.** Check hydration status, evidence of infection, or central cyanosis.
10. **Neck.** Check carotids for bruits, jugular veins for distention, and the neck for tenderness.
11. **Heart.** Is rate fast or slow, regular or irregular? Are extra sounds present, including murmurs, gallops, or rubs?
12. **Chest.** Auscultate for air exchange, breath sound symmetry, decreased or absent breath sounds, including consolidation, egophony, wheezes, prolonged expiration, crepitus of the chest.

13. **Abdomen.** Elderly do not always complain of abdominal pain, especially if steroid-dependent. Check for pulsatile abdominal mass (AAA). Look for surgical scars, listen to bowel sounds and for bruits.

14. **Back.** Check for flank tenderness, ecchymosis, or lesions.

15. **Genitourinary.** Look for evidence of infection, bleeding, or masses.

16. **Rectal.** Check for masses, erythema, tenderness, blood.

17. **Extremities.** Look for trauma, infection, ulcers or nonhealing wounds, clubbing/cyanosis/edema.

18. **Neurologic exam.** Includes memory/attention, cranial nerves, motor and sensory, reflexes, and cerebellar evaluation. If possible, ambulation tests strength, balance, coordination, sensation, and provides an idea of the patient's ability to care for herself. (See this section, 3. Altered Mental Status in the Older Patient, page 301, and Table A-4, Mini Mental Status Exam, page 656.)

B. **Laboratory Data.** Significant electrolyte abnormalities are more likely in older than in younger patients, particularly in the presence of diabetes or diuretics. Anemia, malignancy, and infection of the urinary tract occur with greater frequency. Therefore, liberal use of laboratory tests in the elderly with functional decline is warranted, including drug levels. UA (consider catheter specimen), CBC with Diff, and Lytes are warranted. Consider cardiac enzymes because AMI can present with confusion or change in functional status. Blood, urine, sputum cultures when indicated.

C. **ECG.** Any elderly patient with functional decline.

D. **Radiographic and Other Studies.** Liberal use of CXR (often portable) is warranted, particularly if exam suggests a pulmonary cause. Neuroimaging should be considered, particularly if decline occurred without an otherwise identifiable source.

V. **Plan**

A. **Overall Plan.** Elderly patients with functional decline should be considered for admission, especially those with rapid decline. Individuals living alone may need temporary hospitalization until assisted living can be arranged. Treatable medical conditions resulting in decline likely require hospitalization. Agreement among family members to an outpatient approach and close follow-up is crucial for occasions when this is attempted.

B. **Specific Management Plans.**

1. **Social services consultation.** Always a good idea for elderly patients with a change in functional status. Assistance with meal delivery, preparation, eating (low sodium, soft, high nutritional value), and fluids may be initiated. Social services (and police notification) are needed when elder abuse/neglect is considered.

2. **Infections.** Treat with antibiotics directed at the most likely offending organism(s). Consider local sensitivities and antibiotic resistances. Cultures of blood and urine are helpful, particularly in nosocomial infections.

3. **Cardiovascular.** Treat MI, ACS, dysrhythmias, etc accordingly. Admission is recommended until problem(s) clarified or resolved. Consider enteric-coated aspirin if no contraindication exists.

4. **Pulmonary.** Treat infections, hypoxia, PE, effusions, etc with appropriate medications. Admission is likely if these conditions are the cause of functional decline.

5. **CVA/TIA/seizure.** Neuroimaging likely needed either emergently or urgently. Arrangements should be made if these studies are not done on initial presentation. If no contraindication for enteric-coated aspirin exists, consider its administration.

6. **Metabolic.** Treat accordingly. If hematologic, endocrine, or malignant cause is involved, consult with an appropriate specialist.

7. **Drugs.** Interactions between drugs causing decline warrant removal of one or all offending agents. An appropriate replacement should be initiated. Give instructions to avoid OTC or herbal supplements involved in decline. Toxic levels of drugs, especially due to intentional ingestions, should be treated accordingly, with psychiatric consultation when appropriate.

VI. **ICD-9 Diagnoses:** Adult abuse or adult neglect; Adverse effect of medication (specify med); Alzheimer's dementia; Congestive heart failure—decompensated; Debility—old age or Decline—general, Dementia—senile; Late effect of cerebrovascular disease.

VII. **Problem Case Diagnosis:** UTI resulting in functional decline.

VIII. **Teaching Pearls Question:** Approximately what percentage of elderly patients with bacteremia, pneumonia, UTI, or intraabdominal infection present without a fever?

IX. **Teaching Pearls Answer:** Up to 30% (Ouslander).

REFERENCES

Hebert R. Functional decline in old age. *CMAJ* 1997;157(8):1037–1045.

Ouslander JG. Medical care in the nursing home. *JAMA* 1989;262(18):2582–2590.

Penninx BWJH, Guralnik JM, Ferrucci L, Simonsick EM, Deeg DJH, Wallace RB. Depressive symptoms and physical decline in community-dwelling older persons. *JAMA* 1998;279(21):1720–1726.

Stuck AE, Walthert JM, Nikolaus T, Bula CJ, Hohmann C, Beck JC. Risk factors for functional status decline in community-living elderly people: A systematic literature review. *Soc Sci Med* 1999;48:445–469.

Vita AJ, Terry RB, Hubert HB, Fries JF. Aging, health risks, and cumulative disability. *N Engl J Med* 1998;338:1035–1041.

V. Common Toxicologic Emergency On-Call Problems

1. ACETAMINOPHEN

I. Problem: A young female is brought to the ED with "depression" and having ingested "a lot of pills."

II. Immediate Questions

A. What are the ABCs, vital signs, and mental status? Always assume that such patients intend to do themselves significant harm. Altered mental status should prompt immediate assessment of oxygenation and blood glucose level. All overdose patients require IV access and placement on a monitor, with emergent interventions as indicated clinically.

B. How much acetaminophen was ingested? The usual normal dose is 15 mg/kg. The maximum daily dose is 4 g/day in adults and 90 mg/kg/day in children. The toxic dose after a single acute ingestion is 150 mg/kg, or approximately 7 g in adults. Some people are more susceptible to toxicity: alcoholics, the malnourished, those with AIDS, and anorexics. Children younger than 5 may fare better than adults, but no controlled studies have been done to support this; therefore treatment should not be altered.

C. When was the ingestion? This will be of importance in predicting toxicity and determining the need for *N*-acetylcysteine (NAC) treatment. It is also important to note whether this episode was a single vs multiple ingestions over time, and regular vs an extended-release preparation.

D. Any coingestants, and what medications are possibly available to the patient? Those accompanying the patient (family, paramedics) should be queried as to all medications available to the patient and use of alcohol or illicit drugs. Count remaining pills and subtract from the prescribed amount to estimate ingestion quantity.

III. Differential Diagnosis

A. Polypharmacy overdose.

B. Hepatitis (later stages).

C. Hepatic failure (later stages).

IV. Database

A. Physical Exam Key Points

1. There are no specific findings with acetaminophen overdose. Patients often have minimal GI signs or symptoms of toxicity (nausea, vomiting, anorexia, malaise) with the initial presentation. If presenting in the later stages (≥ 2 days postingestion) symptoms

may be as straightforward as RUQ pain or as complex as fulminant hepatic and multisystem organ failure.

2. Evaluate for evidence of coingestion:
   a. **Vital signs.** Monitor, pulse ox, frequent reassessment.
   b. **Mental status.** Frequent reassessment.
   c. **Dermatologic.** Diaphoresis, anhydrosis, pallor or flushing, bruising, evidence of injection.
   d. **HEENT.** Hypersalivation, excessive dryness.
   e. **Lungs.** Bronchorrhea, wheezing.
   f. **Heart.** Rate, rhythm, regularity.
   g. **Abdomen.** Bowel sounds, urinary retention, tenderness or rigidity.
   h. **Neurologic.** Pupils (size, symmetry, reactivity, nystagmus, dysconjugate gaze), gag reflex, resting motor tone, reflexes, coordination.

B. **Laboratory Data.** The diagnosis of acetaminophen toxicity depends on obtaining a serum acetaminophen level. A level drawn 4–24 h postingestion compared with the "probable toxicity" line on the Rumack–Matthew nomogram is the best predictor of hepatic toxicity, but it should not be relied on with multiple acetaminophen ingestions, chronic ingestions, extended-release formulations, or with overdosages involving anticholinergics or opioids. Baseline measure of hepatic function (glucose, PT, bilirubin) should be obtained. Serum AST and ALT rise within 24 h of ingestion and peak at 48–72 h. Severe toxicity can be defined as AST or ALT greater than 1000 IU/L. Electrolytes and creatinine may reveal anion gap acidosis or renal failure. Consider other studies if H&P or clinical status indicates (aspirin, alcohol, urine drug screen, serum osmolality, HCG, ABG).

C. **Radiographic and Other Studies.** None required for isolated acetaminophen overdose. Studies are directed by the patient's clinical status.

V. Plan

A. **Overall Plan.** A three-stage approach: (1) gut decontamination, (2) N-acetylcysteine (NAC) administration, and (3) supportive care. Patient disposition is dependent on several factors (see B.4.).

B. **Specific Plans.**
   1. **Gut decontamination.** Ipecac-induced emesis is to be avoided due to lack of efficacy and the subsequent delay in administration of activated charcoal and NAC. WBI and gastric lavage is unnecessary due to the rapid absorption of acetaminophen. Activated charcoal 1 g/kg remains the primary method of gut decontamination. There is no evidence that consecutive administration of charcoal and NAC decreases the effectiveness of NAC. There is no need for superloading doses of NAC.
   2. **NAC.** Administer if there is potential toxicity, as suggested by the Rumack–Matthew nomogram, the patient is close to 8 h postinges-

tion, or if the acetaminophen level will not be available within 8 h postingestion. If administered within 8 h, NAC is nearly 100% effective in preventing hepatic toxicity. The standard regimen in the United States for administration NAC is a 72-h protocol that consists of a 140 mg/kg oral loading dose followed by maintenance dosing of 70 mg/kg q4h for 17 doses. The exact mechanism of action is unknown but may involve binding of a toxic metabolite (*N*-acetyl-*p*-benzoquinoneimine, or NAPQI), may directly reduce NAPQI back to acetaminophen, may serve as a glutathione precursor, or be a sulfate precursor. NAC may act as an antioxidant and diminish the classic hepatic toxicity (centrilobular necrosis) even when administered in late acetaminophen toxicity. Administration may be complicated by nausea and vomiting due to the odor and taste of rotten eggs. To improve patient acceptance NAC may be mixed in fruit juice or soft drinks or may be administered by NG tube. Concomitant antiemetic administration may be necessary. IV administration of NAC, common in other countries, is not generally available in the United States. The oral formulation is sterile and can be used intravenously but must be administered through a filter due to particulate matter in the formulation. Anaphylactic reactions to the IV formulation have occurred.

3. **Supportive care.** Initially one should proceed as with all overdoses, assuming a significant coingestant: monitor, IV access, ECG, screening laboratory studies, and other interventions as clinically indicated.

4. **Disposition.** Patients requiring NAC should be hospitalized until completion of therapy. An unmonitored bed is sufficient unless clinical conditions dictate otherwise. Those not at risk for hepatic toxicity should be observed for 4-6 h to exclude potentially toxic coingestants. Consider psychiatric evaluation for all patients with intentional overdose.

VI. ICD-9 Diagnoses: Acetaminophen overdose; State all adverse/toxic effects caused by the drug separately; State intent of poisoning if known (accident, therapeutic use, suicide attempt, assault, undetermined).

VII. Problem Case Diagnosis: Acetaminophen ingestion as suicide gesture.

VIII. Teaching Pearls Question: What is the dose of *N*-acetylcysteine in a patient who has received activated charcoal for acetaminophen ingestion?

IX. Teaching Pearls Answer: There is no evidence that consecutive administration of charcoal and NAC decreases the effectiveness of NAC in vivo. There is no need for superloading doses of NAC.

REFERENCES

Bizovi KE, Aks SE, Paloucek F, Gross R, Keys N, Rivas J. Late increase in acetaminophen concentration after overdose of Tylenol Extended Relief. *Ann Emerg Med* 1996;28(5): 549–551.

Smilkstein MJ. A new loading dose for *N*-acetylcysteine? The answer is no. *Ann Emerg Med* 1994;24(3):538–539.

Smilkstein MJ. Acetaminophen. In Goldfrank LR, Flomenbaum NE, et al (eds). *Goldfrank's Toxicologic Emergencies,* 6th ed. Appleton & Lange 1998:541–564.

Vassallo S, Khan AN, Howland MA. Use of the Rumack-Matthew nomogram in cases of extended-release acetaminophen toxicity. *Ann Intern Med* 1996;125(11):940.

2. ALCOHOLS

I. **Problem:** A young man is brought to the ED after ingesting "alcohol."

II. **Immediate Questions**

A. **What are the ABCs, vital signs, and mental status?** Always assume that overdose patients intend to harm themselves. Altered mental status should prompt immediate assessment of oxygenation, blood glucose level, and consideration to the use of naloxone [Narcan]. In general, all overdose patients require IV access and placement on a monitor, with emergent interventions as indicated clinically.

B. **When was the alcohol ingested?** This will be of importance in predicting toxicity and determining the need for admission versus discharge and further treatment plan.

1. **Methanol** peak plasma levels are reached within 30–60 min following ingestion, although a long latent period (roughly 18–24 h) usually is seen before toxic symptoms develop. Methanol is distributed in the body water, like ethanol, to an extent of about 50–60% of the body weight. Toxic exposure may occur by ingestion, inhalation, or dermal routes.

2. **Isopropyl.** Symptoms typically occur within 30–60 min, with a half-life of the parent compound of 3–16 h.

3. **Acetone,** a major metabolite with similar properties, has a half-life of 7–26 h.

4. **Ethanol** peaks in 30–120 min, with variable kinetics, as do all alcohols.

5. **Ethylene glycol** peaks in 1–4 h, with a half-life of 2.5–4.5 h.

C. **What are the patient's symptoms?**

1. **Methanol** is highly toxic, potentially producing metabolic acidosis, blindness, and death. Toxicity is directly related to the degree of acidosis and thus the time between exposure and specific treatment. Prognosis is poor in patients with coma or seizure and severe metabolic acidosis (pH < 7). Acute poisoning causes initial confusion and ataxia, followed by a 6- to 12-h period with nonspecific malaise, headache, vomiting, abdominal pain, and visual changes. A wide anion gap metabolic acidosis suggests the possibility of methanol overdose. If untreated, methanol poisoning progresses to coma, worsening metabolic acidosis, and finally cardiopulmonary collapse. The most common permanent sequelae following severe poisoning are optic neuropathy, blind-

ness, parkinsonism-like syndromes, toxic encephalopathy, and polyneuropathy.

2. **Isopropyl** ingestion results in CNS depression, ataxia, and upper GI symptoms with occasional hematemesis. Isopropyl poisoning typically results in an elevated osmolar gap without acidosis.

3. **Elevated acetone** may produce false elevations of creatine.

4. **Acute ethanol** poisoning results in CNS depression and rarely hypoglycemia.

5. **Ethylene glycol** ingestion may result in CNS depression, hypocalcemia, and renal failure. An elevated osmolar gap and elevated anion gap acidosis is typically present.

D. **Any coingestants, and what medications are possibly available to the patient?** Those accompanying the patient (family, paramedics) should be queried as to all medications available to the patient and use of alcohol or illicit drugs. Count remaining pills and subtract from the prescribed amount to estimate ingestion quantity. Potential occupational exposures should be sought.

III. **Differential Diagnosis**
   A. **Other Toxic Alcohol Ingestions.** Glycol ethers, all alcohols just described are differentials of one another, etc.
   B. **Septic Syndromes**
   C. **Causes of Lactic Acidosis.** Other poisonings: iron, salicylates, etc.

IV. **Database**
   A. **Physical Exam Key Points**
      1. **GI** symptoms include nausea, vomiting, and abdominal pain. Hematemesis or GI bleeding may suggest chronic ethanol abuse or isopropyl ingestion.
      2. **CNS** symptoms include headache, lethargy, confusion, inebriation, coma, and (rarely) seizures.
      3. **Ophthalmologic** symptoms include alterations of vision, photophobia, "snow blindness," mydriasis, and frank blindness. Papilledema, hyperemia, or pallor may be noted.
      4. **Wood's lamp inspection** for presence of fluorescence may be helpful if ethylene glycol is present.
      5. Evaluate for evidence of coingestion:
         a. **Vital signs.** Monitor, pulse ox, frequent reassessment.
         b. **Mental status.** Frequent reassessment.
         c. **Breath.** Acetone may be present in all but may suggest isopropyl.
         d. **Dermatologic.** Diaphoresis, anhydrosis, pallor or flushing, bruising, evidence of injection.
         e. **HEENT.** Hypersalivation, excessive dryness.
         f. **Lungs.** Bronchorrhea, wheezing.
         g. **Heart.** Rate, rhythm, regularity.
         h. **Abdomen.** Bowel sounds, urinary retention, tenderness or rigidity.

      i. Neurologic. Pupils (size, symmetry, reactivity, nystagmus, dysconjugate gaze), gag, resting motor tone, reflexes, co-ordination.
- **B. Laboratory Data.** Stat serum alcohol panel. Evaluate for the presence of metabolic acidosis. Calculate an osmolar gap with the realization of its severe limitations, such as it is only sensitive early in poisoning and that a normal "gap" does not eliminate the diagnosis. A toxic methanol level would confirm the diagnosis and remains the gold standard. If an osmolar gap is obtained it should be measured by freezing point depression. Electrolytes and creatinine may reveal anion gap acidosis or renal failure. An ABG will more quickly document acid–base status. Elevated acetone may falsely elevate CK. Consider a CK to rule out concomitant rhabdomyolysis. Consider other studies if H&P or clinical status indicate (aspirin, ethanol, urine drug screen, serum osmolality, HCG). An ethanol level is helpful for calculating a corrected osmolar gap, etc.
- **C. Radiographic and Other Studies.** None required for isolated alcohol overdoses. Studies are directed by the patient's clinical status.

V. Plan
- **A. Overall Plan.** Gut decontamination for coingestions (None of the alcohols are significantly absorbed by charcoal); antidote administration (ethanol or 4-methylpyrazole); vitamin supplementation (pyridoxine [B_6], folinic acid, and thiamine); supportive care; and occasional hemodialysis. Patient disposition is dependent on several factors (see d. Disposition).
- **B. Specific Plans**
  1. **Gut decontamination.** Ipecac-induced emesis is to be avoided due to lack of efficacy, and WBI and gastric lavage is unnecessary.
  2. **Activated charcoal.** Activated charcoal at 1 g/kg remains the primary method of gut decontamination. In isolated methanol ingestion it offers no benefit.
  3. **Ethanol administration.** For methanol and ethylene glycol toxicity, administer ethanol if there is potential toxicity, as suggested by the H&P examination prior to laboratory confirmation of toxic methanol levels. Intentional methanol ingestion, altered mental status or visual changes or accidental exposures of greater than a sip warrant institution of ethanol or 4-methylpyrazole. Ethanol has a greater affinity than methanol for alcohol dehydrogenase. Ethanol slows metabolism to formaldehyde and formic acid by competitive inhibition.
     - **a.** The standard regimen is 10% ethanol in D_5W with a loading dose of 10 mL/kg over 30–60 min then maintenance of 1–1.2 mL/kg/h in a nonalcoholic or 1.5–2 mL/kg/h in an alcoholic. During dialysis the maintenance dose should be doubled.
     - **b.** Ethanol metabolism is extremely variable among individuals and requires at least hourly monitoring until steady-state levels are obtained.

    c. Administration may be complicated by nausea, vomiting, CNS changes, and hypoglycemia. Concomitant antiemetic administration may be necessary. Hourly glucose monitoring is recommended.

    d. A goal of a therapeutic range of at 100–150 mg/dL is recommended with continuation of the ethanol infusion until methanol levels are zero.

4. **Methylpyrazole** (4-MP, fomepizole [Antizol]) 15 mg/kg slow infusion over 30 min followed by a maintenance infusion of 10 mg/kg q12h for 4 doses, results in competitive inhibition of alcohol dehydrogenase. It's advantages over ethanol infusion is that there is no need for continuous infusion and no significant CNS changes. The major disadvantage is the increased cost. Doses may have to be increased during dialysis.

    a. **Vitamin supplementation** with folinic acid 1–2 mg/kg IV followed by folic acid 50 mg IV q4h for 1–2 days is recommended for folinic acid is the activated form of folic acid and it is the co-factor required for the conversion of formic acid to carbon dioxide and water for methanol toxicity. Pyridoxine and thiamine are indicated for ethylene glycol toxicity. It is reasonable to administer thiamine to all nonallergic patients with altered mentation.

    b. **Supportive care.** Initially, proceed as with all overdoses, assuming a significant coingestant: monitor, IV access, ECG, screening laboratory studies, and other interventions as clinically indicated. Fluid bolus for dehydration, etc. Sodium bicarbonate for severe metabolic acidosis, in general pH < 7.1. Thiamine 100 mg IV.

    c. **Hemodialysis** has never been proven to change long-term outcomes in human trials, and it is unlikely that any such trials will ever occur. Hemodialysis removes methanol and corrects acidosis as well as decreasing the plasma half-life to approximately 2.3 h. Recommendations regarding the use of hemodialysis are based on case series, etc. In general hemodialysis is recommended for severe acidosis unresponsive to bicarbonate, renal insufficiency, CNS or ophthalmic changes (for methanol toxicity), methanol level > 25 mg/dL or ethylene glycol level > 50 mg/dL. In the setting of ethylene glycol poisoning. Although hemodialysis would be efficacious in the setting of isopropyl and ethanol, good supportive care is all that is typically needed.

    d. **Disposition.** Patients with significant ingestions or who are ill should be admitted. Discharge/medical clearance can be considered if a serum methanol is less than 20 mg/dL, ethylene glycol level < 30 mg/dL, no coingestion with ethanol (ethanol level = zero), no GI bleeding, and no metabolic acidosis or symptoms are present.

VI. **ICD-9 Diagnoses:** Acute alcohol intoxication/drunkenness are different codes from alcohol poisoning or overdose. Alcohol poisoning is used when there is nondependent use or in cases such as suicide attempt; Alcohol abuse; Alcohol dependence; State all adverse/toxic effects caused by the drug separately; State intent of poisoning if known (accident, therapeutic use, suicide attempt, assault, undetermined).

VII. **Problem Case Diagnosis:** Methanol toxicity.

VIII. **Teaching Pearls Question:** Why is folinic acid used instead of folate as an initial dose only in the setting of methanol poisoning?

IX. **Teaching Pearls Answer:** Folic acid is not readily available for a few hours. Folinic acid is almost immediately available and assists in metabolism to no toxic metabolites.

REFERENCES

Brent J, McMartin K, Phillips S, Aaron C, Kulig K. Fomepizole for the treatment of methanol poisoning. *N Engl J Med* 2001;344(6):424–429.

Liu JJ, Daya MR, Carrasquillo O, Kales SN. Prognostic factors in patients with methanol poisoning. *J Toxicol Clin Toxicol* 1998;36(3):175–181.

Swartz RD, Millman RP, Billi JE, Bondar NP, Migdal SD, Simonian SK, et al. Epidemic methanol poisoning: Clinical and biochemical analysis of a recent episode. *Medicine* (Baltimore) 1981;60(5):373–382.

3. AMPHETAMINE OVERDOSE

I. **Problem:** A 38-year-old male is brought to the ED by police officers. The patient was found running around on a busy street. Since his arrest, he has become wildly agitated and requires physical restraints. He is screaming obscenities and attempting to spit on hospital staff. Upon ED arrival the patient's vital signs were BP: 195/100, pulse: 148, RR: 26, temp: 42.0°C. He has widely dilated pupils and multiple needle marks on his arms.

II. **Immediate Questions**

A. **Is the patient's airway intact?**

B. **Are any immediate antidotes indicated?** Bedside glucose testing or empiric dextrose. Empiric naloxone (0.5–2 mg) if opioid toxidrome.

C. **How can control of this agitated patient be achieved to best protect the patient and ED staff members?** Protection of staff with universal precautions and physical restraint of patient. Physical restraint carries inherent risks (hyperthermia, rhabdomyolysis, sudden death). Chemical restraint should be initiated as quickly possible. Parenteral benzodiazepines are the agents of choice. In severe cases, rapid sequence intubation (see Section VIII, Number 15, page 470) may be necessary. Airway and vital signs must be continually reassessed after sedative dosing.

D. Have all abnormal vital signs been addressed? Place patient on monitors and start IV. Apply oxygen for tachypnea or low oxygen saturation. Initially treat cardiovascular instability (hypotension, tachycardia) with IV fluids. Address hyperthermia after agitation is controlled with benzodiazepines.

E. Could amphetamine intoxication be a "red herring"? Other causes of agitation may require emergent intervention and may be difficult to distinguish from sympathomimetic intoxication. Early assessment for trauma and infection should be undertaken.

III. Differential Diagnosis

A. This patient presents with altered mental status (AMS) and a sympathomimetic toxidrome. Diagnosis can be approached by considering AMS and sympathomimetic toxicity separately.

B. AMS/Agitation. Assessment of the altered patient with potential amphetamine toxicity should begin with consideration of other causes of AMS. "AEIOU TIPS" may be a helpful tool for assessment of the patient with AMS:

A—Alcohol
E—Electrolytes
I—Infection
O—Oxygen
U—Uremia
T—Trauma
I—Intoxication
P—Psychiatric
S—Seizures

C. Sympathomimetic toxidrome. Tachycardia, HTN, mydriasis, and diaphoresis indicate possible sympathomimetic intoxication. Violent agitation is common in overdose situations. Examples of agents capable of this syndrome are:

1. Amphetamine
2. Dextroamphetamine
3. Methamphetamine
4. Amphetamine derivatives (MDA, ecstasy)
5. Cocaine
6. Phencyclidine (PCP)

IV. Database

A. Physical Exam Key Points

1. **Mental status.** Amphetamine-intoxicated patients frequently present with **AMS, agitation, psychosis,** and paranoid behavior. Agitation and psychosis may result in high-risk or dangerous behavior.

2. **Vital signs.** Monitor continuously for **hypertensive crisis, cardiovascular instability,** and **hyperthermia.** (Primary causes of morbidity and mortality).

3. **Head/face.** Examine for **traumatic injuries.** Intracranial injury may infrequently resemble amphetamine intoxication.
4. **Neck.** Signs of injury above the scapulae, necessitates evaluation for **C-spine trauma.** Nuchal rigidity may suggest meningitis.
5. **Chest.** Assess breath sounds bilaterally. **Noncardiogenic pulmonary edema** is an infrequent complication of amphetamine toxicity.
6. **Heart.** Auscultate for heart murmurs. Murmurs may suggest **aortic dissection** caused by amphetamine use or **endocarditis** complicating IV drug use.
7. **Abdomen.** Tenderness may indicate **ischemic colitis** or **traumatic injury.**
8. **Skin.** Examine for **abscesses** and **necrotizing fasciitis** in all injection drug abusers.
9. **Neurologic exam.** Focal deficits are unlikely in isolated amphetamine intoxication and should arouse suspicion for **intracranial injury, CVA,** or another cause of AMS.

B. **Laboratory Data.**
1. **Bedside glucose.** Check early.
2. **Electrolytes.** Sodium, Cr, glucose, Ca, and Mg concentrations may aid in determination of the cause of AMS or seizures. Severe **hyponatremia, hypernatremia,** or **hyperkalemia** may be precipitated by amphetamine use.
3. **Total CK.** Test in severe amphetamine intoxication or hyperthermia to identify **rhabdomyolysis.**
4. **Cardiac enzymes.** Serial measurements to identify **MI** in patients with chest pain.
5. **Toxicology screens.** Standard screens detect phenylalkylamine compounds, including most amphetamines, for up to 72 h. Screens cannot confirm or exclude acute intoxication. The usefulness of urine toxicology screening is a source of debate among toxicologists because false-positives and false-negatives frequently occur.
6. **Urine pregnancy test.** All reproductive age females.

C. **Radiographic and Other Studies.**
1. **Head CT.** Obtain in patients with AMS, focal neurologic findings, or severe headache to identify **intracranial hemorrhage, ischemic stroke,** or **traumatic injuries.**
2. **LP.** Recommended for patients with AMS to rule out meningitis. LP may be omitted with rapidly improving mental status. If hemorrhage is a concern, CSF is required to definitively exclude subarachnoid blood even when CT is normal.
3. **CXR.** Obtain for severe intoxication, chest pain, or SOB. Look for signs of **aortic dissection,** pneumothorax, and noncardiogenic pulmonary edema.
4. **ECG.** Obtained for severe intoxication, chest pain, or cardiovascular instability. Examine the ECG for **myocardial ischemia/MI** or **dysrhythmias.**

V. Plan

A. Overall Plan. Support and decontaminate.

1. **Supportive care** is the most important aspect of treatment. The vast majority of patients will survive with good outcome if properly supported. Half of patients presenting to the ED with amphetamine intoxication require no treatment beyond confirmation of diagnosis and observation.

2. **Activated charcoal** if oral amphetamine ingestion presenting within 1–2 h of ingestion. GI absorption of amphetamines is rapid, decontamination therefore is unlikely to benefit patients presenting late. Gastric lavage is not indicated. WBI with PEG solution is indicated when unopened packets containing amphetamine have been swallowed.

B. Specific Plans

1. **CNS**

   a. **Agitation/psychosis.** Early conversion from physical to chemical restraint is important. Parenteral benzodiazepines (diazepam, lorazepam) are the agents of choice.

   b. Seclude victims from external stimuli.

   c. Use of butyrophenone antipsychotics (haloperidol, droperidol) is controversial. Some reports cite effective use of these agents, but others express concern regarding lowering of seizure threshold, extrapyramidal effects, and QT prolongation.

   d. **Seizures.** Seizures are usually responsive to benzodiazepines.

   e. **CVA.** Ischemic or hemorrhagic CVA warrants immediate BP control and management of elevated intracranial pressure. (See Section I, 45. Hypertension, page 136, 65. Stroke/TIA, page 195.)

2. **Cardiovascular**

   a. **Myocardial ischemia/MI.** Patients with chest pain following amphetamine use should receive ECG, cardiac enzyme evaluation, and continuous cardiac monitoring. Administer benzodiazepines as first-line medication to control catecholamine release and tachycardia. Suspected cardiac ischemia/MI is treated with standard therapy: Oxygen, aspirin, nitroglycerin, and morphine.

   b. Pure β-receptor antagonists are contraindicated without concomitant vasodilators because they may precipitate unopposed α stimulation, thereby worsening coronary vasospasm.

   c. Chest pain accompanied by significant ST segment elevation suggesting ischemia warrants primary angioplasty or thrombolytic therapy. Angioplasty is the preferred treatment if available.

   d. **Hypertensive emergency.** Patients with severely elevated blood pressure (> 250/120 mm Hg) and evidence of end-organ damage (neurologic deficit, chest pain, elevated Cr) require

BP control within the first hour after presentation. Benzo-diazepines given initially will often improve BP. Nitroprusside should be instituted if BP remains elevated.

e. Hypotension. Treat hypotension initially with IV fluid. Direct-acting α-receptor agonist (norepinephrine, phenylephrine) preferred for refractory hypotension.

f. Aortic dissection. Aortic dissection requires aggressive BP management.

3. **Systemic.**

   a. Hyperthermia. Check and monitor rectal temperature in sus-pected amphetamine toxicity. Most hyperthermic patients will improve with control of agitation and muscular hyperactivity using benzodiazepines. If chemical sedation does not rapidly improve temperature, active cooling measures should be instituted.

   b. Rhabdomyolysis. Aggressive IV fluid hydration is the most im-portant aspect of treatment. Urine flow may also be augmented with diuretics such as mannitol. Goal of therapy is urine output of 1–2 mL/kg/h. Continue hydration until CK levels are falling and renal insufficiency has resolved.

4. **Infectious.**

   a. **Skin infections.** Administer tetanus prophylaxis and antibi-otics. Abscesses should be incised and drained. Skin infections suspicious for necrotizing fasciitis or gas gangrene require im-mediate surgical consultation. (See Section I, 63. Skin Infec-tions, page 189.)

   b. Endocarditis. Any IV drug user with a new murmur or fever should receive blood cultures, antibiotic coverage, and admission.

VI. **ICD-9 Diagnoses:** Amphetamine overdose; State all adverse/toxic ef-fects caused by the drug separately; State intent of poisoning if known (accident, therapeutic use, suicide attempt, assault, undetermined).

VII. **Problem Case Diagnosis:** Methamphetamine intoxication.

VIII. **Teaching Pearl Question:** What is the key physical examination finding differentiating sympathomimetic toxidrome from anticholinergic toxi-drome?

IX. **Teaching Pearl Answer:** Diaphoresis.

REFERENCES

Albertson TE, Derlet RW, VanHoozen BE. Methamphetamine and expanding complica-tions of amphetamines. *West J Med* 1999;170:214—219.

Callaway CW, Clark RF. Hyperthermia in psychostimulant overdose. *Ann Emerg Med* 1994;24(1):68—76.

Derlet RW, Heischober B. Methamphetamine, stimulant of the 1990s? *West J Med* 1990; 153:625—628.

Derlet RW, Rice P, Horwitz BZ, Lord RV. Amphetamine toxicity: Experience with 127 cases. *J Emerg Med* 1989;7:157–161.

Furst SR, Fallon SP, Reznik GN, Shah PK. Myocardial infarction after inhalation of methamphetamine. *New Engl J Med* 1990;323(16):1147–1148.

Johnson TD, Berenson MM. Methamphetamine-induced ischemic colitis. *J Clin Gastroenterol* 1991;13(6):687–689.

Perez JA, Arsura EL, Strategos S. Methamphetamine-related stroke: Four cases. *J Emerg Med* 1999;17(3):469–471.

Rothrock JF, Rubenstein R, Lyden PD. Ischemic stroke associated with methamphetamine inhalation. *Neurology* 1988;38:589–592.

Shannon M. Methylenedioxymethamphetamine (MDMA, "ecstasy"). *Pediatr Emerg Care* 2000;16(5):377–380.

Waksman J, Taylor RN Jr, Bodor GS, Daly FF, Jolliff HA, Dart RC. Acute myocardial infarction associated with amphetamine use. *Mayo Clin Proc* 2001;76:323–326.

4. ANTICHOLINERGIC POISONING

I. **Problem:** A 17-year-old male and his two friends are found unconscious, unresponsive in the desert. They have apparently consumed an herbal "tea."

II. **Immediate Questions**
   A. **Is the airway intact?** Manage appropriately (See Section VIII, 15. Rapid Sequence Endotracheal Intubation, page 470.)
   B. **What are the vitals and mental status?** Is the patient stable and alert? Apply monitors (cardiac and pulse ox), start IV hydration and oxygen. What is the core temperature? Initiate cooling measures. (See Section I, 46. Hyperthermia, page 139.)
   C. **Was this an accidental or intentional overdose or toxicity?** Are there coingestants or cotoxicities? Is this chronic or acute toxicity? If acute, how much was ingested, and when?
   D. **Does the anticholinergic toxidrome fit the clinical picture?** "Hot as a hare (hyperthermic)," "dry as a bone (dry skin)," "blind as a bat (mydriasis)," "mad as a hatter (delirium)," tachycardia, urinary retention, decreased bowel sounds (ileus), increased respiratory rate.
   E. **Are there any other medical problems?** HTN, diabetes, seizure disorder, cardiac problems, asthma, or pulmonary problems. Medications and allergies.

III. **Differential Diagnosis**
   A. **Hyperthyroidism, Thyroid Storm and Graves's Disease.** Check thyroid, medications, TSH.
   B. **Hypoglycemia.** Check medications, fingerstick blood sugar.
   C. **Meningitis.** Check for rash, antecedent infection, meningeal signs.
   D. **Cardiac Glycoside Toxicity.** Check medications, plant ingestions.
   E. **Status Epilepticus.** Check medications, watch for persistent seizure activity.

    F. Amphetamine Toxicity. Check for street drug use, sweating, urine toxicology.

    G. Antidysrhythmic Toxicity. Check medications, ECG.

    H. Hallucinogen toxicity. Check for history of hallucinogen use, herbal medication use.

IV. Database

    A. Physical Exam Key Points

      1. **Mental status.** Check if patient is alert and oriented (delirious).

      2. **Vital signs.** Check carefully and repeat during evaluation, including core temperature (hyperthermic).

      3. **HEENT.** Check mucous membranes (dry), pupils (dilated).

      4. **Abdomen.** Check for diminished or absent bowel sounds (ileus), distended bladder (urinary retention).

      5. **Neuro.** Check for persistent seizure activity (status epilepticus).

    B. Laboratory Data. None needed if normal mentation and H&P. If delirious, check CBC, electrolytes, UA. Consider urine toxicology, aspirin and acetaminophen levels, blood alcohol level, and pregnancy test. Consider CK and myoglobin if prolonged down time.

    C. Radiographic and Other Studies. Obtain an ECG. Consider head CT, LP, and CXR based on clinical picture.

V. Plan

    A. Overall Plan. Maintain airway, assist ventilation as needed, Insert Foley catheter if delirious or urinary retention evident, treat ingestion of anticholinergic agent (and other substances), treat agitation or seizures, admit to a monitored bed. Aggressively hydrate and cool. May need central line access to administer rapid crystalloid. Aggressive evaporative cooling (See Section I, 46. Hyperthermia, page 139).

    B. Specific Plans

      1. **Antidotes/altering absorption.** Give activated charcoal to decrease absorption. Consider multiple doses. A specific antidote, physostigmine, is indicated only for severe, life-threatening toxicity. It is specifically contraindicated in TCA overdose. *Adult dose:* 0.5–2.0 mg slow IV push; repeat q20min to reverse symptoms. *Pediatric dose:* 0.5 mg slow IV push.

      2. **Basics.** Maintain the ABCs. Place a Foley catheter if delirious or if urinary retention is evident. Hydrate and cool patient.

      3. **Change catabolism.** Not applicable.

      4. **Distribute differently.** Not applicable.

      5. **Enhance elimination.** Not applicable.

VI. ICD-9 Diagnoses:
Anticholinergic overdose; State all adverse/toxic effects caused by the drug separately; State intent of poisoning if known (accident, therapeutic use, suicide attempt, assault, undetermined).

VII. Problem Case Diagnosis:
Jimson weed (*Datura*) toxicity and dehydration.

VIII. Teaching Pearls Question:
How do you differentiate between sympathomimetic toxicity and anticholinergic toxicity on clinical exam?

IX. Teaching Pearls Answer: The skin is diaphoretic in sympathomimetic toxicity and dry in anticholinergic toxicity.

REFERENCES

Bruns J. Toxicity, Anticholinergic. *eMedicine Journal,* June 5 2001, Volume 2, Number 6.
Goldfrank L, Flomenbaum N, Lewin N, Weisman R, Howland MA, Kaul B. Anticholinergic poisoning. *J Toxicol Clin Toxicol* 1982;19(1):17–25.
Wagner R, Keim S. Plant Poisoning, Alkaloids—Tropane. *eMedicine Journal,* November 29 2001, Volume 2, Number 11.

5. BENZODIAZEPINE OVERDOSE

I. **Problem:** A 30-year-old woman, confused and poorly responsive, is brought by paramedics from her home. Roommates called 911, concerned about her "drunken" behavior. She has a history of anxiety and depression.

II. **Immediate Questions**
   A. **Airway intact?** Evidence of emesis? Intubate promptly if respiratory failure (See Section VIII, 15. Rapid Sequence Endotracheal Intubation, page 470).
   B. **Vital signs?** Respirations adequate? Pulse/BP? Hypotensive?
   C. **Level of consciousness?** Gag reflex?
   D. **Timing of possible ingestion?** Last seen, time behavior change noted, reason for presentation to ED (ie, concerns by family, EMS called by strangers, etc).
   E. **Coingestants?** Other depressants, other psychiatric medications, any access to other medications?
   F. **History?** History of previous overdose/suicidality, recent state of mind/mood. Think psychiatric evaluation once medically stable.

III. **Differential Diagnosis**
   A. **Other Drugs/Coingestants.** Such as alcohol, antidepressants, barbiturates, illicit drugs, acetaminophen. Benzodiazepines are often taken with other drugs or medications.
   B. **Stroke.** Or other cause of decreased LOC such as subdural or subarachnoid hemorrhage, head trauma.
   C. **Encephalitis.** Causing decreased LOC.
   D. **Hypoglycemia.** Causing decreased LOC.

IV. **Database**
   A. **Physical Exam Key Points**
      1. **Airway and breathing.** Most common immediate cause of death is respiratory failure. Intubate promptly (See Section VIII, 15. Rapid Sequence Endotracheal Intubation, page 470).
      2. **Neurologic.** Drowsiness, slurred speech, confusion, ataxia. Reported paradoxical reactions of anxiety, aggression, excitement, delirium, are uncommon, but are more common in children.
      3. **Vitals.** Respiratory rate, BP.

B. **Laboratory Data.** Levels are available but are not typically helpful. Ensure lab is testing for any specific suspected agents as not all assays detect all benzodiazepines. Also, as part of routine overdose evaluation, fingerstick glucose, electrolytes, BUN, Cr, and acetaminophen levels. Pregnancy test in any woman of childbearing age.

C. **Radiographic and Other Studies.** ECG may be considered to rule out prolonged QRS from tricyclic coingestion in a patient with decreased LOC. In the presence of respiratory depression, get ABG and CXR.

V. **Plan**

A. **Overall Plan.** Stabilization, respiratory support, resuscitation with fluid (isotonic) support. Routine initial use of dextrose, thiamine, and naloxone should be considered. Decontamination as indicated by clinical condition; should use activated charcoal. Gastric lavage can be considered if coingestants are suspected but presents increased risk due to decreased LOC and respiratory depression. Consult poison center for direction in management, if needed.

B. **Specific Plans.** Flumazenil is a selective antagonist of the CNS effects of benzodiazepines, which should be used very cautiously. It may precipitate withdrawal symptoms with fatal consequences. Although it will reverse the respiratory depression and can prevent the need for intubation, it has a much shorter duration of action than many of the common benzodiazepines. As the antagonist effects wane, a patient may become resedated. In addition, there is a concern about precipitation of seizures or cardiac arrhythmias in patients who have coingested TCAs or other medications, which lower the seizure threshold, and of precipitating withdrawal in patients chronically exposed to benzodiazepines. Bottom line: It isn't necessary to manage benzodiazepine overdoses.

VI. **ICD-9 Diagnoses:** Benzodiazepine overdose; State all adverse/toxic effects caused by the drug separately; State intent of poisoning if known (accident, therapeutic use, suicide attempt, assault, undetermined).

VII. **Problem Case Diagnosis:** Intentional benzodiazepine overdose.

VIII. **Teaching Pearls Question:** Respiratory depression and hypotension are more commonly associated with parenteral administration or oral overdose of benzodiazepines?

IX. **Teaching Pearls Answer:** Be careful with conscious sedation—respiratory depression and hypotension are more commonly associated with parenteral administration.

REFERENCES

Hoffman RS, Goldfrank LR. The poisoned patient with altered consciousness. Controversies in the use of a "coma cocktail." *JAMA* 1995;274(7):562–569.

Longo LP, Johnson B. Addiction: Part I. Benzodiazepines—side effects, abuse risk, and alternatives. *Am Fam Physician.* 2000;61(7):2121–2128.

Mantooth R. Toxicity, Benzodiazepine, *eMedicine Journal,* September 11 2001, Volume 2, Number 9.

Weinbroum AA, Flaishon R, Sorkine P, Szold O, Rudick V. A risk-benefit assessment of flumazenil in the management of benzodiazepine overdose. *Drug Saf* 1997;17(3): 181–196.

6. BETA-BLOCKER OVERDOSE

  I. **Problem:** A 30-year-old presents with bradycardia after an overdose.

  II. **Immediate Questions**

    A. **Is the airway intact?** Manage appropriately (see Section VII, 15. Rapid Sequence Endotracheal Intubation, page 470).

    B. **Is breathing adequate?** Ensure adequate ventilation and oxygenation, clear lungs, check pulse oximeter and supply supplemental oxygen if needed.

    C. **What is the cardiac rhythm? Is the QRS wide or narrow? What is the blood pressure? Is perfusion adequate?** Ensure multiple IV access and begin IV crystalloid boluses for hypotension; reasonable to give trial of atropine for bradycardia, obtain 12-lead ECG.

    D. **Is hypoglycemia present?** Correct with dextrose.

    E. **Access to medications?** Antihypertensives, digoxin, CCBs etc.

    F. **Obtain history** to confirm overdose if possible and rule out primary cardiac or other cause. Consider other medical causes if no clear history to suggest poisoning.

  III. **Differential Diagnosis**

    A. **Toxicologic.** History to suggest intentional or accidental poisoning. (See this section, 7. Calcium Channel blockers, page 334, 8. Cardiac Glycosides, page 339, 11. Cyclic Antidepressants, page 346, 12. Designer Drugs, page 348,)

      1. **Beta-blockers.** Absolute or relative bradycardia (absence of reflex tachycardia) and hypotension, bradycardia unresponsive to atropine, AV blocks, hypoglycemia; QRS widening and convulsions from agents with sodium channel blockade (ie, propranolol).

      2. **CCBs.** Absolute or relative bradycardia and hypotension, bradycardia unresponsive to atropine, AV blocks, hyperglycemia, QRS narrow (unless preexisting BBB); reflex tachycardia with dihydropyridines (ie, nifedipine).

      3. **Digoxin and plants containing cardiac glycosides** (oleander, lily of the valley, foxglove). Bradycardia and hypotension, tachydysrhythmias with AV blocks typical, ST segment depressions, hyperkalemia (acute poisoning), vomiting.

      4. **Sodium channel blockers** (TCAs, diphenhydramine, class I antidysrhythmics, phenothiazines). Bradycardia (with severe poisoning) or tachycardia (more typical) and hypotension, QRS widening, antimuscarinic signs including delirium, convulsions.

5. **Cholinergic agents** (carbamates/organophosphates). Hypotension and bradycardia (may also present with tachycardia) associated with bronchorrhea and other peripheral signs of cholinergic excess (SLUDGE), depressed level of consciousness, QRS normal.
6. **Opioids.** Bradycardia and hypotension (severe poisoning only), hypoventilation, miosis, depressed level of consciousness, all reversible with naloxone, QRS normal (except propoxyphene has sodium channel blockade).
7. **Sedative/hypnotics (benzodiazepines, barbiturates, GHB).** Bradycardia and hypotension (severe poisoning only), hypoventilation, depressed level of consciousness, hypothermia, QRS normal, benzodiazepine effects reversible with flumazenil (Use cautiously if seizure disorder, chronic use of sedative/hypnotic, or coingestion of seizure-producing drug is possible.)
8. **Alpha-agonists (α_1-phenylpropanolamine; α_2-clonidine, oxymetazoline, tetrahydrozoline).** HTN and reflex bradycardia; miosis, hypoventilation, depressed level of consciousness with α_2-agonists

B. **Nontoxicologic.**
   1. **Cardiac.** Heart blocks? Inferior MI? Sinus arrest?
   2. **Hyperkalemia.** QRS prolongation, peaked T waves
   3. **Hypothermia.** Exposure history, check core temperature.
   4. **Hypothyroidism.** Underlying thyroid disease, check core temperature.
   5. **Hypoxia.** Particularly in children.

IV. **Database**
   A. **Physical Exam Key Points**
      1. **Vital signs.** Repeat frequently and reassess with therapy.
      2. **Pulmonary.** Examine frequently, may develop pulmonary edema from fluid therapy because of negative inotropy.
      3. **Cardiac.** Heart rate, pressure, JVD?
   B. **Laboratory Data.** Bedside glucose (fingerstick) if depressed level of consciousness.
   C. **Radiographic and Other Studies.** ECG, CXR, consider echocardiogram, pulmonary artery catheter, electrolytes.

V. **Plan**
   A. **Overall Plan.** Supportive care to maintain tissue perfusion. Patients with hypotension or symptomatic bradycardia should be admitted to the ICU.
   B. **Specific Plans**
      1. **Alter absorption.** Activated charcoal may be beneficial
      2. **Antidote.** Antidote is glucagon begin with 5–10 mg IV and observe for effect, often requires drip (5–10 mg/h); electrical pacing; sodium bicarbonate ampule pushes for QRS prolongation (β-blockers with sodium channel blockade, ie, propranolol).
      3. **Basics.** Airway and breathing management may become necessary for AMS or pulmonary edema.

4. **Vasopressors/inotropes.** Titration required.
   a. **Norepinephrine** or epinephrine (begin 2 μg/min).
   b. **Isoproterenol** (begin 2 μg/min).
   c. **Amrinone** (begin 5 μg/kg/min).
5. **Electrical pacing.** Often will not capture, and when it does perfusion may still not improve if cause is β-blocker or calcium channel blocker, but reasonable to attempt it.
6. **Benzodiazepines.** For convulsions.
7. **Change catabolism.** None.
8. **Distribute differently.** None.
9. **Enhance elimination.** Some agents that have a low volume of distribution and minimal protein binding, such as atenolol and sotalol, may be amenable to hemodialysis.

VI. **ICD-9 Diagnoses:** Beta-blocker overdose; State intent of poisoning if known (accident, therapeutic use, suicide attempt, assault, undetermined); State all adverse/toxic effects caused by the drug separately.

VII. **Problem Case Diagnosis:** Beta-blocker overdose.

VIII. **Teaching Pearls Question:** How does glucagon function as the antidote to β-blocker poisoning?

IX. **Teaching Pearls Answer:** Beta-blockers are antagonists at β_1- or β_2-receptors (or both). Beta-receptor agonism results in activation of adenylate cyclase, which increases production of cyclic-AMP, ultimately resulting in sarcoplasmic reticulum calcium release and myocyte contraction. Glucagon acts on glucagon receptors (distinct from β-receptors) to increase cyclic-AMP production and positive inotropic action.

REFERENCES

Brubacher JR. Beta-adrenergic antagonists. In: Goldfrank LR, Flomenbaum NE, Lewin NA, Weisman RS, Howland MA, Hoffman, RS, eds. *Goldfrank's Toxicological Emergencies.* 6th ed. Appleton and Lange, 1998:809–825.

Kerns W, Kline J, Ford MD. B-blocker and calcium channel blocker toxicity. *Emerg Med Clin North Am* 1994;12:365–390.

7. CALCIUM CHANNEL BLOCKER OVERDOSE

I. **Problem:** A 42-year-old male with a history of depression and hypertension presents after a suicide attempt with mild lethargy, hypotension, and a junctional rhythm.

II. **Immediate Questions**
   A. **Is the airway intact?** Is the patient able to maintain his airway? Manage appropriately (see Section VIII, 15. Rapid Sequence Endotracheal Intubation, page 470).

    B. What are the vital signs and mental status? Apply monitors and pulse ox, obtain ECG, start IV, apply oxygen as needed. Treat hypotension or symptomatic bradycardia now (see V. Plan).

    C. What were the circumstances of the suicide attempt or overdose? What was the time of ingestion? How many tablets were ingested, of what medicine? Other coingestants such as alcohol or illicit drugs? Sustained-release tablets? Interview any witnesses and family members. Obtain any available pill bottles or a list of medicines to which the patient had access (include other family members or friends meds to which patient may have had access). Although not all patients will be forthcoming, most will provide helpful information.

    D. Status since the ingestion? Did the patient vomit? If so, how soon after the ingestion? Were any treatments given (by the patient, family members, or paramedics)? Is patient's mental status declining?

    E. Any PMH, medications, or allergies? Knowledge of medical history/medications can help to direct treatment of suspected ingestants. Old ECGs can be helpful in interpreting subtle abnormalities on the presenting ECG.

    F. Have any forms of decontamination been done? Decontamination is most beneficial if done soon after ingestion. Potential decontamination measures should be started as soon as deemed safe and appropriate. Activated charcoal can be started at home or by paramedics.

III. Differential Diagnosis

A. Nontoxic Causes

    1. MI/cardiac disease/shock. Especially neurogenic shock, anaphylaxis, sepsis, hyperkalemia. Inferior MI can present with identical signs and symptoms.

    2. CNS. CVA, subarachnoid/intracerebral hemorrhage, trauma, hypothermia.

B. Toxic Causes

    1. Bradycardia. Seriously consider β-blockers and digitalis glycosides. Also consider other antiarrhythmics, cholinergic agonists (organophosphates, carbamates, nicotine, myasthenic agents) and α-adrenergic agonists (clonidine).

    2. Hypotension. Consider β-blockers, clonidine, antiarrhythmics, cholinergic agonists, ACE-inhibitors, TCAs and sedative-hypnotic agents, digitalis glycosides.

    3. Altered mental status. Consider sedative-hypnotic agents, TCAs, and multiple others.

IV. Database

A. Physical Exam Key Points

    1. Vital signs. Continuous monitoring is essential. Rhythm, BP, and mental status can change rapidly.

    2. Heart sounds. S_3 or S_4 can give clues to preexisting heart disease.

    3. Neurologic exam. Focal neurologic deficits are rarely toxic in nature. Mental status is classically preserved in CCB toxicity, unlike β-blocker toxicity, in which depressed mental status is typical. However, severe shock due to hypoperfusion can lead to coma or convulsions from any cardiotoxic agent.

4. **Toxidromes.** Examine pupils, abdomen, skin, and vital signs for effects matching classic toxidromes (eg, cholinergic, antimuscarinic, opioid, sedative-hypnotic, withdrawal). There is no specific toxidrome commonly associated with CCB poisoning, other than hypotension with relative preservation of normal ECG complexes.

B. Laboratory Data

1. **Glucose/electrolytes.** CCBs, especially verapamil, often cause hyperglycemia (by indirectly inhibiting insulin release). This can help differentiate these poisonings from β-blocker toxicity that frequently presents with hypoglycemia. Beta-blockers often cause mild hyperkalemia.

2. **Anion gap.** An underlying anion gap is a valuable clue to the underlying abnormality/toxin and can help direct therapy. CCBs do not typically cause an abnormal anion gap.

3. **Acetaminophen level.** Should be drawn on all ingestions because symptoms can be late and nonspecific.

4. **Salicylate level.** Although salicylate ingestion can be suspected in patients with a high anion gap, hypercapnia, hyperthermia, and AMS, consider obtaining a level in unknown ingestions to avoid rapidly occurring and life-threatening complications.

5. **Urine/serum drug screens.** Urine drug screens usually do not change therapy or decision-making in the acute drug overdose setting. Serum levels of CCBs can be obtained, but are usually "send out" tests and are rarely of clinical benefit.

C. Radiographic and Other Studies

1. **ECG.** This test is essential in all poisonings with cardiotoxic potential. Wide complex rhythms are usually not due to CCBs.

2. **CXR.** Noncardiogenic pulmonary edema has been associated with CCB toxicity.

V. Plan

A. Overall Plan. Support and decontaminate!

1. **Activated charcoal.** Activated charcoal binds most drugs within the GI tract and decreases the amount absorbed by the patient. The patient must have an intact airway and mental status to drink activated charcoal. Charcoal is most beneficial if given soon after the ingestion but can still bind toxins even if administration is delayed. The standard dose is 1 g/kg.

2. **WBI.** WBI with PEG-ES (polyethylene glycol electrolyte solution: Go-Lytely) reduces transit time of pills through the GI tract without causing fluid or electrolyte shifts. It can be extremely beneficial, especially when a patient has ingested sustained-release tablets. A standard recommended dose is 0.5 L/h in children and 2 L/h in adolescents and adults. Treatment should be continued until the

rectal effluent is clear, or for 6–8 h. Because large volumes are required, it may be necessary to administer PEG-ES through an NG or feeding tube.

B. **Specific Plans.** Severe CCB poisoning with hypotension and bradycardia is notoriously difficult to treat, and hypotension may be refractory to treatment with standard pressor agents. Although no single therapy has shown consistent benefit in all cases, the following treatments have all proved effective in case reports.

1. **IV fluids.** IV saline is first-line treatment for hypotension and should be used for initial therapy.

2. **Atropine.** Although atropine has often been ineffective in improving bradycardia in severe CCB poisoning, it should be tried for symptomatic bradycardia. The standard dose is 0.5–1.0 mg IV in adults and 0.02 mg/kg IV in children and may be repeated every 2–3 min. Traditionally, the maximum dose is 3 mg (0.04 mg/kg) but higher doses may be necessary.

3. **Calcium.** IV calcium has been reported to improve BP and HR in some cases of CCB toxicity but has not consistently improved parameters in all cases of CCB poisoning. Calcium may work by increasing flow through unblocked cardiac calcium channels. Calcium chloride (13.4 mEq Ca/g) contains over three times more calcium than calcium gluconate (4.3 mEq Ca/g), making it the calcium-containing agent of choice in CCB poisoning. Calcium chloride can damage small veins and cause local necrosis if inadvertently injected into the soft tissues, thus, central line administration should be considered. Calcium can be given as bolus therapy (1–2 g, IV) and, if beneficial, can be given as a continuous infusion (0.2–0.4 mL/kg/h of calcium chloride). Serum calcium should be monitored closely. Patients with moderate toxicity should have serum calcium raised to high normal values (about 10 mg/dL). Severe poisonings may require higher serum levels of calcium to be beneficial. The theoretical risk of cardiac standstill ("stone heart") by administering IV calcium in patients with digitalis glycoside poisoning is unproven and should not delay treatment of severely ill patients with CCB toxicity.

4. **Glucagon.** Glucagon increases intracellular calcium by activating adenylate cyclase, increasing intracellular cAMP and, in turn, stimulating calcium flow through calcium channels. Although it is usually considered an antidote for β-blocker poisoning, glucagon has been reported to improve cardiovascular parameters in some, but not all, cases of CCB poisoning. Large doses of glucagon may be required. An initial bolus of 5–10 mg IV (0.15 mg/kg in children) is recommended. If glucagon is effective in improving HR and BP, a maintenance infusion should be initiated. The rate of the infusion should be titrated to effect.

5. **Pressors.** No single sympathomimetic agent has consistently shown benefit for CCB poisoning, but case reports have sug-

gested occasional success with nearly all agents. The sympath-omimetic agent should be tailored to the predominant symptoms of toxicity. If bradycardia predominates, an agent with mostly β_1 activity would be preferred (epinephrine, norepinephrine). If hypotension is the principal problem, an agent with α_1 activity (and perhaps minimal β_2 activity) could be more useful (norepinephrine, phenylephrine).

    6. Other treatments. When pharmacologic methods fail to improve the patient's condition, manual interventions may be necessary. Transthoracic or IV ventricular pacing may be beneficial. Intraaortic balloon pumps and extracorporeal membrane oxygenation have shown benefit in some cases.

C. Disposition. Extended-release delivery systems have become extremely common in CCB formulations and can result in delayed toxicity after even small (single-tablet or one extra tablet) overdoses, especially in children. All patients suspected of ingesting extended-release CCB formulations should therefore be admitted and observed for 12–24 h to ensure delayed toxicity does not occur. Ingestion of immediate release tablets will reveal symptoms of toxicity within 6–8 h. If patients remain asymptomatic with normal serial ECGs and BP after this period, they can be medically cleared. Any signs of toxicity should prompt admission for extended observation.

VI. ICD-9 Diagnoses: Calcium channel-blocker overdose; State all adverse/toxic effects caused by the drug separately; State intent of poisoning if known (accident, therapeutic use, suicide attempt, assault, undetermined).

VII. Problem Case Diagnosis: CCB overdose.

VIII. Teaching Pearl Question: What is the pathophysiology of CCB overdose?

IX. Teaching Pearl Answer: CCBs block L-type voltage-sensitive slow calcium channels that are located in all types of muscle cells, most notably cardiac (SA node and AV node) and vascular smooth muscle. By impairing the calcium influx into these cells, CCBs cause relaxation and arterial vasodilation in vascular smooth muscle (and resultant hypotension). In heart muscle they cause negative inotropy and inhibit intracardiac conduction (causing bradycardia).

REFERENCES

Belson MG. CCB ingestions in children. *Am J Emerg Med* 2000;18(5):581–586.

Brass BJ. Massive verapamil overdose complicated by noncardiogenic pulmonary edema. *Am J Emerg Med* 1996;14(5):459–461.

Haddad LM. Resuscitation after nifedipine overdose exclusively with intravenous calcium chloride. *Am J Emerg Med* 1996;14(6):602–603.

Papadopoulos J. Utilization of a glucagon infusion in the management of a massive nifedipine overdose. *J Emerg Med* 2000;18(4):453–455.

Proano L. Calcium channel blocker overdose. *Am J Emerg Med* 1995;13:444–450.

Ramoska EA. A one-year evaluation of calcium channel blocker overdoses. Toxicity and treatment. *Ann Emerg Med* 1993;22:196–200.

8. CARDIAC GLYCOSIDE OVERDOSE

I. **Problem:** Medics report that a 58-year-old female cardiac transplant candidate is hypotensive and bradycardic at 30 bpm, and they are unable to pace at a higher rate with the transcutaneous pacer.

II. **Immediate Questions**
   A. **Is the airway intact?** Manage appropriately (See Section VIII, 15. Rapid Sequence Endotracheal Intubation, page 470).
   B. **What are the vitals and mental status?** Is the patient stable and alert? Apply monitors (cardiac and pulse ox), start IV, and oxygen. Place transthoracic pacer leads.
   C. **Was this an accidental or intentional overdose or toxicity?** Are there coingestants or cotoxicities? Is this chronic or acute toxicity? If acute, how much was ingested, and when?
   D. **Are there any associated signs or symptoms?** Visual disturbances (yellow-green color cast, diplopia, blurred vision), weakness, vomiting, SOB, palpitations, seizure, coma, hemodynamic instability, tachyarrhythmias or bradyarrhythmias, heart block, junctional rhythms, VF, or VT.

III. **Differential Diagnosis:** If patient taking digitalis/digoxin and fits clinical picture just described, assume toxicity is high probability.
   A. **Metabolic.** Consider renal failure (acute or chronic) and electrolyte abnormalities (especially potassium and calcium).
   B. **Cardiac Glycoside Plant Poisoning (Foxglove, Oleander).** Consider if patient has had contact with these plants or is using herbal medications.
   C. **Cardiac Glycoside Toad Poisoning (Bufo).** Consider if patient has had contact with *Bufo alvarius* (Colorado River toad or Sonoran Desert toad) or if using *chan su* or Kyushin traditional (herbal) medications (contain toxins from *Bufo bufo gargarizans*).
   D. **CCB Toxicity.** Check medications. (See this section, 7. Calcium Channel Blocker Overdose, page 334)
   E. **Beta-Blocker Toxicity.** Check medications. (See this section, 6. Beta Blocker Overdose, page 332.)
   F. **Other Cardiotoxic Drugs.** Check medications.

IV. **Database**
   A. **Physical Exam Key Points**
      1. **Mental status.** Check if patient is awake and alert.
      2. **Vital signs.** Check carefully and repeat during evaluation.
      3. **Neck.** Check for JVD (CHF).
      4. **Heart sounds.** Check for muffled heart tones (decreased force of contraction, cardiomyopathy).
      5. **Lung sounds.** Check for crackles or wheezes (CHF).
      6. **Neurologic exam.** Check for persistent weakness or confusion (metabolic, CNS toxicity).

   B. **Laboratory Data.** Stat serum digoxin level (may not correlate with degree of toxicity), electrolytes, Cr.

   C. **Radiographic and Other Studies.** ECG. **Repeat if changes in status or rhythm.** If hypoxic or in CHF, CXR. If intentional overdose, consider aspirin and acetaminophen levels, urine toxicology, blood alcohol level, pregnancy test, psychiatric consult.

V. Plan

   A. **Overall Plan.** Maintain airway, assist ventilation as needed, treat hyperkalemia and arrhythmias, treat ingestion of cardiac glycoside (and other substances), admit to a monitored bed.

   B. **Specific Plans**

     1. **Antidotes/altering absorption.** Give activated charcoal if acute ingestion. Give digoxin Fab fragments (Digibind, DigiFab) if significant poisoning or symptomatic arrhythmias, or for prophylaxis if massive ingestion. Dose is based on serum concentration of digoxin or empiric (average 10 vials for acute and 5 vials for chronic intoxication).

     2. **Basics.** Maintain the ABCs.

     3. **Change catabolism.** Not applicable.

     4. **Distribute differently.** Not applicable.

     5. **Enhance elimination.** Not removed by dialysis. Consider repeat doses of activated charcoal.

VI. ICD-9 Diagnoses: Digoxin overdose; State all adverse/toxic effects caused by the drug separately; State intent of poisoning if known (accident, therapeutic use, suicide attempt, assault, undetermined).

VII. Problem Case Diagnosis: Severe chronic digoxin toxicity with acute renal failure and hyperkalemia.

VIII. Teaching Pearls Question: What therapeutic intervention is contraindicated in treating hyperkalemia in the setting of cardiac glycoside toxicity?

IX. Teaching Pearls Answer: Calcium. It may worsen ventricular arrhythmias.

REFERENCES

Brubacher JR, Lachmanen D, Ravikumar PR, Hoffman RS. Efficacy of digoxin specific Fab fragments (Digibind) in the treatment of toad venom poisoning. *Toxicon* 1999; 37(6):931–942.

Brubacher JR, Ravikumar PR, Bania T, Heller MB, Hoffman RS. Treatment of toad venom poisoning with digoxin-specific Fab fragments. *Chest* 1996;110(5):1282–1288.

Lip GY, Metcalfe MJ, Dunn FG. Diagnosis and treatment of digoxin toxicity. *Postgrad Med J* 1993;69(811):337–339.

Olson KR, ed. *Poisoning and Drug Overdose.* 3rd ed. Appleton and Lange, 1999.

Schreiber D, Robertson S. Toxicity, Digitalis. *eMedicine Journal,* May 23 2001, Volume 2, Number 5.

Shumaik GM, Wu AW, Ping AC. Oleander poisoning: Treatment with digoxin-specific Fab antibody fragments. *Ann Emerg Med* 1988;17(7):732–735.

9. CAUSTIC AND CORROSIVE INGESTION

I. **Problem:** A toddler is found crying and drooling next to an opened bottle of drain cleaner.

II. **Immediate Questions**
  A. **What was the route of contact?** Dermal and/or ocular exposures may only need irrigation. Greater potential morbidity if ingested.
  B. **Is the airway intact?** Hoarseness, stridor, or difficulty breathing may portend respiratory failure. Manage appropriately.
  C. **What are the chief complaints?** Chest or abdominal pain suggests possible perforation. Assess need for immediate surgical intervention by physical exam and radiographs.
  D. **What was the substance?**
    1. **Ingestions.**
      a. **Acid or alkali?** Alkali (liquefaction necrosis) causes deeper tissue penetration than acid (coagulation necrosis). Ingested alkalis cause more esophageal injury; acids cause more gastric injury.
      b. **Liquid or solid?** Ingested liquids cause more diffuse injury; solids cause segmental injury.
      c. **Button battery?** Unless lodged in esophagus, most ingested button batteries pass without incident. Caustic injury possible if battery splits.
    2. **Dermal or ocular exposures.**
      a. **Is irrigation with water the best treatment option?** Caustics potentially requiring alternative treatment: hydrofluoric acid, phenol, elemental metals (eg, sodium), solids, and powders.
  E. **Was the exposure intentional?** Larger quantities/worse morbidity with intentional ingestions. Pediatric exposures typically with smaller quantities.

III. **Differential Diagnosis**
  A. **Dermal.** Thermal burn, cellulitis.
  B. **Ocular.** Conjunctivitis, UV keratitis, iritis.
  C. **Ingestion.** Cholinergic toxicity: organophosphates, carbamates.
  D. **Oropharyngeal Infections.** Stomatitis, epiglottitis, diphtheria.
  E. **GI Perforation.** Esophageal rupture, perforated peptic ulcer.

IV. **Database**
  A. **Physical Exam Key Points**
    1. **Airway.** Drooling, stridor. Airway obstruction uncommon but possible if caustic agent aspirated or from glottic edema.
    2. **Oropharynx.** Oral burns and dysphagia are sensitive predictors of esophageal injury; however, lower injury possible without oral burns.

      3. **Abdomen.** Severe pain, peritoneal signs.

      4. **Skin/eyes.** Check for burns. Estimate total BSA burned.

  B. Laboratory Data. Check pH of caustic substance, if possible. Hydrofluoric acid exposures may cause hypocalcemia and hyperkalemia.

  C. Radiographic and Other Studies. CXR or abdominal films to rule out perforation. Localize button batteries by radiograph. Consider urgent endoscopy.

V. Plan

  A. Overall Plan.

    1. **Ingestions.** Unless trivial exposure in minimally symptomatic or asymptomatic patient, endoscopy essential to determine extent of injury and guide therapy. If no oral burns, tolerating food and drink PO, and no abdominal tenderness, consider ED observation and discharge; otherwise admit.

    2. **Dermal.** Copious irrigation, then local burn care. Lower threshold for transfer to burn referral center than for thermal injury.

    3. **Ocular.** Copious irrigation, at least until pH of conjunctival fluid normalizes. Morgan lens helpful. Don't delay irrigation to check visual acuity. Ophthalmologic consult or close ophthalmologic follow-up.

  B. Specific Plans.

    1. **Decontamination** of caustic ingestions controversial.

      a. **Dilution** (water or milk) favored over neutralization.

      b. **Contraindicated.** Induced emesis, gastric lavage, activated charcoal (ineffective; obscures endoscopy).

      c. **Nasogastric aspiration** (not lavage) may be considered in acid ingestions but still carries risk for perforation.

    2. **Endoscopy.** Findings guide therapy. Performed within 48 h of ingestion. If done too early, underestimates injury; if done late, increases risk of perforation. Rating system for esophageal caustic injury:

      a. **1st-degree** (without ulceration). Rarely leads to long-term complications. Usually treated conservatively.

      b. **2nd-degree** (transmucosal burn). May lead to stricture formation. Often treated with steroids ± antibiotics. Both steroids and antibiotics remain controversial.

      c. **3rd-degree** (transmural burn). Frequently lead to strictures and may perforate. Often treated with steroids ± antibiotics; may require surgery.

    3. **Bleach.** Household liquid bleach is an alkaline solution with ~ 5% sodium hypochlorite. Commonly ingested but rarely causes more than superficial injury. Most patients need dilution only (no endoscopy) and can be discharged if stable. **Industrial bleaches may be seriously caustic.**

    4. **Button batteries.** Urgent removal indicated if lodged in esophagus due to risk of pressure ulceration, electrical burn, or caustic injury if battery splits. If below diaphragm, should pass uneventfully.

   5. **Hydrofluoric acid.** Unlike most acids, causes progressive pene-
      trating injury. Binds calcium (and magnesium). Large exposures
      may cause hypocalcemia, hyperkalemia, and metabolic acidosis;
      ECG to screen for significant electrolyte abnormalities. Occupa-
      tional burns to hands and fingers most common. Treat with cal-
      cium to bind fluoride ions; topical, subcutaneous, IV (Bier block),
      or intraarterial routes depending on severity.
   6. **Phenol.** Dilute phenol penetrates skin more easily. Polyethylene
      glycol 300–400 or industrial methylated spirits recommended for
      irrigation but not commonly available in hospitals. Copious water
      irrigation should suffice.
   7. **Elemental metals.** Pure sodium and potassium react explosively
      with water and may ignite on exposure to air. Cover with oil and
      grossly remove particulate matter.
   8. **Caustic solids/powders.** Dissolution in water may increase sur-
      face area contact and skin penetration. Brush off patient prior to
      water irrigation.

VI. **ICD-9 Diagnoses:** Caustic/corrosive exposure; Caustic/corrosive poisoning; State all adverse/toxic effects caused by the drug separately;
   State intent of poisoning/exposure if known (accident, therapeutic use,
   suicide attempt, assault, undetermined).

VII. **Problem Case Diagnosis:** Lye (sodium hydroxide) ingestion.

VIII. **Teaching Pearls Question:** Which commonly ingested alkali household
   cleaning substance causes the least amount of injury and complications?

IX. **Teaching Pearls Answer:** Household bleach (Howell).

REFERENCES

Christesen HB. Prediction of complications following unintentional caustic ingestion in
   children. Is endoscopy always necessary? *Acta Paediatr* 1995;84(10):1177–1182.
Friedman EM, Lovejoy FH. The emergency management of caustic ingestions. *Emerg
   Med Clin North Am* 1984;2(1):77–86.
Homan CS, Maitra SR, Lane BP, Thode HC, Sable M. Therapeutic effects of water and
   milk for acute alkali injury of the esophagus. *Ann Emerg Med* 1994;24(1):14–20.
Howell JM. Alkaline ingestions. *Ann Emerg Med* 1986;15(7):820–825.

10. COCAINE OVERDOSE

 I. **Problem:** A 27-year-old male complains of chest pain.

 II. **Immediate Questions**
    A. **What are the vital signs and mental status?** Is the patient stable
       and alert? Apply monitors (ECG and pulse ox), start IV, apply oxygen.
       Cardiac rhythm? Treat if abnormal.

B. Were other drugs used? Consider multiple toxicities, alcohol toxicity.

C. Onset of symptoms? Chest pain, back pain, SOB, respiratory distress, headache, seizure, focal neurologic deficits, coma.

D. Route of administration? Smoked, snorted, ingested, injected, body packing?

E. Any PMH? Heart disease? Seizure disorder? Stroke? Alcohol withdrawal? Psychiatric? Other street drugs? Medications and allergies?

III. Differential Diagnosis

A. Chest Pain.

1. **Arrhythmia.** Consider VT, PSVT, VF, AF with rapid ventricular response Consider underlying infarction or vasospasm.
2. **MI.** Cocaine accelerates the rate of atherosclerosis and is thrombogenic. J-point elevation on ECG is common in young black men and is not due to ischemia.
3. **Coronary spasm and ischemia.** Frequent. Cocaine induces α-adrenergic-mediated coronary vasospasm.
4. **Chest wall pain.** Check for evidence of ischemia.
5. **Pneumothorax.** Pleuritic pain, common in crack cocaine smokers.
6. **Aortic dissection.** Consider if chest/back pain, elevated BP.

B. Headache, Confusion, Focal, or Global Neurologic Deficit.

1. **Seizure.** Usually brief and self-limited. Status suggests continued drug absorption or hemorrhagic CVA.
2. **Hemorrhagic stroke.** Consider if elevated BP or neurologic deficit.
3. **Hypertensive emergency.** Symptoms resolve after treatment of BP.
4. **Shock—cardiovascular or neurologic.** Consider coingestions and previous diagnoses.

IV. Database

A. Physical Exam Key Points

1. **Mental status.** Confused (AMI, CVA, aortic dissection, coingestants)
2. **Vital signs.** Check carefully and repeat during evaluation.
3. **HEENT.** Check that pupils are equal, reactive (CVA, drugs), and that fundi are without hemorrhage (CVA) Check for evidence of trauma. Check for nasal septum perforation (nasal use).
4. **Heart sounds.** Rub, murmur (endocarditis, pericarditis).
5. **Lung sounds.** Asymmetric (pneumothorax), crackles, or wheezes (CHF, pneumonia).
6. **Abdomen, rectal, and pelvic.** Acute abdomen (bowel infarction), rectal exam (body packing).
7. **Neurologic exam.** Focal deficits (CVA).

B. Laboratory Data. If complete H&P are normal, and patient is asymptomatic, no labs needed. If symptomatic or abnormal physical or co-

ingestants, consider ECG and CXR, electrolytes, CK and cardiac enzymes, blood alcohol level, urine toxicology, and urine pregnancy tests.

    C. Radiographic and Other Studies. If neurologic signs/symptoms present, consider noncontrast CT of the head.

V. Plan

    A. Overall Plan. Treat coma, arrhythmias, seizures, hypotension, and hyperthermia if present. Maintain the airway and intubate if necessary.

    B. Specific Plans.

        1. Antidotes/altering absorption. No antidote available. No gastric decontamination if route of administration was nasal, inhalation, or injection. If ingested, administer activated charcoal. If "body-packing" consider multiple doses of charcoal, WBI, and possible surgical intervention.

        2. Basics. Use esmolol (or propranolol) **and** phentolamine in combination to treat hypertension. Monotherapy with propranolol is no longer recommended. Avoid β-blockers. Use nitrates and CCBs for angina.

        3. Change catabolism. Not applicable.

        4. Distribute differently. Not applicable.

        5. Enhance elimination. Not applicable.

VI. ICD-9 Diagnoses: Cocaine overdose; State all adverse/toxic effects caused by the drug separately; State intent of poisoning if known (accident, therapeutic use, suicide attempt, assault, undetermined).

VII. Problem Case Diagnosis: Crack cocaine use with pneumothorax.

VIII. Teaching Pearls Question: What is the preferred initial treatment of anxiety and tachycardia in patients with cocaine-induced myocardial infarction?

IX. Teaching Pearls Answer: Benzodiazepines. Beta-blocker use may result in unopposed α-adrenergic stimulation.

REFERENCES

Chakko S, Myerburg RJ. Cardiac complications of cocaine abuse. *Clin Cardiol* 1995;18(2): 67–72.

Olson KR, ed. *Poisoning and Drug Overdose.* 3rd ed. Appleton and Lange, 1999.

Pitts WR, Lange RA, Cigarroa JE, Hillis LD. Cocaine-induced myocardial ischemia and infarction: Pathophysiology, recognition, and management. *Prog Cardiovasc Dis* 1997;40(1):65–76.

Qureshi AI, Suri MF, Guterman LR, Hopkins LN. Cocaine use and the likelihood of nonfatal myocardial infarction and stroke: Data from the Third National Health and Nutrition Examination. *Circulation* 200130;103(4):502–506.

11. CYCLIC ANTIDEPRESSANT OVERDOSE

I. **Problem:** A 24-year-old female is brought by ambulance with seizures. Her boyfriend says she's been depressed and they had a fight a few hours ago. He called 911 when he found her mumbling on the couch and not responding.

II. **Immediate Questions**
   A. **Is the airway intact?** Manage appropriately (see Section VIII, 15. Rapid Sequence Endotracheal Intubation, page 470).
   B. **Is their adequate IV access to support circulation?** Consider placing a central line if IV access is minimal or questionable.
   C. **Is there evidence of trauma or a toxidrome?** Anticholinergic, cholinergic, sympathomimetics, or opiates?
   D. **Could this be a suicide attempt?**
   E. **What was the patient's neurologic status prior to the seizure?**
   F. **What is the duration of the seizure?**
   G. **Any PMH?** Is there a history of seizures? Is there any past cardiac disease or surgery? Is there any history of diabetes? Could the patient be pregnant? Any history of neoplasm or renal disease? What medications does she take? Is there a history of drug or alcohol abuse? Was there any mental depression or illness?

III. **Differential Diagnosis**
   A. **Metabolic.** Hypoglycemia, hypocalcemia, hyponatremia.
   B. **Infectious.** Abscess, HIV, meningitis, encephalitis.
   C. **Ingestions.** Cyclic antidepressants, alcohol, lead, strychnine, camphor.
   D. **CNS.** Trauma, neoplasm, arteriovenous malformations, hydrocephalus, hemorrhage, stroke.
   E. **Pregnancy.** Eclampsia, hemorrhage, ectopic pregnancy.

IV. **Database**
   A. **History (critical!)**
      1. Medical problems in past.
      2. Medication use and abuse.
      3. Mental illness and depression.
      4. Evidence of suicidal thoughts.
      5. **Evidence of suicide attempt.** Bottles, notes, or comments. Talk with family, friends, EMS.
   B. **Physical Exam Key Points.**
      1. **Vital signs.** Temperature, hypotension, tachycardia.
      2. **HEENT.** Signs of trauma to the head or face, pupil size/equality/reactivity, airway, evidence of ingestion.
      3. **Neck.** Stiffness, tracheal deviation, trauma.
      4. **Heart.** Rate, rhythm, murmurs.
      5. **Neurologic.** Alertness, response to stimuli, spontaneous movement, GCS.

C. Laboratory Data

1. **Glucose.** Low blood sugar presents in many forms.
2. **ABG.** Will give you an idea of downtime, help direct ventilation/oxygenation needs, and many analyzers will quickly provide electrolytes.
3. **Toxicology, blood alcohol, and pregnancy.** Aspirin and Tylenol levels.
4. **Electrolytes and CBC.**

D. Radiographic and Other Studies

1. **CT scan of the head,** once stabilized, to rule out an intracranial process as the cause **or** result of the event.
2. **ECG to look for tachycardia, or prolongation of QRS.** In TCA overdose the QRS complex widens and tachycardia develops (> 100 ms).

V. Plan

A. Overall Plan. Stabilize the patient by addressing the ABCs while trying to determine the cause of the mental status change and seizures. Determining the cause of mental status changes necessitates a history. While the patient's immediate life threats (ABCs) are being addressed send a nurse to talk with family, friends, and primary physician

B. Specific Plans.

1. **Regardless of cause.** With mental status changes a "cookbook" approach is critical to avoid missing simple, correctable causes. Everyone should receive dextrose, naloxone [Narcan], and thiamin. Assume an ingestion occurred and use lavage and charcoal. A CT scan is almost always indicated (trauma can be a cause or effect).
2. **Metabolic.** Correct abnormality.
3. **Infectious.** Always consider as a cause when no other explanation available. Culture and treat presumptively.
4. **TCA.** Overdoses are characterized by the 4 "C's": convulsions, coma, and cardiovascular collapse. Once the airway is secure, the patient should receive lavaged and be given charcoal. Removal of even a small amount of ingested material may be very beneficial. Additionally with TCAs an anticholinergic effect causes slow emptying of the stomach. Widened QRS and resulting hypotension should be treated with sodium bicarbonate until QRS narrows. Admission, psychiatric consultation, and telemetry are mandatory.
5. **CNS.** Determine cause with CT, and obtain appropriate specialty assistance.
6. **Pregnancy.** Determine by H&P. Treat as per trimester.

VI. ICD-9 Diagnoses: Antidepressant overdose; State all adverse/toxic effects caused by the drug separately; State intent of poisoning if known (accident, therapeutic use, suicide attempt, assault, undetermined).

VII. Problem Case Diagnosis: Elavil overdose.

VIII. **Teaching Pearls Question:** In a 24-year-old that goes into a cardiac arrest with a wide-complex tachycardia, what is the best drug to use?

IX. **Teaching Pearls Answer:** Sodium bicarbonate.

REFERENCES

Bittner M, Joyce DM. Toxicity, Cyclic Antidepressants. *eMedicine Journal* 2:12, 2001.
Clinical Policy for the Initial Approach to Patients Presenting with Acute Toxic Ingestion or Dermal or Inhalation Exposure: *Ann Emerg Med* 1999;33(6):735–761.
Walter FG, Gogarty WS, Callaham M. Antidepressants and monoamine oxidase inhibitors. In Marx JE, Hockberger RS, Walls RM, eds. *Rosen's Emergency Medicine Concepts and Clinical Practice,* Volume II, 2002:1325–1342.

12. DESIGNER DRUG OVERDOSE

I. **Problem:** An agitated and confused teenager is brought to the ED after an all-night dance party.

II. **Immediate Questions**
   A. **What are the vital signs and mental status?** CNS stimulants cause hyperthermia, tachycardia, and HTN, as well as a hyperalert state. CNS depressants can cause bradycardia, respiratory depression, somnolence, and lethargy. Both are known to cause euphoria.
   B. **Was a drug, medication, or mood-altering substance involved?** Often the patient, family, friend or EMS person will be able to divulge this information. It is common for multiple substances to be used in one period.
   C. **If a substance was used, what was the method?** They can be inhaled, taken as a pill, or intravenously injected. The inhalation route includes bagging (spraying a solvent in a bag and then inhaling its contents), huffing (placing a solvent on a rag and covering the mouth and nose), and sniffing.
   D. **Is the patient taking any other medications?** These substances can interact with other medications and produce life-threatening syndromes, such as serotonin syndrome.
   E. **PMH or past psychiatric history?** These are often clues to the diagnosis.
   F. **Are there any overt causes for the patient's AMS?** Signs of trauma or cyanosis may be clues.

III. **Differential Diagnosis**
   A. **Causes of AMS, Not Including Recreational Drugs.** The list includes trauma, infections, organic psychosis, stroke or intracranial space-occupying lesion, electrolyte abnormalities, hypertensive encephalopathy, hypoglycemia, hypoxia, and uremia.
   B. **CNS Stimulants**
      1. **MDMA.** Street names include ecstasy, X, E, Adam, and XTC. Taken orally to "enhance feelings of love" and "emotional close-

ness." Hallucinations can occur at high doses and it is known to cause agitation, psychosis, and hyperthermia.

2. **Methamphetamine.** Known as meth, crank, crystal, and ice. Typically used by insufflation, also by smoking, intravenously, and orally. The patient can be kept awake for days while using this substance. Adverse effects include psychomotor agitation and psychiatric symptoms similar to schizophrenia.

3. **Ephedrine.** Typically found in herbal medications and teas, including *Ma-huang* and "Mormon's tea." This substance is used for its central acting stimulant effect, as a performance-enhancer for athletes, as well as for weight control purposes. Peripheral sympathomimetic signs, such as tachycardia, diaphoresis, tremor, and mydriasis, tend to dominate over CNS signs, requiring massive amounts to be used to gain the stimulant effect.

4. **Ketamine.** Names include K, special K, and vitamin K. This is a derivative of PCP and has a similar clinical presentation. It is similar in popularity within the "club scene." It is used typically by the insufflation method. Adverse reactions include dysphoria, hallucinations, vomiting, and catatonia.

C. **CNS Depressants**

1. **Gamma-hydroxybutyrate (GHB), γ-butyrolactone (GBL) or butanediol (BD).** Typically causes euphoria, drowsiness, dizziness, and, with increasing doses, can cause coma, seizure-like activity, bradycardia, Cheyne-Stokes respirations, and respiratory depression.

2. **Nitrous oxide.** Found in whipping cream chargers or in large cylinders for medical use. Clinical effects are likely secondary to hypoxia. With chronic use a sensorimotor polyneuropathy can develop.

3. **Hydrocarbon inhalation.** Can be used by huffing, bagging, or sniffing. Clinical effects include euphoria, nystagmus, inebriation, lethargy, and coma. Adverse effects include coma, seizures, and arrhythmias.

IV. **Database**

A. **Physical Exam Key Points.** Don't forget to look for signs of trauma.

1. **Vital signs.** These are often markedly altered due to stimulant or depressant effects.

2. **Mental status.** Common findings include agitation, hallucinations, somnolence, lethargy, or coma. Patients may have ideations about hurting themselves or others.

3. **Eyes.** Check the pupils, they tend to dilate with CNS stimulants.

4. **Cardiovascular.** Arrhythmias possible with both stimulants and depressants, especially with hydrocarbon abuse.

5. **Neurologic.** Typically this part of the exam is nonfocal. Ataxia, seizures, and seizure-like activity can occur.

6. **Skin.** Stimulants cause the skin to be warm and moist; with dehydration, these signs may not be reliable. Look for signs of trauma and for needle marks on the patient's body, especially the extremities and neck.

B. **Laboratory Data**

1. **Serum electrolytes, BUN/Cr, glucose.** All patients with AMS should have their blood sugar checked immediately. Serum electrolytes and renal function tests will be helpful. For MDMA users, hyponatremia can occur with excessive physical activity and free water intake. With all stimulants, rhabdomyolysis may occur, baseline renal function tests and CK levels are useful.

2. **UA.** If rhabdomyolysis is suspected, the test may be positive for heme, but RBCs will not be present.

3. **LP.** If the patient is febrile and an infectious cause is suspected.

C. **Radiographic and Other Studies.**

1. **Pulse ox.** Low oxygen saturation could be the cause of the patient's AMS.

2. **Head CT.** This may be warranted for persistent or unexplained mental status changes.

3. **ECG.** If arrhythmias are suspected. The QRS duration should be checked if cyclic antidepressants were taken.

V. **Plan**

A. **Overall Plan.** The mainstay for the majority of cases is supportive. The patient's airway must be maintained and fluid replaced as needed.

B. **Specific Plans**

1. **Coma.** Protect the patient's airway with intubation or other airway protection technique (see Section VIII, 15. Rapid Sequence Endotracheal Intubation, page 470).

2. **Depressant use.** Respiratory support is the first line in treatment of these patients.

3. **Stimulant use.** Agitation may be controlled with benzodiazepines.

4. **Seizures.** Benzodiazepines.

5. **HTN.** May resolve when agitation is controlled; if not, consider vasodilators such as nitroprusside or NTG.

6. **Gastric decontamination and elimination.** Consider activated charcoal for oral ingestions if patient is alert and protecting airway.

VI. **ICD-9 Diagnoses:** MDMA (or whatever specific drug—if known) overdose; State all adverse/toxic effects caused by the drug separately; State intent of poisoning if known (accident, therapeutic use, suicide attempt, assault, undetermined).

VII. **Problem Case Diagnosis:** MDMA and nitrous oxide use.

VIII. **Teaching Pearls Question:** Why are MDMA users at risk for the serotonin syndrome?

IX. **Teaching Pearls Answer:** MDMA has serotonergic activity.

REFERENCES

Goldfrank LR, Flomenbaum NE, Lewin NA, Weisman RS, Howland MA, Hoffman, eds. *Goldfrank's Toxicologic Emergencies.* 6ed. Appleton & Lange, 1998.
Graeme KA. New drugs of abuse. *Emerg Med Clin* 2000;18(4):625–636.
Kurtzman TL, Otsuka KN, Wahl RA. Inhalant use by adolescents. *J Adolesc Health* 2001;28:170–180.

13. IRON OVERDOSE

I. **Problem:** An alert, fearful, 4-year-old child is brought to urgent care by parents 2 h after eating pills "that looked like M&M's."

II. **Immediate Questions**

   A. **ABCs, vital signs?** May deteriorate as toxicity progresses, reflecting hypovolemia, decreased liver function.

   B. **Nature of ingestion?** Iron is found in other forms besides the classic smooth "M&M-like" pill, notably in prenatal and pediatric vitamins.

   C. **Time of ingestion?** Steady-state levels reached in 4 h. After 6 h, binding may yield misleadingly low serum levels.

   D. **Coingestants?** Always think about coingestants. What else could the child have ingested? Did the parents give him anything at home before bringing him in?

   E. **Cause?** Always think about how exposure occurred. Why did child have access to pills? Home safety? Has this happened before?

   F. **Nature of symptoms?** Three reasonable presentations:

   1. Known ingestion, as in this case.

   2. Nausea, diarrhea, especially with hematemesis.

   3. Hyperglycemia with metabolic acidosis—especially with prodrome of GI complaints.

   G. **In which stage of disease is the patient presenting?**

   1. **GI.** Nausea, diarrhea, abdominal pain, hemorrhage with larger ingestions, possible hypovolemia or hyperglycemia.

   2. **Deceptive resolution.** May not occur. Beginning 6 h after ingestion and lasting up to 24 h after ingestion, patients may have a period of improvement, though can have persistent acidosis, hypovolemia, and coagulopathy.

   3. **Metabolic acidosis.** With liver compromise (elevated bilirubin and LFTs, hypoglycemia).

   4. **GI sequelae.** Scarring, gastric outlet obstruction, weeks later.

III. **Differential Diagnosis**

   A. **Gastroenteritis.** GI toxicity likely to present with diarrhea, nausea, possibly hematemesis.

   B. **Diabetic Ketoacidosis.** Hyperglycemia with metabolic acidosis.

   C. **Other Ingestions.** Consider other agents causing GI symptoms, such as salicylates, pesticides, or food-borne toxins, and hepatotoxins such as acetaminophen.

   D. **Coingestants.** Always consider possible coingestants.

IV. **Database**
   A. **Physical Exam Key Points.** Nonspecific, such as possible hypovolemia, abdominal pain.
   B. **Laboratory Data.** Serum iron levels more than 4 h after ingestion. Levels after 6 h may underestimate quantity of ingestion. *Glucose:* > 150 mg/dL may indicate severe toxicity. Low glucose may indicate hepatic dysfunction. *WBC:* > 15K may indicate severe toxicity. *HCT:* May be low due to GI bleed. *Stool:* For occult blood. *Acetaminophen* level: Especially because of hepatotoxic effect. *ABGs, electrolytes, T&C:* For resuscitation/management.
   C. **Radiographic and Other Studies.** Iron tablets, if still present in the GI tract, will be radiopaque and visible on a KUB. Their absence does not preclude severe toxicity.

V. **Plan**
   A. **Overall Plan.** Stabilization, resuscitation with fluid (isotonic) support. Decontamination guided by KUB—gastric lavage if iron in stomach, WBI if evident further down. Pitfalls of decontamination are that iron is gelatinous and can form bezoars (large clumps that may fail to progress through the bowel) and require resection. Always consider coingestants. Does not bind to activated charcoal. Consult poison center/toxicologist.
   B. **Specific Plans.** Chelation with deferoxamine to remove iron via urinary and biliary excretion
      1. **Deferoxamine.** In severe overdose, start IV therapy at 5 mg/kg/h. Increase as blood pressure tolerates to 15 mg/kg/h. Best endpoint is clinical improvement. Avoid administration of greater than 6–8 g/day. *Vin-Rose*-colored urine indicates ferrioxamine excretion but this sign not reliable as endpoint of therapy.

VI. **ICD-9 Diagnoses:** Iron overdose; State all adverse/toxic effects caused by the drug separately; State intent of poisoning if known (accident, therapeutic use, suicide attempt, assault, undetermined).

VII. **Problem Case Diagnosis:** Early stage (asymptomatic) presentation of a child with a strong history for iron ingestion.

VIII. **Teaching Pearls Question:** Is the GI bleeding in iron overdose caused by direct irritation of the GI tract, trauma from vomiting, platelet inhibition by free iron ions, or another mechanism?

IX. **Teaching Pearls Answer:** Direct irritation of the GI tract by iron causes hemorrhagic gastroenteritis, though iron may also cause a coagulopathy.

REFERENCES

Bosse GM. Conservative management of patients with moderately elevated serum iron levels. *J Toxicol Clin Toxicol* 1995;33(2):135–140.
McGuigan MA. Acute iron poisoning. *Pediatr Ann* 1996;25(1):33–38.
Mills KC, Curry SC. Acute iron poisoning. *Emerg Med Clin North Am* 1994;12(2):397–413.
Spannierman C. Toxicity, Iron, *eMedicine Journal,* April 26 2002, Volume 3, Number 4.

14. ORGANOPHOSPHATE POISONING

I. **Problem:** A teenage male presents with agitation, wheezing, copious secretions, and perfuse diaphoresis. He vomits and his emesis smells of hydrocarbons.

II. **Immediate Questions**
   A. **Is the airway intact?** Manage appropriately (see Section VIII, 15. Rapid Sequence Endotracheal Intubation, page 470). Avoid succinylcholine administration.
   B. **What are the vitals and mental status?** Is the patient stable and alert? Apply monitors (ECG and pulse ox), start IV, apply oxygen.
   C. **Does the patient have a classic toxidrome?**
      1. **Cholinergic syndrome?** Profuse diaphoresis, diarrhea, involuntary urination, miosis, bradycardia or tachycardia, bronchorrhea, bronchoconstriction, emesis, lacrimation, salivation, seizures, paralysis, AMS.
      2. **Anticholinergic syndrome?** Dry skin, urinary retention, mydriasis, tachycardia, decreased bowel sounds, dry mouth, AMS, hallucinations.
      3. **Sympathomimetic syndrome?** Diaphoresis, mydriasis, tachycardia, hypertension, AMS.
      4. **Opioid syndrome?** CNS depression, respiratory depression, miosis.
   D. **Did anyone witness the patient's ingestion of the substance?** Interview any witness and inquire as to possible products in the home. Was package of product ingested brought to hospital?
   E. **Any PMH?** History of psychiatric illness, previous suicide attempts, illicit drug use, and any current medications?
   F. **Do clothes smell or contain residue?** If so, double bag clothes, and consider decontamination of patient?

III. **Differential Diagnosis**
   A. **Organophosphate Poisoning or Carbamate Poisoning.**
   B. **Mushrooms.**
   C. **Chemical Warfare Agents (Nerve Agents).**
   D. **Cardiogenic Shock.**
   E. **Septic Shock.**
   F. **Status Asthmaticus.**
   G. **Hydrocarbon Ingestion with Aspiration.**
   H. **Pneumonia.**

IV. **Database**
   A. **Physical Exam Key Points.** Don't forget to completely undress and examine the entire body, including the back.
      1. **General.** Is there a specific smell to the patient?
      2. **Mental status.** Agitated, somnolent, hallucinating, coma.
      3. **Vital signs.** Check carefully and repeat during evaluation.

      4. Mouth. Check for amount of secretions, substance residue.

      5. Nose. Check for secretions.

      6. Eyes. Check pupil size.

      7. Lungs. Check for wheezing, rales, rhonchi.

      8. Heart. Check for heart rate.

      9. Abdomen. Check for bowel sounds

    10. Skin. Check for diaphoresis, flushing.

    12. Neurologic exam. Check pupils for reactivity, reflexes, muscles fasciculations, or flaccidity.

B. Laboratory Data. Check electrolytes, glucose, CBC, acetaminophen level, ABG, plasma cholinesterase level if available.

C. Radiographic and Other Studies. Check CXR if patient in respiratory distress. Check ECG for specific drug effects such as for QRS prolongation (Na-channel blockade) and QT prolongation (K-efflux blockade which predisposes to torsades de pointes and is seen in organophosphate poisoning). If patient is comatose with flaccid paralysis, obtain an EEG because organophosphate-poisoned patients can be in status epilepticus with muscular paralysis.

V. Plan

A. Overall Plan. Cases of suspected organophosphate poisoning should be decontaminated if necessary. Cases of symptomatic organophosphate poisoning should receive atropine in 2-mg doses until respiratory secretions are dry and bronchospasm resolves. Also, pralidoxime should be given in doses of 1 g to symptomatic adults and repeated as necessary. Contact your local poison control center or medical toxicologist.

B. Specific Plans.

    1. Respiratory compromise. Atropine in 2-mg doses repeated every 5 min until control of secretion and bronchospasm occurs.

    2. Muscle fasciculations or flaccid paralysis. Administer pralidoxime 1–2 g and then begin continuous infusion at 500 mg/h until resolution of systems has occurred.

    3. Seizures. Seizures associated with organophosphate or carbamate poisoning should be treated with benzodiazepines (eg, Valium). If seizures cease but the patient has flaccid paralysis, emergent EEG should be performed.

    4. Miosis. If patient develops significant eye pain associated with ciliary spasm, do **not** treat with systemic atropine but rather ophthalmic atropine.

    5. Aspiration pneumonia. Treat supportively.

    6. Dehydration. Administer IV NS as necessary to fluid resuscitate.

VI. ICD-9 Diagnoses: Organophosphate overdose; State all adverse/toxic effects caused by the drug separately; State intent of poisoning if known (accident, therapeutic use, suicide attempt, assault, undetermined)

VII. Problem Case Diagnosis: Acute organophosphate poisoning.

VIII. **Teaching Pearls Question:** Is tachycardia a contraindication to atropine administration in the symptomatic organophosphate poisoned patient?

IX. **Teaching Pearls Answer:** No, tachycardia is common in organophosphate poisoning and its presence is not a contraindication to atropine (Holstege et al).

REFERENCES

Coye MJ, Barnett PG, Midtling JE, Velasco AR, Romero P, Clements CL, et al. Clinical confirmation of organophosphate poisoning by serial cholinesterase analyses. *Arch Intern Med* 1987;147:438–442.

Holstege CP, Kirk M, Sidell FR. Chemical warfare: Nerve agent poisoning. *Crit Care Clin* 1997;13(4):923–942.

Selden BS, Curry SC. Prolonged succinylcholine-induced paralysis in organophosphate insecticide poisoning. *Ann Emerg Med* 1987;16:215–217.

Tafuri J, Roberts J. Organophosphate poisoning. *Ann Emerg Med* 1987;16:193–202.

15. SALICYLATE OVERDOSE

I. **Problem:** A 20-year-old female brought in by EMS with nausea, vomiting, abdominal pain, fever, diaphoresis, tachypnea, and lethargy following an unknown ingestion.

II. **Immediate Questions**

   A. **Is the airway intact? Is there a gag reflex?** Establish and secure airway if indicated.

   B. **What are the vitals (including pulse ox) and mental status?** Is the patient alert and stable? Apply monitors, start IV if not already in place, and give oxygen as needed. Check an immediate fingerstick blood glucose.

   C. **Specifics about the overdose.** What, when, how many, what dose, enteric-coated for delayed absorption? Verifiable (witnesses, pill bottles or fragments)?

   D. **Coingestions.** Any other medications or drugs taken (including alcohol)?

   E. **Treatment prior to admission.** Activated charcoal? Syrup of ipecac (not generally recommended)?

   F. **PMH.** Medications (may be primary cause, or cause interactions or alter typical presentation)? Psychiatric history? Overdoses? LMP? Previous surgeries? Recent illness? Other medical history?

III. **Differential Diagnosis**

   A. **Toxicologic.**

   1. **Salicylism.** Presenting features can include fever, AMS, diaphoresis, nausea, vomiting, abdominal pain, tachypnea and/or hyperpnea, respiratory alkalosis with or without metabolic acidosis, hypokalemia, dehydration, and noncardiogenic pulmonary edema. Can be acute or chronic. Seen with aspirin, oil of win-

tergreen, and some herbal medicines containing these or other salicylates.

2. **Malignant hyperthermia.** Characterized by muscular rigidity and hyperpyrexia following use of certain inhalational anesthetics or succinylcholine in genetically susceptible patients. May recur after initially successful treatment.

3. **Neuroleptic malignant syndrome.** Signs may include AMS; hyperpyrexia, autonomic instability; and lead-pipe muscular rigidity in the setting of usage of lithium or neuroleptic medications, such as prochlorperazine, haloperidol, chlorpromazine (Thorazine), droperidol, or other phenothiazines.

4. **Serotonin syndrome.** Triad of autonomic instability, AMS, and rigidity. May also see mydriasis. Seen after addition or increase in dosage or a serotonergic agent, or addition of another new drug–such as an MAOI–to another serotonergic agent.

5. **Alcohol withdrawal.** Don't forget delirium tremens.

6. **Opiate withdrawal.**

7. **Sympathomimetics.** Cocaine, amphetamine, and other stimulants. May see fever, hypertension, diaphoresis, mydriasis, tachycardia, and agitation.

8. **Anticholinergic poisoning.** Anticholinergic effects can result from many prescription and OTC medications, including antihistamines, antiparkinsonian agents, antipsychotics, antispasmodics, TCAs, and some plants, mushrooms, and certain eye drops, cold remedies, analgesics, and sleeping aids. Look for flushing (red as a beet), pyrexia (hot as a hare), dry skin and mucous membranes (dry as a desert), (blind as a bat) mydriasis and cycloplegia, disorientation, hallucinations (mad as a hatter). Other findings include tachycardia, urinary retention, and decreased or absent bowel sounds.

9. **Other.** Reye's syndrome, theophylline toxicity, caffeine toxicity, acute iron poisoning, sepsis, DKA, meningitis. Lethal catatonia.

B. **Nontoxicologic.** (Remember that history can sometimes be a "red herring.")

1. **Infection.**

2. **Cancer.**

3. **Metabolic derangement.** DKA, addisonian crisis, thyrotoxicosis.

4. **Organophosphate poisoning.**

5. **Intracranial lesion.** Tumor, stroke, meningoencephalitis, abscess.

6. **Inflammatory disorders.** Pericarditis, pancreatitis.

7. **Environmental.** Heat stroke, heat exhaustion.

IV. **Database**

A. **Physical Exam Key Points.** In unknown ingestions, a complete physical exam is essential. Findings may support diagnosis of a toxidrome. Areas of *special* note include:

1. **Vital signs.** Check carefully and repeat frequently, including pulse ox.
2. **HEENT.** Check the pupils for size, symmetry, reactivity, and nystagmus. Check the mouth for chemical burns (eg, erythema, edema).
3. **Lungs.** Check for crackles and wheezes.
4. **Abdomen.** Bowel sounds, rectal bleeding.
5. **Skin.** Check carefully for temperature, color, turgor, and diaphoresis and dryness (axilla and groin are good places to assess).
6. **Neurologic.** Check GCS. Perform mental status exam if patient cooperative.

B. **Laboratory Data.** Labs may be confirmatory or may reveal secondary abnormalities mandating intervention. If history is clear and reliable, fingerstick blood glucose and urine pregnancy test may be all that is required. Also consider electrolytes, BUN, Cr, glucose, CBC, coagulation studies, CPK, ABG, UA, urine tox screen, and quantitative serum salicylate and acetaminophen levels. (Qualitative urine spot tests using either ferric chloride or Trinder's reagent to screen for the presence of salicylate exist.) Low serum uric acid and elevated PT are suggestive of chronic salicylism. LP may be required to rule out meningoencephalitis and subarachnoid hemorrhage, as from a hypertensive bleed.

C. **Radiographic and Other Studies.** If history clear and reliable, none may be required. CXR may show pulmonary edema with severe salicylism. Abdominal radiograph may directly visualize iron pills; some pills in excess may form concretions. Abdominal radiograph may also show GI obstruction or demonstrate free air in bowel perforation. ECG may show QRS widening in TCA overdose. Noncontrast head CT may show hypertensive intracranial hemorrhages in cocaine or other sympathomimetic ingestion and should be performed before LP in patients with focal neurologic signs.

V. **Plan**

A. **Overall Plan.** Initial attention should be focused on immediate life threats with resuscitation provided as needed. Supportive care and diagnostic investigation should proceed simultaneously. Continuous monitoring and frequent reevaluation are important to detect clinical deterioration. Degree of toxicity is best determined by the patient's clinical condition combined with serial salicylate levels, which should be drawn every 1–2 h until the patient's clinical condition stabilizes and levels are declining.

1. **Support and decontaminate!** Establish IV access, provide oxygen, and place the patient on a cardiac monitor. Consider empiric oxygen, thiamine, glucose, and naloxone. If patient presentation is within 1–2 h of ingestion, placing an NG tube may allow removal of contents remaining in the stomach. Activated charcoal 1–2 mL/kg should then be provided, either orally if the patient is alert and cooperative, or via the NG tube.

    2. **Gastric lavage/WBI** using PEG, 2 L/h until clear rectal effluent, may also be indicated. Abdominal radiography may detect pills and pill fragments, although radiolucent materials will not be imaged.

B. Specific Plans.

    1. **Alkalinization of the urine** by bicarbonate infusion (*never* acetazolamide!). Add 3 amp of $NaHCO_3$ to 1 L of D_5W to create an isotonic solution suitable for this task, with potassium added once urine output is ensured. Titrate rate to maintain urine pH at or greater than 7.5 and to maintain arterial blood pH no greater than 7.55. Watch for noncardiogenic pulmonary edema. Invasive hemodynamic monitoring may be necessary in select cases; hyperventilation should be maintained to prevent acute deterioration caused by iatrogenic acute respiratory acidosis. Because of the need to closely monitor volume and neurologic status, electrolytes, salicylate level, and serum and urine pH, ICU placement is generally necessary.

    2. **Provision of adequate (but not excessive) hydration.**

    3. **Potassium replacement and correction** and prevention of hypoglycemia.

    4. **Early consultation with a toxicologist** is advised. Hemodialysis should be considered in those cases of salicylate toxicity that are complicated by clinical deterioration despite supportive care, AMS, pulmonary edema, persistent acidemia, coagulopathy, renal dysfunction, extremes of age, and severe underlying disease.

VI. ICD-9 Diagnoses: Salicylate overdose; State all adverse/toxic effects caused by the drug separately; State intent of poisoning if known (accident, therapeutic use, suicide attempt, assault, undetermined).

VII. Problem Case Diagnosis: Salicylate toxicity (from ingestion of an herbal remedy containing oil of wintergreen).

VIII. Teaching Pearl Question: What is the role of the Done nomogram in salicylate toxicity?

IX. Teaching Pearl Answer: None except perhaps in an acute single salicylate ingestion when the time of ingestion is known, when the ingested product was neither a sustained-release preparation nor oil of wintergreen, and when there is no complicating renal insufficiency or acidemia. The patient's clinical condition and early course should guide clinical therapy, not the salicylate level (Yip et al).

REFERENCES

Weiner AL, Ko C, McKay CA. A comparison of two bedside tests for the detection of salicylates in urine. *Acad Emerg Med* 2000;7(7):834–836.

Yip L, Dart RC, Gabow PA. Concepts and controversies in salicylate toxicity. *Emerg Med Clin North Am* 1994;12(2):351–364.

16. SELECTIVE SEROTONIN REUPTAKE INHIBITOR (SSRI) OVERDOSE

I. **Problem:** A 32-year-old female brought in by ambulance presents with high fever, confusion, and mild tremor.

II. **Immediate Questions**
   A. **Is the airway protected?** Assess airway and breathing. Place pulse oximeter. Start oxygen via nasal cannula. If patient is not protecting airway (apnea, stridorous breath sounds, hypoxia, decreased Sao_2) consider intubation.
   B. **Is patient hemodynamically stable? Temp? Other vitals?** Apply monitors (ECG and pulse ox). Any hypotension/hypertension, bradycardia/tachycardia, arrhythmia, apnea, or hypoxia? If patient has severe hyperthermia (> 41°), consider rapid cooling.
   C. **Course of symptoms?** Onset (rapid vs slow), duration, location (focal vs general), aggravating/relieving factors, and associated symptoms (N/V/rigidity/dry membranes) all provide clues to cause.
   D. **Is there headache or neck stiffness?** Subarachnoid hemorrhage and meningitis are potentially fatal and must be detected early.
   E. **Are there focal neurologic deficits?** Paresis, paresthesias? Focal or general? Unilateral or bilateral?
   F. **Any recent drug ingestion, abuse, or change in medical regimen?** Prescribed medications (antidepressants, antipsychotics, anticholinergics, or antiemetics)? Recreational drugs (amphetamines, cocaine, LSD, PCP)?
   G. **Any PMH? Seizures? Psychiatric disorder?** Hyperthyroidism (Graves's disease or goiter), diabetes, HIV, polycystic kidney disease, or known cerebral aneurysm, previous dystonic reaction?

III. **Differential Diagnosis**
   A. **Metabolic/Endocrine.**
      1. **Hyperthyroidism (thyroid storm).** Consider if history of hyperthyroidism or signs of thyrotoxicosis (diaphoresis, palpitations, weakness, heat intolerance, weight loss).
      2. **Hypoglycemia.** Consider if patient is taking hypoglycemic agents.
   B. **Infectious.**
      1. **Meningitis.** Triad of fever, headache, nuchal rigidity. May have sick contacts.
      2. **Encephalitis.** Fever, headache, nuchal rigidity, along with AMS, seizures, or focal neurologic signs.
      3. **Septicemia.** Consider sources such as cardiac (endocarditis), pulmonary (pneumonia), GI (appendicitis, colitis, perforation), GU (pyelonephritis).
      4. **Tetanus.** Consider if no recent immunization, rigidity.
   C. **Neurologic/Vascular.**
      1. **Intracranial hemorrhage.** Consider recent trauma or ruptured aneurysm.

2. **Dystonic reaction.** Usually localized to specific muscle groups (oculomotor, neck, torso). May be primary or secondary (drug ingestion).

D. Drug-Induced.

1. **Serotonin syndrome.** Triad of AMS, autonomic instability, and neuromuscular hyperactivity. Consider when ingestion of amphetamines, cocaine, lithium, LSD, MAOIs, SSRIs, NSRIs, or TCAs has occurred.

2. **Neuroleptic malignant syndrome.** Characterized by AMS, autonomic instability, hyperpyrexia, and muscular rigidity. Caused by neuroleptics such as phenothiazines (chlorpromazine, prochlorperazine, promethazine) and butyrophenones (droperidol, haloperidol).

3. **Anticholinergic syndrome.** Characterized by mydriasis, tachycardia, dry membranes, fever, and AMS. Atropine, scopolamine, and inhaled anticholinergics can cause anticholinergic syndrome as can antihistamines, neuroleptics, TCAs, and many OTC cough/cold/sleep remedies. Also consider plant and herbal medications.

4. **Malignant hyperthermia.** Caused by inhaled anesthetics and paralytics such as succinylcholine.

5. **Other drugs.** PCP (increased metabolic rate, AMS), strychnine (rigidity).

IV. Database

A. Physical Exam Key Points.

1. **Vital signs.** Check carefully and repeatedly, abnormalities must be addressed immediately.

2. **Mini mental status exam.** Determine degree of confusion and level of consciousness.

3. **Neuromuscular exam.** Assess motor/sensory in cranial and peripheral nerves for focal deficits (CVA, encephalitis, dystonic reaction), pupil symmetry/reactivity/size (ICH, drugs), fundi for papilledema (ICH, encephalitis) nuchal/other muscle groups for rigidity/tenderness (meningitis, neuroleptic malignant syndrome, dystonic reaction, tetanus), and reflexes for hyperreflexia/myoclonus (serotonin syndrome).

4. **Cardiovascular exam.** Assess for murmurs (cardiac source of septicemia).

5. **Pulmonary exam.** Listen for stridor, wheezes, crackles, rales, and decreased breath sounds (pulmonary source of septicemia).

6. **Abdominal exam.** Assess for pain and peritoneal signs (GI source of septicemia).

B. Laboratory Data. *If no source of septicemia is found on H&P:* Perform LP and CSF analysis. Chemistry panel to determine anion gap and glucose level, CBC, urine or serum toxicology screen, UA. CPK if concern for NMS or rhabdomyolysis. Consider blood cultures.

C. Radiographic and Other Studies. *If H&P are normal:* CXR (occult pneumonia) and abdominal radiograph (pills). *If risk factors uncovered in H&P:* CT scan head, ECG.

V. Plan

A. Overall Plan. Ensure ABCs and perform ACLS as indicated. Patients with thyroid storm require ICU admission. All infectious causes of AMS require admission, as will ICH. Drugs causing hyperthermia and AMS should be discontinued and rapid external cooling performed. Specific therapies should be rendered according to syndrome. Admission is dependent on severity and response to ED treatment. Patients with hypoglycemia and dystonic reactions can usually be discharged from ED after treatment.

B. Specific Plans.

1. **Metabolic/endocrine.** Treat hypoglycemia with dextrose. Treat thyroid storm with adrenergic blockade (unless contraindicated), antithyroid medications, and then iodide.

2. **Infectious.** Start empiric antibiotic without delay for meningitis. Antibiotics/antivirals for encephalitis, as directed by clinical suspicion and lab analysis. Treat empirically for septicemia (consider source), regimen to be modified according to culture findings. Benzodiazepines or paralytics, antibiotics, and tetanus immunoglobulin for tetanus. All should be admitted for IV antibiotics and continued supportive care.

3. **Neurologic/vascular.** ICH requires immediate neurosurgical consultation. Anticholinergics for dystonic reactions.

4. **Drug-Induced.** Supportive care, rapid cooling, and activated charcoal (recent ingestion). Benzodiazepines and cyproheptadine or chlorpromazine for serotonin syndrome, propranolol and methysergide have variable efficacy. Dopamine agonists and dantrolene for NMS. Physostigmine for anticholinergic syndrome (if severe and not contraindicated). Dantrolene for malignant hyperthermia.

VI. ICD-9 Diagnoses: SSRI overdose; State all adverse/toxic effects caused by the drug separately; State intent of poisoning if known (accident, therapeutic use, suicide attempt, assault, undetermined).

VII. Problem Case Diagnosis: Serotonin syndrome.

VIII. Teaching Pearls Question: What class of drugs is most likely to precipitate serotonin syndrome when taken with an SSRI?

IX. Teaching Pearls Answer: MAOIs (furazolidone, isocarboxazid, pargyline, phenelzine, procarbazine, tranylcypromine). Meperidine and dextromethorphan (more common than MAOIs) also enhance serotonin levels with SSRIs, predisposing to serotonin syndrome (Mills).

REFERENCES

Graudins A. The serotonin syndrome. In: Harwood-Nuss A, ed. *The Clinical Practice of Emergency Medicine.* Lippincott Williams & Wilkins 2001:1617–1620.

Martin TG. Serotonin syndrome. *Ann Emerg Med* 1996;28(5):520–526

Mills KC. Newer antidepressants and serotonin syndrome. In Tintinalli JE, ed. *Emergency Medicine: A Comprehensive Study Guide.* McGraw-Hill 2000:1072–1079.

Sarko J. Antidepressants, old and new. A review of their adverse effects and toxicity in overdose. *Emerg Med Clin North Am* 2000;18(4):637–654.

VI. Terrorist Attacks

1. GENERAL TERRORISM ASSESSMENT AND RESPONSE

I. Problem: While you are working in your ED, EMS radio reports an explosion and gunfire at a major downtown office building.

II. Immediate Questions
   A. Is my hospital secure and safe?
   B. How do we activate the disaster plan? What happens?
   C. What kind of casualties will we be getting?
   D. How will we get updates?
   E. Where can we get outside help if needed?
   F. Who is in charge?

III. Differential Diagnosis
   A. Accidental vs deliberate explosions.
   B. Nonintentional or planned releases of hazardous materials.
   C. Bioterrorist attacks or natural pandemics.

IV. Database
   A. **Physical Exam Key Points.** Be aware that terrorists as well as victims may come to a hospital, either to cause more damage or for treatment. For blast injury, recognize patterns (ear/lung/gut injury). Recognize toxidromes (eg, cholinergic). Know and use a standard triage system such as START. Dead is dead. Do not work on arrests.
   B. **Laboratory Data.** With multiple victims, only critical labs needed: Hct, T&C. Use pulse ox and noninvasive monitoring to expedite work-up.
   C. **Radiographic and Other Studies.** Probably limited in the immediate response. Maintain spinal immobilization until radiographs obtained or exam is reliable. Empiric treatment and techniques such as bedside US and DPL may replace CT scanning.

V. Plan
   A. **Overall Plan.** Security lockdown to protect hospital. Hospital disaster plan implemented to call in staff and prepare facility. Coordination and communication established with outside agencies. ED ready to rapidly triage and stabilize multiple patients. Rapid discharge of inpatients to open beds especially in ICU.
   B. **Specific Plans.** Prepare for specific types of casualties: blast, crush, general trauma, toxic, radiologic. Prepare for decontamination of patients. Have a plan to rotate staff to allow for replacement and prolonged effort. For biologic attacks, expect days to weeks of effort. Have a plan to obtain backup supplies and meds.

VI. ICD-9 Diagnoses: (As appropriate)

VII. **Problem Case Diagnosis:** Multiple patients with blast and crush injury.

VIII. **Teaching Pearls Question.** What should your first priority be when preparing a hospital to receive victims of a terrorist attack?

IX. **Teaching Pearls Answer.** Self and facility safety and security. Prevent yourself from being a victim of a "second device" or terrorist.

REFERENCES

Macintyre AG, Christopher GW, Eitzen E Jr, Gum R, Weir S, DeAtley C, et al. Weapons of mass destruction events with contaminated casualties: Effective planning for health-care facilities. *JAMA* 2000;283(2):242–249.

Richards CF, Burstein JL, Waeckerle JF, Hutson HR. Emergency physicians and biological terrorism. *Ann Emerg Med* 1999;34(2):183–190.

http://www.cert-la.com/triage/start.htm

Waeckerle JF. Disaster planning and response. *New Engl J Med* 1991;324(12):815–821.

2. BIOLOGICAL TERRORISM

I. **Problem:** A 33-year-old male in excellent health presents to the ED by ambulance with fever, chills, coughing, shortness of breath, hemoptysis, and skin discoloration. He is concerned that he may be a victim of bioterrorism.

II. **Immediate Questions**
   A. **ABCs adequate?**
   B. **How contagious might the patient be?**
   C. **Could this be the index case of a covert bioterrorist attack?**
   D. **Does this patient have any risk factors that might make him vulnerable to such an attack?**
      1. Sexual orientation
      2. Recent travel history
      3. Occupation
      4. Political affiliation
      5. Recent attendance at mass gatherings
      6. Religious affiliation
      7. Typical mode of travel
      8. Ethnicity/race
   E. **Has there been any occurrence or threat anywhere suggestive of a biological attack?**
   F. **Has there been any deviation from the normal health of the community?**
      1. Severe disease manifestations in previously healthy people?
      2. Higher than normal number of patients with fever and respiratory/GI complaints?
      3. Multiple people with similar complaints from a common location?
      4. An endemic disease appearing during an unusual time of year?
      5. Greater than usual EMS runs?

6. Greater number of deaths?
7. Unusual number of rapidly fatal cases?
8. Greater than usual ED census?
9. Greater than usual number of hospitalizations?
10. Greater than usual number of animal illnesses or deaths?
11. Anyone else with similar symptoms?
12. Greater number of patients with severe pneumonia, sepsis, sepsis with coagulopathy, fever and unusual rash, diplopia with progressive weakness.

III. Differential Diagnosis
A. Natural.
1. **Cat scratch fever.**
2. **Meningococcemia.**
3. **Community-acquired pneumonia.**
4. **Atypical pneumonia.**

B. Intentional.
1. **Anthrax (inhalational).** Flu-like prodrome; progressive respiratory distress; hemorrhagic meningitis; hemodynamic instability. *Bacillis anthracis* can be spread as powder, especially if weaponized.
2. **Viral hemorrhagic fever.** Flu-like prodrome; multiple sites of hemorrhage (intracranial, GI, conjunctival); DIC; petechiae, purpura, ecchymosis; GI disturbances; shock; hepatic/renal involvement. Caused by one of at least 18 RNA viruses, eg, yellow fever, Ebola, dengue.
3. **Tularemia.** Flu-like prodrome; cough; chest pain; pneumonia; hemoptysis; pleural effusions; morbilliform rash; pharyngeal ulcers.
4. **Q fever.** Flu-like prodrome; cough; chest pain; pneumonia; neurologic compromise (encephalitis, expressive dysphasia, dysarthria).
5. **Pneumonic plague.** Flu-like prodrome; rapid deterioration with respiratory distress; GI disturbances; ecchymosis, petechiae, purpura, acral gangrene; hemodynamic instability.
6. **Brucellosis.** Flu-like prodrome; respiratory compromise, GI disturbances; hepatosplenic involvement; arthralgias/myalgias; chronic meningoencephalitis.
7. **Ricin.** Flu-like prodrome; dyspnea; pulmonary edema; cyanosis. Derived from castor beans.
8. **Smallpox.** Flu-like prodrome; oral lesions initially followed by macular, papular, vesicular, pustular lesions appearing at same stage and starting on face/arms then on the legs then torso; cough; pulmonary edema; encephalitis; abdominal pain. Tremendously contagious.
9. **Staphylococcal enterotoxin B.** Flu-like prodrome; cough; dyspnea; chest pain; GI disturbances.
10. **T_2-mycotoxin.** Immediate burning of skin; blistering; dermal necrosis; dermal sloughing; mucosal irritation of nose, eyes, mouth; cough; dyspnea; pulmonary edema; bone marrow suppression.

IV. Database

A. Physical Exam Key Points.

1. **Vital signs.** Check for fever (botulism occurs without fever); check vital signs frequently including pulse ox (patients may deteriorate rapidly with bioterrorist agents).

2. **Mental status.** May be altered either due to infection of the CNS (viral encephalitides, anthrax, Q fever, VHF) or result of hypoxemia or hypercarbia secondary to respiratory failure (anthrax, plague).

3. **Neck/nuchal rigidity.** Hemorrhagic meningitis (anthrax), meningitis (tularemia and plague rarely), meningoencephalitis (Q fever, viral encephalitides)

4. **Eyes.** Diplopia (botulism, Q fever), ptosis (botulism), mydriasis (botulism), conjunctival irritation (ricin, T_2 mycotoxin, tularemia), corneal ulcers (smallpox), photophobia (viral encephalitides), conjunctival hemorrhage (VHF).

5. **Respiratory.** Check for stridor (anthrax, plague), wheezes, rales (plague, tularemia, ricin, smallpox, T_2-mycotoxin, Q fever), decreased breath sounds (effusions in anthrax, tularemia), hemoptysis (tularemia, plague, T_2 mycotoxin).

6. **Abdomen.** Tender (anthrax, plague, smallpox, ricin), hepatosplenomegaly (brucellosis, rarely Q fever), GI hemorrhage (ricin, anthrax, plague, T_2 mycotoxin, VHF).

7. **Skin.** Cyanosis (anthrax, plague, botulism, ricin), petechiae, purpura, ecchymosis (plague, VHF), acral gangrene (plague), painless, necrotic ulcers (cutaneous anthrax), bubo (plague), discrete lesions [macules, papules, vesicles, papules] at same stage (smallpox), erythema (T_2 mycotoxin), blisters (T_2 mycotoxin), edema (anthrax, VHF).

B. Laboratory Data.
Gram stain and culture all relevant specimens (eg, blood, CSF, cutaneous lesions). Acquire blood specimens for bacterial and viral cultures, possible ELISA, DFA, and PCR. Hemorrhagic CSF is suggestive of anthrax meningitis.

C. Radiographic and Other Studies.
CXR may show widened mediastinum and bilateral pleural effusions in inhalational anthrax; bilateral lower-lobe infiltrates in plague; diffuse bronchopneumonia with hilar adenopathy and effusions in tularemia.

V. Plan

A. Overall Plan.
Minimizing the spread of infection to others is the primary objective and patient care is a secondary objective. Admission and isolation until organism identified. Consult infectious disease department. Notify local or state public health department. The public health officials will determine whether a bioterrorism event has occurred and are responsible for notifying the CDC and law enforcement.

B. **Specific Plans**
   1. **Isolate patient.** Standard, airborne, droplet, and contact precautions. Revise accordingly as more information becomes available. Mask patient to minimize respiratory contamination. Isolate patient in negative pressure room if possible. Consider N-95 respirators or biological respirators (PAPRs) for those providing direct patient care.
   2. **Patient may require empiric antibiotic therapy** (eg, ciprofloxacin, doxycycline), pressor support.
   3. **Patient care may require aggressive airway management.** (See Section VIII, 15. Rapid Endotracheal Intubation, p 470.)
   4. **Consider prophylactic antibiotic therapy** for those in direct contact with patient (eg, ciprofloxacin, doxycycline).
   5. **Consult infectious disease personnel and infection control department of hospital.**
   6. **Contact local health department.**
   7. **Contact state department of health** (if local authorities are unresponsive).
   8. **Contact local law enforcement.**

VI. **ICD-9 Diagnoses:** Pneumonia, Sepsis, Respiratory failure—as appropriate.

VII. **Problem Case Diagnosis:** Pneumonic plague.

VIII. **Teaching Pearls Question.** What is the incubation period of pneumonic plague?

IX. **Teaching Pearls Answer.** One to six days, usually 2–4 days.

REFERENCES

Eitzen E, Pavlin J, Cieslak T, Christopher G, Culpepper R, eds. *Medical Management of Biological Casualties Handbook.* 4th ed., USAMRIID, 2001.
Inglesby TV, Dennis DT, Henderson DA. Plague as a biological weapon. *JAMA* 2000;283: 2281–2290.
Keim P, Smith KL, Keys C, Takahashi H, Kurata T, Kaufmann A. Molecular investigation of the Aum Shinrikyo anthrax release in Kameido, Japan. *J Clin Microbiol* 2001;39(12): 4566–4567.
McGovern TW, Friedlander AM. "Plague." Part 1, Medical aspects of chemical and biological warfare In: Brig. Gen. R. Zajtchuk, MC, ed. *The Textbook of Military Medicine.* U.S. Army. Office of the Surgeon General, Department of the Army, USA 1997:479–502.
Rega PP. Bio-Terry. *A Stat Manual to Identify and Treat Diseases of Biological Terrorism.* MASCAP, Maumee, Ohio. 2000 (rev. 2001).

3. CHEMICAL TERRORISM

I. **Problem:** EMS calls to notify your ED of a multicasualty HAZMAT incident. Most patients have eye rain, blurry vision, and miosis. A significant minority has these eye signs and symptoms plus nausea, dyspnea, weakness, and fasciculations. One patient is comatose, apneic, and endotracheally intubated. One patient seized and now is in cardiac arrest with CPR and ACLS in progress.

II. Immediate Questions
A. What route of exposure is most common at multicasualty HAZMAT incidents?
B. What toxidrome are these patients manifesting?
C. What agents could cause a multicasualty incident with these signs and symptoms?
D. How would you triage these patients?
E. What are the resuscitation priorities for any patient?
F. What is the poisoning treatment paradigm?
G. Where should decontamination occur?
H. What are the antidotes?
I. What are the indications, contraindications, complications, dosage, and route for each antidote?
J. What bioterrorism agent causes weakness and respiratory arrest, but not fasciculations?

III. Differential Diagnosis
A. Cholinergic Toxidrome Causes.
  1. Organophosphates.
    a. Nerve agents for chemical warfare and chemoterrorism.
    b. Insecticides.
  2. Carbamates.
    a. Insecticides.
    b. Medicinals
  3. Nicotine.
  4. Muscarine-containing mushrooms.
  5. CNS signs mnemonic:
    a.
      Confusion
      Convulsions
      Coma
    b. Remember, Civilian Conservation Corps.
  6. Incidence of signs in moderately poisoned patients in Okumura et al's case series of the Tokyo subway sarin attack.
    a. Ocular signs.
      i. Miosis = 99%.
      ii. Lacrimation = 9%.
    b. Neurologic signs.
      i. Weakness = 37%.
      ii. Fasciculations = 23%.
      iii. Convulsions = 3%.
    c. Cardiopulmonary signs.
      i. Dyspneic respirations = 63%.
      ii. Wheezing = 6%.
      iii. Bradycardia = 4%.

        d. Gastrointestinal signs.
           i. Emesis = 37%.
           ii. Diarrhea = 5%.

IV. Database

A. Physical Exam Key Points.

1. Muscarinic signs mnemonic:

Diarrhea
Urination
Miosis
Bronchospasm, bronchorrhea, bradycardia
Emesis
Lacrimation
Salivation
   a. Remember you need muscles to lift dumbbells.

2. Nicotinic signs mnemonic:

Mydriasis
Tachycardia
Weakness
Hypertension
Fasciculations
   a. Remember, smokers need nicotine every day of the week.

3. CNS signs mnemonic:

Confusion
Convulsions
Coma
   a. Remember, Civilian Conservation Corps.

4. Incidence of signs in moderately poisoned patients in Okumura et al's case series of the Tokyo subway sarin attack.
   a. Ocular signs.
      i. Miosis = 99%.
      ii. Lacrimation = 9%.
   b. Neurologic signs.
      i. Weakness = 37%.
      ii. Fasciculations = 23%.
      iii. Convulsions = 3%.
   c. Cardiopulmonary signs.
      i. Dyspneic respirations = 63%.
      ii. Wheezing = 6%.
      iii. Bradycardia = 4%.
   d. Gastrointestinal signs.
      i. Emesis = 37%.
      ii. Diarrhea = 5%.

B. Laboratory Data.

1. Cholinesterase levels.
   a. Plasma.
   b. Red blood cells.

C. Radiographic and Other Studies.
1. Pulse ox.
2. ABG for dyspneic patients.
3. CXR for dyspneic patients.

V. Plan
A. Overall Plan
1. Isolate the area of the source of exposure and deny entry to the area if not trained in rescue and wearing personal protective equipment that provides respiratory and skin protection.
2. Activate your hospital's disaster plan.
3. Decontaminate patients prior to entering the ED.
4. Simply triage patients into three categories:
   #### a. Mild nerve agent poisoning
   i. *Only* ocular signs and symptoms.
   #### b. Moderate nerve signs and symptoms
   i. Ocular and systemic signs and symptoms but no endotracheal intubation necessary.
   #### c. Severe nerve agent poisoning
   i. Endotracheal intubation necessary.
5. Follow the primary survey and resuscitation mnemonic for all patients:
   Airway with C-spine control
   Breathing
   Cardiovascular
   Disability (nervous system)
   Exposure with environmental control

B. Specific Plans
1. Follow the poisoning treatment paradigm:
   Alter absorption, administer antidotes
   Basics (the primary survey and resuscitation)
   Change catabolism
   Distribute differently
   Enhance elimination
2. Apply the poisoning treatment paradigm in this setting
   #### a. Antidotes/altering absorption.
   i. Remove from exposure.
   ii. Ensure adequate ventilation.
   iii. Strip the patient and wash the skin with detergent and water if there is any possibility of liquid nerve agent contact.
   iv. Atropine: 2 mg (0.05 mg/kg) IV bolus + infusion (0.05 mg/kg/hr)
   v. 2-PAM (pralidoxime): 1 g over 30-min + infusion (10 mg/kg/hr
   vi. Diazepam: 10 mg (0.2 mg/kg) IV

VI. **ICD-9 Diagnoses:** Nerve gas (or name specific agent) poisoning; State intent of poisoning/exposure if known (accident, therapeutic use, suicide attempt, assault, undetermined); State all adverse/toxic effects caused by the drug separately.

VII. **Problem Case Diagnosis:** Nerve agent toxic terrorism by vapor exposure.

VIII. **Teaching Pearl Question.** What is the most common sign after exposure to nerve agent vapor?

IX. **Teaching Pearl Answer.** Miosis (Okumura, et al).

REFERENCE

Okumura T, Takasu N, Ishimatsu S, Miyanoki S, Mitsuhashi A, Kumada K, et al. Report on 640 victims of the Tokyo subway sarin attack. *Ann Emerg Med* 1996;28:129–135. http://ccc.apgea.army.mil/

4. NUCLEAR TERRORISM

I. **Problem:** A bomb explodes in a shopping mall. There are 3 dead and 25 injured at the scene. There are 125 others who are concerned that the bomb may have contained radiation. Some are vomiting at the scene. You have not heard any EMS communications as of yet.

II. **Immediate Questions**
   A. **Is this a simple radiation dispersal problem or a true nuclear (fission) event?** Fission events are associated with higher levels of radiation exposure and induced radiation in which formerly non-radioactive elements are converted to radioactive materials, eg, ^{32}Na, ^{40}K. A surface detonation would involve fallout, which could cause significant beta burns on the skin if left on for prolonged periods (an hour or more). Fallout may look like heavy, dark, or light-colored snowflakes.
   B. **How many casualties are anticipated?** WMD events will possibly involve a large number of casualties, and in particular, may involve large numbers of "worried well" casualties.
   C. **Is the presence of radiation verified?** A credible source should be found to corroborate a radiation event, preferably from a governmental agency or official from plant who oversees radioactive processes. Health or medical physicist from hospital may be listed in radiation disaster plan for important radiologic assistance. Also, radiation safety officer should be part of any radiation disaster plan. Remember, facts change rapidly in such a dramatic event, and initial reports may be inaccurate or confusing.

III. Differential Diagnosis

A. **Radiation Device.** A radiation instrument with an ordinarily legitimate purpose used as a terrorist weapon to expose unsuspecting individuals. Examples would be placement of a radiography source (commonly used to inspect welds, capable of emitting hundreds of rads per hour) in a populated area where people would be exposed (but not contaminated).

B. **Radiation Dispersal Device (RDD).** More commonly known as a "dirty bomb." No fission reaction occurs, only spread of radiation. Such a weapon requires a large radiation source, with uneven distribution to cause death. It is much more likely that an RDD would cause "nuisance radiation" designed to generate fear of long-term effects of increased risk of developing cancer later in life and contamination of buildings and neighborhoods.

C. **Improvised Nuclear Device (IND).** This is a "homemade" nuclear weapon capable of generating fission. Yields are commonly thought to be 0.1 kT (kilotons) to several kilotons. Due to poor construction, such a device would have a low efficiency and a much lower yield than the included nuclear materials would indicate.

D. **Nuclear Weapon.** This government-fabricated weapon is capable of high-efficiency and could have a range from 0.5– 50 kT. Most common estimate is thought to be 1 kT weapon.

E. **Strategic Nuclear Weapon.** This government-fabricated weapon is a fusion (**thermonuclear**) weapon capable of yields from 1 to 50 MT (megatons).

1. **Conventional injury.** No special preparation is required. Manage as for any trauma.

2. **Contamination.** Approach as for trauma. N-95 filter masks may be used if personnel are concerned about particulates. If patients are medically stable, may decontaminate outdoors, but if medically unstable, wait until medical stability is achieved and decontaminate indoors. Self-showering is acceptable if patients are ambulatory. Contaminated runoff going down the drain is acceptable.

3. **Irradiation.** Diagnose by the time to onset of nausea, vomiting, and diarrhea after exposure. The sooner the onset of nausea, vomiting, and diarrhea, the larger the dose. Irradiation can be confirmed with serial CBCs looking at the absolute lymphocyte count. Radiation exposures that do not cause changes in a CBC are more properly termed "**overexposures.**"

4. **Conventional injury with irradiation.** Conventional injury with systemically significant irradiation is synergistic for increased morbidity and mortality. If resources are limited, more severely exposed victims may require an "expectant" classification.

5. **Conventional injury with irradiation** (from detonation).

IV. Database

A. **Physical Exam Key Points.** Look for any obvious dust with a snow-flake appearance. This could be fallout and should be removed immediately. Seriously exposed individuals will experience nausea, vomiting, or diarrhea within 3 h of exposure. Other findings of exposure are skin erythema. Symptoms of high exposure include fever, severe abdominal pain, and an eye-burning sensation. If concern for contamination exists, victims should be surveyed with a radiation survey meter. Any burns seen immediately after exposure will be conventional burns; radiation skin effects (burns, epilation) will occur in 1–3 weeks.

B. Laboratory Data. Serial CBCs taken every 3–6 h confirm significant radiation exposure. A consistent fall in the absolute lymphocyte count over 48 h confirms systemically significant exposure. Absolute lymphocyte count should reach a nadir at 48 h after suspected exposure.

C. Radiographic and Other Studies. Nuclear medicine gamma camera may be used in a rough way to detect internal or external contamination for some radionuclides. (^{125}I ^{201}Tl, ^{57}Co, ^{99m}Tc, ^{111}In, ^{133}Ba, ^{131}I, ^{85}Sr, ^{137}Cs, ^{54}Mn, ^{60}Co.)

V. Plan

A. Overall Plan. The source of the information is key, because radiation exposure and type of device should be determined by credible sources. Establishing the expected number casualties is very important to determining whether disaster plan should be activated. Victims usually self-rescue and present to the nearest ED, without warning. This may be the first indication that a WMD event has occurred.

1. **Next major decision.** Is their need to prepare for contamination? Next decision: Prepare outdoor decontamination area as well as indoor contamination area? Will depend on number and type of casualties. Outdoor decontamination is ideal for the "worried well" individual. Ambulatory victims in no apparent distress may be sent immediately for outdoor decontamination.

   If contamination is thought necessary, a triage station (Table VI–1) should be established outdoors at a common patient entry point for possible diversion either to outdoor decontamination or to a **secondary assessment center.** A second triage center should be established outdoors before hospital entry that is capable of radiation survey. Unstable patients should be isolated with three bedsheets and brought inside for immediate medical treatment. Patients should be stabilized medically before attempting decontamination.

   Preferably, worried well casualties should be sent to a secondary assessment center, an area external to the hospital that is capable of decontamination, shelter, and observation. Those with delayed onset of nausea or vomiting or suspected overexposure could be watched in the secondary assessment center. If contamination is an issue, one or more radiologic emergency areas may be established indoors or outdoors that practice contamination control with traditional "hot," "warm," and "cold" zones. Hot zone

TABLE VI–1. COMBINED-INJURY TRIAGE WHEN RADIATION DOSES ARE KNOWN.[a]

Conventional Triage Categories if Injuries Are Only Trauma	Changes in Expected Triage Category Following Whole-Body Radiation Dose (Gy)		
No radiation exists	< 1.5 (150 rad)	1.5–4.5 (150–450 rad)	> 4.5 (450 rad)
Prodrome onset	< 3 h	1–3 h	< 1 h
Immediate	Immediate	Immediate	Expectant
Delayed	Delayed	Expectant	Expectant
Minimal	Minimal	Expectant	Expectant
Expectant	Expectant	Expectant	Expectant

[a] Decision based on whole-body radiation dose, assuming all casualties are wearing personal dosimeters.
Source: Adapted, with permission, from data in *NATO Handbook on the Concept of Medical Support in NBC.*
Use Table VI–1 when conventional and suspected irradiation is present.

(contaminated zone), warm zone (contamination checkpoint for personnel), cold zone (contamination-free area).

2. **Next decision.** Any systemically significant irradiation? Victims should be categorized by the Chernobyl radiologic triage table (Table VI–2) and have serial CBCs performed. Severe exposures will show fall as quickly as 3 h after exposure. Individuals in lesser triage categories may be have serial CBCs every 6 or even 12 h after exposure. Those with severe hematologic injury should be hospitalized for a prolonged period to observe for of immuno-compromise.

B. **Specific Plans.** Contamination plans should include contingencies for indoor and outdoor decontamination strategies. It should also con-

TABLE VI–2. MODIFIED USSR CHERNOBYL TRIAGE (1986).

	Class 1	Class 2
Prodrome	> 3 h[a]	1–3 h[a]
Lymphs (3–6 days)	600–1000	300–500
TBI dose	1–2 Gy	2–4 Gy
Survival estimate	Probable w/o tx	Possible w/o tx

	Class 3	Class 4
Prodrome	0.5–1 h	< 0.5 h
Lymphs (3–6 days)	100–200	< 100
TBI Dose	4.2–6.3 Gy	6–12, 16 Gy
Survival estimate	Probable w/tx	Not likely

[a] Triage scheme for irradiation injury only.

tain a method for discovering contamination after patient has already presented for care. Such a plan should include placing the patient in a radiologic emergency assistance center (REAC). Consideration should be given to declaring the room the patient occupies an REAC. The areas that the patient has been should be isolated, pending a radiation survey. Any surveyed areas that are subsequently found to be cleared may be returned to normal use. A warm zone, a radiation checkpoint, should be established at the doorway of the REAC for contamination control. Routine operation may then be reinstated (Figure VI–1).

VI. ICD-9 Diagnoses: (As appropriate.)

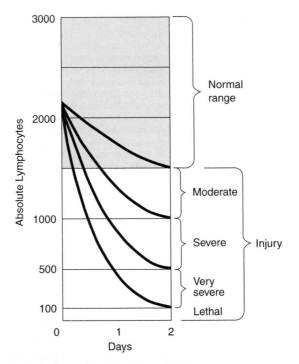

Figure VI–1. Andrews nomogram for confirmation of hematopoietic radiation injury. Absolute lymphocyte counts at 48 h reflect the following: moderate = 1000–1500, severe = 500–1000, very severe = 100–500, lethal = < 100. Prognostic outcome can also be predicted by location and rate of lymphocyte fall for CBCs obtained before 48 h, plotted on the nomogram.

VII. **Problem Case Diagnosis:** Worried well people presented to the ED registration before EMS notification. At that point, the radiation disaster plan was activated, and an REAC was designated where these people were surveyed. They were found free of radiation. The state radiation health department was contacted to verify radiation contamination. Security was augmented and officers began to secure the area. The registration area was isolated until surveyed and found free of radiation. A health physicist was consulted early in the response and further organized survey efforts as triage stations were formed outdoors at a hospital entry/parking lot. A nearby parking deck was established as a secondary assessment center and staffed with hospital personnel. This parking deck was chosen with proximity to restrooms, showers, and entertainment media. The secondary assessment center was supplied with medical charts, soap, hospital gowns, towels, permanent markers, and large plastic and Ziplock bags (for personal effects). The hospital ED received primarily those patients who were seriously ill or obviously injured. One hundred twenty-five worried well presented to the secondary assessment center, and 30 were treated at the ED. Of these, 20 were found to be externally contaminated. When checked with a gamma camera, after external decontamination, none were found to be internally contaminated. Three FBI agents arrived and searched for shrapnel, clothing of the seriously injured, and other evidence. The only radionuclide identified at the scene was ^{192}Ir, a common brachytherapy and radiography source. NCRP Publication 65 was used to determine any immediate actions necessary for treatment. The bomb was thought to be a dirty bomb. The REAC training site (TS) was called for additional radiologic consultation, and it was decided that no other treatment for contamination was necessary. Radiation exposure was thought to be not acutely significant and in the "overexposure" range. All patients received follow-up with a radiation oncologist, who gave them counseling on the ramifications of their exposure. Those who were externally contaminated were also given additional counseling.

VIII. **Teaching Pearls Question(s)**
1. What federal agency is in charge in a terrorist event?
2. What is the most radiosensitive hematopoietic element?

IX. **Teaching Pearls Answer**
1. The FBI. Source: FRP (Federal Response Plan) as part of the Department of Homeland Security.
2. The lymphocyte.

REFERENCES

Andrews GA, Auxier JA, Lushbaugh CC. The importance of dosimetry to the medical management of persons accidentally exposed to high levels of ionizing radiation. In: *Personnel Dosimetry for Radiation Accidents.* International Atomic Energy Agency, 1965, p 13.

Mettler FA, Kelsey CA, Ricks RC, eds. *Medical Management of Radiation Accidents.* CRC Press, 1990, p. 72.

National Council on Radiation Protection and Measurements, *Management of Persons Accidentally Contaminated with Radionuclides,* NCRP Publication No. 65, NCRP Bethesda, MD:1980.

Nishiyama H, Lukes SJ, Saenger EL. Low-level internal radionuclide contamination: Use of gamma camera for detection, *Radiol* 1984;150:235–240.

REAC/TS (Radiological Emergency Assistance Center/Training Site) 865-441-1000 (Ask for REAC/TS response through the operator at Methodist Medical Center.) http://www.orau.gov/reacts/

Walker RI, Cerveny TJ, eds. *Medical Consequences of Nuclear Warfare,* TMM Publications, 1989:11.

VII. Laboratory Diagnosis*

Notes: The ranges of normal values are given below each test, first in conventional units such as metric (eg, milligrams per liter), and then in international units if there is a difference. Reference ranges for each laboratory may vary from the values given; therefore, you should interpret the results of a patient's laboratory value in light of an individual facility's range.

■ ACID-FAST STAIN
Positive: *Mycobacterium* spp. (*tuberculosis* and atypical mycobacteria such as *M avium-intracellulare*), *Nocardia*.

■ ACTH (ADRENOCORTICOTROPIC HORMONE)
8 AM: 20–100 pg/mL or 20–100 ng/L; midnight value: ~ 50% of AM value.
Increased: Addison's disease; ectopic ACTH production (small-cell carcinoma, pancreatic islet cell tumors, thymic tumors, renal cell carcinoma).
Decreased: Adrenal adenoma or carcinoma, nodular adrenal hyperplasia, pituitary insufficiency.

■ ACTH STIMULATION TEST
Used to help diagnose adrenal insufficiency. Cosyntropin (Cortrosyn), an ACTH analogue, is given at a dose of 0.25 mg IM or IV. Collect blood at times 0, 30, and 60 min for cortisol.
Normal response: Basal cortisol of at least 5 μg/dL, an increase of at least 7 μg/dL, and a final cortisol of 16 μg/dL at 30 min or 18 μg/dL at 60 min.
Subnormal/abnormal response: Addison's disease (primary adrenal insufficiency) and secondary adrenal insufficiency: Secondary insufficiency is caused by pituitary insufficiency or suppression by exogenous steroids. An ACTH level and pituitary stimulation tests can be used to differentiate primary from secondary adrenal insufficiency.

■ ALBUMIN, SERUM
3.5–5.0 g/dL or 35–50 g/L.
Decreased: Malnutrition, nephrotic syndrome, CF, multiple myeloma, Hodgkin's disease, leukemia, protein-losing enteropathies, chronic glomerulonephritis, cirrhosis, inflammatory bowel disease, collagen-vascular diseases, hyperthyroidism.

---

*Reproduced, with permission, from Haist SA, Robbins JB, Gomella LG, eds. *Internal Medicine On Call,* 3rd ed. McGraw-Hill, 2002.

■ ALBUMIN, URINE

Normal = < 30 mg/d.

Microalbuminuria 30–300 mg/d (a sign of early renal damage in diabetes mellitus; presence helps identify patients at risk for renal failure, neuropathy, retinopathy, and CAD. Renal function may be preserved with the use of an ACE inhibitor). Microalbuminuria can be detected by determining the albumin-to-creatinine ratio by obtaining a spot urine for albumin and creatinine. Normal is < 30 µg of albumin per milligram of creatinine, and microalbuminuria is defined as 30–300 µg of albumin per milligram of creatinine.

Note: Microalbuminuria can be seen with prolonged exercise, hematuria, fever, or prolonged upright posture.

Nephrotic proteinuria > 3.5 g/d.

■ ALDOSTERONE

Serum—supine: 3–10 g/dL or 0.083–0.28 nmol/L early AM, normal sodium intake; upright: 5–30 g/dL or 0.138–0.83 nmol/L.

Urinary—2–16 µg/24 h or 5.4–44.3 nmol/d.

Increased: Hyperaldosteronism (primary or secondary). Should confirm after oral or IV salt loading.

Decreased: Adrenal insufficiency.

■ ALKALINE PHOSPHATASE

Adult 20–70 U/L.

A γ-glutamyltransferase (GGT) is often useful in determining whether an elevated alkaline phosphatase has its origin from bone or liver. A normal GGT suggests bone origin.

Increased: Increased calcium deposition in bone (hyperparathyroidism), Paget's disease, osteoblastic bone tumors, osteomalacia, pregnancy, childhood, liver disease, and hyperthyroidism.

Decreased: Malnutrition, excess vitamin D ingestion.

■ ALPHA-FETOPROTEIN (AFP)

< 30 ng/mL or < 30 µg/L

Increased: Hepatoma, testicular tumor (embryonal carcinoma, malignant teratoma), spina bifida (in mother's serum).

■ ALT (ALANINE AMINOTRANSFERASE) (SGPT: SERUM GLUTAMIC-PYRUVIC TRANSFERASE)

8–20 U/L.

Increased: Liver disease–liver metastases, biliary obstruction, liver congestion, hepatitis (ALT is more elevated than AST in viral hepatitis; AST is more elevated than ALT in alcoholic hepatitis).

■ AMMONIA
Arterial: 15–45 µg/dL or 11–32 µmol N/L.
Increased: Hepatic encephalopathy, Reye's syndrome.

■ AMYLASE
25–125 U/L.
Increased: Acute pancreatitis, pancreatic duct obstruction (stones, stricture, tumor, sphincter of Oddi spasm), alcohol ingestion, mumps, parotiditis, renal disease, macroamylasemia, cholecystitis, peptic ulcers, intestinal obstruction, mesenteric thrombosis, after surgery (upper abdominal), ovarian cancer, ruptured ectopic pregnancy, and diabetic ketoacidosis.
Decreased: Pancreatic destruction (pancreatitis, cystic fibrosis), liver disease (hepatitis, cirrhosis).

■ ANION GAP
8–12 mmol/L.
Note: The anion gap is a calculated estimate of unmeasured anions and is used to help differentiate the cause of metabolic acidosis.
Increased (High): (> 12 mmol/L): Lactic acidosis, ketoacidosis (diabetic, alcoholic, starvation); uremia; toxins (salicylates, methanol, ethylene glycol, paraldehyde). In addition, dehydration, alkalosis, use of certain penicillins (carbenicillin), and salts of strong acids such as sodium citrate (used as a preservative in packed red blood cells) can cause a mild increase in the anion gap.
Decreased (Low): (< 8 mmol/L): Seen with bromide ingestion, hypercalcemia, hypermagnesemia, multiple myeloma, and hypoalbuminemia.

■ ANTICARDIOLIPIN ANTIBODIES
See Antiphospholipid Antibodies, p 380.

# ■ ANTINEUTROPHIL CYTOPLASMIC ANTIBODIES (ANCAS)
Negative = < 10 EV/mL.
Equivocal = 10–20 EV/mL.
Positive = > 20 EV/mL.
Antibodies to cytoplasmic components of neutrophils, seen in vasculitides.
Two types:

1. **C-ANCA (Cytoplasmic-staining ANCA).** Present in ~ 90% of patients with generalized Wegener's granulomatosis; also seen in rapidly progressive glomerulonephritis and a type of polyarteritis nodosa (microscopic). May be used to follow disease activity; also especially useful in distinguishing active disease from an infectious complication. C-ANCA is not present in other collagen-vascular diseases.

2. **P-ANCA (Perinuclear-staining ANCA).** Seen in a variety of collagen-vascular diseases such as limited Wegener's granulomatosis, polyarteritis nodosa, Goodpasture's syndrome, and other vasculitides; and also seen in several types of glomerulonephritides.

■ ANTINUCLEAR ANTIBODIES (ANA)

Negative: A useful screening test in patients with symptoms suggesting collagen-vascular disease, especially if titer is > 1:160.

Positive: SLE, drug-induced lupus (procainamide, hydralazine, isoniazid, etc), scleroderma, MCTD, RA, polymyositis, JRA (5–20%). Low titers are also seen in non-collagen-vascular disease.

Specific Immunofluorescent ANA Patterns

1. ANA Patterns
   - **Homogenous:** Nonspecific, from antibodies to deoxyribonucleoproteins (DNP) and native double-stranded DNA. Seen in SLE and a variety of other diseases. Antihistone is consistent with drug-induced lupus.
   - **Speckled:** Pattern seen in many connective tissue disorders. From antibodies to extractable nuclear antigens (ENA) including antiribonucleoproteins (anti-RNP), anti-Sm, anti-PM-1, and anti-SS. Anti-RNP is positive in MCTD and SLE. Anti-Sm is found in SLE. Anti-SS-A and anti-SS-B are seen in Sjögren's syndrome and subacute cutaneous lupus. The speckled pattern is also seen with scleroderma.
   - **Peripheral anti-ds DNA Pattern:** From antibodies to native double-stranded DNA and DNP. Seen in SLE.
   - **Nucleolar Pattern:** From antibodies to nucleolar RNA. Positive in Sjögren's syndrome and scleroderma.

2. Other Autoantibodies
   - **Antimitochondrial:** Primary biliary cirrhosis.
   - **Antismooth Muscle:** Low titers are seen in a variety of illnesses; high titers (> 1:100) are suggestive of chronic active hepatitis.
   - **Antimicrosomal:** Hashimoto's thyroiditis.

■ ANTIPHOSPHOLIPID ANTIBODIES

Note: There are two basic categories of antiphospholipid antibody: anticardiolipin and lupus anticoagulant. Both are associated with recurrent arterial or venous thrombosis or fetal demise.

Anticardiolipin antibody. Two forms: IgG, IgM.
IgG normal < 23 U.
IgM normal < 11 U.

Lupus anticoagulant
Negative = normal.
Positive = presence.
Should be suspected with an isolated elevated PTT with no other likely cause.

■ AST (ASPARTATE AMINOTRANSFERASE) (SGOT: SERUM GLUTAMIC-OXALOACETIC TRANSFERASE)

8–20 U/L.

Generally parallels changes in ALT in liver disease.

Increased: Liver disease, AMI, Reye's syndrome, muscle trauma and injection, pancreatitis, intestinal injury or surgery, factitious increase (erythromycin, opiates), burns, brain damage.

Decreased: Beriberi, DM with ketoacidosis, liver disease.

■ B$_{12}$ (VITAMIN B$_{12}$)

140–700 pg/mL or 189–516 pmol/L.

Increased: Leukemia, polycythemia vera.

Decreased: Pernicious anemia, bacterial overgrowth, dietary deficiency (rare—humans normally have 2–3 years of stores), malabsorption, pregnancy.

■ BASE EXCESS/DEFICIT

See Table VII–1, p 381. A decrease in base (bicarbonate) is termed *base deficit;* an increase in base is termed *base excess.*

Excess: Metabolic alkalosis, respiratory acidosis (see Section I, 2. Acid–Base Disorders, p 7).

Deficit: Metabolic acidosis, respiratory alkalosis (see Section I, 2. Acid–Base Disorders, p 7 also see Table VII-2, p 382).

■ BENCE JONES PROTEINS—URINE

Negative: Normal.

Positive: Multiple myeloma, idiopathic Bence Jones proteinuria.

TABLE VII–1. NORMAL BLOOD GAS VALUES.

Measurement	Arterial	Mixed Venous[a]	Venous
pH (range)	7.40 (7.36–7.44)	7.36 (7.31–7.41)	7.36 (7.31–7.41)
pO$_2$ (decreases with age)	80–100 mm Hg	35–40 mm Hg	30–50 mm Hg
pCO$_2$	36–44 mm Hg	41–51 mm Hg	40–52 mm Hg
O$_2$ saturation (decreases with age)	>95%	60–80%	60–80%
HCO$_3^-$	22–26 mmol/L	22–26 mmol/L	22–29 mmol/L
Base difference (deficit/excess)	−2 to +2	−2 to +2	−2 to +2

[a]From right atrium.

Source: Modified and reproduced with permission from Gomella LG, ed. *Clinician's Pocket Reference.* 9th ed. McGraw-Hill; 2002.

■ BICARBONATE (SERUM HCO₃⁻)

22–29 mmol/L.

See Tables VII–1 and VII–2. Also see Carbon Dioxide, Arterial, p 384, for pCO₂ values.

Increased: Metabolic alkalosis, compensation for respiratory acidosis. See Section I, 2. Acid–Base Disorders, p 7.

Decreased: Metabolic acidosis, compensation for respiratory alkalosis. See Section I, 2. Acid–Base Disorders, p 7.

■ BILIRUBIN

Total: < 0.2–1.0 mg/dL or 3.4–17.1 µmol/L;

Direct: < 0.2 mg/dL or < 3.4 µmol/L;

Indirect: < 0.8 mg/dL or < 13.7 µmol/L.

Increased Total: Hepatic damage (hepatitis, toxins, cirrhosis), biliary obstruction (gallstone or tumor), hemolysis, fasting.

Increased Direct (Conjugated): Biliary obstruction (gallstone, tumor, stricture), drug-induced cholestasis, Dubin—Johnson syndrome, and Rotor's syndrome.

Increased Indirect (Unconjugated): Hemolytic anemia (transfusion reaction, sickle cell, collagen-vascular disease), Gilbert's disease, Crigler–Najjar syndrome.

■ BLEEDING TIME

Duke, Ivy: < 6 min; Template: < 10 min.

Increased: Thrombocytopenia, thrombocytopenic purpura, von Willebrand's disease, defective platelet function (aspirin, NSAIDs, uremia).

TABLE VII–2. ACID–BASE DISORDERS WITH APPROPRIATE COMPENSATION.

Disorder	Changes in Normal Values		
	pH	HCO₃⁻	pCO₂
Metabolic acidosis	↓	↓↓	↓
Metabolic alkalosis	↑	↑↑	↑
Acute respiratory acidosis	↓	slight↑	↑↑
Chronic respiratory acidosis	slight↓	↑	↑↑
Acute respiratory alkalosis	↑	slight↓	↓↓
Chronic respiratory alkalosis	slight↑	↓	↓↓

Source: Reproduced with permission from Haist SA, Robbins JB, Gomella LG, eds. *Internal Medicine On Call,* 3rd ed. McGraw-Hill, 2002.

■ BLOOD GAS, ARTERIAL

See Tables VII–1 and VII–2, p 381, 382. For acid–base disorders, see Section I, 2. Acid–Base Disorders, p 7.

■ BLOOD GAS, VENOUS

See Table VII–1, p 381. **Note:** There is little difference between arterial and venous pH and bicarbonate (except with CHF and shock); therefore, the venous blood gas may be occasionally used to assess acid–base status, but venous oxygen levels are significantly lower than arterial levels.

■ BLOOD UREA NITROGEN (BUN)

7–18 mg/dL or 1.2–3.0 mmol urea/L.

Increased: Renal failure, prerenal azotemia (decreased renal perfusion secondary to CHF, shock, volume depletion), postrenal obstruction, gastrointestinal bleeding, hypercatabolic states.

Decreased: Starvation, malnutrition, liver failure (hepatitis, drugs), pregnancy, infancy, nephrotic syndrome, overhydration.

■ BLOOD UREA NITROGEN/CREATININE RATIO

Between 10 and 20:1.

Elevated Ratio (> 20:1): CHF, dehydration, GI bleeding, increased protein intake, drugs such as tetracycline and steroids. Infection (sepsis), high fevers, burns, cachexia.

Decreased Ratio: (< 10:1): Acute tubular necrosis, low-protein diet, starvation, malnutrition, liver disease, SIADH, pregnancy, and rhabdomyolysis.

Note: The ratio may not be appropriate if the patient is in DKA or receiving drugs such as cephalosporin.

The ratio can be altered by interferences in the chemical methods used to measure the creatinine or the BUN, resulting in spurious results. The presence of ketones may seriously elevate the serum creatinine level. Drugs such as cephalosporins, ascorbic acid, and barbiturates may also interfere with the serum creatinine measurement.

■ CALCITONIN

< 100 pg/mL or < 100 g/L.

Increased: Medullary carcinoma of the thyroid, pregnancy, chronic renal insufficiency, Zollinger–Ellison syndrome, pernicious anemia.

■ CALCIUM, SERUM

8.4–10.2 mg/dL (4.2–5.1 mEq/L) or 2.10–2.55 mmol/L;
Ionized: 4.5–4.9 mg/dL (2.2–2.5 mEq/L) or 1.1–1.2 mmol/L.

Note: To interpret a total calcium value, you must know the albumin level. If the albumin is not within normal limits, a corrected calcium can be roughly calculated with the following formula. Values for ionized calcium need no special correction.

Increased: See Section IX, Fluids and Electrolytes, p 479.
Decreased: See Section IX, Fluids and Electrolytes, p 479.

■ CALCIUM, URINE

Average calcium diet: 100–300 mg per 24-h urine.

Increased: Hyperparathyroidism, hyperthyroidism, hypervitaminosis D, distal renal tubular acidosis (type I), sarcoidosis, immobilization, osteolytic lesions (bony metastasis, multiple myeloma), Paget's disease, glucocorticoid excess (either endogenous or exogenous), furosemide.

Decreased: Thiazide diuretics, hypothyroidism, renal failure, steatorrhea, rickets, osteomalacia.

■ CARBON DIOXIDE, ARTERIAL (PCO₂)

36–44 mm Hg. See Tables VII–1 and VII–2, p 381.

Increased: Respiratory acidosis, compensation for metabolic alkalosis. See Section I, 2. Acid–Base Disorders, p 7.

Decreased: Respiratory alkalosis, compensation for metabolic acidosis. See Section I, 2. Acid–Base Disorders, p 7.

■ CARBOXYHEMOGLOBIN

Nonsmoker: < 2%.
Smoker: < 6%.
Toxic: > 15%.

Increased: Smoking, smoke inhalation; exposure to automobile exhaust, faulty heating units with inadequate ventilation.

■ CARCINOEMBRYONIC ANTIGEN (CEA)

Nonsmoker: < 3.0 g/mL or < 3.0 µg/L;
Smoker: < 5.0 g/mL or < 5.0 µg/L.

Increased: Carcinoma (colon, pancreas, lung, stomach), smokers, non-neoplastic liver disease, Crohn's disease, and ulcerative colitis. Test used predominantly to monitor patients for recurrence of carcinoma, especially after colon carcinoma resection.

■ CATECHOLAMINES, FRACTIONATED

Note: Values are variable and depend on the lab and method of assay used. Normal levels listed in Table VII–3 are based on high-performance liquid chromatography technique.

TABLE VII–3. FRACTIONATED CATECHOLAMINES.

Catecholamine	Plasma (Supine)	Urine
Norepinephrine	70–750 pg/mL	14–80 µg/24-h
	414–4435 pmol/L	82.7–473 nmol/L/d
Epinephrine	0–100 pg/mL	0.5–20 µg/24-h
	0–100 pg/mL	2.73–109 nmol/d
Dopamine	<30 pg/mL	65–400 µg/24-h
	<196 pmol/L	424–2612 nmol/d

Source: Reproduced with permission from Haist SA, Robbins JB, Gomella LG, eds. *Internal Medicine On Call,* 3rd ed. McGraw-Hill, 2002.

Increased: Pheochromocytoma, neural crest tumors (neuroblastoma). In extraadrenal pheochromocytoma, norepinephrine may be markedly elevated compared with epinephrine.

■ CATECHOLAMINES, URINE, UNCONJUGATED
> 15 years old: < 100 µg/24 h.
Measures free (unconjugated) epinephrine, norepinephrine, and dopamine.
Increased: Pheochromocytoma, neural crest tumors (neuroblastoma).

■ CBC (COMPLETE BLOOD COUNT, HEMOGRAM)
Note: For normal values, see Table VII–4. For differential, see specific tests.

■ CHLORIDE, SERUM
98–106 mEq/L.
Increased: Metabolic nongap acidosis such as diarrhea, renal tubular acidosis, mineralocorticoid deficiency, hyperalimentation, medications (acetazolamide, ammonium chloride).
Decreased: Vomiting, DM with ketoacidosis, mineralocorticoid excess, renal disease with sodium loss.

■ CHLORIDE, URINE
110–250 mmol per 24-h urine.
See Urinary Electrolytes, p 413.

■ CHOLESTEROL (TOTAL)
140–240 mg/dL or 3.63–6.22 mmol/L.
Desired level: < 200 mg/dL or 5.18 mmol/L.
Increased: Primary hypercholesterolemia (types IIA, IIB, III), elevated triglycerides (types I, IV, V), biliary obstruction, nephrosis, hypothyroidism, diabetes mellitus, pregnancy.

TABLE VII–4. NORMAL CBC VALUES—ADULTS.[a]

WBC	4800–10,800 cells/μL
RBCs	M: 4.7–6.1 × 10^6 cells/μL
	F: 4.2–5.4 × 10^6 cells/μL
Hemoglobin	M: 14–18 g/dL
	F: 12–16 g/dL
Hematocrit	M: 40–54%
	F: 37–47%
MCV	M: 80–94 IL
	F: 81–99 IL
MCH	27–31 pg
MCHC (%)	33–37%
RDW	11.5–14.5
Platelets	150,000–450,000/μL
Differential	
Segmented neutrophils	41–71%
Banded (stab) neutrophils	5–10%
Lymphocytes	24–44%
Monocytes	3–7%
Eosinophils	1–3%
Basophils	0–1%

[a] Refer to hospital reference values.
Source: Modified and reproduced with permission from Gomella LG, ed. *Clinician's Pocket Reference,* 9th ed. McGraw-Hill; 2002.

Decreased: Chronic liver disease, hyperthyroidism, malnutrition (cancer, starvation), myeloproliferative disorders, steroid therapy, lipoproteinemias.

High-Density Lipoprotein (HDL) Cholesterol

Fasting male: 40–60 mg/dL or 0.78–1.81 mmol/L.
Fasting female: 40–60 mg/dL or 0.78–2.07 mmol/L.
Note: HDL highly correlates with the development of CAD; a decreased HDL (< 35 mg/dL) leads to an increased risk, and an increased HDL (> 65 mg/dL) is associated with a decreased risk.
Increased: Estrogen (females), exercise, ethanol.
Decreased: Male gender, β-blockers, anabolic steroids, uremia, obesity, diabetes, liver disease, Tangier disease.

Low-Density Lipoprotein (LDL) Cholesterol

Desired: < 130–160 mg/dL or 3.36–4.14 mmol/L. In the presence of CAD or DM, desired LDL is < 100 mg/dL or 2.58 mmol/L.
Increased: Excess dietary saturated fats, MI, hyperlipoproteinemia, biliary cirrhosis, endocrine disease (diabetes, hypothyroidism).
Decreased: Malabsorption, severe liver disease, abetalipoproteinemia.

Triglycerides

See Triglycerides, p 409.

# ■ COLD AGGLUTININS
Normal = < 1:32.
Increased: *Mycoplasma* pneumonia; viral infections (especially mononucleosis, measles, mumps); cirrhosis; some parasitic infections.

■ COMPLEMENT C3
80–155 mg/dL or 800–1550 ng/L;
> 60 years: 80–170 mg/dL or 80–1700 ng/L.
Note: Normal values may vary greatly depending on the assay used.
Increased: Rheumatic fever, neoplasms (GI, prostate, others).
Decreased: SLE, glomerulonephritis (poststreptococcal and membranoproliferative), vasculitis, severe hepatic failure.
Variable: RA.

■ COMPLEMENT C4
20–50 mg/dL or 200–500 ng/L.
Increased: Neoplasia (GI, lung, others).
Decreased: SLE, chronic active hepatitis, cirrhosis, glomerulonephritis, hereditary angioedema.
Variable: RA.

■ COMPLEMENT CH50 (TOTAL)
33–61 mg/mL or 330–610 ng/L. Tests for complement deficiency in the classical pathway.
Increased: Acute-phase reactants (eg, tissue injury, infections).
Decreased: Hereditary complement deficiencies, any cause of deficiency of individual complement components. See Complement C3, and Complement C4.

■ COOMBS'S TEST, DIRECT
Uses patient's erythrocytes; tests for the presence of antibody or complement on the patient's red blood cells.
Positive: Autoimmune hemolytic anemia (leukemia, lymphoma, collagenvascular diseases, eg, SLE); hemolytic transfusion reaction; sensitization to some drugs (methyldopa, levodopa, penicillins, cephalosporins).

■ COOMBS'S TEST, INDIRECT
More useful for RBC typing. Uses serum that contains antibody from the patient.
Positive: Isoimmunization from previous transfusion, incompatible blood as a result of improper cross-matching.

■ CORTISOL

Serum—8 AM: 5.0–23.0 µg/dL or 138–635 nmol/L; 4 PM: 3.0–15.0 µg/dL or 83–414 nmol/L.

Urine (24-h): 10–100 µg/d or 27.6–276 nmol/d.

Increased: Adrenal adenoma, adrenal carcinoma, Cushing's disease, non-pituitary ACTH-producing tumor, steroid therapy, oral contraceptives.

Decreased: Primary adrenal insufficiency (Addison's disease), Waterhouse–Friderichsen syndrome, ACTH deficiency.

■ CORTROSYN STIMULATION TEST

See ACTH Stimulation Test, p 377.

■ COUNTERIMMUNOELECTROPHORESIS (CIE)

Normal = negative.

CIE is an immunologic technique that allows rapid identification of infectious organisms from body fluids, including serum, urine, CSF, and others. Organisms that can be identified include *Neisseria meningitidis, Streptococcus pneumoniae, Haemophilus influenzae,* and group B streptococcus.

■ C-PEPTIDE

Fasting: = 4.0 g/mL or = 4.0 µg/L;
male > 60 years: 1.5–5.0 g/mL or 1.5–5.0 µg/L;
female: 1.4–5.5 g/mL or 1.4–5.5 µg/L.

Decreased: Diabetes (IDDM), insulin administration, hypoglycemia.

Increased: Insulinoma. Test is useful to differentiate insulinoma from surreptitious use of insulin as a cause of hypoglycemia.

■ C-REACTIVE PROTEIN (CRP)

Normal: < 8 mg/L.

An acute-phase reactant with a relatively short half-life.

Increased: Infections (increase in bacterial infections > increase in viral infections); tissue injury or necrosis (AMI, malignant disease [especially lung, breast, and GI] and organ rejection following transplantation); and inflammatory disorders (RA, SLE, inflammatory bowel disease, and vasculitides).

■ CREATINE PHOSPHOKINASE (CK)

25–145 mU/mL or 25–145 U/L.

Increased: Cardiac muscle (AMI, myocarditis, defibrillation); skeletal muscle (intramuscular injection, hypothyroidism, rhabdomyolysis, polymyositis, muscular dystrophy); cerebral infarction.

CK isoenzymes MM, MB, BB: MB (normal < 6%) increased in AMI (increases in 4–8 h, peaks at 24 h), cardiac surgery; BB not useful.

◼ CREATININE CLEARANCE (CRCL)

Male: 100–135 mL/min or 0.963–1.300 mL/s/m².
Female: 85–125 mL/min or 0.819–1.204 mL/s/m².

A concurrent serum creatinine and a 24-h urine creatinine are needed. A shorter time interval can be used and corrected for in the formula. A quick formula for estimation is also found in Table A–24, Aminoglycoside Dosing, p 678.

To verify if the urine sample is a complete 24-h collection, determine if the sample contains at least 14–26 mg/kg/24 h or 124–230 mmol/kg/d creatinine for adult males; or 11–20 mg/kg/24 h or 97–177 mmol/kg/d for adult females. This test is not a requirement.

Decreased: A decreased CrCl results in an increase in serum creatinine, usually secondary to renal insufficiency. Clearance normally decreases with age. See Creatinine, Serum, Increased, p 389.

Increased: Pregnancy, prediabetic renal failure.

◼ CREATININE, SERUM

Male: 0.7–1.3 mg/dL.
Female: 0.6–1.1 mg/dL.

Increased: Renal failure (prorenal, renal, or postrenal), acromegaly, ingestion of roasted meat, large body mass. Falsely elevated with ketones and certain cephalosporins, depending on assay.

◼ CREATININE, URINE

Male total creatinine: 14–26 mg/kg/24 h or 124–230 µmol/kg/d.
Female: 11–20 mg/kg/24 h or 97–177 µmol/kg/d. See Creatinine Clearance, p 389.

◼ CRYOCRIT

≤ 0.4%. (Negative if qualitative.) Cryocrit, a quantitative measure, is preferred over the qualitative method. It should be collected in nonanticoagulated tubes and transported at body temperature. Positive samples can be analyzed for immunoglobulin class, and light-chain type on request.

> 0.4%. (Positive if qualitative.) *Monoclonal*—Multiple myeloma, Waldenström's macroglobulinemia, lymphoma, chronic lymphocytic leukemia.

Mixed polyclonal or mixed monoclonal—Infectious diseases (viral, bacterial, parasitic), eg, SBE or malaria, SLE, RA, essential cryoglobulinemia, lymphoproliferative diseases, sarcoidosis, chronic liver disease (cirrhosis).

◼ DEXAMETHASONE SUPPRESSION TEST

Used in the differential diagnosis of Cushing's syndrome.

Overnight Dexamethasone Suppression Test

In the rapid version of this test, the patient takes dexamethasone 1 mg PO at 11 PM; a fasting 8 AM plasma cortisol is obtained. Normally, the cortisol level should be < 5 μg/dL or < 138 nmol/L. A value > 5 μg/dL or > 138 nmol/L suggests the diagnosis of Cushing's syndrome; however, suppression may not occur with concomitant obesity, alcoholism, or depression. In these patients, the best screening test is a 24-h urine for free cortisol.

Low-Dose Dexamethasone Suppression Test

After collection of baseline serum cortisol and 24-h urine free cortisol levels, dexamethasone 0.5 mg PO is administered q6h for eight doses. Serum cortisol and 24-h urine for free cortisol are repeated on the second day. Failure to suppress to a serum cortisol of < 5 μg/dL (138 nmol/L) and a urine free cortisol < 30 μg/dL (82 nmol/L) confirms the diagnosis of Cushing's syndrome.

High-Dose Dexamethasone Suppression Test

If the low-dose test is positive, dexamethasone 2 mg PO q6h for eight doses is administered. A fall in urinary free cortisol to 50% of the baseline value occurs in patients with Cushing's disease but not in patients with adrenal tumors or ectopic ACTH production.

■ ERYTHROPOIETIN (EPO)

Normal = 5–30 mU/mL.

There is an inverse relationship between erythropoietin and hematocrit.

Decreased or normal levels: Myelodysplastic syndrome, polycythemia vera, chronic renal disease, early pregnancy, and in preterm infants.

Increased: AZT-treated HIV infection, normocytic anemia, and microcytic anemia.

RIA measurement detects erythropoietin in both the active and inactive forms, whereas the mouse bioassay assesses functional hormones.

■ ETHANOL LEVEL

See Nonantibiotic Drug Levels, Table A–22, p 677.

■ FERRITIN

Male: 15–200 ng/mL or 15–220 μg/L.

Female: 12–150 ng/mL or 12–150 μg/L.

Decreased: Iron deficiency, severe liver disease.

Increased: Hemochromatosis, hemosiderosis, sideroblastic anemia, any inflammatory process (acute-phase reactant).

FIBRIN DEGRADATION PRODUCTS (FDP)
< 10 µg/mL.
Increased: Any thromboembolic condition (DVT, MI, PE); DIC; hepatic dysfunction.

FIBRINOGEN
150–450 mg/dL or 150–450 g/L.
Decreased: Congenital; DIC (sepsis, amniotic fluid embolism, abruptio placentae, prostatic or cardiac surgery); burns; neoplastic and hematologic malignancies; acute severe bleeding; snake bite.
Increased: Inflammatory processes (acute-phase reactant).

FOLATE RED BLOOD CELL
160–640 ng or 360–1450 nmol/mL RBC.
More sensitive for detecting folate deficiency from malnourishment if the patient has started proper nutrition before the serum folate is measured (even one well-balanced hospital meal).
Increased: See Folic Acid (Serum Folate), p 391.
Decreased: See Folic Acid.

FOLIC ACID (SERUM FOLATE)
2–14 ng/mL or 4.5–31.7 nmol/L.
Increased: Folic acid administration.
Decreased: Malnutrition, malabsorption, massive cellular growth (cancer), hemolytic anemia, pregnancy.

FTA-ABS (FLUORESCENT TREPONEMAL ANTIBODY ABSORBED)
Nonreactive.
Positive: Syphilis (test of choice to confirm diagnosis). May be negative in early primary syphilis; may remain positive after adequate treatment.

FUNGAL SEROLOGIES
Negative (< 1:8). Complement-fixation fungal antibody screen that usually detects antibodies to *Histoplasma, Blastomyces, Aspergillus,* and *Coccidioides.*

GAMMA-GLUTAMYLTRANSFERASE (GGT)
Male: 9–50 U/L.
Female: 8–40 U/L. Generally parallels changes in serum alkaline phosphatase and 5'-nucleotidase in liver disease.
Increased: Liver disease (hepatitis, cirrhosis, obstructive jaundice); pancreatitis.

■ GASTRIN

Male: < 100 pg/mL or < 100 ng/L.
Female: < 75 pg/mL or < 100 ng/L.
Increased: Zollinger–Ellison syndrome, pyloric stenosis, pernicious anemia, atrophic gastritis, ulcerative colitis, renal insufficiency, steroid and calcium administration.

■ GLUCOSE

Fasting: 70–105 mg/dL or 3.89–5.83 nmol/L.
2 h postprandial: 70–120 mg/dL or 3.89–6.67 mmol/L.
Increased: See Section I, 23. Diabetic Problems, p 75.
Decreased: See Section I, 23. Diabetic Problems, p 75.

■ GLYCOHEMOGLOBIN (HEMOGLOBIN A$_{1C}$)

4.0–6.0%.
Increased: Poorly controlled DM.

■ GRAM'S STAIN

Rapid Technique

Spread a thin layer of specimen onto glass slide and allow to dry. Fix with heat. Apply gentian violet (15–20 s); follow with iodine (15–20 s), then alcohol (just a few seconds until effluent is barely decolorized). Rinse with water and counterstain with safranin (15–20 s). Examine under oil immersion lens: gram-positive bacteria are dark blue and gram-negatives are red.

Gram-Positive Cocci: *Staphylococcus, Streptococcus, Enterococcus, Micrococcus, Peptococcus* (anaerobic), and *Peptostreptococcus* (anaerobic) spp.

Gram-Positive Rods: *Clostridium* (anaerobic), *Corynebacterium, Listeria,* and *Bacillus.*

Gram-Negative Cocci: *Neisseria, Branhamella, Moraxella, Acinetobacter* spp.

Gram-Negative Coccoid Rods: *Haemophilus, Pasteurella, Brucella, Francisella, Yersinia,* and *Bordetella* species.

Gram-Negative Straight Rods: *Acinetobacter* (*Mima, Herellea*), *Aeromonas, Bacteroides* (anaerobic), *Campylobacter* (comma-shaped) spp, *Eikenella, Enterobacter, Escherichia, Fusobacterium* (anaerobic), *Helicobacter, Klebsiella, Legionella* (small, pleomorphic; weakly staining), *Proteus, Providencia, Pseudomonas, Salmonella, Serratia, Shigella, Vibrio, Yersinia.*

■ HAPTOGLOBIN

26–185 mg/mL.
Increased: Obstructive liver disease; any inflammatory process.
Decreased: Hemolysis (eg, transfusion reaction); severe liver disease.

■ *HELICOBACTER* ANTIBODIES

Normal = negative.

Serologic test to detect antibodies to *Helicobacter pylori* in patients with peptic ulcer disease. High titers of IgG to *Helicobacter* are indicative of *H pylori* infection (sensitivity > 95% and specificity > 95%). More sensitive than biopsy for detecting presence of *H pylori*. It may take 6 months or longer for antibodies to decline appreciably after treatment.

■ HEMATOCRIT

See Table VII–4, p 386, for normal values.
Increased: See Section I, 10. Bleeding Problems, p 32.
Decreased: See Section I, 10. Bleeding Problems, p 32.

■ HEMOGLOBIN

See Table VII–4, p 386, for normal values.
Increased: See Section I, 10. Bleeding Problems, p 32.
Decreased: See Section I, 10. Bleeding Problems, p 32.

■ HEPATITIS TESTS

Table VII–5, p 394.

- **HBsAg:** Hepatitis B surface antigen (formerly Australia antigen). Indicates either chronic or acute infection with hepatitis B. Used by blood banks to screen donors.
- **Total Anti-HBc:** IgG and IgM antibody to hepatitis B core antigen. Confirms either previous exposure to hepatitis B virus (HBV) or ongoing infection. Used by blood banks to screen donors.
- **Anti-HBc IgM:** IgM antibody to hepatitis B core antigen. Early and best indicator of acute infection with hepatitis B.
- **HBeAg:** Hepatitis B$_e$ antigen. When present, indicates high degree of infectiousness. Order *only* when evaluating a patient with *chronic* HBV infection.
- **Anti-HBe:** Antibody to hepatitis B$_e$ antigen. Order with HBeAg. Presence is associated with resolution of active inflammation; but often means virus is integrated into host DNA, especially if host remains HBsAg positive.
- **Anti-HBs:** Antibody to hepatitis B surface antigen. Typically indicates immunity associated with clinical recovery from an HBV infection or previous immunization with hepatitis B vaccine. Order *only* to assess effectiveness of vaccine.
- **HBV-DNA:** Detects presence of viral DNA in serum (pg/mL) quantitatively to confirm infection and assess therapy. Very expensive assay.
- **Anti-HAV:** Total antibody to hepatitis A virus. Confirms previous exposure to hepatitis A virus.

TABLE VII–5. HEPATITIS PANEL TESTING.

Profile Name	Tests	Purpose
■ **Screening**		
Admission: High-risk patients (homosexuals, IV drug users, dialysis patients)	HBsAg Anti-HCV	To screen for chronic or active infection.
All pregnant women	HBsAg	To screen for chronic or active infection.
Percutaneous inoculation	HBsAg Anti-HCV	Test serum of patient (if known) for possible infectivity. Start Hep B vaccination if health care worker not previously immunized.
	Anti-HBs	Determine if vaccinated health care worker is immune and protected.
Pre-HBV vaccine in high-risk patients	HBsAg Anti-HBc	To determine if an individual is infected or already has antibodies and is immune.
■ **Diagnosis**		
Differential diagnosis of acute hepatitis	Anti-HAV IgM HBsAg Anti-HBc IgM Anti-HCV	To differentiate between hepatitis A, hepatitis B and hepatitis C (Anti-HCV may take 4–8 weeks to become positive)
Differential diagnosis of chronic hepatitis (Abnormal LFTs)	HBsAg Anti-HCV (and RIBA or HCV RNA if Anti-HCV is positive)	To rule out chronic hepatitis B or C as a cause of chronically elevated LFTs.
■ **Monitoring**		
Chronic hepatitis B	LFTs HBsAg HBeAg/Anti-HBe Anti-HDV IgM α-fetoprotein HBV DNA	To test for activity, late seroconversion or disease latency in known hepatitis B carrier, superinfection with HDV, development of hepatoma, or resolution of infection after therapy or spontaneously.
Chronic hepatitis C	LFTs HCV RNA α-fetoprotein	To test for activity of hepatitis, likelihood of response to interferon or development of hepatoma
Postvaccination screening	Anti-HBs	To ensure immunity after vaccination
Sexual contact	HBsAg	To monitor sexual partners with acute or chronic hepatitis B

Source: Reproduced with permission from Haist SA, Robbins JB, Gomella LG, eds. *Internal Medicine On Call,* 3rd ed. McGraw-Hill, 2002.

- **Anti-HAV IgM:** IgM antibody to hepatitis A virus. Indicates recent acute infection with hepatitis A virus.
- **Anti-HDV:** Total antibody to delta-agent hepatitis. Confirms previous exposure. Order *only* in patients with known chronic HBV infection.
- **Anti-HDV IgM:** IgM antibody to delta-agent hepatitis. Indicates recent infection. Order *only* in patients with known chronic HBV infection.
- **Anti-HCV:** Antibody against hepatitis C (formerly known as non-A non-B hepatitis). Order to evaluate both acute and chronic hepatitis. Has a low false-positive rate. Used by blood banks to screen donors.
- **Anti-HCV RIBA:** Measures antibody to four separate HCV antigens. Used to confirm positive anti-HCV test.
- **HCV-RNA:** Detects presence of virus by either sensitive RT-PCR or quantitatively by branched DNA. Confirms infection or response to therapy. Very expensive assay.

■ 5-HIAA (5-HYDROXYINDOLEACETIC ACID)
2–8 mg or 10.4–41.6 µmol/24-h urine collection. 5-HIAA is a serotonin metabolite.
Increased: Carcinoid tumors; certain foods (banana, pineapple, tomato).

■ *HISTOPLASMA CAPSULATUM* ANTIGEN, URINE
< 1.0 units/mL
Elevated in disseminated histoplasmosis, less commonly elevated in localized pulmonary *Histoplasma* infections. The most sensitive and rapid diagnostic test available for disseminated histoplasmosis in AIDS patients. After amphotericin B treatment, levels fall to low or nondetectable range. Increase in measurement indicates relapse.

■ HOMOCYSTEINE
5–18 mmol/mL.
Increased: Arteriosclerotic vascular disease, DVT, pregnancy complicated by neural tube defects.
Increases with aging, smoking, and many drugs.

■ HUMAN CHORIONIC GONADOTROPIN, SERUM (HCG BETA SUBUNIT)
< 3.0 mIU/mL;
7–10 days postconception: > 3 mIU/mL; 30 days: 100–5000 mIU/mL;
10 weeks: 50,000–140,000 mIU/mL; > 16 weeks: 10,000–50,000 mIU/mL; thereafter: levels slowly decline.
Increased: Pregnancy, testicular tumors, trophoblastic disease (hydatidiform mole, choriocarcinoma levels usually > 100,000 mIU/mL).

■ HUMAN IMMUNODEFICIENCY VIRUS (HIV) ANTIBODY TEST

Negative: Used in the diagnosis of AIDS and HIV infection and to screen blood for use in transfusion. May be negative in early HIV infection.

ELISA (Enzyme-Linked Immunosorbent Assay)

Used to detect HIV antibody. A positive test is usually repeated and then confirmed by Western blot analysis.

Positive: AIDS, asymptomatic HIV infection, false-positive test.

Western Blot

The technique used as the reference procedure for confirming the presence or absence of HIV antibody, usually after a positive HIV antibody by ELISA determination.

Positive: AIDS, asymptomatic HIV infection.

Note: PCR is becoming a useful tool for detection of the HIV virus. It will be especially useful in very early infection, when antibody may not be present.

■ INTERNATIONAL NORMALIZED RATIO (INR)

See also Prothrombin Time, p 405.

Normal = 1.0.

The INR is used to standardize prothrombin results in patients taking anticoagulants.

- **INR 2–3:** Therapeutic range for most indications, including AF, DVT, PE, and TIA.
- **INR 3.0–4.0:** Prevention of arterial thromboembolism with mechanical valves. This range may also be required in hypercoagulable states, or in recurrent arterial or venous thromboembolic disease.

■ IRON

Males: 65–175 µg/dL or 11.64–31.33 µmol/L.

Females: 50–170 µg/dL or 8.95–30.43 µmol/L.

Increased: Hemochromatosis, hemosiderosis caused by excessive iron intake, excess destruction or decreased production of erythrocytes, liver necrosis.

Decreased: Iron deficiency anemia, nephrosis (loss of iron-binding proteins), anemia of chronic disease.

■ IRON BINDING CAPACITY, TOTAL (TIBC)

250–450 µg/dL or 44.75–80.55 µmol/L.

The normal iron/TIBC ratio is 20–50%; < 15% is characteristic of iron deficiency anemia. An increased ratio is seen with hemochromatosis.

Increased: Acute and chronic blood loss, iron deficiency anemia, hepatitis, oral contraceptives.

Decreased: Anemia of chronic disease, cirrhosis, nephrosis, hemochromatosis.

17-KETOGENIC STEROIDS (17-KGS)
Males: 5–23 mg or 17–80 µmol/24-h urine;
Females: 3–15 mg or 10–52 µmol/24-h urine.
Increased: Adrenal hyperplasia.
Decreased: Panhypopituitarism, Addison's disease, acute steroid withdrawal.

17-KETOSTEROIDS (17-KS)
Males: 9–22 mg or 31–76 µmol/24-h urine;
Females: 6–15 mg or 21–52 µmol/24-h urine.
Increased: Cushing's syndrome, 11- and 21-hydroxylase deficiency, severe stress, exogenous steroids, excess ACTH or androgens.
Decreased: Addison's disease, anorexia nervosa, panhypopituitarism.

■ KOH PREP
Negative: Normal.
Positive: Superficial mycoses (*Candida, Trichophyton, Microsporum, Epidermophyton, Keratinomyces*).

■ LACTATE DEHYDROGENASE (LDH)
45–100 U/L.
Increased: AMI, cardiac surgery, hepatitis, pernicious anemia, malignant tumors, PE, hemolysis, renal infarction.

LACTIC ACID (LACTATE)
4.5–19.8 mg/dL or 0.5–2.2 mmol/L.
Increased: In hypoxia, hemorrhage, circulatory collapse, sepsis, cirrhosis, with exercise.

LEUKOCYTE ALKALINE PHOSPHATASE SCORE (LAP SCORE)
70–140.
Increased: Leukemoid reaction, Hodgkin's disease, polycythemia vera, myeloproliferative disorders, pregnancy, liver disease, acute inflammation.
Decreased: Chronic myelogenous leukemia, pernicious anemia, paroxysmal nocturnal hemoglobinuria, nephrotic syndrome.

LIGASE CHAIN REACTION FOR *NEISSERIA GONORRHOEAE* AND *CHLAMYDIA TRACHOMATIS* FOR URINE

Normal: Not detected.

This is a useful screening test for infections by these agents in populations with a high prevalence. The patient should not have voided 2 h prior to providing specimen.

LIPASE

Variable depending on the method; 10–150 U/L by turbidimetric method.

Increased: Acute pancreatitis; pancreatic duct obstruction (stone, stricture, tumor, drug-induced spasm); fat emboli. Usually normal in mumps.

LUPUS ANTICOAGULANT

See Antiphospholipid Antibodies, p 380.

LYMPHOCYTES, TOTAL

1800–3000/mL.

Used to assess nutritional status. Calculated by multiplying the WBC by the percentage of lymphocytes: < 900, severe; 900–1400, moderate; 1400–1800, minimal nutritional deficit. Lymphopenia is also seen with certain viral infections, including HIV.

MAGNESIUM

1.6–2.4 mg/dL or 0.80–1.20 mmol/L.

Increased: Renal failure, hypothyroidism, magnesium-containing antacids, Addison's disease, severe dehydration.

Decreased: Diuretics, alcoholism, renal disease, diarrhea, endocrine disease, medications, congenital.

MAGNESIUM, URINE

6.0–10.0 mEq/d or 3.00–5.00 mmol/d.

Increased: Hypermagnesemia, diuretics, hypercalcemia, metabolic acidosis, hypophosphatemia.

Decreased: Hypomagnesemia, hypocalcemia, hypoparathyroidism, metabolic alkalosis.

METANEPHRINES, URINE

Total: < 1.0 mg or 0.574 mmol/24-h urine;

Fractionated metanephrines–normetanephrines: < 0.9 mg or 0.517 mmol/24-h urine;

Fractionated metanephrines: < 0.4 mg or 0.230 mg/24-h urine.

Increased: Pheochromocytoma, neural crest tumors (neuroblastoma), false-positives with drugs (phenobarbital, hydrocortisone, others).

■ MONOSPOT
Negative: Normal.
Positive: Mononucleosis.

■ MYOGLOBIN, URINE
Qualitative negative.
Positive: Disorders affecting skeletal muscle (crush injury, rhabdomyolysis, electrical burns, delirium tremens, surgery), AMI.

■ 5′-NUCLEOTIDASE
2–15 U/L.
Increased: Obstructive liver disease.

■ OSMOLALITY, SERUM
275–295 mOsm/kg.
A rough estimation of osmolality is [2(Na) + BUN/2.8 + glucose/18]). The calculation will not be accurate if foreign substances that increase the osmolality (eg, mannitol) are present. If foreign substances are suspected, osmolality should be measured directly.
Increased: Hyperglycemia; alcohol or ethylene glycol ingestion; increased sodium resulting from water loss (diabetes insipidus, hypercalcemia, diuresis); mannitol.
Decreased: Low serum sodium, diuretics, Addison's disease, hypothyroidism, SIADH, iatrogenic causes (poor fluid balance).

■ OSMOLALITY, URINE
Spot 50–1400 mOsm/kg; > 850 mOsm/kg after 12 h of fluid restriction.
The loss of the ability to concentrate urine, especially during fluid restriction, is an early indicator of impaired renal function.

■ OXYGEN, ARTERIAL (PO₂)
See Table VII–1, p 381; see also Section IX, Ventilator Management, p 490.

Decreased:
- **Ventilation-perfusion (V/Q) abnormalities:** COPD, asthma, atelectasis, pneumonia, PE, ARDS, pneumothorax, CF, obstructed airway.
- **Alveolar hypoventilation:** Skeletal abnormalities, neuromuscular disorders, Pickwickian syndrome.
- **Decreased pulmonary diffusing capacity:** Pneumoconiosis, PE, pulmonary fibrosis.
- **Right-to-left shunt:** Congenital heart disease (tetralogy of Fallot, transposition, others).

■ PARATHYROID HORMONE (PTH)

Normal based on relationship to serum calcium, usually provided on the lab report. Also, reference values will vary depending on the laboratory and whether N-terminal, C-terminal, or midmolecule is measured.

PTH midmolecule: 0.29–0.85 ng/mL or 29–85 pmol/L with calcium 8.4–10.2 mg/dL or 2.1–2.55 mmol/L.

Increased: Primary hyperparathyroidism, secondary hyperparathyroidism (hypocalcemic states such as chronic renal failure, others).

Decreased: Hypercalcemia not resulting from hyperparathyroidism and hypoparathyroidism.

■ PARTIAL THROMBOPLASTIN TIME (PTT)

27–38 s.

Prolonged: Heparin use and any defect in the intrinsic clotting mechanism, such as severe liver disease or DIC (includes factors I, II, V, VIII, IX, X, XI, and XII); prolonged use of a tourniquet before drawing a blood sample; hemophilia A and B; lupus anticoagulant; liver disease. Also, elevated in the presence of lupus anticoagulant. See Section I, 10. Bleeding Problems, p 32.

■ PH, ARTERIAL

See Tables VII–1 and VII–2, p 381, 382.

Increased: Metabolic and respiratory alkalosis. See Section I,2. Acid–Base Disorders, p 7.

Decreased: Metabolic and respiratory acidosis. See Section I, 2. Acid–Base Disorders, p 7.

■ PHOSPHORUS

2.7–4.5 mg/dL or 0.87–1.45 mmol/L.

Increased: Hypoparathyroidism, pseudohypoparathyroidism, excess vitamin D, secondary hypoparathyroidism, acute and chronic renal failure, acromegaly, tumor lysis (lymphoma or leukemia treated with chemotherapy), alkalosis, factitious increase (hemolysis of specimen).

Decreased: Renal loss, diarrhea, malnutrition, respiratory alkalosis.

■ PLASMINOGEN

7–17 mg/dL.

Plasminogen activity: 75–140%.

Decreased: Uncommon cause of inherited thrombosis, primary and secondary fibrinolysis, liver disease, after fibrinolytic therapy.

■ PLATELETS

See Table VII–4, p 386.

Platelet counts may be normal in number, but abnormal in function (eg, aspirin therapy); platelet function with a normal platelet count can be assessed by measuring bleeding time.

Increased: Primary thrombocytosis (idiopathic myelofibrosis, agnogenic myeloid metaplasia, polycythemia vera, primary thrombocythemia, chronic myelogenous leukemia). Secondary thrombocytosis (collagen-vascular diseases, chronic infection [osteomyelitis, tuberculosis], sarcoidosis, hemolytic anemia, iron deficiency anemia, recovery from B_{12} deficiency or iron deficiency or heavy ethanol ingestion, solid tumors and lymphomas; after surgery, especially postsplenectomy; response to drugs such as epinephrine, or withdrawal of myelosuppressive drugs).

Decreased: See Section I, 10. Bleeding Problems, p 32.

■ POTASSIUM, SERUM

3.5–5.1 mmol/L.

Increased: See Section IX, Fluids and Electrolytes, p 479.

Decreased: See Section IX, Fluids and Electrolytes, p 479.

■ POTASSIUM, URINE

25–125 mmol/24-h urine; varies with diet. See Urinary Electrolytes, p 413.

■ PROLACTIN

Females: 1–25 ng/mL.

Males: 1–20 ng/mL.

Increased: Pregnancy, nursing after pregnancy, prolactinoma, hypothalamic tumors, sarcoidosis or granulomatous disease of the hypothalamus, hypothyroidism, renal failure, Addison's disease, phenothiazines, butyrophenones (eg, haloperidol [Haldol]).

Decreased: Sheehan's syndrome.

■ PROSTATE-SPECIFIC ANTIGEN (PSA)

< 4 ng/dL.

Most useful as a measure of response to therapy for prostate cancer. Also used for screening for prostate carcinoma. Values > 8.0 ng/dL are associated with carcinoma at the 90% confidence level.

Increased: Prostate cancer, some cases of benign prostatic hypertrophy, prostatic infarction, post ejaculation (returns to normal level in 48 h), vigorous exercise (returns to normal in 48–72 h).

Decreased: Total prostatectomy, response to therapy for prostatic carcinoma.

■ PROTEIN ELECTROPHORESIS, SERUM AND URINE (SERUM PROTEIN ELECTROPHORESIS [SPEP]; URINE PROTEIN ELECTROPHORESIS [UPEP])

Quantitative analysis of the serum proteins is often used in the evaluation of hypoglobulinemia, macroglobulinemia, α_1-antitrypsin deficiency, collagen disease, liver disease, myeloma, and occasionally in nutritional assessment. Serum electrophoresis yields five different bands (see Figure VII–1, p 403; and Table VII–6, p 404). If a monoclonal gammopathy or a low globulin fraction is detected, quantitative immunoglobulins should be checked.

Urine protein electrophoresis can be used to evaluate proteinuria and can detect Bence Jones (light-chain) protein that is associated with myeloma, Waldenström's macroglobulinemia, and Fanconi's syndrome.

■ PROTEIN, SERUM

6.0–7.8 g/dL or 60–78 g/L.

Increased: Multiple myeloma, Waldenström's macroglobulinemia, benign monoclonal gammopathy, lymphoma, sarcoidosis, chronic inflammatory disease.

Decreased: Any cause of decreased albumin or any cause of hypogammaglobulinemia such as common variable hypogammaglobulinemia.

■ PROTEIN, URINE

See also Albumin, Urine, p 378.

< 100 mg/24-h urine;

Spot: < 10 mg/dL (< 20 mg/dL if early-morning collection);

Dipstick: negative.

Increased: Nephrotic syndrome, glomerulonephritis, lupus nephritis, amyloidosis, renal vein thrombosis, severe CHF, multiple myeloma, preeclampsia, postural proteinuria, polycystic kidney disease, diabetic nephropathy, radiation nephritis, malignant HTN.

False-positive: Gross hematuria, very concentrated urine, Pyridium, very alkaline urine.

■ PROTEIN C, PLASMA

Normal = 60–130%.

Decreased: Hypercoagulable states resulting in recurrent venous thrombosis; chronic liver disease; DIC; postoperatively; neoplastic disease and autosomal recessive deficiency.

Figure VII–1. Protein electrophoresis patterns. Examples of (**A**) serum and (**B**) urine protein electrophoresis patterns.

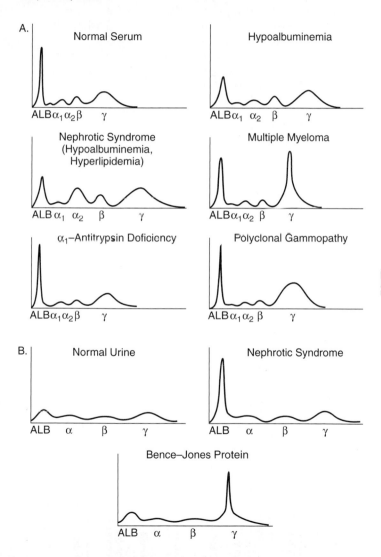

TABLE VII–6. NORMAL SERUM PROTEIN COMPONENTS AND FRACTIONS AS DETERMINED BY ELECTROPHORESIS ALONG WITH ASSOCIATED CONDITIONS.

Protein Fraction	Percentage of Total Protein	Constituents	Increased	Decreased
Albumin	52–68	Albumin	Dehydration (only known cause)	Nephrosis, malnutrition, chronic liver disease
α₁-Globulin	2.4–4.4	Thyroxine-binding globulin, antitrypsin, lipoproteins, glycoprotein, transcortin	Inflammation, neoplasia	Nephrosis, α₁-antitrypsin deficiency (emphysema-related)
α₂-Globulin	6.1–10.1	Haptoglobin, glycoprotein, macroglobulin, ceruloplasmin	Inflammation, infection, neoplasia, cirrhosis	Severe liver disease, acute hemolytic anemia
β-Globulin	8.5–14.5	Transferrin, glycoprotein, lipoprotein	Cirrhosis, obstructive jaundice	Nephrosis
γ-Globulins (immunoglobulins)	10–21	IgA, IgG, IgM, IgD, IgE	Infections, collagen-vascular diseases, leukemia, myeloma	Agammaglobulinemia, hypogammaglobulinemia, nephrosis

Reproduced, with permission, from Gomella LG, ed. *Clinician's Pocket Reference*, 9th ed.: McGraw-Hill: 2002.

■ PROTEIN S, PLASMA
Normal = 60–140%.
Decreased: See Protein C, Plasma. Protein S is a cofactor of protein C; should be ordered along with protein C.

■ PROTHROMBIN TIME (PT)
See International Normalized Ratio (INR), p 396.
11.5–13.5 s.
Evaluates extrinsic clotting mechanism (factors I, II, V, VII, and X).
Prolonged: Drugs such as sodium warfarin (Coumadin), decreased vitamin K, fat malabsorption, liver disease, prolonged use of a tourniquet before drawing a blood sample, DIC, lupus anticoagulant (usually selectively increased PTT). See Section I, 10. Bleeding Problems, p 32.

■ QUANTITATIVE IMMUNOGLOBULINS
IgG: 650–1500 mg/dL or 6.5–15 g/L;
IgM: 40–345 mg/dL or 0.4–3.45 g/L;
IgA: 76–390 mg/dL or 0.76–3.90 g/L;
IgE: 0–380 IU/mL or KIU/L;
IgD: 0–8 mg/dL or 0–80 mg/L.

Increased: Multiple myeloma (myeloma immunoglobulin increased, other immunoglobulins decreased), Waldenström's macroglobulinemia (IgM increased, others decreased), lymphoma, carcinoma, bacterial and viral infections, liver disease, sarcoidosis, amyloidosis, myeloproliferative disorders.
Decreased: Hereditary immunodeficiency, leukemia, lymphoma, nephrotic syndrome, protein-losing enteropathy, malnutrition.

■ RAPID PLASMA REAGIN (RPR)
See VDRL, p 413.

■ RED BLOOD CELL COUNT (RBC)
See Table VII–4, p 386. Also see Hematocrit, p 393.

■ RED BLOOD CELL INDICES
See Table VII–4, p 386.

MCV (Mean Cell Volume)
Increased: Megaloblastic anemia (B$_{12}$, folate deficiency), reticulocytosis, chronic liver disease, alcoholism, hypothyroidism, aplastic anemia.
Decreased: Iron deficiency, sideroblastic anemia, thalassemia, some cases of lead poisoning, hereditary spherocytosis.

MCH (Mean Cellular Hemoglobin)

Increased: Macrocytosis (megaloblastic anemias, high reticulocyte counts).
Decreased: Microcytosis (iron deficiency).

MCHC (Mean Cellular Hemoglobin Concentration)

Increased: Severe and prolonged dehydration; spherocytosis.
Decreased: Iron deficiency anemia, overhydration, thalassemia, sideroblastic anemia.

RDW (Red Cell Distribution Width)

Measure of the degree of homogenicity of RBC size.
Increased: An increase in the RDW suggests two different populations of RBCs, such as a combination of a macrocytic and microcytic anemia or recovery from iron deficiency anemia (microcytosis plus reticulocytosis).

■ RED BLOOD CELL MORPHOLOGY

Poikilocytosis: Irregular RBC shape (sickle, burr).
Anisocytosis: Irregular RBC size (microcytes, macrocytes).
Basophilic stippling: Lead, heavy metal poisoning, thalassemia.
Howell–Jolly bodies: Seen after a splenectomy and in some severe anemias.
Sickling: Sickle cell disease and trait.
Nucleated RBCs: Severe bone marrow stress (hemorrhage, hemolysis), marrow replacement by tumor, extramedullary hematopoiesis.
Target cells: Thalassemia, hemoglobinopathies (sickle cell disease), obstructive jaundice, any hypochromic anemia, after splenectomy.
Spherocytes: Hereditary spherocytosis, immune or microangiopathic hemolysis.
Helmet cells (schistocytes): Microangiopathic hemolysis, hemolytic transfusion reaction, other hemolytic anemias.
Burr cells (acanthocytes): Severe liver disease; high levels of bile, fatty acids, or toxins.
Polychromasia: Appearance of a bluish gray RBC on routine Wright's stain suggests reticulocytes.

■ RETICULOCYTE COUNT

0.5–1.5%.
If the patient's Hct is abnormal, a corrected reticulocyte count should be calculated as follows:
Increased: Hemolysis, acute hemorrhage, therapeutic response to treatment for iron, vitamin B_{12}, or folate deficiency.
Decreased: Infiltration of bone marrow by carcinoma, lymphoma, or leukemia, marrow aplasia, chronic infections such as osteomyelitis, toxins, drugs (> 100 reported), many anemias.

RHEUMATOID FACTOR (RA LATEX TEST)

< 15 IU by microscan kit or < 1:40.

Increased: RA, SLE, Sjögren's syndrome, scleroderma, dermatomyositis, polymyositis, syphilis, chronic inflammation, SBE, hepatitis, sarcoidosis, interstitial pulmonary fibrosis.

SEDIMENTATION RATE (ESR)

- **Wintrobe Scale:** Males: 0–9 mm/h;
- Females: 0–20 mm/h.
- **ZETA Scale:** 40–54%, normal; 55–59%, mildly elevated; 60–64%, moderately elevated; > 65%, markedly elevated.
- **Westergren Scale:** Males < 50 years: 15 mm/h; males > 50 years: 20 mm/h;
- Females < 50 years, 25 mm/h; females > 50 years: 30 mm/h.
- This is a very nonspecific test. The ZETA method is not affected by anemia. The Westergren scale remains the preferred method.

Increased: Infection, inflammation, rheumatic fever, endocarditis, neoplasm, AMI.

■ SGGT (SERUM GAMMA-GLUTAMYLTRANSFERASE)

See Gamma-Glutamyltransferase (GGT), p 391.

■ SGOT (SERUM GLUTAMIC-OXALOACETIC TRANSFERASE) OR AST (SERUM ASPARTATE AMINOTRANSFERASE)

See AST, p 381.

SGPT (SERUM GLUTAMIC-PYRUVIC TRANSFERASE) OR ALT (SERUM ALANINE AMINOTRANSFERASE)

See ALT, p 378.

SODIUM, SERUM

136–145 mmol/L.
Increased: See Section IX, Fluids and Electrolytes, p 479.
Decreased: See Section IX, Fluids and Electrolytes, p 479.

■ SODIUM, URINE

40–210 mmol/24-h urine. See Urinary Electrolytes, p 413.

■ STOOL FOR OCCULT BLOOD (HEMOCCULT TEST)

Negative: Normal.

Positive: Swallowed blood; ingestion of red meat; any GI tract lesion (ulcer, carcinoma, polyp); large doses of vitamin C (> 500 mg/d). See also Section I, 10. Bleeding Problems, p 32.

■ STOOL FOR WBC

Occasional WBCs, usually PMNs.

Increased: *Shigella, Salmonella,* enteropathogenic *Escherichia coli,* pseudo-membranous colitis (*Clostridium difficile*), ulcerative colitis.

■ T_3 (TRIIODOTHYRONINE) RADIOIMMUNOASSAY

120–195 ng/dL or 1.85–3.00 nmol/L.

Increased: Hyperthyroidism; T_3 thyrotoxicosis; exogenous T_4; any cause of increased TBG such as oral estrogens, pregnancy, or hepatitis.

Decreased: Hypothyroidism, euthyroid sick state, any cause of decreased TBG (eg, malnutrition).

■ T_3 RU (RESIN UPTAKE)

24–34%.

Increased: Hyperthyroidism; medications (phenytoin, anabolic steroids, corticosteroids, heparin, aspirin, others); nephrotic syndrome.

Decreased: Hypothyroidism, pregnancy, medications (estrogens, iodine, propylthiouracil, others).

■ T_4 TOTAL (THYROXINE)

5–12 µg/dL or 65–155 nmol/L.

Males: 5–10 µg/dL: 5–10 µg/dL or 65–129 nmol.

Females: 5.5–10.5 µg/dL or 71–135 nmol/L.

Increased: Hyperthyroidism; exogenous thyroid hormone; any cause of increased TBG (eg, estrogens, pregnancy, or hepatitis); euthyroid sick state.

Decreased: Hypothyroidism, euthyroid sick state, any cause of decreased thyroid-binding globulin (eg, malnutrition).

■ THROMBIN TIME

10–14 s.

Increased: Heparin, DIC, elevated fibrin degradation products, fibrinogen deficiency, congenitally abnormal fibrinogen molecules. See Section I, 10. Bleeding Problems, p 32.

■ THYROGLOBULIN

0–60 ng/mL or < 60 µg/L.

Used primarily to detect recurrence of nonmedullary thyroid carcinoma after resection.

Increased: Differentiated thyroid carcinomas (papillary, follicular), thyroid adenoma, Graves's disease, toxic goiter, nontoxic goiter, thyroiditis.
Decreased: Hypothyroidism, testosterone, steroids, phenytoin.

■ THYROID-BINDING GLOBULIN (TBG)

1.5–3.4 mg/dL or 15–34 mg/L.

Increased: Hypothyroidism, pregnancy, medications (oral contraceptives, estrogens), hepatitis, acute porphyria, familial.

Decreased: Hyperthyroidism, medications (androgens, anabolic steroids, corticosteroids, phenytoin), nephrotic syndrome, severe illness, liver failure, malnutrition.

■ THYROID-STIMULATING HORMONE (TSH)

0.7–5.3 mU/mL.

Newer sensitive assays are excellent screening tests for hyperthyroidism as well as hypothyroidism; they allow you to distinguish between a low normal and a decreased TSH.

Increased: Hypothyroidism.

Decreased: Hyperthyroidism. Fewer than 1% of cases of hypothyroidism are from pituitary or hypothalamic disease resulting in a decreased TSH.

■ TRANSFERRIN

220–400 mg/dL or 2.20–4.00 g/L.

Increased: Acute and chronic blood loss, iron deficiency anemia, hepatitis, oral contraceptives.

Decreased: Anemia of chronic disease, cirrhosis, malnutrition nephrosis, hemochromatosis.

■ TRIGLYCERIDES

Males: 40–160 mg/dL or 0.45–1.81 mmol/L.
Females: 35–135 mg/dL or 0.40–1.53 mmol/L; may vary with age.

Increased: Hyperlipoproteinemias (types I, IIb, III, IV, V), hypothyroidism, liver diseases, DM, alcoholism, pancreatitis, AMI, nephrotic syndrome.

Decreased: Malnutrition, congenital abetalipoproteinemia.

■ TROPONIN I

< 0.6 ng/mL or < .6 µg/L.

Increased: In myocardial injury levels > 1.5 ng/mL (1.5 µg/L) is consistent with MI. Sensitivity is similar to CK-MB but more specific. Does not tend to be elevated with skeletal muscle injury nor chronic renal disease as much as the CK-MB. False-positives can be seen in clotted specimens and in the presence of heterophil antibodies. Elevated within 4–8 h of myocardial injury with peak at 12–16 h, but remains elevated for 5–9 days.

■ TROPONIN T

< 0.1 ng/mL or < .1 µg/L.

Increased: In myocardial injury but also in muscle disease such as muscular dystrophy. Not as valuable in assessing acute myocardial injury though it parallels troponin I. Its importance may be in risk stratification of cardiac patients (determining those patients with unstable angina who are more likely to have a cardiac-related death).

■ TRYPTASE

5.6–13.5 µg/L.

Increased: Diseases of mast cell activation such as anaphylaxis or mastocytosis.

Released in a slower manner than histamine and more stable so that it can be detected for a longer period of time than histamine. In anaphylaxis, histamine peaks in 5 min and returns to normal in less than 1 h. Tryptase peaks in 1–2 h and returns to normal after a few hours.

■ URIC ACID

Males: 4.5–8.2 mg/dL or 0.27–0.48 mmol/L.
Females: 3.0–6.5 mg/dL or 0.18–0.38 mmol/L.

Increased: Gout; renal failure; destruction of massive amounts of nucleoproteins (tumor lysis after chemotherapy, leukemia or lymphoma); toxemia of pregnancy; drugs (especially diuretics); hypothyroidism; polycystic kidney disease; parathyroid diseases.

Decreased: Uricosuric drugs (salicylates, probenecid, allopurinol), Wilson's disease, Fanconi's syndrome, pregnancy.

■ URINALYSIS, ROUTINE

Appearance

- **Normal:** Yellow, clear, straw-colored
- **Pink/red:** Blood, hemoglobin, myoglobin, food coloring, beets
- **Orange:** Pyridium, rifampin, bile pigments
- **Brown/black:** Myoglobin, bile pigments, melanin, cascara bark, iron, nitrofurantoin, metronidazole, sickle cell crisis
- **Blue:** Methylene blue, *Pseudomonas* UTI (rare), hereditary tryptophan metabolic disorders
- **Cloudy:** UTI (pyuria), blood, myoglobin, chyluria, mucus (normal in ileal loop specimens), phosphate salts (normal in alkaline urine), urates (normal in acidic urine), hyperoxaluria
- **Foamy:** Proteinuria, bile salts

pH

(4.6–8.0)

Acidic: High-protein diet; methenamine mandelate; acidosis; ketoacidosis (starvation, diabetic); diarrhea; dehydration.

Basic: UTI, involving *Proteus;* renal tubular acidosis; diet (high vegetable, milk, immediately postprandial); sodium bicarbonate or acetazolamide therapy; vomiting; metabolic alkalosis; chronic renal failure.

Specific Gravity

Normal: 1.001–1.035.

Increased: Volume depletion, CHF, adrenal insufficiency, DM, SIADH, increased proteins (nephrosis). If markedly increased (1.040–1.050), suspect artifact, excretion of radiographic contrast medium, or some other osmotic agent.

Decreased: Diabetes insipidus, pyelonephritis, glomerulonephritis, water load with normal renal function.

Bilirubin

Negative dipstick.

Positive: Obstructive jaundice, hepatitis, cirrhosis, CHF with hepatic congestion, congenital hyperbilirubinemia (Dubin–Johnson syndrome).

Blood (Hemoglobin)

Negative dipstick.

Positive: Hematuria (See Section I, 70. Urinary Tract Problems, p 208.); free hemoglobin (from trauma, transfusion reaction, or lysis of red blood cells); or myoglobin (crush injury, burn, or tissue ischemia).

Glucose

Negative dipstick.

Positive: DM; other endocrine disorders (pheochromocytoma, hyperthyroidism, Cushing's syndrome, hyperadrenalism); stress states (sepsis, burns); pancreatitis; renal tubular disease; medications (corticosteroids, thiazides, birth control pills); false-positive with vitamin C ingestion.

Ketones

Negative dipstick.

Positive: Starvation, high-fat diet, alcoholic and DKA, vomiting, diarrhea, hyperthyroidism, pregnancy, febrile states.

Leukocyte Esterase

Negative dipstick.

Positive: Infection (test detects five or more WBC/HPF or lysed WBCs).

Microscopy

Note: Many laboratories will no longer perform urine microscopy on a routine basis when the dipstick is negative and the gross appearance is normal.

- **RBCs:** (Normal: 0–3/hpf.) Trauma, UTI, prostatic hypertrophy, genitourinary tuberculosis, nephrolithiasis, malignant and benign tumors, glomerulonephritis.
- **WBCs:** (Normal: 0–4/hpf.) Infection anywhere in the urinary tract, genitourinary tuberculosis, renal tumors, acute glomerulonephritis, radiation damage, interstitial nephritis (analgesic abuse). (Glitter cells represent WBCs lysed in hypotonic solution.)
- **Epithelial cells:** (Normal: occasional.) Acute tubular necrosis, necrotizing papillitis.
- **Parasites:** (Normal: none.) *Trichomonas vaginalis, Schistosoma haematobium.*
- **Yeast:** (Normal: none.) *Candida albicans* (especially in diabetics and immunosuppressed patients, or if a vaginal infection is present).
- **Spermatozoa:** (Normal: after intercourse or nocturnal emission.)
- **Crystals:** Normal:

  Acid urine: Calcium oxalate (small square crystals with a central cross), uric acid.
  Alkaline urine: Calcium carbonate, triple phosphate (resemble coffin lids).
  Abnormal: Cystine, sulfonamide, leucine, tyrosine, cholesterol, or excessive amounts of the crystals noted earlier.

- **Contaminants:** Cotton threads, hair, wood fibers, amorphous substances (all usually unimportant).
- **Mucus:** (Normal: small amounts.) Large amounts suggest urethral disease. Ileal loop urine normally has large amounts.
- **Hyaline cast:** (Normal: occasional.) Benign hypertension, nephrotic syndrome.
- **RBC cast:** (Normal: none.) Acute glomerulonephritis, lupus nephritis, SBE, Goodpasture's disease, vasculitis, malignant hypertension.
- **WBC cast:** (Normal: none.) Pyelonephritis or interstitial nephritis.
- **Epithelial cast:** (Normal: occasional.) Tubular damage, nephrotoxin, viral infections.
- **Granular cast:** (Normal: none.) Results from breakdown of cellular casts, leads to waxy casts.
- **Waxy cast:** (Normal: none.) End stage of a granular cast; evidence of severe chronic renal disease, amyloidosis.
- **Fatty cast:** (Normal: none.) Nephrotic syndrome, DM, damaged renal tubular epithelial cells.
- **Broad cast:** (Normal: none.) Chronic renal disease.

Nitrite
Negative dipstick.
Positive: Bacterial infection (a negative test does not rule out infection).

Protein

See also Albumin, Urine, p 378.
Negative dipstick.
Positive: See Protein, Urine, p 402.

Reducing Substance

Negative dipstick.
Positive: Glucose, fructose, galactose.
False-positives: Vitamin C, antibiotics.

Urobilinogen

Negative dipstick.
Positive: Bile duct obstruction, suppression of gut flora with antibiotics.

■ URINARY ELECTROLYTES

These "spot urines" are of limited value because of large variations in daily fluid and salt intake. Results are usually indeterminate if a diuretic has been given. Sodium is most useful in the differentiation of volume depletion, oliguria, or hyponatremia. Chloride is useful in the diagnosis and treatment of metabolic alkalosis. Urinary potassium levels are often used in the evaluation of hypokalemia.

- **Chloride < 10 mmol/L:** Chloride-sensitive metabolic alkalosis. See Section I, 2. Acid–Base Disorders, p 7.
- **Chloride > 20 mmol/L:** Chloride-resistant metabolic alkalosis. See Section I, 2. Acid–Base Disorders, p 7.
- **Potassium < 10 mmol/L:** Hypokalemia, from extrarenal losses.
- **Potassium > 10 mmol/L:** Renal potassium wasting (diuretics, brisk urinary output).
- **Sodium < 20 mmol/L:** Volume depletion, hyponatremic states, prerenal azotemia (CHF, shock, others), hepatorenal syndrome, edematous states.
- **Sodium > 40 mmol/L:** Acute tubular necrosis, adrenal insufficiency, renal salt wasting, SIADH.
- **Sodium > 20–40 mmol/L:** Indeterminate.

■ URINARY INDICES

Table VII–7. These indices are used in determining the cause of oliguria. See Section I, 70. Urinary Tract Problems, p 208.

■ VANILLYLMANDELIC ACID (VMA), URINE

2–7 mg/dL or 10.1–35.4 mmol/d.
VMA is urinary metabolite of both epinephrine and norepinephrine.
Increased: Pheochromocytoma; neural crest tumors (neuroblastoma, ganglioneuroma). False-positive with methyldopa, chocolate, vanilla, others.

■ VDRL TEST (VENEREAL DISEASE RESEARCH LABORATORY) OR RAPID PLASMA REAGIN (RPR)

Normal: Nonreactive.
Good screening test for syphilis. Almost always positive in secondary syphilis but frequently becomes negative in late syphilis. Also, in some

TABLE VII–7. URINARY INDICES IN ACUTE RENAL FAILURE ACCOMPANIED BY OLIGURIA: DIFFERENTIAL DIAGNOSIS OF OLIGURIA.

Index	Prerenal	Renal (ATN)
Urine osmolality	>500	<350
Urinary sodium	<10–20	>30–40
Urine/serum creatinine	>40	<20
Fractional excreted sodium[a]	<1	>1
Renal failure index[b]	<1	>1

[a] Fractional excreted sodium $= \dfrac{\text{(urine/serum sodium)}}{\text{(urine/serum creatinine)}} \times 100$

[b] Renal failure index $= \dfrac{\text{(urine sodium} \times \text{serum creatinine)}}{\text{(urine creatinine)}}$

Modified and reproduced with permission from Gomella LG, ed. *Clinician's Pocket Reference,* 9th ed. McGraw-Hill; 2002.

patients with HIV infection, the VDRL can be negative in primary and secondary syphilis.

Positive (reactive): Syphilis, SLE, pregnancy and drug addiction. If reactive, confirm with FTA-ABS (false-positives may occur with bacterial or viral illnesses).

■ WHITE BLOOD CELL COUNT

See Table VII–3, p 385.
Increased: See Section I, 61. Sepsis, p 183.
Decreased: See Section I, 12. Cancer Problems, p 38.

■ WHITE BLOOD CELL DIFFERENTIAL

See Table VII–4, p 386. Many hospitals are now performing differentials on automated machines. The newer automated differentials can differentiate neutrophils, lymphocytes, monocytes, eosinophils, and basophils. A manual differential must be done to discriminate between segmented and banded neutrophils.

Neutrophils

40–70% segmented neutrophils, 5–10% banded neutrophils.
Increased: Exercise, pain, stress, infection, burns, drugs, thyrotoxicosis, steroids, malignancy, chronic inflammatory disease (vasculitis, collagen-vascular disease, colitis), lithium, epinephrine, asplenia, idiopathic.
Decreased: Congenital, immune-mediated, drug-induced, infectious (viral, rickettsial, parasitic).

Lymphocytes

Normal: 24–44%.

Increased: Measles; German measles (rubeola); mumps, whooping cough (*Bordetella pertussis*); smallpox; chickenpox (varicella-zoster); influenza; viral hepatitis; infectious mononucleosis (Epstein-Barr virus); virtually any viral infection; acute and chronic lymphocytic leukemias.

Decreased: Following stress, burns, trauma; normal finding in 22% of population; uremia; some viral infections (including HIV).

Lymphocytes, Atypical

Normal: 0–3%.

> 20%: Infectious mononucleosis (Epstein–Barr virus), CMV infection, viral hepatitis, toxoplasmosis.

3–20%: Viral infections (mumps, rubeola, varicella), rickettsial infections, tuberculosis.

Monocytes

Normal: 3–7%.

Increased: SBE, brucellosis (*Brucella*), typhoid fever (*Salmonella typhi*), kala-azar (visceral leishmanlasls), trypanosomiasis (*Trypanosoma*), rickettsial infection, ulcerative colitis, sarcoidosis, Hodgkin's disease, monocytic leukemias, collagen-vascular diseases.

Decreased: Myelodysplasia, aplastic anemia, hairy cell leukemia, cyclic neutropenia, thermal injuries, collagen-vascular diseases.

Eosinophils

Normal: 0–3%.

Increased: Allergies, parasites, skin diseases, malignancy, drugs, asthma, Addison's disease, collagen-vascular diseases. (A handy mnemonic is **NAACP:** **N**eoplasm, **A**llergy, **A**ddison's disease, **C**ollagen-vascular diseases, **P**arasites).

Decreased: After steroids; ACTH; after stress (infection, trauma, burns); Cushing's syndrome.

Basophils

Normal: 0–1%.

Increased: Chronic myeloid leukemia; rarely, in recovery from infection and from hypothyroidism.

Decreased: Acute rheumatic fever, lobar pneumonia, after steroid therapy, thyrotoxicosis, stress.

■ WHITE BLOOD CELL MORPHOLOGY

- **Auer rod:** Acute myelogenous leukemias.
- **Döhle bodies:** Severe infection, burns, malignancy, pregnancy.

- **Hypersegmentation:** Megaloblastic anemias, iron deficiency, myeloproliferative disorders, drug-induced.
- **Toxic granulation:** Severe illness (sepsis, burns, high temperature).

■ ZINC

60–130 µg/dL or 9–20 µmol/L.

Increased: Atherosclerosis, CAD.

Decreased: Inadequate dietary intake (parenteral nutrition, alcoholism); malabsorption; increased needs such as pregnancy or wound healing; acrodermatitis enteropathica.

REFERENCES

Burtis CA, Ashwood ER. *Tietz's Textbook of Clinical Chemistry.* 3rd ed. WB Saunders,1999.

Coudrey L. The troponins. *Arch Intern Med* 1998;158:1173–1180.

Jurado R, Mattix H. The decreased serum urea nitrogen-creatinine ratio. *Arch Intern Med* 1998;115:2509–2511.

Pettijohn TL, Doyle T, Spiekerman AM, Watson LE, Riggs MW, Lawrence ME. Usefulness of positive troponin-T and negative creatine kinase levels in identifying high-risk patients with unstable angina pectoris. *Am J Cardiol* 1997;80:510–511.

Tchetgen MB, Song JT, Strawderman M, Jacobsen SJ, Oesterling JE. Ejaculation increases the serum prostate-specific antigen concentration. *Urology* 1996;47:511–516.

VIII. Procedures

1. ABSCESS DRAINAGE

Indications

1. Treatment of a soft-tissue, localized collection of purulence.
2. Drainage of a submucosal collection of purulence (ie, peritonsillar, rectal abscess).

Contraindications

1. Abscess when pain control is difficult to achieve in the ED.
2. Large abscess that needs extensive debridement and, therefore, prolonged analgesia and anesthesia.
3. Location near neurovascular bundles where delicate dissection is better performed in the operating theater.

Materials: Suture tray (forceps, hemostat, scissors, 4×4s, drape), 11- or 15-blade scalpel, antiseptic solution such as povidone–iodine, packing material (thin packing strip gauze, ¼ in. or smaller, either plain or povidone–iodine), 1% lidocaine ± epinephrine, 10- and 30-mL syringes, small- and large-gauge needles, and 500 mL of sterile saline or water.

Procedure
General

1. Obtain informed consent.
2. For patients at high risk for endocarditis or septicemia (prosthetic cardiac valves, congenital cardiac malformations, history of rheumatic fever, acquired valvular dysfunction, IV drug users, or immunocompromised patients) administer prophylactic antibiotics (cefazolin 1 g IV, 30 min prior).
3. Scrub skin with antiseptic solution and drape in a sterile fashion.
4. Obtain local anesthesia in one of three ways using lidocaine (max 4 mg/kg, lidocaine with epinephrine 7 mg/kg) with or without epinephrine (systemic analgesia and sedation may be necessary):
   a. Regional block, if anatomically appropriate.
   b. Field block via circumferential SC infiltration.
   c. Local infiltration of SC tissue overlying abscess (simply inject lidocaine into SC tissue at the dome of the abscess, blanching will spread evenly in an outward direction).
5. Incise the skin overlying the fluctuant area in a simple linear fashion with the 11- or 15-blade scalpel in a direction parallel to the lines of skin tension to a length equal to that of the size of the abscess cavity and to a depth that penetrates into the abscess cavity.
6. Drain the purulence.
7. Probe the depth of the abscess with a 4×4-covered hemostat to define depth of cavity, break up loculations, and express additional purulence

with gentle compression. Sharp curettage is unnecessary. Avoid use of gloved finger due to risk of retained needle fragments from IV drug use.

8. Irrigate cavity under high pressure with 500 mL of sterile saline or water.
9. Pack loosely with strip gauze.
10. Apply absorbent dry gauze dressing over the packed abscess.

Unique Abscesses

1. **Bartholin's gland:** Make a stab incision the width of the scalpel blade to insert the catheter to the mucosal aspect of the gland, puncture the abscess cavity with a hemostat, drain purulence, insert the catheter, fill catheter with 3–4 mL of water (catheter causes fistulization and replaces packing).
2. **Breast:** Superficial abscesses are drained in the typical fashion with an incision radial to the areola. Intramammary and retromammary abscesses necessitate operative treatment.
3. **Perirectal:** Only localized, superficial perianal abscesses may be drained in the previously mentioned manner. Ischiorectal, intersphincteric, high intramuscular, and pelvirectal abscesses require surgery.
4. **Sebaceous cyst (infected):** Requires excision of pearly white capsule by grasping edges with hemostats and core removal by sharp dissection. All other steps remain the same.

Complications: Artery or vein damage resulting in hemorrhage, nerve damage with residual local numbness, scarring, poor wound healing in patients with diabetes or peripheral vascular disease and systemic bacteremia.

REFERENCES

Biderman P, Hiatt JR. Management of soft-tissue infections of the upper extremity in parenteral drug abusers. *Am J Surg* 1987;154:526–528.

Folstad SG. Soft tissue infections. In: Tintinalli JE. *Emergency Medicine—A Comprehensive Study Guide.* 5th ed. McGraw-Hill, 2000.

Meislin HW, Guisto JA. Soft tissue infections. In: Marx JE. *Rosen's Emergency Medicine: Concepts and Clinical Practice.* 5th ed. Mosby Inc, 2002:1944–1957.

Shulman ST, Amren DP, Bisno AL, Dajani AS, Durack DT, Gerber MA, et al. Prevention of bacterial endocarditis. *Circulation* 1984;70:1123A–1127A.

2. ARTERIAL LINE PLACEMENT

Indications

1. Frequent arterial sampling required.
2. Invasive hemodynamic monitoring required.

Contraindications

1. Poor collateral circulation.
2. Coagulopathy (relative contraindication).

Materials: Two-inch long, 20-gauge or smaller Angiocath or Arrow kit, arm-board, sterile dressing, sterile gloves, mask, gown, sterile towels, povidone–iodine, lidocaine, 25-gauge needle, syringe, 3-0 suture, needle driver or straight needle, arterial line setup (transducer, tubing, pressure bag with heparinized saline).

Radial Artery

Procedure

1. Obtain consent (unless implied emergency consent applies).
2. Verify presence of collateral circulation with Allen test. Have patient make fist while occluding both the radial and ulnar arteries. Open fist and release pressure on ulnar artery. The hand should flush with color within 5 s. If hand does not reprofuse, then test contralateral artery for placement.
3. Hyperextend wrist over gauze rolls and tape to arm board. Locate radial pulse at its most superficial location. Prep out area with povidone–iodine and drape with sterile towels. Gown and glove.
4. Make a small skin wheal of lidocaine with 25-gauge needle at puncture site.
5. Place Angiocath or Arrow needle in dominant hand with the bevel facing upward, and locate arterial pulse with the other. Advance needle at a 30–45-degree angle to skin until flash is seen in hub of needle. Now advance entire assembly 1–2 mm. Advance the catheter over the needle and remove needle. Apply pressure proximal to catheter to control bleeding and attach to pressure tubing.
6. Arrow Angiocath systems use the Seldinger technique. Use same steps as above until flash in needle hub is seen. Then advance wire smoothly until it is completely through catheter unit. Stop if resistance is met, and reposition catheter. Success is often enhanced by dropping the angle of the catheter and attempting again to thread the wire. Once wire is easily fully extended, pass catheter over the needle and withdraw needle–wire unit. Apply pressure proximal to catheter to control bleeding and attach to pressure tubing.
7. Suture catheter in place with 3-0 suture and apply sterile dressing.
8. Instruct nurse to zero the transducer and begin monitoring (Figure VIII–1).

Complications: Infection, thrombosis of artery, hemorrhage, distal emboli, pseudoaneurysm formation.

3. ARTHROCENTESIS

Indications

1. Diagnosis of cause of joint fluid.
2. Pain relief from an acute hemarthrosis or a tense effusion.
3. Local instillation of medications in acute and chronic inflammatory arthritides.

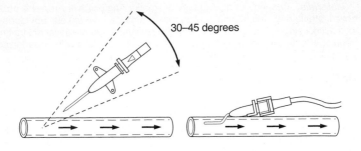

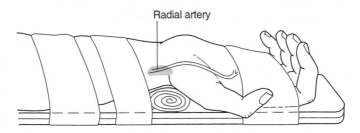

Figure VIII–1. Technique of redial artery catheterization. (Reproduced, with permission, from Gomella TL, ed. Arterial access. In: *Neonatology.* 5th ed. McGraw-Hill, 2003.)

Contraindications

1. Presence of infection overlying the site to be punctured.
2. Bacteremia (relative).

Materials: Sterile gloves, povidone–iodine solution, alcohol sponges, sterile towel (with center perforation), vapor coolant (eg, fluormethane solution), 1 or 2% lidocaine, sterile gauze dressings, sterile syringe (20 mL) Luer-Lok needles (18, 20, 22, and 25 gauge), plain test tubes, test tubes with liquid anticoagulant, contact microbiology lab to determine their preference for transporting fluid for bacterial, fungal, acid-fast bacillus (AFB) culture, and Gram's stain.

General

Procedure

1. Obtain consent.

2. Select punctures site. In most instances, the approach is via the extensor surfaces of joints, because most major vessels and nerves are found in flexor surfaces. Also, the synovial pouch is usually more superficial on the extensor side of a joint.
3. Clean area with iodinated solution, such as povidone-iodine three times. Allow area to dry because the bactericidal effects of iodine are both concentration- and time-dependent. Remove iodine solution with alcohol wipe. Place sterile perforated drape over the joint.
4. Anesthetize the area with 1 or 2% lidocaine using a 22- or 25-gauge needle. Infiltrate the skin down to the area of the joint capsule but do not enter joint space. Alternatively, a vapor coolant may be used topically just before needle insertion.
5. Attach a syringe to an 18- to 22-gauge needle. Insert the needle at the desired anatomic point, through the skin and SC tissue, and into the joint space. Remove as much fluid as possible.
6. For corticosteroid injection, remove the syringe from the needle, leaving the needle in the joint space. Attach the steroid-containing syringe to the needle. Pull back on the plunger to ensure that the needle is not in a vein. Inject the steroid. Forty milligrams of methylprednisone is used for large-sized joints such as the knee and 20 mg for medium-sized joints, such as the ankle or wrist.
7. After aspiration or steroid injection is completed, remove the needle and apply pressure and then a sterile dressing.
8. Send fluid for cell count with differential, crystal analysis, Gram's staining, bacterial culture, and synovial fluid glucose measurement.

A. Specific Sites
Knee Joint

1. **Landmarks:** Medial surface of the patella at the middle or superior portion of the patella
2. **Position:** Knee is fully extended. Relaxation of the quadriceps muscle greatly facilitates needle placement. The foot is kept perpendicular to the floor.
3. **Needle insertion:** Insert posterior to the medial portion of the patella into the patellar–femoral groove. Direct the needle slightly inferiorly and posteriorly (Figure VIII–2).

Wrist Joint

1. **Landmarks:** The dorsal radial tubercle (Lister's tubercle) is an elevation found in the center of the dorsal aspect of the distal end of the radius. The extensor pollicis longus tendon runs in a groove on the radial side of the tubercle. The tendon can be palpated by active extension of the wrist and thumb.
2. **Position:** Wrist is flexed 20–30 degrees and ulnar deviated. Traction is applied to the hand.

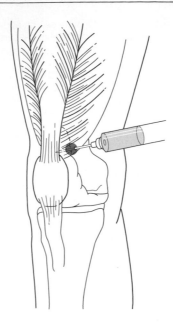

Figure VIII–2. Arthrocentesis of the knee. (Reproduced, with permission, from Haist SA, Robbins JB, Gomella LG, eds. *Internal Medicine on Call.* 3rd ed. McGraw-Hill, 2002.)

3. **Needle insertion:** A 22-gauge needle is inserted dorsally, just distal to the dorsal tubercle and on the ulnar side of the extensor pollicis longus tendon. The anatomic snuff box, located more radially, should be avoided (Figure VIII–3).

Ankle Joint

1. **Landmarks:** The medial malleolar sulcus, which is bordered medially by the medial malleolus and laterally by the anterior tibial tendon. The tendon can be easily identified by active dorsiflexion of the foot.
2. **Position:** With the patient lying supine on the table, the foot is plantar flexed.
3. **Needle insertion:** Insert at a point just medial to the anterior tibial tendon and directed into the hollow at the anterior edge of the medial malleolus. The needle has to be inserted 2–3 cm to penetrate the joint space (Figure VIII–4).

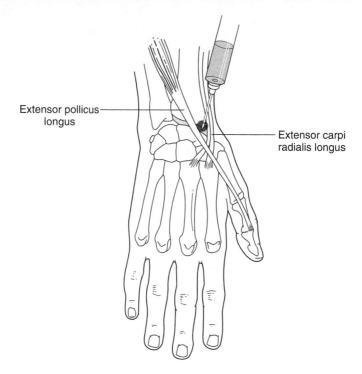

Extensor pollicus longus

Extensor carpi radialis longus

Figure VIII–3. Arthrocentesis of the wrist. (Reproduced, with permission, from Haist SA, Robbins JB, Gomella LG, eds. *Internal Medicine on Call.* 3rd ed. McGraw-Hill, 2002.)

Elbow Joint

1. **Landmarks:** With the elbow extended, the depression between the radial head and the lateral epicondyle of the humerus is palpated.
2. **Position:** With the palpating finger still touching the radial head, the elbow is flexed to 90 degrees. The forearm is pronated, and the palm is placed down flat on a table.
3. **Needle insertion:** A 22-gauge needle is inserted from the lateral aspect just distal to the lateral epicondyle and is directed medially.

Complications: Infection, bleeding.

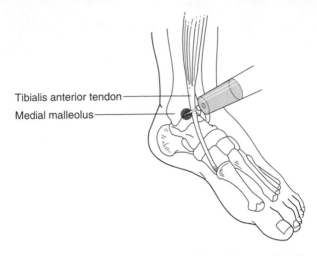

Tibialis anterior tendon
Medial malleolus

Figure VIII–4. Arthrocentesis of the ankle. (Reproduced, with permission, from Haist SA, Robbins JB, Gomella LG, eds. *Internal Medicine on Call.* 3rd ed. McGraw-Hill, 2002.)

REFERENCE

Lefor AT, Gomella LG. Arthrocentesis. In: Lefor AT, Gomella LG (eds). *Surgery on Call.* 3rd ed. Lange Medical Books/McGraw-Hill, 2001:356–360.

4. BEDSIDE ULTRASOUND

Trauma Ultrasound (FAST—Focused Assessment with Sonography for Trauma)

Indications: To identify pericardial, intraperitoneal, or intrathoracic fluid in

1. Blunt abdominal trauma (BAT).
2. Penetrating thoracic/abdominal trauma.
3. Unexplained hypotension in patients (trauma and nontrauma).
4. Dyspnea with suspected pleural/pericardial effusion.
5. To verify fetal cardiac activity in the pregnant trauma patient.

Contraindications: Only relative contraindication is the immediate need for laparotomy or interventional procedure (eg, thoracotomy)

Materials: Ultrasound gel, ultrasound machine with a transducer (curvilinear; microcurvilinear; or small-footprint, phased-array transducer with frequencies between 2.5 and 5.0 MHz are acceptable; however, 3.0 or 3.5 MHz is the most common).

Procedure: The FAST exam, in its simplest form, uses four primary sonographic windows to evaluate the patient (Figure VIII–5). I recommended that these windows be viewed in sequence. This may decrease error rates if physicians evaluate patients with a standardized technique; furthermore, the following sequence is presented to exclude immediate life threats in order of severity (pericardial effusion/impending tamponade, and hemoperitoneum/hemothorax). It is recommended the heart be imaged first. With the patient supine, set the ultrasound depth to 20–24 cm, then optimize the image as needed.

1. **View 1:** Examine the **heart** in a subxiphoid/subcostal window with the transducer directed under the xiphoid process toward the left shoulder in a horizontal plane. The transducer indicator should point to the patient's right (Figures VIII–5A, VIII–5B).
   a. Move the probe to identify the four chambers of the heart and surrounding pericardium
   b. Confirm cardiac activity and look for an anechoic (black) region between the pericardium and the myocardium, indicating a pericardial effusion.
   c. A parasternal long axis view is an option when visualization with the subxiphoid view is inadequate. (See Cardiac Ultrasound section, p 428.)
2. **View 2:** Examine the **right upper quadrant** (Morison's pouch); the transducer indicator is aimed toward the head in a coronal plane (in a line from the axilla to the ipsilateral hip, Figure VIII–5C). Transducer is directed as a coronal section through the body in the midaxillary line. Start between the tenth and twelfth ribs initially, then move cephalad, or caudal to complete the evaluation. Tilt the transducer anterior and posterior to scan completely through Morison's pouch. Be sure to identify the inferior tip of the liver (Figures VIII–5B, VIII–5D).
   a. Identify the liver and right kidney interface. This region is known as Morison's pouch. An anechoic collection or region between the liver and right kidney, adjacent to these organs or in the subdiaphragmatic recess is consistent with free fluid and hemoperitoneum.
   b. Evaluate the right supradiaphragmatic recess for hemothorax.
3. **View 3:** Examine the **left upper quadrant** (splenorenal space); the transducer indicator is aimed toward the head in a coronal plane (in a line from the axilla to the ipsilateral hip). Transducer is directed as a coronal section through the body in the posterior-axillary line. Start between the ninth and eleventh ribs initially, then move cephalad, or caudal to complete the evaluation. Tilt the transducer anterior and posterior to scan completely through the splenorenal space. Be sure to identify the inferior tip of the spleen and the inferior pole of the left kidney (this will usually require moving the transducer caudally. See Figures VIII–5A, VIII–5E).
   a. Identify the spleen and left kidney interface. This region is a physiologic potential space. An anechoic collection about the region or between the spleen and left kidney is consistent with free fluid and hemoperitoneum.
   b. Evaluate the left diaphragmatic recess and the left subdiaphragmatic recess.

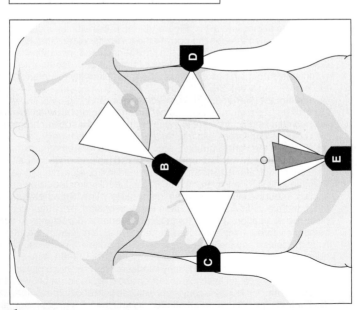

Figure VIII–5. FAST-Focused assessment with sonography for trauma.

A. Anatomic map, indicating transducer placement for the respective sonograms.

B. Subxiphoid cardiac: Abnormal, positive for a pericardial effusion. (Note the anechoic area between the liver and the right ventricle and atrium.)

C. Right upper quadrant: Abnormal with free fluid (Morison's pouch).

D. Left upper quadrant (splenorenal): Abnormal. Note the anechoic fluid surrounding the spleen and midkidney.

E. Suprapubic sagittal view: Abnormal with fluid in the pouch of Douglas.

Key: L = liver; PE = pericardial effusion; FL = fluid; K = kidney; SP = spleen; B = bladder; U = uterus.

(Courtesy of Paul R. Sierzenski, MD, RDMS, Christiana Care Health System, Newark, Delaware)

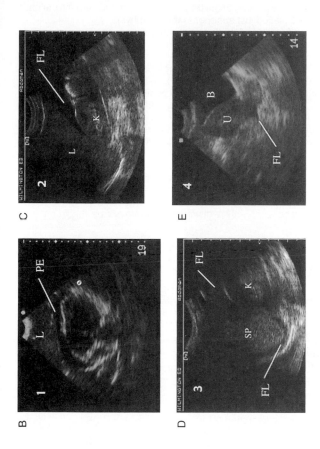

Figure VIII-5. FAST-Focuses assessment with sonography for trauma. **A.** Anatomic map, indicating transducer placement for the respective sonograms. **B.** Subxiphoid cardiac: Abnormal, positive for a pericardial effusion. (Note the anechoic area between the liver and the right ventricle and atrium.) **C.** Right upper quadrant: Abnormal with free fluid (Morison's pouch). **D.** Left upper cuadrant (splenorenal): Abnormal. Note the anechoic fluid surrounding the spleen and midkidney. **E.** Suprapubic sagittal view: Abnormal with fluid in the pouch of Douglas. *Key*: L = liver; PE = pericardial effusion; FL = fluid; K = kidney; SP = spleen; B = bladder; U = uterus. (Courtesy of Paul R. Sierzenski, MD, RDMS, Christiana Care Health System, Newark, Delaware)

4. **View 4:** Examine the **pelvis** (suprapubic window) in both the sagittal and transverse planes. Ideally the bladder is full to aid visualization, if a Foley is in place it may be clamped (See Figures VIII–5A, VIII–5E).

   a. *Sagittal View (Longitudinal)*: Transducer is placed about 1 cm above the symphysis pubis with the transducer indicator toward the patient's head, and placed just superior to the symphysis.

      i. Identify the bladder (triangular in shape in this view when fully distended), uterus (pear-shaped, if present), and rectum. An anechoic region occurs between the bladder and uterus, between the uterus and rectum, or loops of bowl floating superior/posterior to the bladder (Figure VIII–5E).

   b. *Transverse View:* From the sagittal position rotate the probe 90 degrees counterclockwise so the transducer indicator points to the patient's right.

      i. Identify the bladder (rectangular in this view when fully distended), uterus (oval hyperechoic structure, if present) and rectum. Identify the bladder (triangular in shape in this view when fully distended), uterus (oval-shaped, if present), and rectum. An anechoic region occurs between the bladder and uterus, between the uterus and rectum, or loops of bowl floating superior/lateral to the bladder.

5. Clean the transducer with a disinfectant approved by the transducer manufacturer.

Complications: No clear complications from the procedure itself.

REFERENCE

Salen PN, Melanson SW, Heller MB. The focused abdominal sonography for trauma (FAST) examination. Considerations and recommendations for training physicians in the use of a new clinical tool. *Acad Emerg Med* 2000;7:162–168.

Cardiac Ultrasound (Echo)

Indications: To identify the presence or absence or cardiac activity or pericardial effusion in/for

1. Penetrating thoracic/abdominal trauma.
2. Unexplained hypotension.
3. Dyspneic patients.
4. Acute myocardial infarction (AMI).
5. Suspected proximal aortic dissection.
6. Ultrasound guided cardiac procedures (transvenous pacing or pericardiocentesis).

Contraindications: Only relative contraindication is the immediate need for interventional procedure (eg, thoracotomy).

Materials: Ultrasound gel, ultrasound machine with a transducer (microcurvilinear, small phased array, or a mechanical sector transducer with frequencies between 2.0 and 4.0 MHz are acceptable; however, 2.0–2.5 MHz is most common.).

Procedure: By convention cardiac ultrasound images are oriented on the right of the display screen (which will effectively be the patient's left). This may be a significant cause of initial confusion for many who have not performed echocardiography. Most ultrasound systems today include cardiac presets that automatically reverse the orientation to the right of the display screen. The following section describes a sonographic approach for a correctly oriented image using standard cardiac orientation.

1. **View 1:** Examine the heart in a **subxiphoid/subcostal window** with the transducer directed under the xiphoid process toward the left shoulder in a horizontal plane. The transducer indicator should point to the patient's right (Figures VIII–6A, VIII–6B).
   a. Move the probe to identify the four chambers of the heart and surrounding pericardium.
   b. Confirm cardiac activity and look for an anechoic (black) or hypoechoic region between the pericardium and the myocardium, indicating a pericardial effusion.
2. **View 2:** Examine the heart in a **parasternal long axis** with the patient supine or in the left lateral decubitus (LLD) position. Transducer is placed in the third, fourth, or fifth left parasternal intercostal spaces with the transducer indicator oriented toward the right clavicle or shoulder. In a line from the right shoulder to the left antecubital fossa (Figures VIII–6B, VIII–6C.
   a. Identify the left atrium, left ventricle, aortic valve, aortic root, aortic outflow tract, and the surrounding echogenic pericardium
   b. Confirm cardiac activity and look for an anechoic (black) region between the pericardium and the myocardium, indicating a pericardial effusion.
   c. An aortic root measurement greater than 3.8 cm is abnormal and should be suspect for either aortic dissection or aneurysm.
3. **View 3:** Examine the heart in the **parasternal short axis;** from the parasternal long axis position, rotate the transducer 90 degrees clockwise (to the patient's left). You may just place the transducer in the third, fourth, or fifth left parasternal intercostal space in a line connecting the left clavicle/shoulder and the right hip (Figures VIII–6B, VIII–6C).
   a. Identify the left ventricle (circular), right ventricle (crescent-shaped), and surrounding pericardium.
   b. Confirm cardiac activity and look for an anechoic (black) region between the pericardium and the myocardium, indicating a pericardial effusion.
4. **View 4:** Examine the heart with the **four-chamber apical** view; place the transducer over the cardiac apex or the point of maximal intensity (PMI) with the beam directed toward the right clavicle/shoulder in a plane coronal to the heart. The transducer indicator is directed toward the left axilla (Figures VIII–6D).

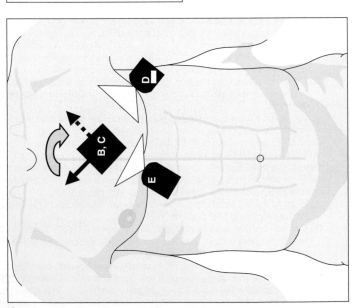

Figure VIII–6. Cardiac ultrasound-Echo.
A. Anatomic map, indicating transducer placement for the respective sonograms.
B. Parasternal long axis (PSLAX): Normal PSLAX cardiac view.
C. Parasternal short axis (PSSAX): Normal PSSAX view, showing the left ventricle at the level of the papillary muscles.
D. Four-chamber apical (4CA): Abnormal 4CA, showing a pericardial effusion.
E. Subxiphoid: See Figure VIII–5B. FAST exam.
Key: RV = right ventricle; LV = left ventricle; LA = left atrium; Root = proximal aortic root; PE = pericardial effusion; RA = right atrium.

(Courtesy of Paul R. Sierzenski, MD, RDMS, Christiana Care Health System, Newark, Delaware)

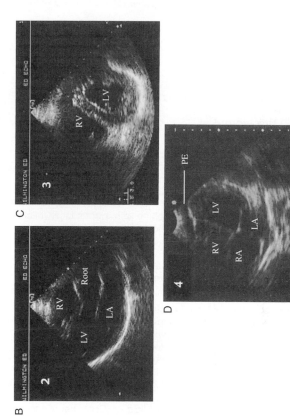

Figure VIII-6. Cardiac ultrasound-Echo. **A.** Anatomic map, indicating transducer placement for the respective sonograms. **B.** Parasternal long axis (PSLAX): Normal PSLAX cardiac view. **C.** Parasternal short axis (PSSAX): Normal PSSAX view, showing the left ventricle at the level of the papillary muscles. **D.** Four-chamber apical (4CA): Abnormal 4CA, showing a pericardial effusion. **E.** Subxiphoid: See Figure 8-5B. FAST exam. *Key:* RV = right ventricle; LV = left ventricle; LA = left atrium; Root = proximal aortic root; PE = pericardial effusion; RA = right atrium. (Courtesy of Paul R. Sierzenski, MD, RDMS, Christiana Care Health System, Newark, Delaware)

a. Identify the left ventricle, right ventricle, left atrium, right atrium, and surrounding pericardium.
b. Confirm cardiac activity and look for an anechoic (black) region between the pericardium and the myocardium, indicating a pericardial effusion.
5. Clean the transducer with a disinfectant approved by the transducer manufacturer.

Complications: No clear complications from the procedure itself.

REFERENCE

Blaivas M. Incidence of pericardial effusion in patients presenting to the emergency department with unexplained dyspnea. *Acad Emerg Med* 2001;8:1143–1146.

Gallbladder (GB) Ultrasound

Indications

1. Right upper quadrant pain.
2. Jaundice/icterus.
3. Epigastric pain.

Contraindications: None
Materials: Ultrasound gel, ultrasound machine with a transducer (microcurvilinear, small-phased array or a mechanical sector transducer with frequencies between 2.5 and 5.0 MHz are acceptable; however, 3.0–3.5 MHz is most common.)
Procedure: The gallbladder must be evaluated in a minimum of two planes. This is primarily a sagittal and a transverse view. An oblique view may be added or necessary for evaluation.

1. Patient is supine or in the left lateral decubitus position (right lateral decubitus, semierect, and standing positions may be helpful).
2. Examine the gallbladder in the sagittal plane. Place the transducer in the subxiphoid region with the probe indicator directed toward the patient's head and move along the right costal margin to approximately the midclavicular line. Identify the gallbladder by the following landmarks of the portal vein/triad and the main lobar fissure (if it is visualized) (Figure VIII–7A).
3. Identify the liver, portal vein (PV), common bile duct (CBD), hepatic artery (HA), gallbladder (GB), and the main lobar fissure (MLF) (spanning these two structures), and look for the following:
   a. **Gallstones:** Bright oval to round hyperechoic structure(s) within the gallbladder that often have a posterior shadow on ultrasound (Figure VIII–7B).
   b. **Pericholecystic fluid:** An anechoic stripe is evident that borders the outer gallbladder wall and should be visualized in two views. (This fluid is often, but not necessarily circumferential).

    c. Thickened gallbladder wall: A GB wall > 4.0 mm is considered abnormal.

    d. Sonographic Murphy's sign: Tenderness of the gallbladder when compressed under direct visualization with the ultrasound transducer.

    e. Dilated common bile duct (CBD): A CBD with an internal diameter greater than 4.0 mm is dilated; however, age variations exist.

4. Scan through the GB completely from its medial to lateral boarders.
5. Examine the GB in the transverse plane; from the sagittal plane rotate the transducer 90 degrees counterclockwise so that the transducer indicator points to the patient's right. Scan through the GB from proximal to distal (Figures VIII–7C–E).
6. Clean the transducer with a disinfectant approved by the transducer manufacturer.

Complications: No clear complications from the procedure itself.

REFERENCES

Liang FC. Ultrasonography of the acute abdomen. *Radiol Clin North Am* 1992;30: 389–400.

Spitz HB. Non-pelvic abdominal ultrasound: An overview for emergency physicians. *J Emerg Med* 1984;1:509–520.

Abdominal Aorta

Indications

1. Abdominal, back, or flank pain.
2. Pulsatile abdominal mass.
3. Hypotensive patient with abdominal pain or distention.
4. Syncope.

Contraindications: None

Materials: Ultrasound gel, ultrasound machine with a transducer (curvilinear, microcurvilinear array, small-phased array, or a mechanical sector transducer with frequencies between 2.5 and 5.0 MHz are acceptable; however, 3.0–3.5 MHz is most common.)

Procedure: Because aortic aneurysms can be either fusiform (most common) or saccular, it is essential that the aorta ultrasound include a sagittal and transverse plane evaluation. Clearly the transverse plane is critical and is often the first view obtained in the emergency setting.

1. Patient is supine.
2. Examine the aorta in the **transverse plane.** Place the transducer in the subxiphoid region with the probe indicator directed toward the patient's right, and slowly move along the path of the aorta to its bifurcation (near the umbilicus; Figure VIII–8A).

    a. Identify the liver, aorta, inferior vena cava (IVC), superior mesenteric artery (SMA), splenic vein (SV), and the "spinal stripe" at the level of the proximal to mid aorta (Figure VIII–8B).

(*text continues on page 438*)

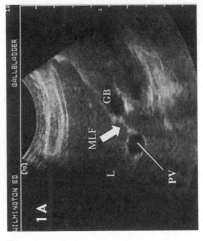

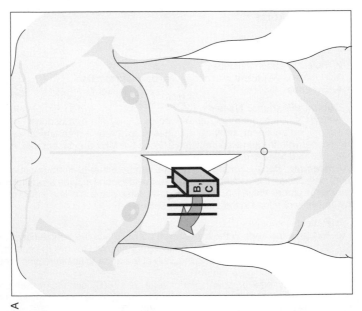

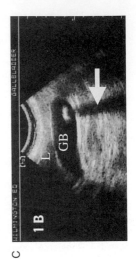

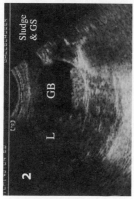

E

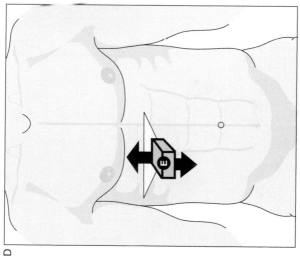

D

Figure VIII–7. Gallbladder ultrasound.
A. Anatomic map, indicating transducer placement for sonograms B and C.
B. Sagital gallbladder sonogram, showing key gallbladder landmarks of the portal vein and the hyperechoic main lobar fissure *(arrow).*
C. Sagital gallbladder: Abnormal, showing echogenic gallstone with classic posterior acoustic shadowing *(arrow).*
D. Anatomic map, indicating transducer placement for sonogram E.
E. Transverse gallbladder sonogram: Abnormal, showing echogenic sludge and nonshadowing gallstones within the gallbladder.
Key: L = liver; MLF = main lobar fissure; GB = gallbladder; PV = portal vein; GS = gallstones.

(Courtesy of Paul R. Sierzenski, MD, RDMS, Christiana Care Health System, Newark, Delaware)

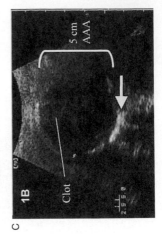

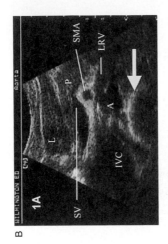

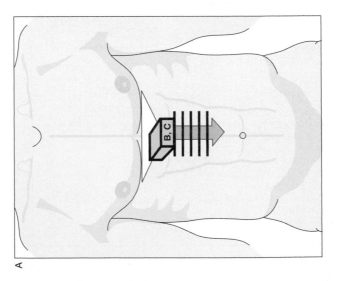

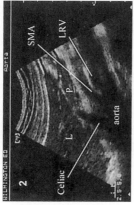

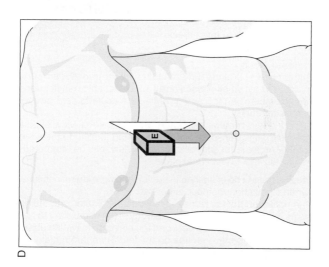

Figure VIII–8. Abdominal aorta.

A. Anatomic map, indicating transducer placement for sonograms B and C.

B. Transverse midabdominal aorta: Normal, showing the liver, splenic vein, SMA, LRV, aorta, IVC, and spinal stripe with shadow (*arrow*).

C. Transverse distal abdominal aorta: Abnormal, showing 5.0-cm AAA with thrombus.

D. Anatomic map, indicating transducer placement for sonogram E.

E. Sagittal proximal aorta: Normal, showing the liver, celiac artery, pancreas, LRV, SMA, and aorta.

Key: L = liver; P = pancreas; SV = splenic vein; A = aorta; LRV = left renal vein; IVC = inferior vena cava; AAA = abdominal aortic aneurysm; SMA = superior mesenteric artery.

(Courtesy of Paul R. Sierzenski, MD, RDMS, Christiana Care Health System, Newark, Delaware)

b. Identify the IVC, aorta, and spinal stripe at the mid and distal aorta.
c. A proximal, mid, and distal abdominal aorta measurement should be made. Aorta measurements of greater than 3.0 cm are suggestive of an aneurysm. Examine the aorta through the level of its bifurcation (Figure VIII–8C).

3. Examine the aorta in the **sagittal plane;** Place the transducer in the epigastrium with the transducer indicator oriented toward the patient's head. Move down the abdominal aorta to the bifurcation (Figure VIII-8D, E).
4. Clean the transducer with a disinfectant approved by the transducer manufacturer.

Complications: No clear complications from the procedure itself.

REFERENCE

Reynolds T, Santos T, Weidemann J, Langenfeld K, Warner MG. The evaluation of the abdominal aorta: A "how to" for cardiac sonographers. *J Am Soc Echocardiogr* 1990;3:336–346.

Renal Ultrasound

Indications

1. Renal colic.
2. Abdominal pain in the elderly to differentiate renal colic from AAA.
3. Hematuria.
4. Costovertebral angle (CVA) tenderness.
5. Flank pain.

Contraindications: None

Materials: Ultrasound gel, ultrasound machine with a transducer (curvilinear, microcurvilinear array, small-phased array, or a mechanical sector transducer with frequencies between 2.5 and 5.0 MHz are acceptable; however, 3.0–3.5 MHz is most common.)

Procedure: The kidneys may be evaluated with the coronal view used in the trauma FAST exam; this transducer position is often familiar to the sonographers. An anterior or posterior sagittal or oblique view may be attempted if the kidney is not visualized in the coronal plane.

1. Patient is supine or may be examined in the left and right lateral decubitus positions when a posterior approach is desired.
2. Examine the right then the left kidney. Transducer indicator is to the patient's head as a coronal plane through the body in the midaxillary to posterior axillary line. Begin scanning between the eleventh to twelfth ribs on the right and the ninth to eleventh ribs on the left. Scan through the kidney from anterior to posterior by pivoting the transducer from posterior to anterior (Figure VIII–9A,B).
   a. Identify the liver, right kidney, renal cortex (with pyramids), and central renal sinus.

   b. Identify the spleen, left kidney, renal cortex (with pyramids), and central renal sinus (Figure VIII–9C).
   c. Hydronephrosis: Dilatation of the renal sinus with dark black, anechoic fluid within the bright renal sinus.
   d. Renal calculi: Bright hyperechoic oval/round structures within the cortex or renal sinus (posterior shadowing is often present).
   e. Renal cyst: Anechoic, round or oval structure often at the periphery of the renal cortex with a thin wall; few or no internal echoes and posterior acoustic enhancement (Figure VIII–9C).
   f. Renal masses: If other views are necessary or pathology is identified, try an anterior approach with the transducer sagittal (indicator toward the head) and transverse (indicator toward the patient's right). The posterior oblique view with the transducer placed at the ninth through twelfth rib space at the lateral scapular line may also be used.
3. Clean the transducer with a disinfectant approved by the transducer manufacturer.

Complications: None

Pelvic Ultrasound

Indications

1. Pelvic/abdominal pain.
2. Vaginal bleeding (pregnant or nonpregnant patient).
3. Suspected pregnancy.

Contraindications: Suspected premature rupture of membranes is a relative contraindication to endovaginal ultrasound.

Materials: Ultrasound gel, ultrasound machine with a transducer (curvilinear, microcurvilinear array, small-phased array, or a mechanical sector transducer with frequencies between 2.5 and 5.0 MHz are acceptable; however, 3.0–3.5 MHz is most common.). Transvaginal ultrasound is performed with an endovaginal or endocavitary transducer of at least 5.0 MHz. A barrier transducer cover is required, which is often a manufacture sheath or a latex condom. Gel is required between the transducer and the cover to eliminate any air gap.

Procedure: The primary goal in pelvic ultrasound is to effectively rule out an ectopic pregnancy by identifying an intrauterine pregnancy. A full and thorough evaluation of the uterus is required; then and only then should the ovaries be evaluated. Pelvic ultrasound may include both a transabdominal as well as a transvaginal component. In the transabdominal ultrasound the bladder is used as a sonographic window and is ideally full. The transvaginal ultrasound is ideally performed with the bladder empty because when fully distended the bladder may displace the uterus and pelvic organs. Both approaches include a long and a short axis view.

1. Patient is supine.
2. Patient is supine.

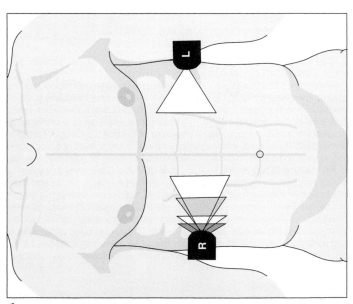

Figure VIII–9. Renal ultrasound.
A. Anatomic map, indicating transducer placement for the sonograms.
B. Coronal comparison of kidneys: Abnormal; note the dilatation in the sinus of the kidney labeled with hydronephrosis compared with the dense hyperechoic sinus of the normal kidney.
C. Left kidney: Abnormal, large 7.0-cm renal cyst at the inferior pole of the kidney, showing classic findings of a smooth wall, anechoic fluid, and posterior acoustic enhancement.

(Courtesy of Paul R. Sierzenski, MD, RDMS, Christiana Care Health System, Newark, Delaware)

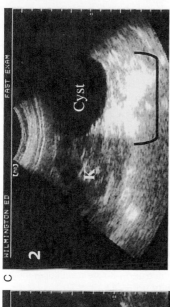

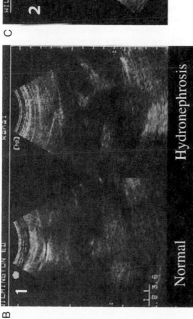

Figure VIII–9. Renal ultrasound. **A.** Anatomic map, indicating transducer placement for the sonograms. **B.** Coronal comparison of kidneys: Abnormal; note the dilatation in the sinus of the kidney labeled with hydronephrosis compared with the dense hyperechoic sinus of the normal kidney. **C.** Left kidney: Abnormal, large 7.0-cm renal cyst at the inferior pole of the kidney, showing classic findings of a smooth wall, anechoic fluid, and posterior acoustic enhancement. (Courtesy of Paul R. Sierzenski, MD, RDMS, Christiana Care Health System, Newark, Delaware)

3. Examine the **pelvis** (suprapubic window) in both the sagittal and transverse planes. Ideally the bladder is full to aid visualization; if a Foley is in place it may be clamped.
   a. *Sagittal View (Longitudinal)*: Transducer is placed about 1 cm above the symphysis pubis with the transducer indicator toward the patient's head and placed just superior to the symphysis (Figure VIII–10A, B).
      i. Identify the bladder (triangular in shape in this view when fully distended), uterus (pear-shaped), and rectum. An anechoic region between the bladder and uterus, between the uterus and rectum, or loops of bowl floating superior/posterior to the bladder may be evident.
   b. *Transverse View:* From the sagittal position rotate the probe 90 degrees counterclockwise so the transducer indicator points to the patient's right (Figure VIII–10C).
      i. Identify the bladder (rectangular in this view when fully distended), uterus (oval hyperechoic structure, if present), and rectum. Identify the bladder (triangular in shape in this view when fully distended), uterus (oval-shaped), and rectum. An anechoic region between the bladder and uterus, between the uterus and rectum, or loops of bowl floating superior/lateral to the bladder may be evident.
4. Examine the pelvis with the transvaginal approach: Place a small amount of ultrasound gel between the transducer tip and the transducer cover.
   a. *Sagittal Plane:* Begin in the sagittal plane with the transducer indicator directed up to the ceiling (Figure VIII–10D, E).
      i. Identify the bladder (triangular), uterus, endometrial stripe, rectum, and the vesicouterine and rectouterine pouches (pouch of Douglas)
      ii. Follow the endometrial stripe to the cervix, then return to the fundus and scan through to the later horns of the uterus.
      iii. Look for a gestational sac, intrauterine pregnancy, etc.
   b. *Coronal Plane:* From the sagittal plane rotate the transducer 90 degrees counterclockwise so the transducer indicator points to the patient's right.
      i. Identify the bladder (triangular), uterus, endometrial stripe, rectum, and the vesicouterine and rectouterine pouches (pouch of Douglas).
      ii. Scan through the uterus from the fundus to the cervix
      iii. Look for a gestational sac, intrauterine pregnancy, etc.
5. **Ovaries:** Only after you have evaluated the uterus and its contents, should you attempt to evaluate the ovaries. This can be performed in the longitudinal or the coronal plane. The iliac vessels will be your landmark, with the ovary classically noted to be anterior and medial to the vessel. Evaluate the ovary in two planes (Figure VIII–10A and D).
6. Clean the transducer with a disinfectant approved by the transducer manufacturer.

Complications: No clear complications from the procedure itself.

REFERENCES

Blaivas M, Sierzenski P, Plecque D, Lambert M. Do emergency physicians save time when locating a live intrauterine pregnancy with bedside ultrasonography? *Acad Emerg Med* 2000;7:988–993.

Choi H, Blaivas M, Lambert MJ. Gestational outcome in patients with first-trimester pregnancy complications and ultrasound-confirmed live intrauterine pregnancy. *Acad Emerg Med* 2000;7:200—203.

5. CENTRAL VENOUS LINE PLACEMENT

Indications

1. Rapid fluid administration required.
2. Vasopressive medication administration.
3. Total parenteral nutrition.
4. Invasive hemodynamic monitoring, eg, Swan–Ganz catheter.
5. Hemodialysis.
6. Lack of alternative access.

Contraindications

1. Known severe atherosclerotic disease at vessel site (relative contraindication).
2. Coagulopathy (relative contraindication).

Materials: Sterile gown and gloves, mask, sterile towels, povidone–iodine, lidocaine, 25-gauge needle, syringe, 3-0 suture, needle driver or straight needle. Commercial catheter kits: single-lumen units—Cordis (for large volume administration and PA catheter placement), Shiley (for hemodialysis), and triple-lumen units (for low to moderate flow rates and additional access ports). These commercial kits will contain all necessary needles, scalpel, guidewires, sheaths, and dilators. Please note that when opening multiple kits, guidewires are of varying lengths and are not necessarily interchangeable.

Right Internal Jugular Vein Approach

(Left side is not recommended as a first approach because laceration of the thoracic duct, left brachiocephalic vein, or superior vena cava is possible)

Procedure

1. Obtain consent (unless implied emergency consent applies).
2. Patient should be connected to ECG monitoring unit.
3. Place patient in Trendelenburg position.
4. Identify landmarks: (Figure VIII–11). Three common sites, but most favor the middle approach: anterior or medial to sternocleidomastoid muscle belly; middle between the two heads of the sternocleidomastoid muscle; posterior or lateral to the sternocleidomastoid muscle belly. Further description here will detail the middle approach.
5. Prep out neck with povidone–iodine and drape with sterile towels.

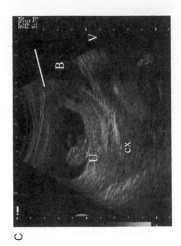

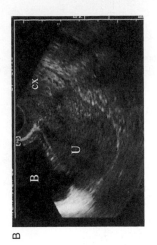

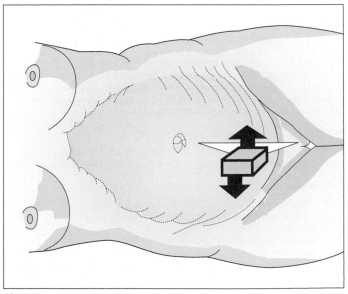

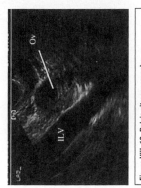

E

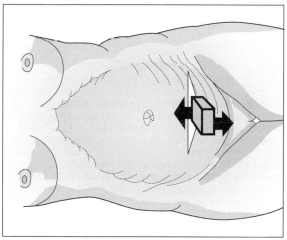

D

Figure VIII-10. Pelvic ultrasonography.
A. Anatomic map, indicating transducer placement for sonograms B and C.
B. Endovaginal sagittal ultrasound: Ultrasound of nonpregnant patient, showing the key identifying landmarks of the bladder and cervix to verify the structure identified is the uterus.
C. Transabdominal sagittal ultrasound of pregnant patient, showing bladder, uterus with intrauterine pregnancy. Identifying landmarks of vagina, cervix, and bladder.
D. Anatomic map, indicating transducer placement for sonogram E.
E. Sagittal left ovary: Normal. Note the classic relation of the ILV to the ovary with peripheral follicles.
Key: B = bladder; cx = cervix; U = uterus; V = vagina; ILV = iliac vein; Ov = ovary.
(Courtesy of Paul R. Sierzenski, MD, RDMS, Christiana Care Health System, Newark, Delaware)

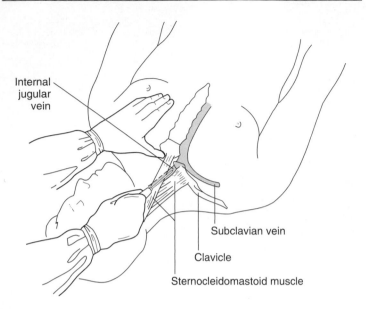

Internal
jugular
vein

Subclavian vein

Clavicle

Sternocleidomastoid muscle

Figure VIII–11. The technique for internal jugular vein catheterization, central approach (Reproduced, with permission, from Lefor AT, Gomella LG, eds. *Surgery on Call,* 3rd ed. McGraw-Hill, 2001:344.)

6. Open commercial catheter kit. Familiarize yourself with contents.
7. Preflush lumen(s) of the catheter with saline and close all ports except the distal port (if using a triple-lumen catheter).
8. Cordis units should have the dilator placed inside of the sheath prior to vein insertion.
9. Load the large-bore, thin-walled needle onto the 10-mL syringe with gentle pressure only (pressure that is too firm makes this needle difficult to remove, which often leads to the needle becoming dislodged from the vein after successful cannulation).
10. Make a small wheal of lidocaine at planned puncture site with 25-gauge or smaller needle.
11. Initial location of the internal jugular vein can be confirmed with a small-gauge finder needle. This creates less trauma for the patient but is often omitted because of the frequent emergent nature of gaining central access.
12. Direct the thin-walled needle at the apex of the triangle between the two heads of the sternocleidomastoid. The needle should be aimed at the ipsilateral nipple and at a 15–30-degree angle to the skin.

13. Once through the skin, aspirate as the needle is advanced to determine if cannulation is successful. Nonpulsatile dark venous blood should be easily withdrawn into the syringe. Be certain if unsuccessful at first pass to slowly withdraw the needle as a flash of blood may be seen on the return path.
14. Remove the syringe from the needle. Venous blood should continue to flow (air embolism can occur here if the patient is not in Trendelenburg position); the guidewire is then advanced through the lumen of the needle.
15. The wire should easily pass through the needle. Watch the ECG monitor for signs of ventricular irritation. If irritation occurs, withdraw the wire until arrhythmias cease.
16. While maintaining constant control of the guidewire, withdraw the needle over the guidewire.
17. Enough wire should be left outside of the patient to accommodate the length of the catheter.
18. With a stabbing motion use the scalpel to make a small nick in the skin where the guidewire enters.
19. Feed the guidewire through the dilator of the Cordis unit or the distal lumen of the triple-lumen catheter. Maintain constant control of the wire at the skin site until the end of the guidewire exits the proximal end of the catheter.
20. The distal end of the wire is now held firmly while the catheter is advanced over it though the skin into the vessel. The larger Cordis catheter may require a rotatory movement to enable it to dilate and pass through the dermis and SC tissue.
21. The guidewire is now removed from the catheter. For Cordis catheters, the wire and dilator are removed together in one assembly.
22. Aspirate blood from the distal port to again confirm correct placement.
23. Flush the catheter with saline.
24. Suture catheter in place with 3-0 suture and cover with a sterile dressing.
25. A CXR should be obtained to rule out pneumothorax and to confirm placement. The tip of catheter should be seen at the junction between the superior vena cava and the right atrium.

Subclavian Vein Approach (right or left)

(Left approach is preferred for floating a Swan–Ganz catheter.)

Procedure

1. Obtain consent (unless implied emergency consent applies).
2. Patient should be connected to ECG monitoring unit.
3. Place patient in Trendelenburg position.
4. A small rolled-up towel placed between the scapulae and gentle arm distraction with external rotation of the humerus may aid in successful cannulation of vein.
5. Identify landmarks see Figure VIII–12. Prep out subclavian area and neck simultaneously (facilitates secondary approach to the neck should subclavian attempt prove unsuccessful).

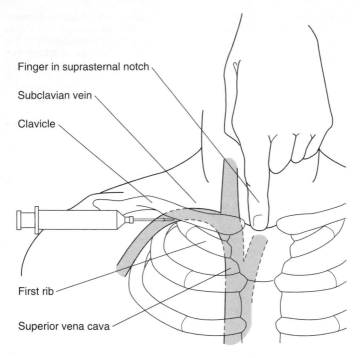

Finger in suprasternal notch

Subclavian vein

Clavicle

First rib

Superior vena cava

Figure VIII–12. The technique for subclavian vein catheterization. (Reproduced, with permission, from Gomella LG. ed. *Clinician's Pocket Reference,* 9th ed. McGraw-Hill, 2002:259.)

6. Follow steps 6 through 10 for internal jugular line placement.
   Place nondominant hand on sternal notch.
7. Direct thin-walled needle toward sternal notch while passing above the first rib and below the clavicle. Bevel of needle should be caudally directed, which facilitates easy passage of the guidewire into the SVC and decreases an inadvertent wire passage into the jugular vein.
8. Follow steps 13 through 25 for internal jugular line placement.

Femoral Vein Approach (right or left)

Procedure
(Safest approach with no risk of pneumothorax)

1. Obtain consent (unless implied emergency consent applies).
2. Place patient supine and slightly flex hip and externally rotate femur.
3. Prep out area and drape with sterile towels.

4. Identify landmarks: NAVL—nerve, artery, vein, lymphatics in lateral to medial orientation.
5. Follow steps 6 through 10 for internal jugular line placement.
   With nondominant hand on femoral artery, direct thin-walled needle just medial to the arterial pulse, while maintaining 45-degree angle to the skin. The needle bevel should be directed cephalad.
6. Once through the skin, aspirate as the needle is advanced to determine if cannulation is successful Nonpulsatile dark venous blood should be easily withdrawn into the syringe. Be certain if unsuccessful at first pass to slowly withdraw the needle because a flash of blood may be seen on the return path.
7. Remove the syringe from the needle. Venous blood should continue to flow; the guidewire is then advanced through the lumen of the needle.
8. Follow steps 16 through 25 for internal jugular line placement.

Complications: Pneumothorax, hemothorax, arterial puncture, air embolus, infection, hemorrhage, distal emboli.

REFERENCES

Conahan TJ 3rd, Schwartz AJ, Geer RT. Percutaneous catheter introduction: The Seldinger technique. *JAMA* 1977;237:446–447.
Sznajder JI, Zvoibil ГП, Dittermann H, Welner P, Bursztein S. Central vein catheterization: Failure and complication rates by three percutaneous approaches. *Arch Intern Med* 1986;146:259–261.

6. CRICOTHYROTOMY

Surgical Cricothyrotomy

Indications

1. Need for definitive airway control.
2. Failure of or contraindication to orotracheal and nasotracheal intubation.

Contraindications
No absolute contraindications. Relative contraindications include

1. Coagulopathy.
2. Anterior neck hematoma.
3. Overlying infection.
4. Fractured larynx.
5. Possible tracheal transection.

Materials

1. Scalpel with No. 11 blade.
2. Tracheal hook.
3. Trousseau dilator.
4. No. 4 Shiley cuffed tracheostomy tube with obturator.

5. Povidone–iodine antiseptic solution.
6. 4 × 4 gauze pads
7. 3-0 silk suture material.

Procedure

1. Palpate the thyroid and cricothyroid cartilages.
2. Prepare the neck in sterile fashion.
3. Locate the cricothyroid membrane. Begin palpation in the sternal notch and work cephalad in the midline. The cricothyroid membrane is the depression just cephalad to the cricoid cartilage. Some prefer to locate the membrane by starting at the thyroid notch, then palpating down the midline to the first depression.
4. Make a vertical incision in the midline from the thyroid cartilage extending caudally 3–4 cm.
5. Using blunt dissection, locate the cricothyroid membrane.
6. Place the tracheal hook through the cricothyroid membrane, holding traction on the inferior margin of the thyroid cartilage. Do not relax the traction on this cartilage.
7. Make a horizontal incision through the cricothyroid membrane.
8. Dilate the space using the Trousseau dilator, especially in the vertical dimension, and remove the dilator.
9. Pass the Shiley No. 4 tube through the space, passing the tube posteriorly through the space, then inferiorly.
10. Remove the tracheal hook carefully.
11. Inflate the balloon.
12. Suture the flanges in place.
13. Remove the obturator and replace it with the inner cannula and connect to ventilation source.

Complications

1. Improper placement.
2. Inadequate ventilation.
3. Hemorrhage.
4. Aspiration.
5. Infection.
6. Barotrauma.

Needle Cricothyrotomy

Indications: Patient younger than 8 years old.
Contraindications

1. Same as for surgical cricothyrotomy.
2. Complete upper airway obstruction.

Materials

1. 14- or 16-gauge angiocatheter.
2. 3- or 5-mL syringe.

3. Hemostat.
4. Normal saline.
5. 30-psi oxygen source and tubing.
6. Povidone–iodine antiseptic solution.
7. 4 × 4 gauze pads.
8. 3-0 silk suture material.
9. Towel roll.

Procedure

1. If it is not contraindicated, place towel roll under patient's shoulders and lower neck to maximize exposure of neck.
2. Identify the cricothyroid membrane. Begin palpation in the sternal notch and work cephalad in the midline. The cricothyroid membrane is the depression just cephalad to the cricoid cartilage. Some prefer to locate the membrane by starting at the thyroid notch, then palpating down the midline to the first depression.
3. Attach the angiocatheter to the syringe. Aspirate 1–2 mL of NS into the barrel of the syringe.
4. Prepare the anterior midline neck in sterile fashion. Locate the cricothyroid membrane again. Stabilize the thyroid cartilage with the thumb and middle fingers of the nondominant hand. Place the index finger of the nondominant hand on the cricothyroid membrane.
5. Advance the angiocatheter through the skin and cricothyroid membrane into the larynx while maintaining negative pressure on the syringe. The appearance of bubbles in the barrel of the syringe should confirm proper location of the assembly.
6. Once into the larynx, advance the catheter over the needle in a caudad fashion. Remove the needle and syringe, being careful to stabilize the catheter in place.
7. Suture the catheter in place. Attach the catheter directly to the wall oxygen supply or jet ventilation source.

Complications: Same as for surgical cricothyrotomy.

REFERENCES

Bramwell KJ. Needle cricothyrotomy. In: Rosen P, Chan TC, Vilke GM, Sternbach G, eds. *Atlas of Emergency Procedures.* Mosby, 2001:22–23.
Peak DA, Roy S. Needle cricothyrotomy revisited. *Pediatr Emerg Care* 1999;15(3):224–226.
Walls RM. Cricothyrotomy. In Rosen P, Chan TC, Vilke GM, Sternbach G, eds. *Atlas of Emergency Procedures.* Mosby, 2001:24–29.

7. EYE AND NOSE PROCEDURES

Eye

A. Eye Irrigation
Indications: Chemical or foreign body in eye.
Contraindication: Globe perforation.

Materials: Saline (liter bag), IV tubing, basin or trough to catch run off, topical anesthetic.

Procedure

1. Anesthetize eyes with topical anesthetic.
2. Assemble IV tubing and bag.
3. Assist patient with eye opening (may require lid retractors).
4. Open IV tubing wide.
5. Gently irrigate eyes making sure to include the cul-du-sac under lids.
6. Wash lids and lashes to remove adherent material.
7. A nasal cannula placed on nasal bridge will allow bilateral irrigation.
8. Morgan lens—Placed under lids after topical anesthesia is applied, this special device with tubing attached allows for constant bilateral irrigation.

B. Foreign Body and Rust Ring Removal

Indication: Foreign body either in cul-du-sac under lid, adherent to cornea or embedded in cornea.

Contraindication: Globe perforation.

Materials: Topical anesthetic, eye irrigation solution, cotton-tipped applicator, Tb syringe and needle, Alger brush.

Procedure

1. Apply topical anesthesia.
2. **Irrigation:** Use squeeze bottle to irrigate foreign body out; may require cotton-tipped applicator to remove.
3. **Applicator:** Moisten tip with topical anesthetic, use cotton tip to scrape foreign body out; may cause a larger abrasion.
4. **Tb syringe:**
   a. Using slit lamp magnification.
   b. Rest hand on patient's cheek.
   c. Visualize needle tip and foreign body.
   d. Slowly advance needle with bevel down until touches cornea adjacent to foreign body.
   e. Scoop out foreign body.
   f. Visualize to ensure complete removal.
5. **Alger brush:** This device is essentially a small electric burr that allows material adherent to the cornea to be debrided under controlled conditions.
   a. Start device by spinning burr by hand (some devices have a button that must be held down).
   b. Rest hand on patient's cheek.
   c. Have patient fix gaze on object over the examiner's shoulder.
   d. Visualize burr and foreign body under slit lamp.
   e. Slowly remove adherent material in a circular motion.
   f. Visualize cornea to ensure complete removal.

C. Intraocular Pressure

Indications: Suspicion of elevated intraocular pressure as in glaucoma and iritis.

Contraindications: Perforated globe, infection.

Methods

1. **Schiötz tonometer**
   a. Apply topical anesthesia.
   b. Clean device footplate with alcohol.
   c. Put 7.5-g weight in place.
   d. Zero device on hard surface in case.
   e. Place patient in supine position.
   f. Hold open lids without placing pressure on globe.
   g. Rest tonometer on center of cornea and read scale.
   h. Use chart that is provided with device to obtain intraocular pressure.
   i. Clean device footplate with alcohol.
2. **Tono-Pen**
   a. Apply topical anesthesia.
   b. Apply condom on tip of device.
   c. Depress button until two parallel lines are displayed and a beep occurs.
   d. Have the patient stare at a fixed position.
   e. Gently tap the device on the center of the cornea. With each valid reading a small chirp will occur. Continue repeatedly tapping on the cornea until a longer beep is heard.
   f. The intraocular pressure will be displayed on the screen.
   g. Remove and discard the condom. Replace with a new condom for storage.

Nose

A. *Cautery:* See epistaxis discussion.
B. *Anterior Packing:* See epistaxis discussion.
C. *Posterior Packing:* See epistaxis discussion.
D. *Drainage of Septal Hematoma*

Indications: Trauma has caused a hematoma to form between the perichondrium and cartilage of the nasal septum. It is important to remove the hematoma to prevent pressure necrosis of the cartilage and subsequent saddle deformity of the nose.
Contraindications: Untreated coagulopathy.
Materials: Topical anesthetic, No. 15 or 11 blade on scalpel, small Frazier tip suction, sterile rubber band drain, anterior nasal packing.

Procedure

1. Apply topical anesthesia.
2. Make an elliptical incision from posterior to anterior over the hematoma, removing a small amount of skin to prevent premature closure.
3. Suction out clot with small Frazier tip suction.
4. Place rubber band drain.
5. Pack anterior nasal vault as in anterior epistaxis.
6. Start oral antibiotics (cefazolin, amoxicillin/clavulanate, TMP-SMZ).
7. Reexamine every 24 h until hematoma has resolved.

E. Nasal Foreign Body Removal

Indication: Impacted foreign body in nose.
Contraindications: Uncooperative patient, airway obstruction.

1. **Baropressure method**
   a. Occlude unaffected nostril with your hand.
   b. Forcefully blow in child's mouth (or have parent try).
   c. Often the object will be propelled from the nose.
2. **Direct method**
   a. Apply topical anesthetic and vasoconstrictor.
   b. Have assistant restrain child's head. Conscious sedation may be required to safely remove the foreign body.
   c. Remove with bayonet forceps, alligator forceps, wire loop, or right-angle hook.
3. **Balloon catheter method**
   a. Apply topical anesthetic and vasoconstrictor.
   b. Have assistant restrain child's head. Conscious sedation may be required to safely remove the foreign body.
   c. Pass No. 10 or 12 French Foley catheter until balloon is past foreign body.
   d. Inflate with 2–3 mL of air.
   e. Withdraw catheter slowly until the foreign body is pushed more anterior in the nose.

Complications

1. Epistaxis—typically minor.
2. Laceration of nasal mucosa—typically minor.
3. Barotrauma of pulmonary system—pneumothorax, pneumomediastinum, perforation of TM are possible but not reported.
4. Failure to remove foreign body, which often requires ENT consultation and at times a trip to the OR.

8. INTRAOSSEOUS LINE PLACEMENT

Indications

1. To administer drugs, fluids, blood during resuscitation when vascular access cannot be obtained rapidly.
2. To obtain vascular access in critically ill children when peripheral venous access is difficult or impossible.

Contraindications

1. Fracture or severe injury to site.
2. Overlying cellulitis or infection.
3. Previous unsuccessful intraosseous attempts in same bone.
4. Known osteogenesis imperfecta or osteopetrosis.

Materials: Intraosseous needle (15- or 18-gauge needle with stylet, prefer-ably bone marrow aspiration needle or specially made intraosseous needle), povidone–iodine wipe, alcohol wipe, two 10-mL syringes (one with NS), tape, 4×4 gauze pads, gloves.

Procedure

1. Find landmarks (flat portion of anterior medial tibia, 1–3 cm below prox-imal tibial tuberosity), alternative sites are above medial malleolus, dis-tal femur, anterior superior iliac spine.
2. Position patient supine with hip flexed and abducted, knee flexed. Place fin-gers of nondominant hand on lateral sides of leg adjacent to insertion site to stabilize knee from above. Do not place fingers behind the insertion site.
3. Put on gloves, prep area with povidone–iodine wipe, alcohol wipe.
4. Insert needle at 90-degree angle with rotating, back-and-forth "screwing" motion and steady pressure on flat portion of tibia; use palm of hand for leverage.
5. Stop insertion when a "pop" is felt; needle is now stable and perpendic-ular to bone.
6. Remove stylet, attach 10-mL syringe, attempt to aspirate blood and bone marrow (may not be possible, even with successful placement).
7. Attach 10-mL syringe with NS, flush; if syringe flushes easily without ex-travasation, secure flange of needle to leg using tape and gauze pads.
8. If syringe does not flush easily, insertion is not successful; remove nee-dle and reattempt in opposite leg.
9. All medications administered through IO line should be followed by 5-mL saline flush. Volume bolus can be administered using 60-mL syringes pushed manually or pressure bag.

Complications: Bent needle, missed placement (sliding off bone, pene-trating through posterior cortex, soft-tissue placement), fracture, osteomyelitis, compartment syndrome, extravasation of drugs

REFERENCES

Iserson KV, Criss E. Intraosseous infusions: A usable technique. *Am J Emerg Med* 1986;4(6):540–542.

Mattera CJ. Take aim—hit your IO target. A comprehensive approach to pediatric in-traosseous infusion, including site selection, needle insertion & ongoing assessment. *J Emerg Med Serv* 2000;25(4):38–48.

9. LACERATION AND WOUND CARE

Indications: Primary objectives include preserving viable tissue, restoring tissue continuity and function, optimizing development of wound strength, min-imizing risk of infection, and optimizing cosmetic outcome.

Contraindications: Wound closure is contraindicated in wounds > 6 h old, or > 12 h old on the face, puncture wounds, and most animal and human bites.

Materials

1. Suture kit, including local anesthetic, 1 or 2% lidocaine, with or without epinephrine, suture material.
2. Irrigation materials, including NS or sterile water, syringe with splash guard.
3. Skin preparations, including povidone–iodine and a cleansing soap such as chlorhexidine.
4. Instruments, including needle driver, small scissors, forceps, and curved hemostat.
5. Gauze pads (4×4).
6. Sterile towels and gloves.

Procedures

1. **Evaluation:** All wounds need to be adequately evaluated. Examine type of wound and look for associated injuries, including blood vessel, nerve, or tendon injury. Joint wounds need to be examined closely for penetration into joint capsule. Always assess neurovascular status and function of area before and after repair.
2. **Wound preparation**
   a. **Disinfection of surrounding skin:** *Povidone–iodine* is possibly "wound-toxic" and should not come in contact with open wound, but can be used to disinfect surrounding area.
      Poloxamer 188/chlorhexidine is good for cleansing of skin and wound; however, it has no antibacterial activity.
   b. **Debridement:** Obvious devascularized and mutilated tissue should be excised in attempt to provide a clean, viable wound edge.
   c. **Hair removal:** Shaving area shown to increase risk of infection. Hair can be cleansed similar to skin; if hair removal necessary, it can be cut. Avoid shaving/cutting eyebrows.
   d. **Irrigation:** Copious irrigation necessary to adequately clean wound. High-pressure/high-volume irrigation most effective in cleaning wounds; however, it can cause some tissue edema, which decreases resistance to infection and should be used in significantly contaminated wounds. Low-pressure irrigation can be used in "clean" wounds. Additional mechanical scrubbing assists in dislodging particulate matter.
3. **Anesthesia:** Most agree anesthesia should be provided before irrigation and debridment to optimize patient comfort and provide adequate wound preparation.
   a. **Topical:** These agents are useful in decreasing pain associated with laceration repair and are particularly helpful in pediatric patients and some facial lacerations where infiltration may obscure cosmetic landmarks.
   b. **Local agents and technique:** Lidocaine 1% and 2% most commonly used; when combined with epinephrine it can help prolong duration

of action, reduce amount of anesthetic necessary, and promote venostasis. Lidocaine with epinephrine should be avoided in digits, tip of nose, penis, or ears due to lack of collateral blood flow and theoretical risk of ischemic injury. Pain of local anesthesia administration can be reduced by using a smaller needle (less than 25 gauge), slow rate of infiltration, by injecting through wound instead of intact skin, buffering with sodium bicarbonate, and warming the anesthetic.

c. **Nerve blocks:** Useful for large lacerations, heavily contaminated wounds, and areas difficult to infiltrate locally such as the fingers and plantar aspect of foot.

d. **Sedation:** Should be considered in pediatric patients with larger lacerations or wounds in cosmetically important areas.

4. **Suture techniques and type:** Three types of wound closure:

a. **Primary:** If wound less than 6–8 h old (less than 12 h old for facial wounds) and can be adequately prepared and reapproximated.

b. **Secondary:** Wound basically heals on its own ("secondary intention"). Used in wounds that present after 8 h, heavily contaminated wounds, or punctures.

c. **Delayed primary:** Primary closure of wounds that were heavily contaminated or presented late, but require closure for cosmetic or functional purposes. Closure typically done 48–72 h after initial injury.

Tension is of primary importance in wound repair because it can worsen scarring and cause wound necrosis and dehiscence. Use techniques that reduce the tension on the wound, and employ deep, absorbable sutures, vertical mattress sutures, or multiple simple interrupted sutures. Skin sutures should be last step to achieve the best cosmetic appearance and **not** to be used to "pull" wound margins together.

Wound edges tend to invert with healing, so repair must concentrate on everting the margin of the wound with repair. This is best accomplished by introducing the suture needle through the skin at a 90-degree angle.

Select the smallest diameter suture that provides adequate strength in closing the wound. All suture types vary in strength, infection propensity, inflammation potential, and rates of absorption. Absorbable suture should not only be used in deep or subcutaneous buried suturing but also considered in areas where suture removal is difficult, such as fingertips or inside the mouth.

d. **Alternatives**

i. **Tape:** Wound tape cannot evert edge or close deep structures. Should only be considered in superficial or partial-thickness wounds with little tension.

ii. **Staples:** Markedly decrease time required in wound repair and provides a strong closure. Provides a cosmetically acceptable repair in areas such as scalp, torso, and extremities. Should not be used on face or cosmetically important areas, or areas requiring close approximation to maintain function.

   iii. Adhesive "skin glue": Provides benefit of minimal pain or trauma
   to patient and less time required in wound repair. If extensive irrigation or debridment required, local anesthesia is still indicated.
   Glue has low tensile strength, particularly in the first 48 h and
   should not be used in area with significant tension.
5. **Wound care**
   a. **Dressings:** Most clinicians recommend a wound dressing to cover
   the wound for at least the first 24–36 h after repair. Usually includes
   a thin film of antibiotic ointment followed by a nonadherent dressing
   and finally a dry, sterile gauze dressing. Splints should be considered
   if the wound crosses a joint and is at risk for increased tension.
   Wound checks should be done at 24–48 h in patients with bite wounds,
   heavily contaminated wounds, and hand wounds. Current recommendations for facial wounds include gentle cleansing with soap and
   water to minimize or remove eschar formation followed by a thin film
   of antibacterial ointment two to three times a day. Scars contain no
   melanin, so light-skinned patients should be advised to avoid excessive sun exposure to the wound
   b. **Antibiotics:** Consider antibiotic prophylaxis in high-risk wounds:
   heavily contaminated, animal and human bites, hand wounds, immunosuppression of patient.
   c. **Tetanus:** Update tetanus status as indicated and consider tetanus
   immune globulin in those inadequately immunized. Wounds at increased risk for tetanus include crush injuries, stellate lacerations,
   and heavily contaminated wounds.
   d. **Suture removal:** Timing is important because if removed too early
   wound may dehisce and late removal may worsen scarring.

Suture Removal Times

Scalp: 8–10 days
Facial: 3–5 days
Chest/abdomen: 8–10 days
Back: 12–14 days
Arm/hand: 8–10 days
Fingertip: 10–12 days
Lower extremity: 8–12 days
Joint extensor surface: 10–14 days

6. **Special wounds**
   a. **Puncture wounds:** By definition, puncture wounds are deeper than
   they are wide and are typically caused by an object that may contain
   significant enough bacteria to seed the deep tissue. These wounds
   should not be closed because they are difficult to adequately irrigate
   and cleanse.
   b. **Animal bites:** Animals typically cause puncture and shearing wounds
   with subsequent inoculation of bacteria into the wound. The primary
   consideration should be adequate irrigation and debridement of de-

vitalized tissue. Puncture wounds should not be closed. In wounds requiring closure to maintain function; deep, absorbable sutures should be avoided. Cat bites are considered to have higher risk of infection due to nature of bite and increased incidence of *Pasteurella multocida*. High-risk bites in which antibiotics should be considered include hand wounds, facial wounds in infants, puncture or crush wounds, immunosuppressed patients (including diabetics, alcoholics, elderly), and cat bites.

c. **Human bites:** Treat the same as animal bites; however, hand wounds have a high incidence of infection. Always explore hand wounds thoroughly for evidence of extension into joint capsule or tendon injury.

d. **Facial wounds:** Patients will be much more concerned regarding cosmetic outcome in facial wounds. Take additional time to identify skin landmarks (ie, vermilion border) and reapproximate carefully. Minimize tension on the wound with deep sutures and use smallest diameter suture possible (6-0 nylon).

Complications: Wound infection; continued bleeding; dehiscence; abscess formation; loss of normal function of area; unrecognized nerve, vascular, or tendon injury.

REFERENCE

Edlich RF, Rodeheaver GT, Morgan RF, Berman DE, Thacker JG. Principles of emergency wound management. *Ann Emerg Med* 1988;17:1284–1302.

10. LUMBAR PUNCTURE

Indications
Diagnostic

1. Infection (bacterial, mycobacterial, viral, fungal, protozoan).
2. Subarachnoid hemorrhage (SAH).
3. Inflammatory diseases (Guillain–Barré, MS, certain vasculitides).
4. Leptomeningeal carcinomatosis.

Therapeutic

1. Spinal anesthetics.
2. Alleviation of intrathecal pressure (pseudotumor cerebri).
3. Introduction of contrast, steroids, antibiotics, or chemotherapeutic agents.

Contraindications

1. Local infection/cellulitis at site of puncture.
2. Known or suspected elevation in intracranial pressure (tumor, bleeding, edema, abscess).
3. Severe coagulopathy or thrombocytopenia.
4. Degenerative joint disease of the spine (relative).

Materials: Sterile lumber puncture tray with the following: two drapes (one fenestrated/one unfenestrated), gauze, povidone–iodine, 1% lidocaine ampule, 20-gauge needle, anesthesia needle, spinal needle, manometer with tubing and stopcock, four CSF collection tubes, adhesive bandage. Sterile gloves, gown, and mask.

Procedure

1. Obtain informed consent from patient after explaining risks and benefits.
2. Position patient for optimal access either on side in fetal position with back perpendicular to gurney, or seated and flexed forward at the hips with thorax and shoulder rolled forward over support (Figure VIII–13).
3. Adjust gurney and stool to desired height.
4. Placing your hands on patient's left and right posterior superior iliac crests, imagine a straight line running between them. The L3-L4 interspace should be where this line intersects the spinal column. You **must** be below the L1-L2 interspace (point at which spinal cord becomes cauda equina). This is your site of needle insertion. You may mark it with the hub of a needle cover or a permanent marker.
5. Open sterile tray without contaminating contents.
6. Don your mask, sterile gloves (and gown if used).
7. Prepare all necessary equipment. Draw up lidocaine, uncap CSF collection tubes and place upright in numerical order, connect manometer to tubing and stopcock.
8. Pour povidone–iodine into basin without compromising sterile field.
9. Place unfenestrated drape at base of patient's back atop the gurney. Take care not to contaminate your gloves (this can be done by folding the drape over the gloves while tucking it under the patient.
10. Now, using the sponge sticks or gauze moistened with povidone–iodine, scrub the previously delineated puncture site at the L3-L4 interspace, starting at the proposed puncture site and scrubbing in firm concentric circles from that site outward. Take care not to allow the solution to drip from superior aspects of the field downward, as this will contaminate your puncture site.
11. Fill the syringe with 1% lidocaine, affix a small-gauge needle, and raise a small skin wheal in the marked interspace. Then advance the needle into the deeper subcutaneous tissues while injecting anesthetic and aiming for the umbilicus. You should only use approximately 50% of the lidocaine for this.
12. Next inject the remainder of the lidocaine into the deeper subcutaneous tissues in a fan-like distribution to anesthetize the recurrent spinal nerves in this area.
13. Examine the spinal needle to ensure that the stylet will freely advance and withdraw. Then check that the notch on the stylet is facing upward.
14. Insert the spinal needle, following the previous puncture direction while slowly advancing the needle into the interspace. This should be performed with the needle remaining parallel to the bed (perpendicular to the skin) and advancing toward the umbilicus. If you feel bony resistance, gently withdraw and aim slightly more cephalad.

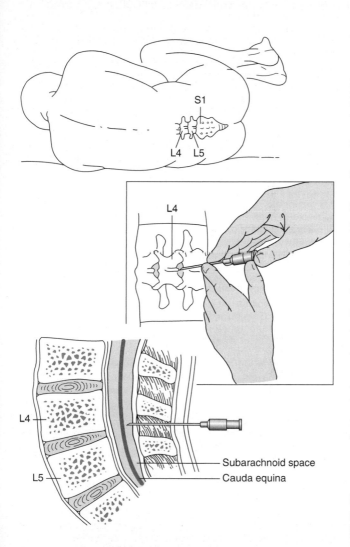

Figure VIII–13. When you are performing a lumbar puncture, place the patient in the lateral decubitus position and locate the L4–L5 interspace. Control the spinal needle with two hands and enter the subarachnoid space. (Reproduced, with permission, from Haist SA, Robbins JB, Gomella LG, eds. *Internal Medicine on Call.* 3rd ed. McGraw-Hill, 2002:416.)

15. Frequently withdraw the stylet, checking for CSF flow as you advance through the ligaments.
16. A "pop" indicates that the ligamentum flavum and dura mater have probably been penetrated, and withdrawing the stylet should reveal CSF flowing outward.
17. If measuring opening pressures, the manometer/tubing/stopcock apparatus should be snugly affixed to the spinal needle as the CSF exits. The opening pressure is measured as the point at which the meniscus ultimately rises (normal = 5–20 cm H_2O in a patient with relaxed neck and legs; 10–28 cm H_2O in a patient with neck and legs flexed). The CSF tubes can then be filled by opening the spigot of the stopcock and filling each tube with approximately 1 mL of the CSF.
18. If not measuring opening pressures, you may simply fill each tube with 1 mL of CSF as it exits the spinal needle. Take care to fill the tubes, as they are numbered, in sequential order.
19. Once the tubes have been filled and capped, you can replace the stylet and withdraw the spinal needle in a smooth, single motion. The patient's back may now be cleaned and a bandage applied.
20. Label the CSF tubes and send for analysis: (1) cell count, Gram's stain. (2) protein/glucose. (3) culture and sensitivity. (4) hold (for repeat cell count, or other analyses).

Complications: Headache, bleeding/bruising, infection ranging from local cellulitis to meningitis, mild local backache, transient sciatic-type sharp pain radiating into leg or groin, exacerbation of previous spinal column complaints (eg, root compression syndromes).

REFERENCE

Carson D, Serpell M. Choosing the best needle for diagnostic lumbar puncture. *Neurology* 1996;47(1):33–37.

11. PARACENTESIS

Indications

1. Diagnosis of cause of ascites.
2. Therapeutic drainage of massive ascites for symptomatic relief (eg, respiratory and abdominal discomfort).

Contraindications

1. Clinically evident fibrinolysis or DIC.
2. Markedly distended bowel (relative).
3. Pregnancy (relative).

Materials: 20-mL syringe, 1.5-in. needles: 22 gauge for diagnostic taps and 16 or 18 gauge for therapeutic taps. Obese patients may require spinal needles (ie, 3.5-in. needles); specimen tubes, 1% lidocaine, vacuum bottles, phlebotomy tubing, povidone–iodine, drapes, sterile gloves, mask.

Procedure

1. Unless ascites is unquestionably present on physical examination, an ultrasound should be obtained before proceeding with the procedure.
2. Obtain consent.
3. Have patient empty bladder before paracentesis.
4. Place the patient supine with the head of the bed or examining table slightly elevated. Primary preferred site is infraumbilical midline through linea alba. Preferred alternative site is in either lower quadrant, approximately 4–5 cm cephalad and medial to the anterior superior iliac spine (lateral to the rectus sheath). Patients with lesser amounts of fluid may be placed in a lateral decubitus position with introduction of the needle into the midline or dependent lower quadrant. The rectus muscle should be avoided because of the presence of the superior and inferior epigastric vessels. Avoid sites of surgical scars.
5. Observe sterile technique. Use drapes, povidone–iodine, sterile gloves, mask. Apply povidone–iodine to skin area.
6. Inject lidocaine into skin and SC tissues.
7. Attach needle to the syringe and insert through the abdominal wall. The needle should be advanced slowly at 5-mm increments. After each small advancement, aspirate for a few seconds while the needle is stationary, then advance, then aspirate, and so on until the peritoneum is entered and fluid is aspirated.
8. Aspirate the amount of fluid needed for tests (30–50 mL). For a therapeutic tap, a 16- or 18-gauge needle can be connected to vacuum bottles with phlebotomy tubing. Large volume (up to 5 L) can be safely removed over a period of 60–90 min.
9. Order studies on fluid:
   a. **Routine:** Cell count, albumin, culture in blood culture bottles.
   b. **Optional:** Total protein, glucose, lactate dehydrogenase, amylase, Gram's stain, cytology, TB smear and culture.

Complications: Abdominal wall hemorrhage, precipitous fall in BP or electrolyte imbalance following rapid removal of large amounts of fluid, persistent fluid leakage, peritonitis, perforated viscus.

12. PERITONEAL LAVAGE (DIAGNOSTIC PERITONEAL LAVAGE)*

Indications

1. Evaluation of intraabdominal trauma (bleeding, perforation).
2. Acute peritoneal dialysis.

Contraindications: None are absolute. Relative contraindications include multiple abdominal procedures, pregnancy, and any coagulopathy.

---

*Reproduced, with permission, from Lefor AT, Gomella LG, Wiebke EA, Fraker DL, eds. *Surgery On Call,* 3rd ed. McGraw-Hill, 2001.

Materials: Prepackaged diagnostic peritoneal lavage or peritoneal dialysis tray.

Procedure

1. For a diagnostic peritoneal lavage (DPL), a Foley catheter and an NG tube must be in place. Prep the abdomen from above the umbilicus to the pubis. Wear gloves and mask.
2. The site of choice is in the midline 1–2 cm below the umbilicus. Avoid the site of old surgical scars (danger of adherent bowel). When a subumbilical scar or pelvic fracture is present, a supraumbilical approach is preferred.
3. Infiltrate the skin with 1% lidocaine with epinephrine. Incise the skin in the midline vertically and expose the fascia.
4. Pick up the fascia and either incise it or puncture it with the trocar and peritoneal catheter. Caution is needed to avoid puncturing any viscera. Use one hand to hold the catheter near the skin and to control the insertion while the other hand applies pressure to the end of the catheter. After entering the peritoneal cavity, remove the trocar and direct the catheter inferiorly into the pelvis.
5. For a diagnostic lavage, gross blood indicates a positive tap. If no blood is encountered, instill 10 mL/kg (about 1 L in adults) of RL or NS into the abdominal cavity.
6. Gently agitate the abdomen to distribute the fluid, and after 5 min drain off as much fluid as possible into a bag on the floor (minimum fluid for a valid analysis is 200 mL in an adult). Send the fluid for analysis (amylase, bile, bacteria, food fibers, hematocrit, cell count). See Table VIII–1, page 465 for the diagnosis of the fluid.
7. Remove the catheter and suture the skin. When the catheter is inserted for pancreatitis or peritoneal dialysis, suture it in place.
8. A negative DPL does not rule out retroperitoneal trauma. A false-positive DPL can be caused by a pelvic fracture.

Complications: Infection, bleeding, perforated viscus.

13. PROCEDURAL SEDATION IN ADULTS

Indications

1. Pain control and sedation for therapeutic interventions (significant pain or anxiety).
2. Immobility for diagnostic studies and minor procedures (pediatrics).
3. **Definitions**
   a. **Conscious sedation:** A minimally depressed level of consciousness that retains the patient's ability to maintain a patent airway independently and continuously and to respond appropriately to physical stimulation and verbal commands.
   b. **Deep sedation:** A controlled state of depressed consciousness or unconsciousness from which the patient is not easily aroused and is unable to respond purposefully to physical stimulation or verbal command. This may be accompanied by a partial or complete loss

TABLE VIII–1. DIAGNOSTIC PERITONEAL LAVAGE FINDINGS THAT SUGGEST INTRAABDOMINAL TRAUMA.

Positive	20 mL gross blood on free aspiration (10 mL in children)
	>100,000 RBC/μL
	>500 WBC/μL (if obtained > 3 hours after the injury)
	>175 units amylase/dL
	Bacteria on Gram's stain
	Bile (by inspection or chemical determination of bilirubin contents)
	Food particles (microscopic analysis of strained or spun specimen)
Intermediate	Pink fluid on free aspiration
	50,000–100,000 RBC/μL
	in blunt trauma
	100–500 WBC/μL
	75–175 units amylase/dL
Negative	Clear aspirate
	<100 WBC/μL
	<75 units amylase/dL

RBC = red blood cells; WBC = white blood cells.
Reproduced, with permission, from Macho JR, Lewis FR Jr. Krupski WC: Management of the injured patient. In: *Current Surgical Diagnosis & Treatment*, 11th ed. Way LW, ed. McGraw-Hill, 2003.

of protective reflexes and an inability to maintain a patent airway independently.

   c. General anesthesia: A controlled state of unconsciousness accompanied by a loss of protective reflexes, including loss of the ability to maintain a patent airway independently or to respond purposefully to physical stimulation or verbal command.

Contraindications

1. Inadequate operator experience, equipment, or time to correct airway and hemodynamic complications that may result from patient entering a depth of sedation *at least one level deeper than the planned level of sedation.*
2. Inadequate NPO time (relative to urgency of procedure and necessity of sedation).
3. Lack of appropriate institutional privileges for agents/depth of sedation.
4. Class III or IV anesthesia patients (these are high-risk patients and an anesthesiologist should be involved in these sedations).

Materials: Appropriate monitoring (pulse ox, continuous ECG, automatic BP cuff, trained observer/recorder—RN or technician), IV access if indicated, working suction, BVM and appropriate airway equipment (oral airways, intubation equipment), medications and appropriate "rescue" drugs, adjunctive oxygen (nasal cannula, blow-by, nonrebreather), defibrillator, ACLS medication cart.

Common Medications: Incremental dosages in the following table refer to common initial doses, not total. After time to onset, these dosages may be repeated to appropriate level of sedation. Individual responsiveness to dosages may vary.

Medication	Incremental Dose	Onset	Duration	Complication	Rescue
Ketamine	4 mg/kg IM	5–15 min	60–90 min	Laryngospasm	BVM
	0.5–2 mg/kg IV	30–60 s	5–10 min	Paralysis	
Versed	0.05–0.1 mg/kg IV	2–3 min	30–60 min	Apnea	Flumazenil
Fentanyl	0.5–1 µg/kg IV	2–3 min	45–60 min	Apnea	Naloxone
Propofol	0.5 mg/kg IV	15–30 s	4–8 min	Apnea, hypotension	BVM, IVF
Etomidate	0.1 mg/kg IV	60–90 s	10–15 min	Myoclonus, apnea, vomiting	Versed, BVM

BVM = bag, valve, mask; IVF = intravenous fluid.

Procedure

1. Discuss risks and benefits of sedation as well as alternatives with patient/ guardian and obtain informed consent. Include risks of apnea, aspiration, and death.
2. Evaluate risk for patient: Consider NPO time (6–8 h solids, 2–3 h clears, 3 h solids for ketamine), airway anatomy, underlying cardiac or pulmonary disease, history of alcohol or drug abuse (increased medication requirements and increased risk of apnea).
3. Set-up monitors and rescue equipment. Have suction running, BVM plugged into oxygen, check for appropriate size of mask and oral airway.
4. Calculate drug dosages, especially in children. Know amounts in milligrams and milliliters for both sedation medications and any rescue medications.
5. Place patient on supplemental oxygen.
6. Titrate medication to effect—don't rely on set amounts. Know the approximate time to onset and duration of each medication. Administer in step-wise amounts and wait until peak onset of medication before giving additional dosages to avoid oversedation and apnea.
7. Determine when patient is at desired level of sedation for procedure as evaluated by responsiveness to painful and verbal stimuli and ability to protect airway.
8. Monitor patient's ventilation, oxygenation, hemodynamic stability, and airway reflexes.
9. Initiate procedure.
10. Administer maintenance dosages of medication as necessary during procedure. Be cautious of oversedation—when pain stimulus from procedure ends, the patient may become suddenly oversedated.
11. Monitor patient until he or she is clearly becoming less sedated and is able to protect airway.
12. RN or technician monitors patient until he or she is at baseline mental status.
13. Give appropriate discharge instructions regarding sedation.

Complications: Apnea, respiratory depression, laryngospasm, hypotension, myoclonus, inadequate sedation, death.

REFERENCES

American College of Emergency Physicians. Clinical policy for procedural sedation and analgesia in the emergency department. *Ann Emerg Med* 1998;31:663–667.

American Society of Anesthesiology. Practice guidelines for sedation and analgesia by non-anesthesiologists. *Anesthesiology* 2002;96:1014–1017.

14. PROCEDURAL SEDATION IN CHILDREN

Indications

1. Facilitate therapeutic procedures.
2. Obtain high-quality diagnostic information.
3. Decrease stress levels of patient, family, and medical provider.

Contraindications—absolute and relative

1. Young infants < 6 months—find someone experienced with sedation in these patients.
2. Airway instability, compromise.
3. Cardiac disease, instability.
4. Neurologic compromise.
5. Use of other sedating medications.
6. Non-hospital-based setting.
7. Lack of proper personnel and monitoring equipment.
8. Lack of consent from parents.
9. Class III and IV anesthesia patients.

General Principles

1. Decide what is causing patient distress (anxiety or pain) and treat that symptom.
2. Use the least amount of sedation to get the job done.
3. Avoid mixing agents from many drug classes.
4. Shorter acting meds usually preferred.
5. Routes of administration.
    a. Painless preferred (PO, IN, PR).
    b. Intranasal (IN) dosing made easier with atomizer syringe tips.
    c. IM route used less often than in past.
    d. IV access is gold standard, allows titration of sedation depth and duration.
6. Gain experience with a small number of agents.
7. Ask for anesthesia department's help and advice.
8. Read your hospital's sedation protocols and regulations regarding NPO status.

Materials

1. Personnel
    a. Physician performing procedure should not be the one monitoring the patient.

  b. Other team members should record meds, monitor patient, assist with airway.
2. Equipment.
  a. Pulse ox, suction, intubation supplies.
  b. Positive pressure O_2 delivery system (BVM).
  c. For deeper levels of sedation, CR and BP monitors.
  d. Reversal agents (naloxone, flumazenil) available.
3. Medications
  a. Midazolam: Most commonly used pediatric sedative, administered via many routes. Produces anxiolysis and amnesia. Starting doses include 0.01 mg/kg IV, 0.4 mg/kg IN, 0.5 mg/kg PO. Duration 30–45 min.
  b. Ketamine: Produces trance-like dissociated state characterized by unresponsiveness, open eyes, and nystagmus. Increases HR, BP, RR, and ICP (contraindicated with head trauma). Dose 2 mg/kg IV, 4–5 mg/kg IM. Give with atropine or glycopyrrolate in small children to dry secretions. Produces 15–30 min of deep sedation, 45 min of cranky drowsiness after that.
  c. Fentanyl: Opioid providing profound analgesia and minimal sedation; side effects include nausea and facial pruritus. Starting dose 1–2 µg/kg IV, titrate well. Rapid pushes of high doses may cause chest wall rigidity.
  d. Etomidate: Commonly used for RSI, recent studies reveal use in pediatric procedural sedation. Limited experience thus far. 0.1 mg/kg IV produces deep sedation for 10–20 min. Airway failure, emesis and myoclonus are chief concerns.
  e. Propofol: Potent sedative/general anesthetic for careful IV administration. Recent studies reveal its potential in pediatric procedural sedation. Limited experience thus far. 0.5–1.0 mg/kg IV produces deep sedation for 10–20 min. Must be very cautious to avoid airway failure and hypotension.
  f. Barbiturates: Uncommonly used except rectally for scans.
  g. Chloral hydrate: Rarely used, no analgesia or anxiolysis, duration long for ED setting.
  h. Demerol-phenergan-thorazine mixture ("dem compound," "DPT shot," "cardiac cocktail"): Outmoded IM cocktail producing longer acting and less predictable sedation than modern agents.
  i. Nitrous oxide: Not often available, but an excellent choice for older, more cooperative children. Usually self-administered (patient holds mask) in a 50:50 mix with oxygen.

Procedure

1. Obtain history of previous sedation, allergies, last oral intake.
2. Perform physical exam to determine patency of airway and degree of patient distress.
3. Obtain and document informed consent (may be verbal). Parental presence at bedside always helps.

4. If using PO or IN route, administer medication while patient is on parent's lap. Move patient to bed as medication takes effect.
5. Position patient in "airway-friendly" position—-small shoulder roll helps keep patient in "sniffing" position; keep head midline.
6. Use appropriate monitoring: pulse ox at a minimum, HR and BP monitoring for deeper levels of sedation.
7. Do not wait for patient to desaturate, place all on oxygen.
8. IV meds should be given via slow push.
9. During procedure, and until patient recovers, monitor the patient's vital signs and physiologic status.
10. After procedure, allow patient to awaken with parents at bedside.

Complications

1. Respiratory depression
   a. Most commonly seen as falling oxygen saturations, do not let it progress. Stop procedure, rescue the patient.
   b. Simplest initial treatment may be pain stimulus (pinch, sternal rub) to get patient to take a deep breath.
   c. Place patient on supplemental oxygen if not already on it.
   d. Give breaths via BVM until patient recovers.
2. Airway compromise.
   a. Upper airway many be compromised in the sedated patient—apparent as "snoring" breath sounds.
   b. Treat by repositioning airway, extending neck, jaw thrust.
3. Emesis.
   a. Stop procedure, roll patient on side and suction immediately.
   b. Many modern medications produce emesis only rarely. Emesis caused by ketamine usually occurs during recovery phase, when patient is not deeply sedated.
4. Emergence reactions.
   a. Patients receiving ketamine may awaken in an agitated, disoriented, and dysphoric state. This happens with teenagers and adults more than in young children. Minimize occurrence by allowing patient to emerge in a calm supportive environment with dim lights, decreased noise, and parents at the bedside. Could be due to lack of analgesia when significant pain is present.
5. Paradoxical reactions.
   a. About 5% of small children may become excited and agitated when treated with medications affecting their mental status. Initially reported with midazolam but can occur with other sedatives. Could be due to undersedation (ketamine especially) or lack of analgesia.
6. **Allergic reactions**
   a. Rarely seen but possible, standard treatment required. Opioids (especially morphine) release histamine and are associated with transient pruritus and rash that does not require treatment.

REFERENCES

Krauss B, Green S. Sedation and analgesia for procedures in children. *New Engl J Med* 2000;342:938–945.
Krauss B, Shannon M, Damian F, Fleisher G. *Guidelines for Pediatric Sedation.* American College of Emergency Physicians, 1995.

15. RAPID SEQUENCE ENDOTRACHEAL INTUBATION

Indications

1. Acute respiratory failure.
2. Hypoxemia unresponsive to supplemental high-flow oxygen.
3. Inability to protect the airway.
4. Overall management of critically ill patients.

Contraindications

1. Predicted difficult airway.
2. Cardiopulmonary arrest.

Materials: Laryngoscope handle and blades, endotracheal tubes, paralytic agent, induction agent, adjunctive medications, suction, nonrebreather face mask, BVM, stethoscope, end tidal CO_2 detector, rescue devices for failed airway including cricothyrotomy kit.

Procedure

1. Assess patient for difficulty of intubation, difficulty of mask ventilation, and difficulty of cricothyrotomy.
2. Explain to patient that he will be put to sleep, have a breathing tube put in, and placed on a ventilator.
3. Prepare and check all equipment, recruit assistants to administer medications, hold cricoid pressure, maintain in-line immobilization if necessary.
4. Preoxygenate patient for 5 min on 15 L/min nonrebreather face mask.
5. Pretreat patient to mitigate side effects from intubation.
   a. Lidocaine 1 mg/kg for patients with increased intracranial pressure.
   b. Fentanyl 2–3 µg/kg if hemodynamically stable and increased ICP, ischemic heart disease, or aneurysm is present (slow IVP over 2 min).
   c. Atropine 0.02 mg/kg if patient younger than 10 years old.
   d. Defasciculate with vecuronium 0.01 mg/kg if using succinylcholine and patient has an increased ICP.
6. Simultaneously administer paralytic agent (succinylcholine 2 mg/kg) and induction agent (etomidate 0.3 mg/kg) rapid IVP. If a contraindication to succinylcholine exists (muscular dystrophy, history of malignant hyperthermia, known hyperkalemia, subacute stroke, spinal cord injuries and burns), use a nondepolarizing paralytic agent such as rocuronium 1 mg/kg.
7. Have assistant apply cricoid pressure and maintain it until patient is successfully intubated and tube placement is confirmed. Have another assistant maintain cervical immobilization if there is potential for a cervical injury.

8. Perform laryngoscopy, expose glottis, and pass endotracheal tube between the vocal cords.
9. Confirm tube placement by several means: auscultate chest for breath sounds, auscultate epigastrium for absence of gastric sounds, inspect chest for symmetric chest expansion, use end tidal CO_2 detector, use esophageal detector device.
10. Place patient on a ventilator and institute mechanical ventilation with settings appropriate for the patient's clinical state.
11. Obtain portable CXR to confirm appropriate position of the tip of the endotracheal tube (midtrachea).
12. Administer sedative agent as needed to keep patient comfortable. Consider administering a long-acting paralytic agent if clinically indicated.

Complications: Dental trauma, laryngeal trauma, dysrhythmias, pneumothorax, pneumomediastinum, aspiration, inadvertent esophageal intubation, malignant hyperthermia, failed airway, oxygen desaturation, brain death, cardiac arrest.

REFERENCES

Gerardi M J, Sachetti AD, Cantor RM, Santamaria JP, Gausche M, Lucid W, et al. Rapid sequence intubation of the pediatric patient. *Ann Emerg Med* 1996;28:55–74.
Walls RM. Rapid-sequence intubation in head trauma. *Ann Emerg Med* 1993;22: 1008–1013.

16. THORACENTESIS

Indications

1. Diagnosis of cause of pleural effusion.
2. Therapeutic drainage of pleural effusion.
3. Instillation of sclerosing agent.

Contraindications

1. Presence of lung mass, parenchyma, or abscess obstructing access to fluid (relative).
2. Bleeding disorder (relative).

Materials: Thoracentesis kit or minor surgery tray plus 20-mL syringe; 20-gauge, 1.5-in. needle; 14-gauge Angiocath needle; three-way stopcock; specimen tubes; 1% lidocaine; povidone–iodine; occlusive dressing.

Procedure

1. Ensure density on CXR is in fact a pleural effusion—get a **lateral decubitus** view.
2. Obtain consent.
3. Find landmarks and aspiration site with patient sitting upright but protected from fall in case of syncope. If not ultrasound-guided, percuss fluid level on posterolateral back (usually sixth through eighth space) posterior

axillary line. If unable to percuss fluid level easily, refer to radiology department for US or CT-guided procedure.
4. Apply povidone–iodine to skin area (10 cm^2).
5. Inject lidocaine into skin and SC tissues. Also around **superior** margin of rib (~ 5–10 mL lidocaine total).
6. Attempt aspiration of pleural fluid with 20-gauge needle **superior** to rib (Figure VIII–14). If not successful, reassess fluid-level location. If unable to locate, consider referral to radiology department for US or CT-guided procedure. If fluid aspirated easily, continue.
7. Insert kit thoracentesis needle or 14-gauge Angiocath at same location as fluid aspirated (**superior** to rib). Leave plastic catheter in place. Attach three-way stopcock and aspirate fluid with syringe. Place 1–2 mL in each specimen tube. Therapeutic drainage can be facilitated with extra tubing and fluid containers (vacuum bottles or sterile plastic thoracentesis bags). **Do not drain more than** 1500 mL of fluid.
8. Patient should do a Valsalva's maneuver as needle is removed. Apply occlusive dressing.
9. Order upright expiratory CXR to rule out pneumothorax. Order studies on fluid (Table VIII–2):
    a. **Lavender-top:** pH, specific gravity, cell count with Diff.
    b. **Red-top:** Protein, glucose, LDH.
    c. **Sterile 10-mL container:** Gram's stain and cultures (aerobic and anaerobic).

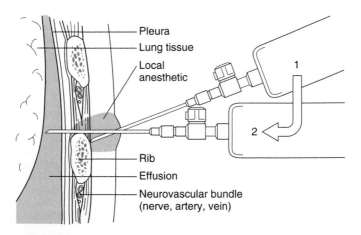

Figure VIII–14. In a thoracentesis, the needle is passed over the top of the rib to avoid the neuro-vascular bundle. (Reproduced, with permission, from Gomella LG. ed. *Clinician's Pocket Reference,* 9th ed. McGraw-Hill, 2002:305.)

TABLE VIII–2. DIFFERENTIAL DIAGNOSIS OF PLEURAL FLUID.

Lab Value	Transudate	Exudate
Specific gravity	<1.016	>1.016
Protein (pleural fluid)	<2.5 g/100 mL	>3 g/100 mL
Protein ratio (pleural fluid-to-serum ratio)	<0.5	>0.5
LDH ratio (pleural fluid-to-serum ratio)	<0.6	>0.6
Pleural fluid LDH	<200 IU	>200 IU
Fibrinogen (clot)	No	Yes
Cell count and differential	Low WBC count	WBC count > 2500/mL; suspect an inflammatory exudate (early polys, later monos)

Transudate: Nephrosis, congestive heart failure, cirrhosis.
Exudate: Infection (parapneumonic, empyema, tuberculosis, viral, fungal, parasitic), malignancy, peritoneal dialysis, pancreatitis, chylothorax.
Grossly bloody tap: Trauma, pulmonary infarction, tumor, and iatrogenic causes.
pH: The pH of pleural fluid is usually > 7.3. If between 7.2 and 7.3, suspect tuberculosis or malignancy or both. If < 7.2, suspect an empyema.
Glucose: Normal pleural fluid glucose is two-thirds serum glucose. If the pleural fluid glucose is much, much lower than the serum glucose, then consider empyema or rheumatoid arthritis (0–16 mg/100 mL) as the cause of the effusion.
Triglycerides and positive Sudan stain: Chylothorax.
LDH = lactic dehydrogenase, WBC = white blood cells; polys = polymorphonuclear leukocytes; monos = monocytes.
Modified and reproduced with permission from Gomella LG, Lefor AT, eds. *Surgery On Call*, 3rd ed. McGraw-Hill; 2002.

    d. If malignancy suspected, order cytology screen (heparinized green-top).
    e. Other optional studies: Fungal cultures, AFB smears and culture, amylase, and Sudan stain (chylothorax).

    Complications: Pneumothorax, hemothorax, infection, parenchymal laceration (lung, liver, spleen, kidney), infection, vasovagal reaction.

REFERENCE

Klein JS, Schultz S, Heffner JE. Interventional radiology of the chest: Image-guided percutaneous drainage of pleural effusions, lung abscess, and pneumothorax. *Am J Roentgenol* 1995;164:581–588.

17. THORACOSTOMY TUBE PLACEMENT

Indications

1. Clinically significant pneumothorax, hemothorax, hemopneumothorax.
2. Other fluid collections in pleural space, eg, empyema, recurrent pleural effusions, chylothorax.

Contraindications: (all relative)

1. Multiple pleural adhesions or blebs.
2. Coagulopathy.
3. Indications for emergency thoracotomy.
4. Recurrent pneumothoraces requiring surgery.

Materials: Chest tube tray, 1% lidocaine with epinephrine, chest tubes (28–36 French for adults or 16–24 French for peds), sterile gloves, povidone–iodine, water seal apparatus, autotransfusion apparatus (if hemothorax is suspected), 0 or 1-0 silk sutures, petroleum gauze, wide adhesive tape.

Procedure

1. Obtain informed consent if procedure is not emergent.
2. Consider IV analgesia/sedation if hemodynamically stable.
3. Place on O_2 by nasal cannula and titrate oxygen to maintain oxygen saturations > 95%.
4. Position patient (supine).
   a. **Axillary insertion (preferred):** Raise head of bed 30–60 degrees, restrain patient's ipsilateral hand above his or her head and contralateral hand at the side.
   b. **Midclavicular insertion:** Restrain both hands at sides.
5. Identify a location for tube placement.
   a. Fourth or fifth intercostal space anterior to midaxillary line.
   b. Second intercostal space midclavicular line.
   c. Alternative sites may be used in an emergency.
6. Use universal precautions: sterile gloves, gown, mask, and eye protection.
7. Prepare operative site with povidone–iodine and place sterile drapes.
8. Estimate length of tube to be inserted by using incision site to apex of lung and place clamp at this distance. All tube fenestrations must be within the pleural space.
9. Cut the tip of the extrathoracic end of tube squarely to facilitate connections.
10. Grasp the intrathoracic end with a curved clamp, locking it with the tip of the tube protruding from the jaws.
11. Inject local anesthetic to skin overlying rib below desired intercostal space. (The rib inferior to this may be chosen, with the intention of tunneling superiorly to desired intercostal space.)(Figure VIII–15)
    a. Start with skin weal and proceed to SC tissues, periosteum, parietal pleura.
    b. Advance (while aspirating) over rib into pleural space—air or fluid should return.
12. Use scalpel to make 2–4-cm transverse incision through skin overlying the rib.
13. Extend incision via blunt dissection with a Kelly clamp down to the fascia overlying the intercostal muscles. Then, tunnel superiorly by advancing with the clamp closed and then pulling back with points spread.
14. With points closed, apply pressure over the rib to the desired intercostal space and advance Kelly clamp through intercostal muscles and into the pleural space. A rush of air or fluid should occur.

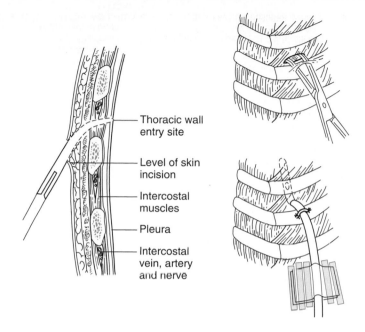

Thoracic wall entry site

Level of skin incision

Intercostal muscles

Pleura

Intercostal vein, artery and nerve

Figure VIII–15. Chest tube technique, demonstrating the location of the neurovascular bundle and the creation of the subcutaneous tunnel. (Reproduced, with permission, from Gomella TL, ed. Chest tube placement. In: *Neonatology.* 5th ed. McGraw-Hill, 2003.)

15. Spread points of the Kelly clamp and pull outward, widening the defect.
16. Insert gloved finger through incision and into the pleural space. Palpate lung, sweep finger in all directions, checking for adhesions.
17. With finger still in place, grasp intrathoracic end of chest tube preloaded into curved clamp and insert it through skin incision, advancing superiorly through defect in chest wall using finger as a guide.
18. Release clamp, advance tube (still using finger to guide) superiorly, medially, and posteriorly until clamp that represents desired length arrives at chest wall.
19. Remove clamp. A properly placed tube should have air movement/ condensation with respiration.
20. Place a "stay" suture with 0 or 1-0 silk on the lateral margin of the skin. After tying, use the long tails to wrap firmly several times around the tube and the tie firmly to prevent tube slippage.
21. Close the remaining skin defect with a horizontal mattress or purse string suture, using the long tails to once again wrap around the tube and secure it. This suture may be tied using double throw "surgeon's

TABLE VIII–3. MOST PROCEDURES CAN BE ACCOMPLISHED WITH COMMERCIALLY AVAILABLE KITS, IN THE EVENT THESE KITS ARE NOT AVAILABLE, THE FOLLOWING GUIDELINES ARE PROVIDED AND REFERRED TO IN EACH PROCEDURE SECTION WHERE APPROPRIATE.

Minor Procedure tray
- Sterile gloves
- Sterile towels/drapes
- 4 × 4 gauze sponges
- Povidone–iodine (Betadine) prep solution
- Syringes 5, 10, 20 mL
- Needles 18, 20, 22, 25 gauge
- 1% lidocaine (with or without epinephrine)
- Adhesive tape

Instrument tray
- Scissors
- Needle holder
- Hemostat
- Scalpel and blade (No. 10 for adult. No. 15 for children or delicate work)
- Suture of choice

Reproduced, with permission, from Lefor AT, Gomella LG, eds. *Surgery On Call,* 3rd ed. McGraw-Hill, 2001.

knots" and finally tied in a bow. Upon removal of the tube, the suture can be pulled tight to close the defect.
22. Ask for assistance to attach tube to water seal apparatus.
23. Place petroleum gauze at junction of the tube and skin. Cover this with plain gauze with a Y-cut so that the tube runs through the center of the pad. Repeat, with Y-cut 90 degrees rotated.
24. Tape dressing and tube securely.
25. Ask patient to cough—bubbles in water seal apparatus indicate patency.
26. Obtain CXR.

Complications: Infection, bleeding, great vessel injury, nerve injury, diaphragmatic perforation, visceral injury (lung, liver, spleen, GI), incorrect tube position, air leaks, subcutaneous/mediastinal emphysema, reexpansion pulmonary edema/hypotension.

18. VENOUS CUTDOWN*

Indication: Venous access when percutaneous puncture is not practical.
Materials: A prepackaged cutdown tray or minor procedure tray and instrument tray (Table VIII–3) with silk suture (3-0, 4-0), and a catheter of choice (eg, Medicut, Angiocath).

*Reproduced, with permission, from Lefor AT, Gomella LG, Wiebke EA, Fraker DL, eds. *Surgery On Call,* 3rd ed. McGraw-Hill, 2001.

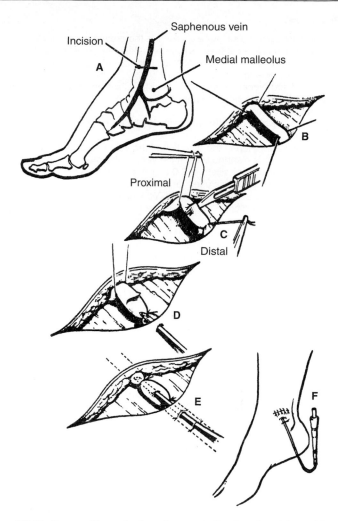

Figure VIII–16. Venous cutdown using the saphenous vein. Here the catheter is inserted through a separate stab wound. (Reproduced with permission from Gomella LG, ed. *Clinician's Pocket Reference.* 5th ed. Appleton-Century-Crofts, 1986)

Procedure

1. The most common site for a cutdown is the greater saphenous vein. The best location for a cutdown is approximately one finger breadth anterior and superior to the medial malleolus (Figure VIII–16). Other sites on the foot, hand, or arm can be used.
2. Apply a tourniquet proximal to the site. Children may need to be restrained. Prep the skin with antiseptic solution, drape the patient, and put on sterile gloves.
3. Infiltrate the skin over the vein with 1% lidocaine. Incise the skin transversely.
4. Spread the incision in the direction of the vein with a hemostat until the excess tissue is cleaned off. Lift the vein off the posterior tissues.
5. Pass two chromic or silk ties (3-0 or 4-0) behind the vein. Tie off the distal vein. The upper tie is used for traction.
6. Make a transverse nick in the vein. You may need a catheter introducer ("banana") to hold open the lumen of the vein.
7. Insert the plastic catheter or IV cannula into the vein and tie the proximal suture to secure it in place. The catheter may also be inserted through a separate stab wound and then passed into the vein.
8. Attach the fluid, release the tourniquet, and close the skin with a silk or nylon suture. Apply a sterile dressing.

Complications: Infection, bleeding, arterial injury, nerve injury, false lumen passage.

IX. Fluids and Electrolytes

1. INTRODUCTION

Understanding fluid and electrolyte imbalances and how to effectively treat them is an essential part of emergency medicine.

2. PREHOSPITAL

Intravenous access and hydration are key components to prehospital care; however, IV fluids should never take priority over transporting the patient to the hospital for definitive care. Crystalloid solutions, such as normal saline (NS) or lactated Ringer's (LR), should be initiated while performing other critical tasks such as intubation or during transport in the ambulance.

3. EMERGENCY DEPARTMENT FLUID MANAGEMENT

As in prehospital management, isotonic crystalloid fluids are the preferred initial fluids for correcting intravascular fluid deficits seen, for example, in dehydration, hypovolemia, hemorrhagic or septic shock, and burns (Table IX–1). In cases of hemorrhage, give approximately 3–4 times the volume of the estimated blood loss. For example if loss = 400 mL of blood, give 1.5 L of NS or LR.

There is no evidence that colloid solutions improve the outcome for volume resuscitation.

General Notes

1. Avoid hypotonic solutions in pediatrics because may precipitate cerebral edema.
2. Excessive NS boluses can cause hyperchloremic acidosis. Switch to LR after 2–4 L.
3. Maintenance fluids should include $\frac{1}{2}\frac{1}{4}$ NS for adults and $\frac{1}{4}$ NS if patient is younger than 2 years.
   Add dextrose solutions if no parenteral or oral nutrition.
4. In treating DKA add D_5W to the solution when serum glucose level is less than 250.

4. SELECTED ELECTROLYTE EMERGENCIES

A. Hypercalcemia

Definition: Serum calcium > 14 mg/dL or ionized calcium greater than 3.5 mmol/L

TABLE IX–1. COMPOSITION OF COMMONLY USED CRYSTALLOIDS

	Na (mEq/L)	K (mEq/L)	Cl (mEq/L)	HCO$_3$ (mEq/L)	Kcal	Glucose (g/L)
LR	130	4	109	28	9	—
NS	154	—	154	—	—	—
½ NS	77	—	77	—	—	—
D$_5$W	—	—	—	—	170	50
D$_5$ ½ NS	77	—	77	—	170	50

Differential Diagnosis

1. Hyperparathyroidism
2. Malignancies
3. Diuretics
4. Antacids
5. Immobilization
6. Sarcoidosis
7. Endocrinopathies

Signs & Symptoms: Symptoms may be nonspecific, such as polyuria, polydipsia, constipation, nausea, or mental status changes. Patient may also have pain associated with renal calculi or bone pain.

ED Studies

1. Repeat calcium and check other electrolytes.
2. Albumin: Serum levels are indicative of albumin-bound calcium.
3. ABG: Acidosis causes less albumin: calcium binding.
4. Bun/Cr: Check renal function.
5. UA: Hematuria could suggest nephrolithiasis.
6. CXR: May show evidence of malignancy or sarcoidosis.
7. ECG: May see prolonged PR interval and shortened QT interval.

ED Treatment

1. Fluid hydration with NS is the key intervention.
2. Saline diuresis promotes calcium excretion.
3. Furosemide (Lasix) at dose of 20–80 mg IV q2–4h promotes calcium excretion as long as volume status is adequate.
4. Calcitonin, diphosphonates, or steroids may be used, but effects are not immediate.
5. Dialysis may be used as a last resort.

B. Hypocalcemia

Definition: Serum calcium < 8.0 mg/dL or 2 mmol/L

Differential Diagnosis

1. Parathyroid hormone deficiency (ie, surgical excision during thyroidectomy or irradiation).
2. Decreased parathyroid activity.
3. Vitamin D deficiency from malnutrition, malabsorption, or defective metabolism (eg, in renal or liver disease).
4. Calcium loss or sequestration (ie, pancreatitis, hyperphosphatemia, osteoblastic disease).

Signs & Symptoms: Muscle twitches from spasm to tetany (remember Chvostek's and Trousseau's signs?), hyperreflexia, mental status changes, and ECG changes. Watch for laryngeal spasm and seizure in rare cases.

ED Studies

1. Serum electrolytes: Look for other correctable electrolyte abnormalities.
2. Serum albumin or ionized calcium: Determine true calcium level.
3. BUN/Cr
4. Lipase: If suspect pancreatitis.
5. ECG: QT prolongation, inverted T waves, arrhythmias.

ED Treatment

1. Calcium chloride: 100 mg/mL in 10-mL vial (total 1 g; a 10% solution, contains 273 mg of Ca.). Give 5–10 mL IV slowly, not to exceed 1 mL/min.
2. Calcium gluconate: 1 g in 10-mL ampoule contains 93 mg of Ca. Give 10–20 mL IV slowly.

C. Hyperkalemia

Definition: Serum potassium > 5.5 mEq/L

Differential Diagnosis

1. Renal failure.
2. Pseudohyperkalemia: Hemolyzed blood specimen.
3. Acidosis: Example would include DKA in which the potassium is shifted out of the cells in exchange for hydrogen ions.
4. Drugs: Examples include potassium-sparing diuretics, heparin, digitalis toxicity, NSAIDS, and ACE inhibitors.
5. Tissue breakdown.
6. Endocrinopathies: Adrenal insufficiency.
7. Succinylcholine.

Signs & Symptoms: Weakness, tingling, hyperreflexia, and ECG changes.

ED Studies

1. ECG: Starts with peaked T waves that progress to widening of the QRS complex and flattening of the p waves, then the QRS blends with the T wave forming the sine wave. Ultimately ventricular fibrillation and asystole may follow.
2. Repeat electrolytes to ensure not falsely elevated potassium.
3. BUN/Cr.
4. ABG.
5. Serum CK: If suspect rhabdomyolysis.
6. CBC with platelets.
7. Digoxin level if indicated.

ED Treatment

1. 10% Calcium chloride: Give 5–10 mL IV. Onset of action in 1–3 min. Duration of action approximately 30–60 min.
2. Sodium bicarbonate: Give 1 mEq/kg IV. Onset 5–10 min. Duration 1–2 h.
3. Insulin and glucose: Give 1 amp D_{50} with 10 units of regular insulin (approximately 1 U of insulin for every 2.5 g of glucose.) Onset 30 min. Duration 4–6 h.
4. Nebulized albuterol: Give 10–20 mg nebulized medication over 15 min.
5. Furosemide: 40–80 mg IV boluses.
6. Kayexalate: 15–50 g PO or PR with sorbitol.
7. Dialysis.

Note: Calcium, bicarbonate, insulin/glucose, and albuterol are only temporizing measures until the potassium is excreted from the body.

D. Hypokalemia

Definition: Serum potassium < 3.5 mEq/L.

Differential Diagnosis: Deficits typically caused by GI losses, renal losses. or transcellular shifts.

1. GI: GI tract is rich in potassium, particularly the lower GI tract. Large losses of potassium can occur with diarrhea. Vomiting can cause hypokalemia secondary to the metabolic alkalosis and subsequent renal excretion of potassium.
2. Renal: Diuretics, renal tubular acidosis, primary aldosteronism, Cushing's syndrome, hyperreninemic states.
3. Cellular shifts: Alkalosis is an example.

Signs and Symptoms: Weakness, hyporeflexia, paresthesias, paralysis, nausea, vomiting, diarrhea, and arrhythmia.

ED Studies

1. ECG: May show various arrhythmias including PVCs, PACs, VT, or VF. A characteristic U wave may be present.

2. Electrolytes: A concomitant hypomagnesia may be present.
3. ABG.
4. Urine Lytes: If cause is unclear, renal losses may be present.
5. Dig level: Hypokalemia may potentiate dig toxicity.

ED Treatment

1. KCL administered IV. Should not exceed 10 mEq/h in a peripheral IV and 20 mEq/h in a central line. For every 40 mEq of KCL there is an estimated 0.5 rise in plasma potassium.
2. KCL orally may be used for mild, asymptotic hypokalemia. Generally given 20–80 mEq/day.

E. Hypernatremia

Definition: Serum sodium > 145 mEq/L.

Differential Diagnosis

1. Renal losses can occur with any osmotic diuresis such that caused by diuretics, hyperglycemia, mannitol, urea, or postobstructive diuresis. Also consider central or nephrogenic diabetes insipidus, which is a loss of free water.
2. Extrarenal losses can include insensible loss of water greater than sodium seen with fevers, burns, or GI losses.
3. Increases in total body sodium can be seen with steroids, primary aldosteronism, Cushing's syndrome, and administration of hypertonic solutions.

Signs and Symptoms: Look for evidence of hypovolemia, such as orthostatic changes or dry mucous membranes. Also may have neuromuscular irritability, including tremors, rigidity, hyperreflexia, and seizures, as well as altered mental status changes such as lethargy and coma.

ED Studies

1. Urine sodium
   a. Urine [Na] > 20 mmol/L usually indicates water loss greater than sodium loss (ie, osmotic diuresis) or increase total body sodium (ie, hypertonic fluids).
   b. Urine [Na] < 20 mmol/L usually seen in cutaneous or GI losses.
   c. Urine [Na] variable with pure free water loss.
2. Urine osmolality and serum osmolality.
   a. Urine osmolality > 700 mOsm/L may indicate insufficient water intake with or without extrarenal losses.
   b. Urine osmolality < serum osmolality suggests central or nephrogenic DI.
   c. Urine osmolality between 700 mOsm/L and serum osmolality may suggest osmotic diuresis or renal failure.
3. CT of head may be indicated in possible cases of an intracranial process causing central DI.

ED Treatment

1. Calculate free water deficit = [(plasma Na /140) − 1] × lean body weight (kg) × 0.04.
2. Start fluid replacement with D_5W, ½ NS, or ¼ NS. Give ½ of free water deficit in first 12 h and the remainder over next 24 h.
3. Fluid replacement should be slow, correcting Na by 12 mEq/L/day to avoid cerebral edema (may replace faster at 1 mEq/L/h if hypernatremia known to be acute).
4. Diuretics with free water or dialysis removes Na.

F. Hyponatremia

Definition: Serum sodium < 130 mEq/L, typically symptomatic < 120 mEq/L.

Differential Diagnosis

1. Isoosmolar (plasma Osm 275–290): Hyperlipidemia, paraproteinemia.
2. Hyperosmolar (plasma Osm > 290): Mannitol, hyperglycemia.
3. Hyposmolar (plasma Osm < 275).
    a. Euvolemic with urinary Osm> 100: SIADH, hypothyroidism, thiazides, NSAIDs, renal failure, adrenal insufficiency.
    b. Euvolemic with urinary Osm < 100: Psychogenic polydipsia.
    c. Hypovolemic: GI losses, burns fevers, third spacing (urinary Na < 10 mEq/L). Diuretics, salt-wasting nephropathies, decreased aldosterone (urinary Na > 10).
    d. Hypervolemic: CHF, nephrotic syndrome, cirrhosis (urinary Na < 10). Chronic renal failure (urinary Na > 20).

Signs and Symptoms: Stigmata of volume changes (ie, CHF, orthostatic hypotension, poor skin turgor, etc.), nausea, malaise, headache to late findings of coma, seizure, and respiratory arrest. Symptoms occur typically when Na < 115 or with rapid decline.

ED Studies

1. Electrolytes.
2. BUN/Cr,
3. Plasma and urine osmolality.
4. Urine sodium.
5. TSH and LFTs if indicated.

ED Treatment

1. Treat underlying condition.
2. If euvolemic (ie, SIADH), fluid restriction or, if severe, use 3% NaCl. Rate of correction should be approximately 2.0 mEq/L/h for first 3–4 h, not to

exceed 12 mEq/L in 24 h. Too rapid of correction may cause central pontine myelinolysis.

3. Loop diuretics impair free water retention. May add with hypertonic solutions.

REFERENCES

Dolich MO, Cohn SM. Solutions for volume resuscitation in trauma patients. *Curr Opin Crit Care* 1999;5:523–528.

Jackson J, Bolte R. Risks of intravenous administration of hypotonic fluids in pediatric patients in the ED and prehospital setting. *Am J Emerg Med* 2000;18:269–270.

Kapoor M, Chan GZ. Fluid and electrolyte abnormalities. *Crit Care Clin* 2001;17(3):503–529.

X. Blood Component Therapy*

RED BLOOD CELL TRANSFUSIONS

The blood supply in the United States has never been safer; however, transfusion with blood should be carefully considered and avoided whenever possible. Transfusions are indicated when:

1. Symptoms from acute blood loss have failed to respond to crystalloid infusions.
2. Symptoms from a chronic anemia have not improved with other therapeutic interventions.

Clinicians should not establish empiric, automatic transfusion thresholds.

ANEMIA

(See also Section I, 10. Bleeding Problems, p 32).

When confronted with a chronic anemia, the clinician must consider whether the Hgb and Hct accurately reflect the RBC mass. The RBC mass is more important with respect to oxygen transport than the measured Hct or Hgb; however, a low Hgb or Hct usually reflects a low RBC mass. An increased plasma volume may result in a dilutional change in the Hgb and make an anemia appear more severe. Increased plasma volume may occur in CHF, pregnancy, and paraproteinemia.

Acute Blood Loss: In the setting of acute blood loss and hypotension, blood volume and tissue perfusion must be restored, as well as oxygen-carrying capacity being improved. You should use electrolyte solutions or colloids initially. Blood losses of 500–1000 mL in an adult do not usually require blood transfusion unless an underlying anemia or another medical condition is present requiring added oxygen-carrying capacity.

RBC Products: Availability and Indications

1. **Whole blood.** Few conditions are indications for transfusion of whole blood today, except for transfusion for the massively bleeding patient when volume and oxygen-carrying capacity can be supplied in one product. Stored whole blood is not an adequate replacement for platelets or labile coagulation factors.
2. **Packed RBCs.** This product, which is basically a unit of whole blood with two thirds of the plasma removed, has become the standard RBC product for most transfusions.

---

*Reproduced, with permission, from Haist SA, Robbins JB, Gomella LG, eds. *Internal Medicine On Call*, 3rd ed. McGraw-Hill, 2002.

3. **Leukocyte-poor RBCs.** In this product, 70–90% of the leukocytes have been removed by a variety of techniques. Leukocyte-poor RBCs are used in patients with a history of repeated febrile reactions to standard packed RBC transfusions. These reactions are usually due to leukocyte antigens. Leukocyte-poor RBCs are indicated for patients expected to require extensive blood product support.

4. **Washed RBCs.** Virtually all plasma and nonerythrocyte cellular elements are removed in this product. Washed cells are indicated in patients with febrile reactions to leukocyte-poor RBCs, in patients with allergic reactions to plasma components (IgA deficiency), and in patients with paroxysmal nocturnal hemoglobinuria when exposure to complement may exacerbate the hemolytic process.

5. **Frozen stored RBCs.** Used primarily for autologous transfusion for elective surgery and to maintain availability of units for patients with alloantibodies to high-incidence blood group antigens.

6. **CMV-negative products.** Patients undergoing organ and bone marrow transplantation require aggressive immunosuppressive therapy to ensure engraftment and avoid graft rejection. If these patients or candidates for organ or bone marrow transplantation are CMV-negative prior to their transplant, CMV-negative blood products will minimize the risk of CMV infection complicating their transplantation course.

Complications: See Section I, 69. Transfusion Reaction, p 206.

PLATELET TRANSFUSIONS

(See also Section I, 10. Bleeding Problems, p 32).

Indications: Platelet transfusions are indicated for any patient with a major bleeding event involving a qualitative or quantitative platelet disorder. Prophylactic platelet transfusions are most commonly indicated in settings of decreased platelet production, such as aplastic anemia, acute leukemia, or chemotherapy, or radiation-induced bone marrow suppression. In these settings, many institutions empirically give transfusions to patients with platelet counts < 10,000. Individuals with fever, mucosal ulcerations, and planned invasive procedures are frequently supported with platelets to maintain counts > 20,000.

Individuals with thrombocytopenia on the basis of platelet destruction (either via antibodies or consumption) rarely benefit from prophylactic transfusion. In general, transfusion with ongoing platelet destruction is indicated only when greater than expected bleeding of a microvascular nature is present.

The efficacy of platelet transfusion in the setting of platelet dysfunction is not well documented. Desmopressin (DDAVP) should be considered in this circumstance. Patients with lifelong quantitative or qualitative platelet disorders should not be transfused prophylactically solely on the basis of platelet count, bleeding time, or other platelet function studies. Overuse of platelets increases the risk of alloimmunization and subsequent inadequate response to platelet transfusions. Likewise, patients with ITP should not be prophylactically transfused.

Complications

1. **Transmission of viral infections**
2. **Reactions to plasma components, RBCs, and WBCs.** Reactions to RBC antigens rarely cause a hemolytic transfusion reaction. They can cause alloimmunity and a potential for problems such as the use of Rh-positive platelets in an Rh-negative female. The patient should receive intravenous anti-D globulin (RhoGAM) if she is of childbearing age.
3. **Possible transmission of bacterial infections.** This potential problem is caused by extended storage time and or incorrect temperature of platelet concentrates.
4. **Development of alloimmunization.** This problem eventually develops in two thirds of patients receiving multiple transfusions of platelets. May necessitate the use of HLA-matched platelets to achieve adequate post-transfusion counts.

PLASMA COMPONENT THERAPY

The following is a list of commonly available plasma products and selected remarks about indications and complications.

Fresh-Frozen Plasma

1. Contains all factors, but titers of factors VIII and V decline with long-term storage. Can be used for replacement of factor deficiencies, but problems include long turnaround time because of the need for thawing, and the potential volume of plasma needed to correct certain factor deficiencies.
2. Other side effects include urticaria, fever, nausea, headaches, and pruritus. These can usually be treated or prevented with antihistamines and antipyretics.
3. Transmission of viral infections is less likely than with the factor concentrates.

Single-Donor Plasma

1. Collected from one donor unit of whole blood. Levels of factors V and VIII decline appreciably with storage; single-donor plasma should not be used to replace these factors.
2. Risk of hepatitis and other infections is equivalent to the risk associated with transfusing a unit of whole blood.

Cryoprecipitate

1. Contains high levels of factor VIII, von Willebrand's factor, and fibrinogen. Useful in factor VIII deficiency, von Willebrand's disease, fibrinogen disorders, and uremic bleeding.

2. Contains insignificant amounts of other coagulation factors. Most frequently used for hypofibrinogenemia related to conditions that cause consumptive coagulopathy. Therefore, most patients receiving cryoprecipitate will require other blood components.

Factor VIII Concentrate

1. Various preparations are available. Only genetically engineered preparations should be used so as to avoid transmitting HIV and viral hepatitis.
2. Use is limited to patients with factor VIII deficiency.

Vitamin K-Dependent Factor Concentrates

1. Contains factors II, VII, IX, and X; protein C; and protein S. Useful in these specific factor deficiencies and in patients with factor VIII inhibitors.
2. Risk of hepatitis and thromboembolic disease exists because of the presence of activated factors in some preparations.

Gamma Globulin: Many different forms of IV and IM gamma globulins are available for a wide variety of indications and reactions.

1. **Indications**
   a. Nonspecific immunoglobulin for non-B hepatitis prophylaxis. Hepatitis B immunoglobulin is used for prophylaxis for hepatitis B. Specific immunoglobulins can also be used for postexposure prophylaxis for varicella and rabies.
   b. Prophylactic or therapeutic intravenous use for inherited or acquired humoral immune deficiencies.
   c. Treatment of acute and chronic immune ITP.
2. **Reactions.** The following are adverse effects that might result from the administration of gamma globulin.
   a. **Anaphylactoid reaction.** An immediate reaction attributed to complement activation. Symptoms and signs may include flushing, chest tightness, dyspnea, fever, chills, nausea, vomiting, hypotension, and back pain. These reactions are uncommon with the currently available preparations but can occur with both IV and IM administration. Therapy consists of discontinuation of the infusion and use of diphenhydramine (Benadryl), steroids, epinephrine, and vasopressors if necessary.
   b. **Inflammatory reaction.** This is characteristically a delayed reaction. Signs and symptoms may include headache, malaise, fever, chills, and nausea. The reaction disappears with discontinuation of gamma globulin therapy.

REFERENCES

Practice strategies for elective red blood cell transfusion. American College of Physicians. *Ann Intern Med* 1992;116:403–407.

Fresh-Frozen Plasma, Cryoprecipitate, and Platelet Administration Practice Guidelines Development Task Force of the College of American Pathologists. Practice parameter for the use of fresh-frozen plasma, cryoprecipitate, and platelets. *JAMA* 1994;271:777–781.

Goodnough LT, Brecher ME, Kanter MH, AuBuchon JP. Transfusion medicine—blood transfusion. *N Engl J Med* 1999;340:438–447.

XI. Ventilator Management*

1. INDICATIONS & SETUP

I. Indications

  A. Ventilatory Failure. A $Paco_2 > 50$ mm Hg indicates ventilatory failure; however, many patients experience chronic ventilatory failure with renal compensation (retaining HCO_3^-). The absolute pH is often a better guide to determining the need for ventilatory assistance than $Paco_2$. A significant acidemia suggests an acute respiratory acidosis or acute decompensation of a chronic respiratory acidosis. A respiratory acidosis with a rapidly falling pH or an absolute pH < 7.24 is an indication for ventilatory support.

    The prototype of pure ventilatory failure is the drug overdose patient in whom there is a sudden loss of central respiratory drive with uncontrolled hypercarbia. Patients with sepsis, neuromuscular disease, and chronic obstructive pulmonary disease (COPD) may have hypercarbic ventilatory failure.

  B. Hypoxemic Respiratory Failure. Inability to oxygenate is an important indication for ventilatory support. A $Pao_2 < 60$ mm Hg on > 50% inspired fraction of oxygen (Fio_2) constitutes hypoxemic respiratory failure. Newer nomenclature uses the Pao_2/Fio_2 (P/F) ratio to characterize hypoxemia. A P/F ratio < 200 is consistent with acute respiratory distress syndrome (ARDS), whereas a ratio between 200 and 300 is termed **acute lung injury.** Although these patients can sometimes be treated with higher Fio_2 delivery systems, such as partial or nonrebreather masks, or continuous positive airway pressure (CPAP) delivered by mask, they are at high risk for cardiopulmonary arrest. They should be closely monitored in an ICU if they are not intubated. Worsening of the respiratory status necessitates prompt intubation and ventilatory support.

    The prototype disease for hypoxemic respiratory failure is ARDS, in which the high shunt fraction leads to refractory hypoxemia.

  C. Mixed Respiratory Failure. Most patients have failure of both ventilation and oxygenation. The indications for ventilatory support remain the same as listed earlier.

    An example of mixed respiratory failure occurs in the COPD patient with an acute exacerbation. Bronchospasm alters the ventilation–perfusion ratio (V/Q) relationships, leading to worsening hypoxemia. Bronchospasm and accumulated secretions lead to a high work of breathing and consequent hypercarbia.

---

*Reproduced, with permission, from Haist SA, Robbins JB, Gomella LG, eds. *Internal Medicine On Call*, 3rd ed. McGraw-Hill, 2002.

D. Neuromuscular Disease with Respiratory Failure. This is actually a subcategory of ventilatory failure but deserves separate mention because it requires different management. Hypercarbia occurs just before arrest; thus, clinical data other than ABGs are needed. Patients with myasthenia gravis, Guillain–Barré syndrome, and muscular dystrophy are at risk of respiratory failure.

1. Respiratory rates > 24/min are an early sign of respiratory failure. A progressive rise in the respiratory rate or sustained respiratory rates > 35/min are indications for ventilatory support.

2. Abdominal paradox indicates dyssynergy of chest wall muscles and diaphragms and impending respiratory failure. It is manifested by inward movement of the abdominal wall during inspiration rather than the normal outward motion.

3. A vital capacity < 15 mL/kg is associated with acute respiratory arrest as well as an inability to clear secretions. Similarly, a negative inspiratory force < −25 cm H_2O implies impending respiratory arrest.

   Guillain–Barré syndrome is the prototypic neuromuscular disease in which the preceding criteria require strict attention. A patient with Guillain–Barré syndrome should be closely observed and followed with frequent vital capacity (VC) measurements. A rapidly falling VC, or VC < 1000 mL, requires respirator support.

II. Partial Ventilatory Assistance

A. CPAP (Continuous Positive Airway Pressure) may be administered by full face mask or nasal mask. Pressures of 5–15 cm H_2O may be used to recruit alveoli and improve oxygenation for refractory hypoxemia. CPAP has proven efficacy in respiratory failure due to pulmonary edema as well as in acute exacerbations of COPD. (It is thought to decrease work of breathing by splinting airways open and thus counteracting intrinsic positive end-expiratory pressure [PEEP].)

B. BiPAP (Bidirectional Positive Airway Pressure) may provide significant ventilatory assistance in patients with chronic neuromuscular diseases, COPD, or pneumonia; or for patients in whom intubation is not an option. Initial settings would be IPAP (inspiratory pressure) 12 cm; EPAP (expiratory pressure) 4 cm; patient assist mode and backup rate, 12 breaths per minute. IPAP can then be titrated upward to increase the effective tidal volume. An experienced respiratory therapist is vital to the success of BiPAP. Starting at very low pressures and providing proper mask fit and a lot of reassurance are mandatory for success. Conventional ventilators can also be used to provide noninvasive ventilation via a face mask interface.

C. CPAP or BiPAP requires intensive respiratory therapy support for titration of O_2 and pressure as well as adjustments of the mask because leaks are common. Necrosis of the bridge of the nose may occur.

D. Contraindications. Rapidly progressive respiratory failure, coma (inability to protect the airway), vomiting, pneumothorax, and gastric distension. Partial ventilatory support should be administered only in an ICU or step-down unit.

III. Tracheal Intubation

(See Section VIII, 15. Rapid Sequence Endotracheal Intubation, p 470.) Endotracheal intubation is actually the most difficult and complication-ridden part of ventilator initiation. Skill and experience are required for correct placement. Aspiration, esophageal intubation, and right mainstem bronchus intubation are common complications. Bilateral breath sounds always need to be confirmed by chest auscultation in each axilla. An immediate postintubation portable CXR should be obtained. An inline CO_2 sensor can be used for rapid confirmation of tracheal intubation. Intubation can be accomplished by three routes:

A. Nasotracheal Intubation. This can be accomplished blindly and in an awake patient. Intubation requires experience and adequate local anesthesia. Complications include intubation of the esophagus, nosebleeds, kinking of the endotracheal tube (ETT), and postobstructive sinusitis. A smaller ETT is usually required for nasotracheal versus orotracheal intubation; this leads to a higher work of breathing because of increased resistance, difficulties with adequate suctioning, and higher ventilation pressures. Nasotracheal ETTs are more comfortable than orotracheal ETTs; they are less damaging to the larynx because they are better stabilized in the airway. This type of intubation should be avoided in the presence of facial trauma.

B. Orotracheal Intubation. Placement of orotracheal tubes requires normal neck mobility to allow hyperextension of the neck for direct visualization of the vocal cords. Larger ETTs can be placed via this route. Adequate local anesthesia or sedation is necessary for safe placement without aspiration.

C. Tracheostomy. Tracheostomy is a surgical procedure most often done acutely for upper airway obstruction; however, in patients who require more than 14–21 days of ventilatory support, a tracheostomy is recommended. Tracheostomy tubes facilitate the weaning process by decreasing tube resistance because the tube is shorter and has a wider radius. Patients can eat with a tracheostomy and find the tubes more comfortable than those used for tracheal intubation.

IV. Ventilator Setup

A. The Ventilator. Contemporary ventilators are volume-cycled, pressure-targeted, or time-cycled. Elaborate alarm systems are present to alert personnel to problems such as inadequate minute ventilation or tidal volume, high peak pressure, and disconnection of the ETT.

Effective ventilation is measured by changes in $Paco_2$. Minute ventilation (V_e) can be calculated by tidal volume × breath rate. Thus, ventilation may be adjusted by changing the breath rate, the tidal volume, or both. Tidal volumes > 10 mL/kg may cause overdistension of alveoli and increase the risk of pneumothorax. Recent ARDS research suggests that a tidal volume of 5 mL/kg ideal body weight (IBW) is optimal.

(It is thought that excessive stretch may lead to increased inflammatory response and alveolar leak.) Most initial tidal volumes are therefore set at 5–8 mL/kg IBW.

Oxygenation is adjusted by changing Fio_2. Prolonged $Fio_2 > 60\%$ may cause pulmonary fibrosis. Thus, down-adjustment to "safe levels" sufficient to maintain O_2 saturation $> 90\%$ should be attempted as indicated by ABGs. If an O_2 saturation $> 90\%$ cannot be maintained when decreasing the $Fio_2 < 60\%$, other means to increase oxygenation such as PEEP should be used.

The mode of ventilation should be specified:

1. **Assist control (AC) mode** allows the patient to trigger machine breaths once a threshold of inspiratory flow or effort is made. Each breath is a full machine breath. AC mode also supplies a backup rate in cases of apnea or paralysis. It is typically used in pulmonary edema states (both cardiogenic and noncardiogenic) as well as after cardiopulmonary resuscitation.

2. **Intermittent mandatory ventilation (IMV)** provides a set number of machine breaths per minute and allows the patient to make spontaneous breaths as well. Synchronized intermittent mandatory ventilation (SIMV) allows synchronization of the IMV breaths with patient efforts. As the rate is turned down, the patient assumes more and more of the work of breathing. Typically SIMV is used in patients with obstructive airways disease (COPD or asthma).

3. **CPAP** allows completely spontaneous respirations while the patient is still connected to the ventilator. A set amount of continuous pressure may be applied as well (0–30 cm H_2O). It is almost always used in conjunction with pressure support.

4. **Pressure support.** Pressure support is an inspiratory boost given to augment spontaneous respiratory efforts. Thus, in CPAP mode or in SIMV, pressure support can be used to overcome the work of breathing imposed by the ventilatory system (endotracheal tube, tubing, demand valves) when a patient takes a spontaneous breath. Typically, an 8- to 10-cm pressure boost is used. Pressure support can also be used at higher levels during ventilator weaning (see 4. Weaning, p 505).

5. **Pressure control.** Recent-model ventilators may be set to operate in a pressure-limited mode rather than volume-targeted. A set pressure boost is maintained for a measured time period in this mode. The primary goal is an improvement in oxygenation—often at the expense of ventilation (clearance of CO_2). Another goal is the limitation of peak airway pressures below 40 cm H_2O and thus minimization of barotrauma or overstretching of the lung. Pressure control is primarily used in ARDS. Often inverse ratio ventilation (increasing inspiratory time) is done simultaneously. Because this stimulates a breath-holding maneuver, it feels unnatural to patients, and they usually require deep sedation or paralysis in this

mode. **Caution:** Pressure control should be used *only under supervision of ICU-trained faculty or fellows.*

6. **Airway pressure release ventilation (APRV)** is very similar to pressure control; however, the patient is able to breathe throughout the machine cycles. Thus, deep sedation and paralysis can be avoided. Typical settings might be
   - P: high 30 s
   - T (time): high 3 s
   - P: low 8 s
   - T: low 0.5 s

   APRV is used primarily in patients with ARDS.

7. **Initial ventilator settings** should be dictated by the underlying condition as well as by previous blood gas results. An example of the initial settings for a 70-kg patient after respiratory arrest would be
   - Fio_2 1.0 (100%)
   - AC mode
   - Rate 18
   - Tidal volume 560 mL

   An attempt should be made to supply the patient with at least as much minute ventilation as was required prior to intubation. Thus, a patient with pulmonary edema, ARDS, or neuromuscular disease may require a minute ventilation rate of 14–22 L/min. The AC mode will generally be more comfortable and will alleviate the work of breathing to a large extent. Sample settings might be
   - Fio_2 1.0
   - AC mode
   - Rate 22
   - Tidal volume 550 mL

   The patient with COPD, on the other hand, should not be overventilated initially. Such patients may have a chronically high bicarbonate levels because of renal compensation, and overventilation may cause a severe alkalosis. (A pH > 7.55 is felt to be severely arrhythmogenic as well as moving the oxyhemoglobin curve to the right, which impedes oxygen release to the tissues.) Sample settings might be
   - Fio_2 0.5 (50%)
   - SIMV mode
   - Pressure support 10 cm
   - Rate 12
   - Tidal volume 600 mL

B. **Additional Setup Requirements**
   1. **Restrain the patient's hands** because the natural reaction to the ETT on awakening is to pull it out.
   2. **Place an NG tube** to decompress the stomach or to continue essential oral medications.

3. **Obtain a stat portable CXR** to confirm ETT placement and to reassess any underlying pulmonary disease. The tip of the ETT should be 3–4 cm above the carina.
4. **Treat any underlying pulmonary disease** (maximize bronchodilators in status asthmaticus or vasodilators and diuretics in pulmonary edema).
5. **Consider prophylactic measures.** Heparin 5000 U SC q12h may reduce the incidence of PE while the patient is on bed rest. Stress ulceration bleeding can be prevented by the use of any of the following: antacids; H_2 antagonists (cimetidine, ranitidine); sucralfate (Carafate); or tube feedings (enteral nutrition).
6. **Order other medications as needed,** such as morphine for pain and lorazepam (Ativan) for agitation.

2. ROUTINE MODIFICATION OF SETTINGS

ABGs should be monitored and adjusted to a normal pH (7.37–7.44) and a Pao_2 > 60 mm Hg on less than 60% O_2. Tachypnea should be investigated for adequacy of ventilation or for any other cause (eg, fever) prior to sedating the patient.

I. **Adjusting Pao_2**
A. **To Decrease:** Inspired fraction of oxygen (Fio_2) should be decreased in increments of 10–20% every 30 min. The "rule of sevens" states that there will be a 7-mm Hg fall in Pao_2 for each 1% decrease in Fio_2.
B. **To Increase**
1. **Ventilation** has some effect on Pao_2 (as shown by the alveolar air equation); therefore, correction of the respiratory acidosis will improve oxygenation.
2. **PEEP** can be added in increments of 2–4 cm H_2O. PEEP recruits previously collapsed alveoli, holds them open, and restores functional residual capacity (FRC) to a better physiologic level. It counteracts pulmonary shunts and will raise Pao_2. PEEP increases intrathoracic pressure and may thus impede venous return and decrease cardiac output. This is particularly true in the presence of volume depletion and shock. Consult your ICU staff or fellow if high PEEP is needed or if the BP drops with PEEP adjustment.

II. **Adjusting $Paco_2$**
A. **To Decrease**
1. Increase the rate or tidal volume.
2. Check for leaks in the system.
3. Decrease CO_2 production by treating fever, minimizing shivering, and controlling agitation.
B. **To Increase**
1. Decrease the rate.

2. You may have to switch from AC to SIMV mode to eliminate patient-driven central hyperventilation. Remember, every breath is a full machine breath in AC mode!

3. An old and effective method is to place increased exhalation tubing to increase deadspace. The patient is then rebreathing his or her CO_2.

3. TROUBLESHOOTING

3A. Agitation

I. **Problem:** The ventilator patient becomes agitated, struggles constantly, tries to pull out all tubes, and actively fights the respirator.

II. **Immediate Questions**

A. Is the patient still properly connected? Hypoxemia or hypercarbia resulting from disconnection of the respirator may result in agitation. A patient who can speak is probably no longer intubated.

B. Review the ventilator flow and pressure waveforms. Look for auto-PEEP. Failure of the expiratory flow to flatten at zero indicates airtrapping, or auto-PEEP. This may cause increased work of breathing and agitation (an experienced respiratory therapist will be able to measure it for you and then apply external PEEP to counterbalance it). A double dip on the inspiratory flow curve usually indicates the patient has air hunger and wants a higher peak flow.

C. What were the most recent ABGs? Again, hypoxemia or hypercarbia can cause agitation. Adjusting the settings can correct either problem.

D. What does the CXR show? Atelectasis from mucous plugging or pneumothorax can occur spontaneously in asthma or as a result of barotrauma and can result in hypoxemia or hypercarbia. The endotracheal tube touching the carina almost always causes coughing or agitation.

E. What is the underlying diagnosis? What are the current medications and IV fluids? Agitation may be related to the underlying diagnosis or to a medication and is unrelated to the patient's respiratory status. Cimetidine (Tagamet) and narcotics can cause confusion, especially in the elderly. Multiple metabolic disturbances (eg, hyponatremia and hypernatremia) can lead to confusion and possibly agitation. (See Section I, 3. Altered Mental Status, p 11.)

F. What are the ventilator settings? The ventilator setting may have been set incorrectly, resulting in hypoxemia or hypercarbia. A high sensitivity setting may make it impossible for the fatigued patient to trigger a breath. Barotrauma resulting in pneumothorax is associated with high PEEP settings, high tidal volumes, and peak inspiratory pressures > 45 cm.

III. Differential Diagnosis
A. Causes of Respiratory Decompensation
1. **Worsening of underlying pulmonary disease**
2. **Pneumothorax**
3. **Endotracheal tube displacement.** The tube may be outside the trachea, high in the glottis, or down the right mainstem bronchus.
4. **Mucous plugs.** May result in atelectasis and hypoxemia.
5. **Ventilator malfunction**
6. **PE.** Immobilization is a major risk for PE.
7. **Aspiration**
8. **Inadequate oxygenation or respiratory muscle fatigue**

B. Sepsis
C. ICU Psychosis
D. Medications.
Multiple medications such as digoxin (Lanoxin), lidocaine, theophylline, imipenem-cilastatin (Primaxin), diazepam (Valium) and other benzodiazepines, meperidine and other narcotics, and cimetidine may cause psychosis, especially in high doses or with decreased clearance states.

E. Electrolyte Imbalance.
Hyponatremia, hypernatremia, hypercalcemia, hypocalcemia, and hypophosphatemia can cause confusion, which can lead to agitation.

IV. Database
A. Physical Exam Key Points
1. **Endotracheal tube.** Carefully check the patency, position, and function of the ETT.
2. **Vital signs.** Tachypnea may suggest hypoxemia. Tachycardia and hypertension can result from agitation or be associated with respiratory failure or an underlying problem such as MI. Hypotension may be due to auto-PEEP, volume depletion, sepsis, cardiogenic shock, tension pneumothorax, or massive PE. An elevated temperature suggests sepsis, ventilator-associated nosocomial pneumonia, or PE. Tachycardia, tachypnea, and fever may be associated with PE or MI. A pulsus paradoxus > 16 mm Hg implies severe respiratory distress or pericardial tamponade.
3. **HEENT.** Check for distended neck veins suggesting pericardial tamponade or CHF. Tracheal deviation may be caused by a tension pneumothorax.
4. **Chest.** Auscultate for bilateral breath sounds. Absent breath sounds on one side suggests pneumothorax or an improperly placed ETT. Bilaterally absent breath sounds can be secondary to either bilateral pneumothoraces or severe respiratory failure.
5. **Extremities.** Check for cyanosis.
6. **Skin.** Palpate for subcutaneous emphysema, which can result from a very high PEEP or may be seen in asthmatics.

B. Laboratory Data

1. **ABGs.** To rule out hypoxemia and hypercarbia as well as severe acidosis or alkalosis.
2. **Electrolyte panel.** Including calcium and phosphorus.

C. Radiographic and Other Studies.
A CXR to rule out atelectasis and pneumothorax and to evaluate underlying pulmonary pathology.

V. Plan

A. Emergency Management

1. **Examine the patient** as outlined earlier. Carefully check the ETT function, ventilator connections, and chart.
2. **Suction the patient vigorously.** This confirms tube patency and clears out any mucous plugs.
3. **Bag the patient manually** to check for ease of ventilation. Marked difficulty can be seen with tension pneumothorax or mucus plugging. If auto-PEEP is suspected, use a slower rate and decrease the tidal volume. This allows trapped gas time to escape and thus will allow decreased intrathoracic pressure and increased venous return back to the heart.
4. **Obtain ABGs, electrolyte panel, and stat CXR.**
5. **If the patient appears cyanotic** or "air hungry," turn the Fio_2 to 1.0 and the ventilator mode to AC.
6. **If hypotension and unilaterally absent breath sounds** are found concomitantly, consider chest tube insertion for tension pneumothorax. Patients on ventilators can rapidly die of tension pneumothoraces.
7. **If you suspect ICU psychosis,** reassure the patient. Have a family member help reorient the patient. Often a familiar voice will work wonders! Ask the nurses to move the patient to a room with a window; this environmental feature has been shown to reduce ICU psychosis.
8. **Check the ventilator settings.** Perhaps too much effort is required to open the valves or to initiate a breath. Ask the respiratory therapist to lower the triggering sensitivity to 0.5 or 1.0 cm H_2O. Experiment with adding a little more pressure support for patient comfort.
9. **If everything else is stable** and the patient is endangering himself or herself, sedate the patient. Haloperidol (Haldol) 0.5–2.0 mg IM or IV and lorazepam (Ativan) 0.5–2.0 mg IV are the currently recommended agents.

3B. Hypoxemia

I. Problem: The respirator patient requires > 60% Fio_2 to maintain a Pao_2 > 60 mm Hg.

II. Immediate Questions

A. What is the sequence of ABGs? In other words, is this an acute or a slowly developing change? A rapid deterioration implies an immediate life-threatening process such as a tension pneumothorax or a massive PE.

B. What is the underlying diagnosis? A patient with long-bone fractures may develop fat embolus syndrome, a patient with sepsis may develop ARDS, or a patient with head injury might develop neurogenic pulmonary edema.

C. What are the ventilator settings? Has a change been made recently? An error may have been made with the ventilator settings, or recent changes may have been made too aggressively in an attempt to wean the patient from the ventilator. Some patients are very sensitive to PEEP changes.

III. Differential Diagnosis

A. Shunts Secondary to Alveolar Filling or by Obstructed Bronchi with Consequent Collapse
   1. **Pneumonia**
   2. **Pulmonary contusion**
   3. **Atelectasis.** The ETT may be placed too far in the right mainstem bronchus, or mucous plugs may be present.
   4. **ARDS or cardiogenic pulmonary edema**

B. Cardiac Level Shunt. An acute ventricular septal defect, especially in the setting of an AMI, may develop. Sudden pulmonary hypertension may occasionally lead to a patent foramen ovale and physiologic shunt at the atrial level. A tip-off to this is a worsening shunt and PaO_2 as PEEP is increased.

C. Shunts Secondary to Pneumothorax

D. Ventilation–Perfusion (V/Q) Mismatch
   1. **Bronchospasm**
   2. **PE**
   3. **Aspiration.** Still possible, even when an ETT is in place.

E. Inadequate Ventilation
   1. **Ventilator disconnection or malfunction**
   2. **Incorrect settings.** Has the patient recently been changed to IMV, which has resulted in hypoventilation?
   3. **Sedatives.** These can result in hypoxemia secondary to hypoventilation. Sedatives should be used cautiously, especially during weaning. Patients on ventilators may develop atelectasis due to failure to sigh or cough when sedated.
   4. **Neuromuscular disease.** Hypophosphatemia or aminoglycosides can cause neuromuscular weakness, which can cause hypoxemia secondary to hypoventilation and lack of sighing.

IV. Database

A. Physical Exam Key Points
   1. **ETT.** Confirm proper ETT position and listen for any leaks.
   2. **Vital signs.** Tachypnea implies worsening of the respiratory status. Tachycardia can be associated with a variety of conditions, including PE, sepsis, MI, and worsening of underlying pulmonary pathology. Fever can be seen with PE, MI, or an infection.

3. **Neck.** Stridor suggests upper airway obstruction.
4. **Chest.** Check for bilateral breath sounds, signs of consolidation, or new onset of wheezing. Unilateral breath sounds suggests a pneumothorax or possibly displacement of the ETT in one of the mainstem bronchi. Palpate the chest for new subcutaneous emphysema, which can occur in asthmatics or as a result of high PEEP.
5. **Heart.** New murmurs or a new S_3 or S_4 may be seen with an MI. A new systolic murmur may suggest a ventricular septal defect (VSD) or mitral regurgitation secondary to papillary muscle rupture.
6. **Extremities.** Check nailbeds for cyanosis from worsening pulmonary status. Also check legs for unilateral edema or other signs of phlebitis that point to PE.
7. **Skin.** Check for new rashes, which may suggest a drug or anaphylactic reaction.

B. **Laboratory Data**
1. **Repeat ABGs or check oximetry** to assess accuracy of initial ABGs and progression of deterioration.
2. **Sputum appearance and Gram's stain** may direct antibiotic therapy if pneumonia is present.
3. **A Swan–Ganz catheter** must be in place to measure mixed venous oxygen saturation (Svo_2). Svo_2 is a direct reflection of oxygen delivery to the tissues and extraction of oxygen. The pulmonary artery catheter can also be used to determine the presence of an intracardiac shunt.

C. **Radiographic and Other Studies**
1. **Stat CXR.** To rule out atelectasis and pneumothorax, and to evaluate underlying pulmonary disease.
2. **Electrocardiogram.** An evolving MI may be evident. New right-axis deviation, RBBB, P pulmonale, or an S wave in lead I, a Q wave in lead III, and a T wave in lead III ($S_1Q_3T_3$) suggest PE; however, these characteristic findings are often absent. Sinus tachycardia is the most common electrocardiographic finding with PE.
3. **V/Q scan.** If clinical suspicion is high for PE.
4. **Swan–Ganz catheter.** To measure pulmonary capillary wedge pressure (PCWP) and to exclude a cardiac shunt as well as to measure cardiac output and maximum O_2 consumption.

V. **Plan**
A. **Suction.** Vigorously suction the patient to prove patency of the ETT and dislodge mucous plugs.
B. **Treat Underlying Disorders**
1. **Insert chest tube** for pneumothorax.
2. **Reassess choice of antibiotic agents.** A pneumonia secondary to *Legionella* infection requires erythromycin (1 g IV q6h) or another macrolide.
3. **Consider more vigorous chest physical therapy** or even bronchoscopy for recalcitrant mucous plugging or atelectasis.

   4. **Maximize bronchodilators** if bronchospasm is the problem. Corticosteroids such as hydrocortisone 125 mg or methylprednisolone 60 mg should be added and given IV q6h. Aerosolized albuterol should be given at least q4h.
   5. **Cardiogenic pulmonary edema** should be vigorously treated with afterload reduction and diuresis.

C. **Optimize Ventilator Settings**
   1. **Correct any hypoventilation.** This may mean giving up on weaning, and using the AC mode with the patient essentially controlled on a high minute ventilation.
   2. **Increase Fio_2 to 100%.** Your first priority is to prevent anoxic brain or cardiac damage. You may then reduce the Fio_2 as other maneuvers further improve the Pao_2.
   3. **PEEP will recruit unused, collapsed, or partially collapsed alveoli to overcome pulmonary shunts.** It should be added in 2–4 cm of H_2O increments while cardiac output and BP are monitored.
   4. **Oxygen consumption ($\cdot VO_2$)** can be markedly reduced by administering a neuromuscular blocking agent as a last resort. Remember to provide adequate analgesia and sedation as well. Nerve stimulation studies should be done routinely to monitor the neuromuscular blockade; otherwise, these agents should be used for $\_< 24$ h.

D. **Optimize Hemodynamics**
   1. **Consider Swan–Ganz placement** when high levels of PEEP are in use, when shock of unclear cause is present, when a cardiac shunt is suspected, or when volume status is unclear.
   2. **Correct volume excess** because it will obviously worsen CHF and ARDS.
   3. **Volume depletion** will likewise alter both cardiac output and V/Q ratios and may adversely affect oxygen delivery. A drop in BP with the addition of PEEP almost always results from volume depletion.
   4. **Correct anemia** so as to maximize O_2 delivery. Oxygen delivery to tissue depends on the hemoglobin as well as the cardiac output and Sao_2. If ARDS is present, RBC transfusions should either be washed or administered through leukocyte removal filters to prevent an exacerbation of the ARDS secondary to the transfusion.
   5. **Correct low cardiac output** to maximize O_2 delivery. Inotropic agents (eg, dobutamine) and agents for afterload reduction (eg, IV nitroglycerin or nitroprusside) can be used.

E. **Prone Positioning.** If the primary lung disorder is ARDS or acute lung injury, consider prone positioning of the patient. Up to 70% of patients will have a dramatic response. However, the nursing and respiratory therapy staff need experience in this technique because ETT dislodgement and unusual pressure sores may occur. Patients are left prone for 6–12 h, flipped back supine for 1–2 h, and then the cycle is repeated.

3C. Hypercarbia

I. **Problem:** The patient's $Paco_2$ remains > 40 mm Hg. $Paco_2$ is a direct reflection of both CO_2 production and alveolar ventilation. $Paco_2$ increases when V/Q mismatch worsens or deadspace increases.

II. **Immediate Questions**
   A. **What is the sequence of ABGs? In other words, is this an acute or a slowly developing change?** Rapid deterioration implies an immediate life-threatening process, such as a tension pneumothorax or a massive PE.
   B. **What is the underlying diagnosis?** Worsening of underlying pulmonary disease (pneumonia, atelectasis, or bronchospasm) can cause hypoventilation. CHF can cause V/Q mismatch and CO_2 retention.

III. **Differential Diagnosis**
   A. **Inadequate Minute Ventilation (V_e)**
      1. **Too low a rate, inadequate tidal volume, or both**
      2. **Patient tiring during SIMV or weaning**
      3. **ETT leak**
      4. **Worsening bronchospasm**
      5. **PE.** Keep in mind that immobilization is a major risk factor.
   B. **Increased CO_2 Production**
      1. **High-carbohydrate feedings**
      2. **Increased metabolism.** Causes include hyperthyroidism, fever, sepsis, and high work of breathing as well as rewarming after surgical procedures (a common but frequently overlooked cause of CO_2 production).
   C. **Oversedation.** Decreases central ventilatory drive.

IV. **Database**
   A. **Physical Exam Key Points**
      1. **ETT.** Check ETT position and look for a leak.
      2. **Vital signs.** Tachycardia can be associated with fever, sepsis, worsening bronchospasm, PE, and hyperthyroidism. Tachypnea can be seen with PE, worsening bronchospasm, or sepsis. Fever suggests infection but can also be seen with hyperthyroidism and PE.
      3. **Chest.** Auscultate for new wheezes and look for inequality of breath sounds.
      4. **Heart.** Listen for a new loud P_2, which suggests a PE.
      5. **Extremities.** Check patient's legs for unilateral edema or other signs of thrombophlebitis.
      6. **Musculoskeletal exam.** Check for signs of respiratory fatigue such as abdominal paradox or accessory muscle use.
   B. **Laboratory Data**
      1. **ABGs.** Repeat ABGs or check oximetry to assess accuracy of initial values and progression of deterioration.
      2. **CBC with Diff.** An increased WBC with an increase in banded neutrophils suggests an infection or sepsis.

    C. Radiographic and Other Studies. With a CXR, proper ETT position can be ensured and new pulmonary infiltrates can be ruled out.

V. Plan

    A. Check Position and Functioning of ETT. If there is a persistent leak, replace the tube.

    B. Verify Proper Ventilator Function. Check with particular care for leaky connections.

    C. Drugs. Verify that the ordered sedatives are the drugs actually given, and note time of last dose. If the patient is oversedated, you can either increase the minute ventilation (V_e); or reverse sedation with naloxone (Narcan) 0.4 mg IV for narcotics or flumazenil (Romazicon) 1.0 mg IV over 5 min for benzodiazepines.

    D. Look for a Source of Sepsis. Adjust antibiotics as indicated. Lower $V \cdot O_2$ by treating fever with acetaminophen (Tylenol) or a cooling blanket.

    E. Review Ventilator Settings. If the tidal volume is too low, deadspace ventilation will be present. Correct this condition by increasing the tidal volume. If the patient is tiring on a low SIMV rate, switch to either a higher rate or change to AC mode.

    F. Review the Patient's Nutrition Regimen. If the patient is critically ill with bronchospasm or ARDS, you may be forced to reduce CO_2 production by decreasing the percentage of carbohydrates in tube feedings or IV hyperalimentation fluid.

3D. High Peak Pressures

  I. Problem: The ventilator peak pressures remain consistently above 50 cm H_2O.

  II. Immediate Questions

    A. Is this a new problem or has it developed progressively? The answer to this question will be readily available on the respiratory therapy bedside flow sheet.

    B. What is the underlying diagnosis? Severe status asthmaticus or ARDS can cause high ventilatory peak pressures.

    C. What are the most recent ABGs? A decrease in the pO_2 or an increase in the pCO_2 may point to a worsening of the underlying pulmonary disease.

    D. Has ETT function or position changed? Is it possible to suction the patient? The tube could be kinked or plugged by secretions.

  III. Differential Diagnosis

    A. ETT

        1. **Too small or obstructed** by secretions.

        2. **Kinked,** especially if placed nasotracheally.

        3. **Migration** down the right mainstem so that the entire tidal volume flows into one lung. This condition also increases coughing and anxiety.

B. **Incorrect Ventilator Settings**
1. **High tidal volume.** Tidal volumes > 10 mL/kg may increase distension pressure tremendously.
2. **High PEEP.** PEEP should always be used at the lowest possible level.
3. **High minute ventilation.** A high minute ventilation may lead to the phenomenon of auto-PEEP, in which the patient has inadequate time to exhale, leading to "stacked breaths." Auto-PEEP may cause hypotension because of high intrathoracic pressure decreasing venous return.
C. **Worsening Lung Disease.** Lung compliance decreases in all of the following:
1. **Severe status asthmaticus**
2. **ARDS**
3. **Cardiogenic pulmonary edema**
4. **Interstitial lung disease**
D. **Uncooperative or Agitated Patient**
1. **Biting the ETT**
2. **Fighting the ventilator**
3. **Coughing**
E. **Abdominal Distension.** The recently described abdominal compartment syndrome can lead to both inability to ventilate and hypotension. It is diagnosed by measuring intravesicular (bladder) pressure and may result from severe ascites or intraabdominal hemorrhage causing increased abdominal cavity pressure.
F. **Tension Pneumothorax.** It is always imperative to exclude this as a cause of new onset of high peak pressures because death can occur quickly.

IV. **Database**
A. **Physical Exam Key Points**
1. **ETT.** Check position to rule out migration down the right mainstem bronchus; check patency of the ETT.
2. **Vital signs.** Tachycardia and tachypnea can occur with worsening of the underlying pulmonary disease and with agitation. Hypotension and tachycardia are seen with tension pneumothorax, severe auto-PEEP, and the abdominal compartment syndrome.
3. **HEENT.** An increase in jugular venous distension (JVD) implies CHF. Tracheal deviation can be seen with tension pneumothorax.
4. **Chest.** Absent breath sounds, especially with hypotension, and unilateral hyperresonance to percussion point to tension pneumothorax. Rales suggest CHF.
5. **Heart.** An S_3 over the apex implies left ventricular dysfunction and CHF.
6. **Abdomen.** Examine for tenderness and distension.
7. **Extremities.** New cyanosis is consistent with worsening of underlying pulmonary disease. Edema will be seen with biventricular or right-sided heart failure.
8. **Skin.** Check for subcutaneous emphysema, which can be associated with barotrauma or with severe asthma.

    B. Laboratory Data
       1. ABGs. Repeat ABGs or check oximetry to assess accuracy of initial values and progression of deterioration.
       2. CBC with Diff. An increased WBC with an increase in banded neutrophils suggests an infection or sepsis.
  C. Radiographic and Other Studies. Use a stat portable CXR to check ETT position, rule out kinking, rule out pneumothorax, and assess any change in underlying pulmonary disease.
  D. Ventilator. Ask the respiratory therapist to measure auto-PEEP or check for it via the waveforms. **View the peak airway pressure pattern.** A rapid rise and fall suggests a kinked or obstructed ETT. Check the patient's mouth to be sure the patient is not biting the tube. Suction the ETT to make sure it is not occluded and leading to artificially high pressures.

V. Plan
  A. Try to Suction the Patient. If the patient is biting down, insert an oral airway or sedate the patient. If the patient is not biting down on the ETT but the suction tube will not go down the ETT, the ETT is kinked or blocked, possibly by a mucus plug, and must be replaced.
  B. Use an Ambu Bag and Confirm Equal Breath Sounds. Unequal breath sounds may result from a tension pneumothorax or from improper positioning of the ETT. Reposition the ETT if necessary. On an average-sized person, an oral ETT should not be in farther than 24 cm at the lip; however, there is considerable variability among patients, and the CXR should always be reviewed. If there is considerable resistance to bagging, a tension pneumothorax, auto-PEEP, or a mucus plug may be present.
  C. Place a Chest Tube if a pneumothorax is present.
  D. Adjust the Ventilator. Try to reduce the PEEP to the minimum needed for adequate oxygenation. Try reducing high tidal volumes to 5 mL/kg body weight. Increase Fio_2 as needed to ensure adequate oxygenation.
  E. Sedation may have to be increased.
  F. Consider Switching to APRV or Pressure Control Modes. These modes exquisitely control high peak pressures while often improving oxygenation as well.

4. WEANING

I. Requirements: Once the underlying cause of respiratory failure has been corrected, it is time for the most arduous task of all, weaning the patient from the respirator.
  A. Stabilization. The underlying disease is under optimum control.
  B. Initiation of Weaning. The process is begun in the early morning. Patients prefer to rest at night rather than work at breathing. Desirable conditions are
    1. $Pao_2 > 60$ mm Hg on no PEEP; and $Fio_2 = 0.5$
    2. Minute ventilation < 10 L/min

3. **Negative inspiratory force more negative than –20 cm H$_2$O**
4. **Vital capacity > 800 mL**
5. **Tidal volume > 300 mL**
6. **Rapid shallow breathing index < 90 (60-s breath rate/tidal volume in liters).** This is the most predictive indicator of success.

II. **Weaning Techniques**
   A. **T-Piece (or T-Tube Bypass).** The patient is taken off the respirator for a limited period of time, and the ETT is connected to a constant flow of O$_2$ (usually 40%). If the patient tolerates breathing independently for 2 h, he or she is extubated immediately. In research studies, this technique has been the most rapid.

   This technique, however, has important drawbacks. No alarms are available because the patient is totally disconnected from the ventilator. The technique is time-consuming for the respiratory therapists and nurses. Perhaps most important, it is much more work for the patient than breathing spontaneously without an ETT. This is due to the relatively small diameter of the tube. (Remember that resistance increases by the fourth power of the radius of a tube.) T-tube trials are thus usually limited to 2-h trials or less.

   B. **SIMV.** In this method, fewer and fewer machine breaths are given as the patient begins taking spontaneous breaths in the intervals. For example, a patient breathing at a rate of 14 in AC mode is switched to SIMV mode, rate 14. The rate is then decreased to 10, to 6, to 4, and then to 0. Most physicians either place the patient on CPAP mode at this juncture or observe the patient briefly on a T-piece.

   This method has several theoretical advantages over T-piece weaning. Backup alarms, including automatic rates in case of apnea, are in place. A graded assumption of work is done, allowing respiratory muscle "retraining"; however, this method has never been proven clearly superior to T-piece weaning. Moreover, there is still a high work of breathing because of the ETT resistance as well as the inherent resistance of the SIMV circuit valves.

   One way to decrease the work of breathing with the SIMV weaning technique is to add pressure support (PS) to the system. **Pressure support** is a positive pressure boost that is initiated when a certain liter flow rate during inspiration is sensed by the respirator. It then supplies a set amount of positive pressure (and by Boyle's law, it also supplies some tidal volume). A PS level of 8–12 cm will overcome the increased work caused by the ETT resistance.

   C. **CPAP and PS.** In this method, the patient is switched to the spontaneous breathing mode, which in some ventilators is the CPAP mode. In current usage, CPAP is equivalent to PEEP, except that it is used exclusively in spontaneously breathing mode. Anywhere from 0 to 30 cm H$_2$O pressure may be used, but generally the lowest level possible (usually 05 cm H$_2$O) is preferred. PS may be used concomitantly to augment the patient's spontaneous breaths. It can then be progressively decreased as the patient increases tidal volumes. For example, PS levels of 25, then 20, then 15, and finally 10 can be used while monitoring the patient's breath rate, tidal volumes, and ABGs.

This method requires an alert, cooperative patient who is breathing spontaneously; if those conditions do not pertain, why wean anyway? Machine backup functions remain in place in case of apnea or other inadequate parameters.

D. Extubation to BiPAP. Patients with advanced lung disease may never reach standard weaning criteria. Extubation to partial ventilatory support is often successful. It decreases risk of ventilator-associated pneumonia and saves the patient from having a tracheostomy tube.

III. Timing: Deciding when to extubate the patient is part of the art of medicine. Still, the fulfillment of certain criteria ensures success. The following weaning parameters (as discussed earlier) are acceptable:
   A. Respiratory rate is < 30/min.
   B. ABGs show a pH > 7.35 and adequate oxygenation on 50 L FiO_2.
   C. The patient is awake and alert.
   D. A normal gag reflex is present.
   E. The stomach is not distended.

IV. Postextubation Care: After extubation, it is important to encourage the patient to cough frequently and forcefully. Respiratory therapy treatments should be continued. Incentive spirometry should be used several times an hour while the patient is awake to encourage deep breathing. The patient must be carefully observed for stridor, respiratory muscle fatigue, or other signs of failure. Oxygen should be given at the same level or at a level slightly higher than was given via the respirator prior to intubation. The ABGs should be checked 2–4 h after extubation to confirm adequate ventilation and oxygenation.

REFERENCES

Albert RK. Prone ventilation (ARDS). *Clin Chest Med* 2000;21:511–517.

Glauser FL, Polatty C, Sessler CN. Worsening oxygenation in the mechanically ventilated patient: Causes, mechanisms and early detection. *Am Rev Respir Dis* 1988;138:458–465.

Luce JM, Pierson DJ, Hudson LD. Intermittent mandatory ventilation. *Chest* 1981;79: 678–685.

Marcy TW, Marini JJ. Respiratory distress in the ventilated patient. *Clin Chest Med* 1994;15:55–73.

Raoof S, Khan FA. *Mechanical Ventilation Manual*. American College of Physicians Press, 1998.

Slutsky AS. ACCP consensus conference-Mechanical ventilation. *Chest* 1993;104: 1833–1859.

Tobin MJ. Mechanical ventilation. *N Engl J Med* 1994;330:1056–1061.

XII. Commonly Used Medications

This section is a quick reference to commonly used medications. You should be familiar with all of the doses, indications, contraindications, side effects, and drug interactions of the medications that you prescribe. Such detailed information is beyond the scope of this manual and can be found in the package insert, *Physicians' Desk Reference* (PDR), or the American Hospital Formulary Service.

Drugs in this section are listed in alphabetic order by generic names. The listed uses include both labeled indications and common off-label uses on the basis of recommendations of our editorial board. Some of the more common trade names are listed for each medication. Where no pediatric dose is provided, the implication is that the use of the agent is not well established in this age group or is infrequently used. Drugs under the control of the Drug Enforcement Agency (Schedule 2–5 controlled substances) are indicated by the symbol [C].

Drugs used in emergency cardiac care are preceded with the acronym *ECC.* The dosing regimens shown in this section are those recommended in guidelines from the American Heart Association and the International Liaison Committee on Resuscitation (*Circulation* 2000;(Suppl 1):102.) and the 2000 *Handbook of Emergency Cardiovascular Care for Health Care Providers* published by the American Heart Association, Dallas, TX 2000 (www.cpr-ecc.americanheart.org). These doses may be slightly different from other recommended doses listed for the individual drugs.

CLASSIFICATION

ALLERGIC DISORDERS

Antihistamines

Cetirizine
Chlorpheniramine
Clemastine fumarate
Desloratadine
Cyproheptadine

Diphenhydramine
Fexofenadine
Hydroxyzine
Loratadine

Miscellaneous Agents

Budesonide

Cromolyn

ANTIDOTES

Acetylcysteine
Charcoal
Deferoxamine
Digoxin immune FAB
Dimercaprol

Edetate disodium
Ethanol
Flumazenil
Fomepizole
Ipecac syrup

Methylene blue
Mesna
Naloxone
Penicillamine

Physostigmine
Pralidoxime
Sorbitol
Succimer

ANTIMICROBIAL AGENTS

Antibiotics

Aminoglycosides

Amikacin
Gentamicin
Neomycin

Streptomycin
Tobramycin

Cephalosporins, First Generation

Cefadroxil
Cefazolin

Cephalexin

Cephalosporins, Second Generation

Cefaclor
Cefotetan
Cefoxitin

Cefprozil
Cefuroxime
Loracarbef

Cephalosporins, Third Generation

Cefdinir
Cefepime → 4th Gen
Cefixime
Cefmetazole
Cefonicid
Cefoperazone
Cefotaxime
Cefpodoxime

Ceftazidime
Ceftibuten
Ceftizoxime
Ceftriaxone
Cefuroxime
Cephapirin
Cephradine

Fluoroquinolones

Ciprofloxacin
Ciprofloxacin and hydrocortisone otic
Gatifloxacin
Levofloxacin
Lomefloxacin

Moxifloxacin
Norfloxacin
Ofloxacin
Sparfloxacin

Macrolides

Azithromycin
Clarithromycin

Dirithromycin
Erythromycin

Penicillins

Amoxicillin
Amoxicillin-clavulanate
Ampicillin
Ampicillin-sulbactam
Cloxacillin
Dicloxacillin
Mezlocillin
Nafcillin
Oxacillin

Penicillin G aqueous
Penicillin G benzathine
Penicillin G procaine
Penicillin V
Piperacillin
Piperacillin-tazobactam
Ticarcillin
Ticarcillin-clavulanate

Tetracyclines

Doxycycline

Tetracycline

Miscellaneous Agents

Aztreonam
Clindamycin
Cortisporin, otic
Fosfomycin
Imipenem-cilastatin
Linezolid
Meropenem
Metronidazole

Mupirocin
Nitrofurantoin
Quinupristin/dalfopristin
Rifampin
Silver nitrate
Trimethoprim-sulfamethoxazole
Vancomycin

Antifungals

Amphotericin B
Amphotericin B cholesteryl
  sulfate complex
Amphotericin B lipid complex
Amphotericin B liposomal
Ciclopirox
Clotrimazole

Econazole
Fluconazole
Itraconazole
Ketoconazole
Miconazole
Nystatin

Antimycobacterials

Ethambutol
Isoniazid
Pyrazinamide

Rifampin
Rifapentine
Rifater

Antiretrovirals

Abacavir
Amprenavir
Combivir
Delavirdine
Didanosine
Efavirenz
Indinavir
Lamivudine

Nelfinavir
Ritonavir
Nevirapine
Saquinavir
Stavudine
Zalcitabine
Zidovudine

Antivirals

Acyclovir
Amantadine
Famciclovir
Foscarnet
Ganciclovir
Interferon alpha-2B and ribavirin

Interferon alfacon-1
Oseltamivir
Ribavirin
Rimantadine
Valacyclovir
Zanamivir

Miscellaneous Agents

Pentamidine

Silver sulfadiazine

ANTINEOPLASTIC AGENTS

Alkylating Agents

Altretamine
Carboplatin

Cisplatin

Nitrogen Mustards

Chlorambucil
Cyclophosphamide

Ifosfamide
Melphalan

Nitrosoureas

Carmustine

Antibiotics

Bleomycin sulfate
Dactinomycin
Daunorubicin

Doxorubicin
Idarubicin
Plicamycin

Antimetabolites

Cytarabine
Cytarabine liposomal
Fludarabine
Fluorouracil

Mercaptopurine
Methotrexate
6-Thioguanine

Hormones

Anastrozole
Bicalutamide
Goserelin
Leuprolide acetate

Megestrol acetate
Nilutamide
Tamoxifen acetate

Mitotic Inhibitors

Etoposide
Teniposide
Vinblastine

Vincristine
Vinorelbine

Miscellaneous Agents

Aldesleukin
Aminoglutethimide
BCG
Dacarbazine
Docetaxol

Hydroxyurea
Levamisole
Mitoxantrone
Paclitaxel

CARDIOVASCULAR AGENTS

Alpha$_1$-Adrenergic Blockers
Doxazosin   Terazosin
Prazosin

Angiotensin-Converting Enzyme Inhibitors
Benazepril   Moexipril
Captopril   Perindopril
Enalapril and enalaprilat   Quinapril
Fosinopril   Ramipril
Lisinopril   Trandolapril

Angiotensin-II Receptor Antagonists
Candesartan   Losartan
Eprosartan   Telmisartan
Irbesartan   Valsartan

Antiarrhythmic Agents
Adenosine   Lidocaine
Amiodarone   Mexiletine
Atropine   Moricizine
Digoxin   Procainamide
Disopyramide   Propafenone
Esmolol   Quinidine
Flecainide   Sotalol
Ibutilide   Tocainide

β(Beta)-Blockers
Acebutolol   Labetalol
Atenolol   Metoprolol
Atenolol and chlorothiazide   Nadolol
Betaxolol   Penbutolol
Bisoprolol   Pindolol
Carteolol   Propranolol
Carvedilol   Timolol
Esmolol

Calcium Channel Antagonists
Amlodipine   Nicardipine
Bepridil   Nifedipine
Diltiazem   Nimodipine
Felodipine   Nisoldipine
Isradipine   Verapamil

Centrally Acting Antihypertensive Agents
Clonidine   Guanethidine
Guanabenz   Guanfacine
Guanadrel   Methyldopa

Diuretics

Acetazolamide
Amiloride
Bumetanide
Chlorothiazide
Chlorthalidone
Ethacrynic acid
Furosemide
Hydrochlorothiazide
Hydrochlorothiazide and amiloride

Hydrochlorothiazide and spironolactone
Hydrochlorothiazide and triamterene
Indapamide
Mannitol
Metolazone
Spironolactone
Torsemide
Triamterene

Inotropic Agents

Amrinone
Digoxin
Dobutamine
Dopamine
Epinephrine

Isoproterenol
Milrinone
Norepinephrine
Phenylephrine

Lipid-Lowering Agents

Atorvastatin
Cholestyramine
Colestipol
Colesevelam
Fenofibrate
Fluvastatin

Gemfibrozil
Lovastatin
Niacin
Pravastatin
Simvastatin

Vasodilators

Epoprostenol
Fenoldopam
Hydralazine
Isosorbide dinitrate
Isosorbide mononitrate

Minoxidil
Nitroglycerin
Nitroprusside
Tolazoline

CENTRAL NERVOUS SYSTEM AGENTS

Antianxiety Agents

Alprazolam
Buspirone
Chlordiazepoxide
Clorazepate
Diazepam
Doxepin

Hydroxyzine
Lorazepam
Meprobamate
Oxazepam
Prazepam

Anticonvulsants

Carbamazepine
Clonazepam
Diazepam
Ethosuximide
Fosphenytoin

Gabapentin
Lamotrigine
Levetiracetam
Lorazepam
Oxcarbazepine

Pentobarbital
Phenobarbital
Phenytoin
Tiagabine

Topiramate
Valproic acid
Zonisamide

Antidepressants

Amitriptyline
Amoxapine
Bupropion
Citalopram
Desipramine
Doxepin
Fluoxetine
Fluvoxamine
Imipramine
Maprotiline

Mirtazapine
Nefazodone
Nortriptyline
Paroxetine
Phenelzine
Sertraline
Trazodone
Trimipramine
Venlafaxine

Antiparkinsonian Agents

Amantadine
Benztropine
Bromocriptine
Carbidopa/levodopa
Entacapone

Pergolide
Pramipexole
Procyclidine
Selegiline
Trihexyphenidyl

Antipsychotics

Chlorpromazine
Clozapine
Fluphenazine
Haloperidol
Lithium carbonate
Mesoridazine
Molindone
Loxapine

Olanzapine
Perphenazine
Prochlorperazine
Risperidone
Thioridazine
Thiothixene
Trifluoperazine

Sedative Hypnotics

Chloral hydrate
Diphenhydramine
Estazolam
Flurazepam
Hydroxyzine
Midazolam
Pentobarbital
Phenobarbital

Propofol
Quazepam
Secobarbital
Temazepam
Triazolam
Zaleplon
Zolpidem

Miscellaneous Agents

Nimodipine

Tacrine

ENDOCRINE SYSTEM AGENTS

Antidiabetic Agents
Acarbose
Acetohexamide
Chlorpropamide
Glimepiride
Glipizide
Glyburide
Glucagon
Insulin

Metformin
Miglitol
Pioglitazone
Repaglinide
Rosiglitazone
Tolazamide
Tolbutamide

Hormones and Synthetic Substitutes
Cortisone
Desmopressin
Dexamethasone
Fludrocortisone acetate
Glucagon

Hydrocortisone
Methylprednisolone
Prednisolone
Prednisone
Vasopressin

Hypercalcemia Agents
Calcitonin
Etidronate

Gallium nitrate
Plicamycin

Osteoporosis Agents
Alendronate
Calcitonin

Raloxifene
Risedronate

Thyroid/Antithyroid
Levothyroxine
Liothyronine
Methimazole

Potassium iodide
Propylthiouracil
Thyroid

MISCELLANEOUS AGENTS

Demeclocycline

Diazoxide

GASTROINTESTINAL SYSTEM AGENTS

Antacids
Alginic acid
Aluminum carbonate
Aluminum hydroxide
Aluminum hydroxide with
  magnesium carbonate
Aluminum hydroxide with
  magnesium hydroxide

Aluminum hydroxide with magnesium
  hydroxide and simethicone
Calcium carbonate
Magaldrate
Simethicone

Antidiarrheals
Bismuth subsalicylate
Diphenoxylate with atropine
Kaolin/pectin

Lactobacillus
Loperamide
Octreotide

Antiemetics

Buclizine
Chlorpromazine
Dimenhydrinate
Dolasetron
Dronabinol
Droperidol
Granisetron
Meclizine

Metoclopramide
Ondansetron
Prochlorperazine
Promethazine
Scopolamine
Thiethylperazine
Trimethobenzamide

Antiulcer Agents

Cimetidine
Famotidine
"GI Cocktail"—Maalox/Mylanta +
　viscous lidocaine (Donnatal)
Lansoprazole
Misoprostol
Nizatidine
Omeprazole
Pantoprazole
Rabeprazole

Ranitidine
Sucralfate
Anti-*Helicobacter pylori*
Bismuth subsalicylate + metronidazole
　+ tetracycline
Lansoprazole + amoxicillin +
　clarithromycin
Ranitidine bismuth citrate +
　clarithromycin

Cathartics/Laxatives

Bisacodyl
Docusate calcium
Docusate potassium
Docusate sodium
Glycerin suppositories
Lactulose

Magnesium citrate
Magnesium hydroxide
Mineral oil
Polyethylene glycol-electrolyte soln
Psyllium
Sorbitol

Enzymes

Pancreatin

Pancrelipase

Miscellaneous Agents

Alosetron
Dexpanthenol
Dicyclomine
Hyoscyamine
Hyoscyamine, atropine,
　scopolamine and phenobarbital
Infliximab

Mesalamine
Metoclopramide
Misoprostol
Olsalazine
Propantheline
Sulfasalazine
Vasopressin

HEMATOLOGIC MODIFIERS

Anticoagulants

Ardeparin
Dalteparin
Danaparoid
Enoxaparin
Heparin

Lepirudin
Protamine
Tinzaparin
Warfarin

Antiplatelet Agents
Abciximab
Aspirin
Clopidogrel
Eptifibatide

Reteplase
Ticlopidine
Tirofiban

Antithrombic Agents
Alteplase, recombinant (TPA)
Aminocaproic acid
Anistreplase
Aprotinin
Dextran 40

Reteplase
Streptokinase
Tenecteplase
Urokinase

Hemopoietic Stimulants
Epoetin alfa (erythropoietin)
Filgrastim (G-CSF)

Oprelvekin
Sargramostim (GM-CSF)

Volume Expanders
Albumin
Dextran 40

Hetastarch
Plasma protein fraction

Miscellaneous Agents
Antihemophilic factor VIII
Cilostazol
Desmopressin

Lepirudin
Pentoxifylline

IMMUNE SYSTEM AGENTS

Immunomodulators
Interferon alfa

Immunosuppressives
Antithymocyte globulin (ATG)
Azathioprine
Basiliximab
Cyclosporine
Daclizumab

Muromonab-CD3
Mycophenolate mofetil
Sirolimus
Steroids
Tacrolimus

Vaccines/Serums/Toxoids
BCG vaccine
Cholera vaccine
CMV Immune globulin
Diphtheria
Haemophilus B conjugate
Hepatitis A vaccine
Hepatitis B immune globulin
Hepatitis B vaccine
Immune globulin, IV
Influenza vaccine
Japanese encephalitis vaccine

Lyme disease vaccine
Measles, mumps and rubella
   vaccine
Meningococcal vaccine
Plague vaccine
Pneumococcal vaccine, polyvalent
Pneumococcal 7-valent conjugate
Polio vaccine
Rabies vaccine
Rabies immune globulin
RHO immune globulin

RSV immune globulin
Tetanus immune globulin
Tetanus toxoid

Varicella immune globulin
Varicella vaccine
Yellow fever vaccine

MUSCULOSKELETAL SYSTEM AGENTS

Antigout Agents
Allopurinol
Colchicine

Probenecid
Sulfinpyrazone

Muscle Relaxants
Aspirin and meprobamate
Baclofen
Carisoprodol
Chlorzoxazone
Cyclobenzaprine
Dantrolene

Diazepam
Metaxalone
Methocarbamol
Orphenadrine
Quinine sulfate
Tizanidine

Neuromuscular Blockers
Atracurium
Cisatracurium
Mivacurium
Pancuronium
Pipecuronium

Rapacuronium
Rocuronium
Succinylcholine
Vecuronium

Miscellaneous Agents
Edrophonium
Leflunomide

Methotrexate

OB/GYN AGENTS

Contraceptives
Levonorgestrel implants

Norgestrel

Estrogen Supplements
Esterified estrogens
Esterified estrogens with
  methyltestosterone
Estradiol
Estradiol transdermal

Estrogen, conjugated
Estrogen, conjugated with
  methyltestosterone
Ethinyl estradiol

Vaginal Preparations
Urea
Miconazole
Nystatin

Terconazole
Tioconazole

Miscellaneous Agents
Gonadorelin
Leuprolide
Magnesium sulfate
Medroxyprogesterone

Methylergonovine
Oxytocin
Terbutaline

OPTHALMIC AGENTS

Acetazolamide
Apraclonidine
Artificial tears
Atropine
Bacitracin and polymyxin B
  (Polysporin)
Betaxolol
Brimonidine
Brinzolamide
Carteolol
Ciprofloxacin
Cromolyn
Cyclopentolate
Diclofenac
Dorzolamide
Dorzolamide and timolol
Dipivefrin
Echothiophate iodine
Erythromycin
Fomivirsen
Gentamicin
Homatropine
Ketorolac
Ketotifen
Latanoprost
Levobunolol
Levocabastine
Lodoxamide

Naphazoline and antazoline
Naphazoline and pheniramine
Nedocromil
Neomycin, bacitracin and polymyxin-B
Neomycin, polymyxin-B and
  dexamethasone
Neomycin, polymyxin-B and
  hydrocortisone
Neomycin, polymyxin-B and
  prednisolone
Norfloxacin
Ofloxacin
Olopatadine
Phenylephrine
Pilocarpine
Pemirolast
Prednisolone
Proparacaine
Rimexolone
Sulfacetamide
Tetracaine
Timolol
Tobramycin
Tobramycin and dexamethasone
Tropicamide
Trifluridine
Vidarabine

OTIC AGENTS

Acetic acid/aluminum acetate
Antipyrine and benzocaine
Carbamide peroxide
Ciprofloxacin/hydrocortisone

Neomycin, polymyxin-B and
  hydrocortisone
Ofloxacin otic
Triethanolamine polypeptide oleate

PAIN RELIEVERS

Local Anesthetics
Antipyrine and benzocaine
Anusol
Capsaicin
Cocaine
Bupivacaine
Dibucaine

Fluori-Methane
Lidocaine
Lidocaine/prilocaine
Lidocaine 5% patch
Mepivacaine

Migraine Headache Medications

Acetaminophen with butalbital
   +/- caffeine
Almotriptan
Butalbital, aspirin and caffeine
Naratriptan

Rizatriptan
Serotonin 5-HT$_1$ Receptor Agonists
   (See Table A–35, Page 687)
Sumatriptan (Imitrex)
Zolmitriptan (Zomig)

Narcotics

Opioids

Alfentanil
Buprenorphine
Butalbital, aspirin, and codeine
Butorphanol
Codeine
Dezocine
Fentanyl
Fentanyl transdermal
Fentanyl transmucosal
Hydrocodone
Hydrocodone and acetaminophen
Hydrocodone and aspirin
Hydromorphone

Levorphanol
Meperidine
Methadone
Morphine
Nalbuphine
Oxycodone and acetaminophen
Oxycodone and aspirin
Oxymorphone
Propoxyphene
Propoxyphene and acetaminophen
Propoxyphene and aspirin
Pentazocine
Sufentanil

Nonnarcotic Opioids

Acetaminophen
Acetaminophen with codeine
Aspirin
Aspirin with codeine

Butalbital and acetaminophen
Butalbital and aspirin
Tramadol

Nonsteroidal Antiinflammatories

Aspirin
Celecoxib
Diclofenac
Diflunisal
Etodolac
Fenoprofen
Flurbiprofen
Ibuprofen
Indomethacin
Ketoprofen
Ketorolac

Meclofenamate
Meloxicam
Nabumetone
Naproxen
Naproxen sodium
Oxaprozin
Piroxicam
Rofecoxib
Salsalate
Sulindac
Tolmetin

RESPIRATORY TRACT AGENTS

Antitussives and Decongestants

Acetylcysteine
Benzonatate
Codeine

Dextromethorphan
Guaifenesin
Guaifenesin and codeine

Guaifenesin and dextromethorphan
Guaifenesin and pseudoephedrine
Hydromorphone and guaifenesin

Hydrocodone and homatropine
Hydrocodone and pseudoephedrine
Pseudoephedrine

Bronchodilators

Albuterol
Albuterol and ipratropium
Aminophylline
Bitolterol
Ephedrine
Epinephrine
Isoetharine

Isoproterenol
Levalbuterol
Metaproterenol
Pirbuterol
Salmeterol
Terbutaline
Theophylline

Respiratory Inhalants

Acetylcysteine
Beclomethasone
Budesonide
Cromolyn sodium
Flunisolide

Fluticasone
Ipratropium
Nedocromil
Triamcinolone acetonide

Miscellaneous Agents Leukotriene Inhibitors

Beractant
Montelukast

Zafirlukast
Zileuton

STEROIDS

Systemic

Betamethasone
Cortisone
Dexamethasone
Hydrocortisone

Methylprednisolone acetate
Methylprednisolone succinate
Prednisone
Prednisolone

Topical

Alclometasone dipropionate
Amcinonide
Augmented betamethasone
Betamethasone dipropionate
Betamethasone valerate
Clobetasol propionate
Clocortolone pivalate
Desonide
Desoximetasone
Dexamethasone
Diflorasone diacetate
Fluocinolone acetonide

Fluocinonide
Flurandrenolide
Fluticasone propionate
Halcinonide
Halobetasol
Hydrocortisone
Hydrocortisone acetate
Hydrocortisone butyrate
Hydrocortisone valerate
Mometasone furoate
Prednicarbate
Triamcinolone

DIETARY SUPPLEMENTS

Calcium chloride
Calcium acetate
Calcitriol

Cholecalciferol
Cyanocobalamin (vitamin B_{12})
Ferrous sulfate

Folic acid
Iron dextran
Leucovorin
Magnesium oxide
Magnesium sulfate

Phytonadione (vitamin K)
Potassium supplements
Pyridoxine (vitamin B_6)
Sodium bicarbonate
Thiamine (vitamin B_1)

URINARY TRACT AGENTS

Ammonium aluminum sulfate
Belladonna and opium suppositories
Bethanechol
Dimethyl sulfoxide (DMSO)
Flavoxate
Hyoscyamine
Methenamine mandelate
Nalidixic acid
Neomycin–polymyxin bladder irrigant

Nitrofurantoin
Oxybutynin
Pentosan polysulfate
Phenazopyridine
Potassium citrate
Potassium citrate and citric acid
Sodium citrate
Trimethoprim

Benign Prostatic Hyperplasia
Doxazosin
Finasteride

Tamsulosin
Terazosin

PROCEDURAL SEDATION

Etomidate
Fentanyl
Ketamine

Methohexital
Midazolam
Propofol

MISCELLANEOUS AGENTS

Isotretinoin
Lindane
Megestrol acetate
Naltrexone
Nicotine gum
Nicotine nasal spray
Nicotine transdermal

Permethrin
Pyrethrin/piperonyl butoxide
Sibutramine
Sildenafil
Sodium polystyrene sulfonate
Witch hazel

GENERIC DRUGS

■ Abacavir (Ziagen)
Uses: HIV infection
Dose: Adults. 300 mg bid. *Peds.* 8 mg/kg bid
Notes: Hypersensitivity manifested as fever, rash, fatigue, GI and respiratory symptoms reported. Stop drug immediately and do not rechallenge. Lactic acidosis and hepatomegaly/steatosis reported

■ Abciximab (ReoPro) (see Cover)
Uses: Prevention of acute ischemic complications in patients undergoing PTCA. **ECC.** ACS without ST elevation

Dose: 0.25 mg/kg administered 10–60 min prior to PTCA, then 0.125 µg/kg/min (10 mg/min) cont inf for 12 h. **ECC.** ACS with PCI in 24 h: 0.25 mg/kg IV bolus up to 1 h before, then 0.125 µg/kg/IV

Notes: Used concomitantly with heparin; may cause allergic reactions

■ Acarbose (Precose)
Uses: Type 2 DM
Dose: 25–100 mg PO tid with meals
Notes: May be taken concomitantly with sulfonylureas

■ Acebutolol (Sectral)
Uses: HTN; ventricular arrhythmias, angina
Dose: 200–400 mg, PO bid

■ Acetaminophen (Tylenol, others)
Uses: Mild pain, headache, fever
Dose: Adults. 650–1000 mg PO or PR q4–6h. **Peds.** 10 mg/kg/dose PO or PR q4–6h

Notes: Overdose causes hepatotoxicity and is treated with *N*-acetylcysteine; charcoal is not usually recommended; no antiinflammatory or platelet-inhibiting action

■ Acetaminophen with Codeine (Tylenol No. 1, No. 2, No. 3, No. 4; others) [C]
Uses: No. 1, No. 2, No. 3 for mild-to-moderate pain; No. 4 for moderate-to-severe pain; antitussive

Dose: Adults. 1–2 tabs q3–4h PRN. **Peds.** Acetaminophen 10–15 mg/kg/dose; codeine 0.5–1.0 mg/kg/dose q4–6h (useful elixir dosing guide: 3–6 years, 5 mL/dose; 7–12 years, 10 mL/dose)

Notes: Caps contain 325-mg acetaminophen, tabs, 300 mg; codeine in No.1: 7.5 mg, No.2: 15 mg, No.3: 30 mg, No.4: 60 mg; 5-mL elixir contains 120-mg acetaminophen, 12-mg codeine plus alcohol

■ Acetaminophen + Butalbital +/- Caffeine (Fioricet, Medigesic, others) [C]
Uses: Mild pain; HA, especially associated with stress
Dose: 1–2 tabs or caps PO q4/6h PRN

■ Acetazolamide (Diamox)
Uses: Diuresis, glaucoma, alkalinization of urine, refractory epilepsy
Dose: Adults. Diuretic: 250–375 mg IV or PO q24h in ÷ doses. *Glaucoma:* 250–1000 mg PO qd in ÷ doses. *Peds. Epilepsy:* 8–30 mg/kg/24h PO in 4 ÷ doses. *Diuretic:* 5 mg/kg/24h PO or IV. *Alkalinization of urine:* 5 mg/kg/dose PO bid–tid. *Glaucoma:* 20–40 mg/kg/24h PO in 4 ÷ doses
Notes: Contra in renal failure, sulfa hypersensitivity; follow Na^+ and K^+; watch for metabolic acidosis

■ Acetic Acid and Aluminum Acetate (Otic Domeboro)
Uses: Otitis externa
Dose: 4–6 gtt in ear(s)

■ Acetohexamide (Dymelor)
Uses: Management of non-insulin-dependent DM
Dose: 250–1500 mg qd

■ Acetylcysteine (Mucomyst)
Uses: Mucolytic agent as adjuvant therapy for chronic bronchopulmonary diseases and CF; as tid antidote to acetaminophen hepatotoxicity within 24 h of ingestion
Dose: Adults & Peds. Nebulizer: 3–5 mL of 20% soln diluted with equal volume of water or NS administered tid–qid. *Antidote:* PO or NG; 140 mg/kg diluted 1:4 in carbonated beverage as loading dose, then 70 mg/kg q4h for 17 doses
Notes: Watch for bronchospasm when used by inhal in asthmatics; activated charcoal adsorbs acetylcysteine when given PO for acute APAP ingestion

■ Acyclovir (Zovirax)
Uses: Herpes simplex and herpes zoster viral infections
Dose: Adults. Topical: Apply 0.5-in. ribbon q3h. *Oral:* Initial genital herpes: 200 mg PO q4h while awake; 5 caps/d for 10 d. Chronic suppression: 400 mg PO bid–tid. Intermittent therapy: As for initial treatment, except treat for 5 days at the earliest prodrome. *Herpes zoster:* 800 mg PO 5 ×/d. *IV:* 5–10 mg/kg/dose IV q8h. *Peds.* 5–10 mg/kg/dose IV or PO q8h or 750 mg/m2/24h ÷ q8h.
Notes: Adjust dose in renal insufficiency

■ Adenosine (Adenocard) (See Cover)
Uses: Paroxysmal SVT, including that associated with Wolff–Parkinson–White syndrome
Dose: Adults. 6 mg rapid IV, repeated in 1–2 min at 12 mg IV if no response. *ECC.* 6 mg over 1– 3 s, then 20 mL NS bolus, elevate extremity; repeat 12 mg in 1–2 min PRN. *Peds.* 0.03–0.25 mg/kg IV bolus; repeat higher dose in 1–2 min

if no response; **ECC.** 0.1 mg/kg rapid IV push, follow with > 5 mL NS flush; 0.2 mg/kg for second dose)

Notes: Doses > 12 mg are not recommended; caffeine and theophylline antagonize the effects of adenosine

■ Albumin (Albuminar, Buminate, Albutein, others)

Uses: Plasma volume expansion for shock resulting from burns, surgery, hemorrhage, or other trauma

Dose: *Adults.* 25 g IV initially; subsequent infusions should depend on clinical situation and response. *Peds.* 0.5–1.0 g/kg/dose; infuse at 0.05–0.1 g/min

Notes: Contains 130–160 mEq Na$^+$/L.

■ Albuterol (Proventil, Ventolin)

Uses: Treatment of bronchospasm in reversible obstructive airway disease; prevention of exercise-induced bronchospasm

Dose: *Adults.* 2–4 inhals q4–6h; 1 Rotocaps inhaled q4–6h; 2–4 mg PO tid–qid. *Peds.* 2 inhals q4–6h; 0.1–0.2 mg/kg/dose PO, to max dose of 2–4 mg PO tid

■ Albuterol and Ipratroprium (Combivent)

Uses: Management of COPD
Dose: 2 inhals qid

■ Aldesleukin [IL-2] (Proleukin)

Uses: Treatment of metastatic renal cell carcinoma, melanoma, and colorectal cancer

Dose: 600,000 IU/kg (0.037 mg/kg) administered every 8 h by a 15-min infusion for 14 doses. After 9 d of rest, repeat schedule for another 14 doses, for a max of 28 doses per cycle.

Notes: Administer only in a hospital with an ICU and an available specialist; may cause severe hypotension and "capillary leak syndrome," resulting in reduced organ perfusion

■ Alendronate (Fosamax)

Uses: Treatment and prevention of osteoporosis, and Paget's disease
Dose: *Osteoporosis treatment:* 10 mg/d PO. *Prevention:* 5 mg/d PO. *Paget's disease:* 40 mg/d PO

Notes: Should take 30 min before meals to avoid GI upset.

■ Alfentanil (Alfenta) [C]

Uses: Adjunct in the maintenance of general anesthesia.
Dose: *Adults & Peds* older than 12 y: 8–75 mg/kg IV infusion; total dose depends on the duration of the operative procedure

■ Allopurinol (Zyloprim, Lopurin)
Uses: Gout, treatment of hyperuricemia of malignancy, uric acid urolithiasis
Dose: Adults. Initial 100 mg PO qd; usual 300 mg PO qd. *Peds.* Use only for treating hyperuricemia of malignancy in children; 10 mg/kg/24h ÷ q6–8h (max 600 mg/24h)
Notes: Aggravates acute gout episode, do not begin until acute episode resolves

■ Alosetron (Lotronex)
Uses: Irritable bowel syndrome
Dose: 1 mg bid
Notes: May be taken without regard to food intake

■ Alprazolam (Xanax) [C]
Uses: Anxiety and panic disorders; anxiety associated with depression
Dose: 0.25–2 mg PO tid
Notes: Reduce dose in elderly and debilitated patients

■ Alteplase, Recombinant [TPA] (Activase)
Uses: Acute MI, PE, stroke; *ECC.* Acute MI in adults. ST-segment elevation of 1 mm or more in at least two contiguous leads in the setting of AMI. *Adjuvant therapy:* 60–325 mg aspirin chewed as soon as possible. Begin heparin immediately and continue for 48 h if alteplase is used
Dose: 100 mg IV over 3 h. *ECC Adult:* Dose based on patient weight, not to exceed 100 mg. *Approved dose regimens for AMI patients:* (1) Accelerated infusion: 1. 15 mg bolus; 2. then 0.75 mg/kg over next 30 min (not to exceed 50 mg); 3. then 0.50 mg/kg over next 60 min (not to exceed 35 mg). (2) Three-h infusion: (a) 60 mg in first hour (initial 6–10 mg as a bolus; (b) then 20 mg/h for 2 additional hours. *Acute ischemic stroke:* (1) 0.9 mg/kg (maximum 90 mg) infused over 60 min; (2) 10% of total dose as initial IV bolus over 1 min; (3) Give remaining 90% over the next 60 min
Notes: May cause bleeding.

■ Altretamine (Hexalen)
Uses: Palliative treatment of ovarian cancer
Dose: 260 mg/m^2/d PO ÷ q6h, for 14–21 consecutive days of a 28-d cycle
Notes: May cause neurologic and hematologic toxicity

■ Aluminum Carbonate (Basaljel)
Uses: Hyperacidity (peptic ulcer, hiatal hernia, etc); supplement to management of hyperphosphatemia in renal disease
Dose: Adults. 2 caps or tabs or 10 mL (in water) q2h PRN. *Peds.* 50–150 mg/kg/24h PO ÷ q4–6h

■ Aluminum Hydroxide (Amphojel, ALTernaGEL, Alu-Cap, Alu-Tab)
Uses: See Aluminum Carbonate
Dose: Adults. 10–30 mL or 2 tabs/caps PO q4–6h. *Peds.* 5–15 mL PO q4–6h
Notes: Can be used in renal failure; may cause constipation

■ Aluminum Hydroxide with Magnesium Carbonate (Gaviscon)
Uses: Hyperacidity (peptic ulcer, hiatal hernia, etc)
Dose: Adults. 15–30 PO pc and hs. *Peds.* 5–15 mL PO qid or PRN
Notes: Doses qid are best given after meals and hs; may cause hypermagnesemia

■ Aluminum Hydroxide with Magnesium Hydroxide (Maalox)
Uses: Hyperacidity (peptic ulcer, hiatal hernia, etc)
Dose: Adults. 10–60 mL or 2–4 tabs PO qid or PRN. *Peds.* 5–15 mL PO qid or PRN
Notes: Doses qid are best given after meals and hs; may cause hypermagnesemia in renal insufficiency

■ Aluminum Hydroxide with Magnesium Trisilicate (Gaviscon-2)
Uses: Hyperacidity
Dose: Chew 2–4 tabs qid and hs

■ Aluminum Hydroxide with Magnesium Hydroxide and Simethicone (Mylanta, Mylanta II, Maalox Plus)
Uses: Hyperacidity with bloating
Dose: Adults. 10–60 mL or 2–4 tabs PO qid or PRN. *Peds.* 5–15 mL PO qid or PRN
Notes: May cause hypermagnesemia in renal insufficiency; Mylanta II contains twice the amount of aluminum and magnesium hydroxide as Mylanta

■ Amantadine (Symmetrel)
Uses: Treatment or prophylaxis of influenza A viral infections; Parkinsonism
Dose: Adults. Influenza A: 200 mg PO qd or 100 mg PO bid. *Parkinsonism:* 100 mg PO qd–bid. *Peds.* 1–9 y: 4.4–8.8 mg/kg/24h to a max of 150 mg/24h ÷ qd–bid; *> 9 y:* same as adults.
Notes: Reduce dose in renal insufficiency

■ Amikacin (Amikin)
Uses: Treatment of serious infections caused by gram-negative bacteria.
Dose: Adults & Peds. 15 mg/kg/24h ÷ q8–12h or based on renal function; refer to Aminoglycoside dosing (Table A–24, page 676).
Notes: May be effective against gram-negative bacteria resistant to gentamicin and tobramycin; monitor renal function carefully for dose adjustments; monitor serum levels (see Table A–23, page 676).

■ Amiloride (Midamor)
Uses: HTN and CHF
Dose: 5–10 mg PO qd
Notes: Hyperkalemia may occur; monitor serum potassium levels

■ Aminocaproic Acid (Amicar)
Uses: Excessive bleeding resulting from systemic hyperfibrinolysis and urinary fibrinolysis
Dose: Adults & Peds. 100 mg/kg IV, then 1 g/m^2/h to max of 18 g/m^2/d or 100 mg/kg/dose q8h.
Notes: Administer for 8 h or until bleeding is controlled; Contra in DIC; not for upper urinary tract bleeding; oral form rarely used.

■ Aminoglutethimide (Cytadren, Elipten,)
Uses: Adrenal cortex carcinoma, Cushing's syndrome, and prostate cancer
Dose: 750–1500 mg/d in ÷ doses plus dexamethasone 2–5 mg/d or hydrocortisone 20–40 mg/d
Notes: Toxicity includes adrenal insufficiency ("medical adrenalectomy"), hypothyroidism, masculinization, hypotension, vomiting, rare hepatotoxicity, rash, myalgia, and fever

■ Amino-Cerv pH 5.5 Cream
Uses: Mild cervicitis, postpartum cervicitis/cervical tears, postcauterization, postcryosurgery, and postconization
Dose: 1 applicator intravaginally qhs for 2–4 wk.
Notes: Contains 8.34% urea, 0.5% sodium propionate, 0.83% methionine, 0.35% cystine, 0.83% inositol, benzalkonium chloride.

■ Aminophylline
Uses: Asthma and bronchospasm; apnea of prematurity
Dose: Adults. Acute asthma: Load 6 mg/kg IV, then 0.4–0.9 mg/kg/h IV cont inf. *Chronic asthma:* 24 mg/kg/24h PO or PR ÷ q6h. ***Peds.*** Load 6 mg/kg IV, then 1.0 mg/kg/h IV cont inf
Notes: Individualize dose; signs of toxicity include nausea, vomiting, irritability, tachycardia, ventricular arrhythmias, and seizures; follow serum levels care-

fully; aminophylline is about 85% theophylline (see Table A–22, page 675); erratic absorption with rectal doses

■ Amiodarone (Cordarone)

Uses: Recurrent VF or hemodynamically unstable VT

Dose: Adults. Load: 800–1600 mg/d PO for 1–3 wk. Maint: 600–800 mg/d PO for 1 mo, then 200–400 mg/d. IV: 15 mg/min for 10 min, then 1 mg/min for 6 h; Maint dose of 0.5 mg/min cont inf. **ECC. Adults.** Max cumulative **Dose:** 2.2 g IV/24 h.

Cardiac arrest: 300 mg IV push. Consider repeating 150 mg IV push in 3–5 min. Max cumulative **Dose:** 2.2 g IV/24 h). *Wide-complex tachycardia (stable):* Rapid inf: 150 mg IV over 10 min (15 mg/min); every 15 min PRN. Slow inf: 360 mg IV over 6H (1 mg/min). Maint inf: 540 mg IV over 18H (0.5 mg/min). **Peds.** 10–15 mg/kg/24h ÷ q12h PO for 7==10 d, then 5 mg/kg/24h ÷ q12h or qd (infants and neonates may require a higher loading dose). **ECC.** Refractory pulseless VT, VF: 5 mg/kg rapid IV bolus. *Perfusing supraventricular and ventricular arrhythmias:* Load: 5 mg/kg IV/IO over 20–60 min (repeat, max 15 mg/kg/day).

Notes: Average half-life is 53 d; potentially toxic effects leading to pulmonary fibrosis, liver failure, and ocular opacities, as well as exacerbation of arrhythmias; IV concentrations of > 0.2 mg/mL should be administered via a central catheter

■ Amitriptyline (Elavil)

Uses: Depression, peripheral neuropathy, chronic pain, cluster and migraine headaches

Dose: Adults. Initially, 50–100 mg PO qhs; may increase to 300 mg qhs. **Peds.** Not recommended if younger than 12 y unless for chronic pain: 0.1 mg/kg qhs initially, then advance over 2–3 wk to 0.5–2 mg/kg qhs

Notes: Strong anticholinergic side effects; may cause urinary retention and sedation

■ Amlodipine (Norvasc)

Uses: HTN, chronic stable angina, and vasospastic angina

Dose: 2.5–10 mg PO qd

■ Ammonium Aluminum Sulfate (Alum)

Uses: Hemorrhagic cystitis

Dose: 1–2% soln used with constant bladder irrigation with NS

Notes: Can be used safely without anesthesia and in the presence of vesicoureteral reflux. Encephalopathy has been reported; obtain aluminum levels, especially in patients with renal insufficiency. Alum soln often precipitates and occludes catheters

■ Amoxapine (Asendin)
Uses: Depression and anxiety
Dose: Initially, 150 mg PO qhs or 50 mg PO tid; increase to 300 mg daily
Notes: Reduce dose in elderly patients; taper slowly when discontinuing therapy

■ Amoxicillin (Amoxil, Larotid, Polymox, Others)
Uses: Treatment of susceptible gram-positive bacteria (streptococci), and gram-negative bacteria (*Haemophilus influenzae, Escherichia coli, Proteus mirabilis*)(ie, SBE prophylaxis, otitis media, respiratory, skin and UTIs).
Dose: *Adults.* 250–500 mg PO tid. *Peds.* 25–100 mg/kg/24h PO ÷ q8h; 200 mg–400 mg PO bid (equivalent to 125 mg–250 mg tid).
Notes: Cross-hypersensitivity with penicillin; may cause diarrhea; skin rash is common; many hospital strains of *E coli* are resistant.

■ Amoxicillin/Potassium Clavulanate (Augmentin)
Uses: Treatment of infections caused by β-lactamase-producing strains of *H influenzae, Staphylococcus aureus,* and *E coli.*
Dose: *Adults.* 250–500 mg as amoxicillin PO q8h or 875 mg q12h. *Peds.* 20–40 mg/kg/d as amoxicillin PO ÷ q8h.
Notes: Do not substitute two 250-mg tabs for one 500-mg tab or an overdose of clavulanic acid will occur; may cause diarrhea and GI intolerance. This is a combination of a β-lactamase antibiotic and a β-lactamase inhibitor.

■ Amphotericin B (Fungizone)
Uses: Severe, systemic fungal infections (eg, *Candida* spp, histoplasmosis, etc.); bladder irrigation for fungal infections
Dose: *Adults & Peds.* Test dose of 1 mg, then 0.25–1.5 mg/kg/24h IV over 4–6 h. Doses often range from 25 to 50 mg qd or qod. Total dose varies with indication. *Bladder irrigation:* 50 mg in 1-L sterile water irrigated over 24 h; used for 2–7 d or until culture is negative
Notes: Severe side effects with IV infusion; monitor renal function; hypokalemia and hypomagnesemia may be seen from renal wasting; pretreat with acetaminophen and antihistamines (Benadryl) to help minimize adverse effects such as fever; topical and oral forms are available

■ Amphotericin B Cholesteryl (Amphotec)
Uses: Invasive fungal infection in persons refractory or intolerant to conventional amphotericin B
Dose: *Adults & Peds.* Test dose of 1.6 mg–8.3 mg, over 15–20 min, followed by a dose of 3–4 mg/kg/d. Infuse at a rate of 1 mg/kg/h
Notes: Do NOT use in-line filter, final concentration, 0.6 mg/mL

■ Amphotericin B Lipid Complex (Abelcet)

Uses: Invasive fungal infection in persons refractory or intolerant to conventional amphotericin B.

Dose: 5 mg/kg/d IV administered as a single daily dose; infuse at a rate of 2.5 mg/kg/h

Notes: Filter soln with a 5-mm filter needle; do not mix in electrolyte-containing solns. If infusion exceeds 2 h, gently mix contents of the bag

■ Amphotericin B Liposomal (Ambisome)

Uses: Invasive fungal infection in persons refractory or intolerant to conventional amphotericin B

Dose: Adults & Peds. 3–5 mg/kg/d, infused over 60–120 min

■ Ampicillin (Amcill, Omnipen)

Uses: Treatment of susceptible gram-negative (*Shigella, Salmonella, E coli, H influenzae, P mirabilis*) and gram-positive (streptococci) bacteria

Dose: Adults. Between 500 mg and 2 g PO, IM, or IV q6h. *Peds.* Neonates < 7 d: 50–100 mg/kg/24h IV ÷ q8h. *Term infants:* 75–150 mg/kg/24h ÷ q6–8h IV or PO, *Infants >1 mo and children:* 100–200 mg/kg/24h ÷ q4–6h IM or IV; 50–100 mg/kg/24h ÷ q6h PO up to 250 mg/dose. *Meningitis:* 200–400 mg/kg/24h ÷ q4–6h IV.

Notes: Cross-hypersensitivity with penicillin; can cause diarrhea and skin rash; many hospital strains of *E coli* are now resistant

■ Ampicillin/Sulbactam (Unasyn)

Uses: Treatment of infections caused by β-lactamase-producing organisms of *S aureus, Enterococcus* spp, *H influenzae, P mirabilis,* and *Bacteroides* species

Dose: Adults. 1.5–3.0 g IM or IV q6h. *Peds.* Dosed by ampicillin content 100–200 mg ampicillin/kg/d 150–300 mg Unasyn ÷ q6h; max daily dose, 8 g ampicillin (12 g Unasyn)/d

Notes: 2:1 ratio of ampicillin/sulbactam; adjust dose in renal failure; observe for hypersensitivity reactions

■ Amprenavir (Agenerase)

Uses: HIV infection

Dose: Adults. 1200 mg bid. *Peds.* 20 mg/kg bid or 15 mg/kg tid up to 2400 mg/d

Notes: CDC recommends HIV-infected mothers not breast-feed due to risk of transmission of HIV infant, oral soln contra in *Peds* <4 y

■ Amrinone (Inocor) (see Cover)

Uses: Short-term management of CHF

Dose: Adults & Peds. Initially give IV bolus of 0.75 mg/kg over 2–3 min followed by Maint dose of 5–10 mg/kg/min. **ECC. Adults.** (1)0.75 mg/kg, over 10–15 min (do not mix with dextrose); (2) then 5–15 µg/kg/min titrated to effect; (3) Hemodynamic monitoring preferred. **ECC. Peds.** Load: 0.75–1.0 mg/kg IV over 5 min; may repeat twice (max: 3 mg/kg). Cont inf: 5 to 10 µg/kg/min IV

Notes: Not to exceed 10 mg/kg/d; incompatible with dextrose-containing solns; monitor for fluid and electrolyte changes and renal function during therapy

■ Anastrozole (Arimidex)

Uses: Treatment of breast cancer following tamoxifen.

Dose: 1 mg/d

Notes: No detectable effect on adrenal corticosteroids or aldosterone; may increase cholesterol levels

■ Anistreplase (Eminase) (See Cover)

Uses: Treatment of AMI

Dose: ECC. 30 units IV over 2–5 min

Notes: Use 2 peripheral IV lines, one exclusively for thrombolytic administration. May not be effective if readministered more than 5 d after anistreplase, streptokinase, or streptococcal infection because of production of antistreptokinase antibody

■ Antihemophilic (AHF) Factor [Factor VIII] (Monoclate-P)

Uses: Treatment of classic hemophilia A with factor VIII deficiency

Dose: Adults & Peds. 1 AHF U/kg increases factor VIII concentration in the body by approximately 2%. Units required = Body weight (kg) × (desired factor VIII increase as % normal) × (0.5). Prophylaxis of spontaneous hemorrhage: 5% normal. Hemostasis following trauma or surgery: 30% normal. Head injuries, major surgery, or bleeding: 80–100% normal. Patient's percentage of normal level of factor VIII concentration must be ascertained before dosing for these calculations. Typical dosing is 20–50 U/kg/dose given q12–24h

Notes: Not effective in controlling bleeding of patients with von Willebrand's disease; derived from pooled human plasma

■ Antipyrine and benzocaine (Auralgan)

Uses: Temporary relief of painful inflammatory conditions of the ear (serous otitis media, swimmers ear, otitis externa); aid to cerumen removal

Dose: Adults & Peds. Fill ear canal and place cotton plug to retain; repeat q1–2 h PRN; cerumen apply tid–qid for 2–3 d

■ Antithymocyte Globulin [ATG] (Atgam)
Uses: Management of allograft rejection in renal transplant patients
Dose: Adults. 10–30 mg/kg/d. *Peds.* 5–25 mg/kg/d
Notes: Do not administer to a patient with a history of severe systemic reaction to any other equine gamma globulin preparation; discontinue treatment if severe unremitting thrombocytopenia or leukopenia occurs

■ Apraclonidine (Lopidine)
Uses: Glaucoma
Dose: 1–2 gtt of 0.5% tid

■ Aprotinin (Trasylol)
Uses: Reduction or prevention of blood loss in patients undergoing CABG
Dose: High-Dose: 2 million KIU load, 2 million KIU for the pump prime dose, followed by 500,000 KIU/h until surgery ends. *Low-Dose:* 1 million KIU load, 1 million KIU for the pump prime dose, followed by 250,000 KIU/h until surgery ends. Max total dose of 7 million KIU
Notes: 1 KIU 5 0.14 mg of aprotinin

■ Ardeparin (Normiflo)
Uses: Prevention of DVT and PE following knee replacement
Dose: 35–50 U/kg SQ q12h. Begin the day of surgery and continue for <14 d
Notes: Laboratory monitoring not necessary

■ Artificial Tears [OTC] (Tears Naturale, others)
Uses: Dry eyes
Dose: 1–2 gtt tid–qid

■ Aspirin (Bayer, St. Joseph, Others)
Uses: Mild pain, HA, fever, inflammation, prevention of emboli, and prevention of MI
Dose: Adults. Pain, fever: 325–650 mg q4–6h PO or PR. *RA:* 3–6 g/d PO in ÷ doses. *Platelet inhibitory action:* 81–325 mg PO qd. *Prevention of MI:* 81–325 mg PO qd. *ECC.* In the acute setting, administer to all patients with ACS 160–325 mg PO (chewing preferred ASAP onset of ACS) *Peds.* CAUTION: Use linked to Reye's syndrome; avoid use with viral illness in children. *Antipyretic:* 10–15 mg/kg/dose PO or PR q4h up to 80 mg/kg/24h. *RA:* 60–100 mg/kg/24h PO ÷ q4–6h (monitor serum levels to maintain between 15 and 30 mg/dL); avoid use with CrCl < 10 mL/min and in severe liver disease; avoid or limit alcohol intake

Notes: GI upset and erosion are common adverse reactions; discontinue use 1 wk before surgery to avoid postop bleeding complications

Aspirin with Codeine (Empirin No. 1, No. 2, No. 3, No. 4) [C]
Uses: Relief of mild-to-moderate pain
Dose: Adults. 1–2 tabs PO q3–4h PRN. *Peds.* Aspirin 10 mg/kg/dose; codeine 0.5–1.0 mg/kg/dose q4h
Notes: Codeine in #1: 7.5 mg, #2:mg, #3 30 mg, #4: 60 mg

Aspirin with Meprobamate (Equagesic) [C]
Uses: Treatment of musculoskeletal disease in patients with signs of tension or anxiety
Dose: Adults. 1 tab PO tid–qid

Atenolol (Tenormin)
Uses: HTN, angina, post MI, antiarrhythmic, acute alcoholic withdrawal
Dose: Adults. HTN and angina: 50–100 mg PO qd. *AMI:* 5 mg IV × 2 doses, then 50 mg PO bid, *ECC.* All patients with suspected MI; may reduce chance of VF and reduce damage. (1) 5 mg slow IV (over 5 min); (2) In 10 min, second dose 5 mg slow IV; (3) In 10 min, if tolerated, start 50 mg PO, then 50 mg PO bid

Atenolol and Chlorthalidone (Tenoretic)
Uses: HTN
Dose: 50–100 mg PO qd

Atorvastatin (Lipitor)
Uses: Elevated cholesterol and triglycerides along with dietary modifications
Dose: Initial dose 10 mg daily, may be increased to 80 mg/d
Notes: May cause myopathy, monitor LFT regularly

Atracurium (Tracrium)
Uses: Adjunct to anesthesia to facilitate endotracheal intubation
Dose: Adults & Peds. 0.4–0.5 mg/kg IV bolus, then 0.08–0.1 mg/kg every 20–45 min PRN
Notes: Patient must be intubated and on controlled ventilation. Use adequate amounts of sedation and analgesia

Atropine
Uses: Preanesthetic, symptomatic bradycardia, asystole; organophosphate poisoning, bronchodilator, mydriatic and cycloplegic for eye exam, uveitis, reversal of neuromuscular blockade with neostigmine or edrophonium

Dose: Adults. Preanesthetic: 0.3–0.6 mg IM/IV/SQ. *Ophthalmic:* 1–2 gtt qid or 1/4 in. of 1% oint; refraction, administer 1 h before exam. ***ECC.*** First drug for symptomatic bradycardia (but not Mobitz II). Second drug (after epinephrine or vasopressin) for asystole or bradycardic PEA. *Asystole or PEA:* 1 mg IV push. Repeat every 3–5 min (if asystole persists) to 0.03–0.04 mg/kg max. *Bradycardia:* 0.5–1.0 mg IV every 3–5 min as needed; max 0.03–0.04 mg/kg. *Endotracheal:* 2–3 mg in 10 mL NS. ***Peds.*** *Preanesthetic:* 0.01 mg/kg/dose SQ/IM/IV (max 0.4 mg). ***ECC. Peds.*** IV: 0.02 mg/kg. Min single dose: 0.1 mg, max: 0.5 mg. Max adolescent single dose: 1.0 mg. May double for second IV dose. Max child total dose: 1.0 mg. Max adolescent total dose: 2.0 mg. Endotracheal: 0.02 mg/kg (larger doses than IV may be required)
Notes: Can cause blurred vision, urinary retention, dry mucous membranes

■ Azathioprine (Imuran)
Uses: Adjunct for the prevention of rejection following organ transplantation; RA; systemic lupus erythematosus
Dose: Adults & Peds. 1–3 mg/kg IV or PO daily
Notes: May cause GI intolerance; inj should be handled with appropriate precautions

■ Azithromycin (Zithromax)
Uses: Treatment of acute bacterial exacerbations of COPD, mild community-acquired pneumonia, pharyngitis, otitis media, skin and skin structure infections, nongonococcal urethritis, and PID. Treatment and prevention of *Mycobacterium avium* complex (Mac) infections in HIV-infected persons
Dose: Adults. PO: Respiratory tract: 500 mg on the first day, followed by 250 mg PO qd for 4 more days. *Nongonococcal urethritis:* 1 g as a single dose. *Prevention of Mac:* 1200 mg PO once a week. IV: 500 mg for at least 2 d, followed by 500 mg PO for total of 7–10 d. ***Peds.*** *Otitis media:* 10 mg/kg PO on day 1, then 5 mg/kg/d on days 2–5. *Pharyngitis:* 12 mg/kg/d PO for 5 d
Notes: Should be taken before meals

■ Aztreonam (Azactam)
Uses: Infections caused by aerobic gram-negative bacteria where β-lactam may not be useful, including *Enterobacter, H influenzae, Pseudomonas* sepsis, UTI, skin infections, intraabdominal and gynecologic infections
Dose: Adults. 1–2 g IV/IM q6–12h. ***Peds.*** *Premature infants:* 30 mg/kg/dose IV q12h. *Term infants, children:* 30–50 mg/kg/dose q6–8h
Notes: Not effective against gram-positive or anaerobic bacteria; may be given to penicillin-allergic patients

■ Bacitracin and polymyxin B (Polysporin)
Uses: Blepharitis, conjunctivitis, and prophylactic treatment of corneal abrasions
Dose: Apply q3–4h

■ Baclofen (Lioresal)
Uses: Spasticity secondary to severe chronic disorders such as MS or spinal cord lesions
Dose: 5 mg PO tid initially, increase every 3 d to max effect; max dose 80 mg/d
Notes: Caution in patients with seizure disorder and neuropsychiatric disturbances

■ Basiliximab (Simulect)
Uses: Prevention of acute organ transplant rejections
Dose: *Adults.* 20 mg IV 2 h prior to transplant, then 20 mg IV 4 d posttransplant. *Peds.* 12 mg/m^2 up to a max. of 20 mg 2 h prior to transplant, then the same dose IV 4 d posttransplant.
Notes: Murine/human monoclonal antibody

■ BCG [Bacillus Calmette–Guérin] (TheraCys, Tice BCG)
Uses: BCG vaccination not recommended in US adults; consider in high-risk children who are PPD-negative to 5 TU and cannot receive INH prophylaxis; bladder carcinoma
Dose: Bladder cancer, contents of 1 vial prepared and instilled in bladder for 2 h. Repeat once wkly for 6 wk; repeat 3 wkly doses 3, 6, 12, 18, and 24 mo after initial therapy
Notes: Contra <14 d after transureathral resection of bladder tumor, history of BCG sepsis, immunosuppression, steroid use

■ Beclomethasone (Beconase, Vancenase Nasal Inhalers)
Uses: Allergic rhinitis refractory to conventional therapy with antihistamines and decongestants
Dose: *Adults.* 1 spray intranasally bid–qid. *Peds.* 6–11 y: 1 spray intranasally tid.
Notes: Nasal spray delivers 42 mg/dose

■ Beclomethasone (Beclovent Inhaler, Vanceril Inhaler)
Uses: Chronic asthma
Dose: *Adults.* 2–4 inhals tid–qid (max 20/d). *Peds.* 1–2 inhals tid–qid (max 10/d)
Notes: Not effective for acute asthmatic attacks; may cause oral candidiasis

■ Belladonna and Opium Suppositories (B & O Supprettes) [C]
Uses: Treatment of bladder or rectal spasms; moderate-to-severe pain

Dose: Insert 1 suppository rectally q4–6h PRN. (15A = 30 mg powdered opium; 16.2 mg belladonna extract. 16A = 60 mg powdered opium; 16.2 mg belladonna extract)

Notes: Anticholinergic side effects; caution subjects about sedation, urinary retention, constipation

■ Benazepril (Lotensin)
Uses: HTN
Dose: 10–40 mg PO qd
Notes: May cause symptomatic hypotension in patients taking diuretics; may cause a nonproductive cough

Benzonatate (Tessalon Perles)
Uses: Symptomatic relief of nonproductive cough
Dose: 100 mg PO tid
Notes: May cause sedation

Benztropine (Cogentin)
Uses: Treatment of Parkinson's disease and drug-induced extrapyramidal disorders
Dose: 1–6 mg PO, IM, or IV in ÷ doses
Notes: Anticholinergic side effects

■ Bepridil (Vascor)
Uses: Treatment of chronic stable angina, HTN and CHF
Dose: 200–400 mg PO daily (adjust dose after 10 d)
Notes: May cause serious ventricular arrhythmias, including torsade de pointes and agranulocytosis

■ Beractant (Survanta)
Uses: Prevention/treatment of respiratory distress syndrome (RDS) in premature infants.
Dose: 4 mL/kg intratracheally; up to 4 doses in the first 48 h of life at least 6 h apart; additional therapy based on clinical response

Betamethasone and clotrimazole, topical (Lotrisone)
Uses: Topical treatment of fungal skin infections
Dose: Apply bid
Notes: Combination antifungal and antiinflammatory

Betamethasone, systemic (Celestone, others)
Uses: Steroid replacement, antiinflammatory, immunosuppressive
Dose: 0.6–7.2 mg/d PO ÷ bid–tid; up to 9 mg/d IM; intraarticular 0.5–2.0 mL

Betamethasone, Topical (Diprolene, Diprolene AF, Valisone, Others)
Uses: Topical steroid therapy of dermatosis (psoriasis, seborrhea, atopic, allergic and neuro dermatitis)
Dose: Apply to lesion up to tid
Notes: Betamethasone dipropionate and augmented (Diprolene) available in 0.05% gel, oint or lotion; betamethasone valerate (Valisone) available as cream 0.01%, 0.1%, lotion and oint 0.1%

Betaxolol (Kerlone)
Uses: HTN, ocular for glaucoma
Dose: 10–20 mg PO, qd; ophthalmic: 1–2 gtt of soln or suspension bid

Bethanechol (Urecholine, Duvoid, various)
Uses: Neurogenic atony of the bladder with urinary retention, acute postoperative and postpartum functional (nonobstructive) urinary retention.
Dose: Adults. 10–50 mg PO tid–qid or 5 mg SQ tid–qid and PRN. *Peds.* 0.3–0.6 mg/kg/24h PO ÷ tid–qid
Notes: Contra in bladder outlet obstruction, asthma, CAD; do not administer IM or IV

Bicalutamide (Casodex)
Uses: Treatment of advanced prostate cancer in combination with LHRH analogue
Dose: 50 mg PO qd
Notes: Follow LFTs; can cause gynecomastia

Bicarbonate, see Sodium bicarbonate

Bisacodyl (Dulcolax, others)
Uses: Constipation, bowel prep
Dose: Adults. 5–10 mg PO or 10 mg rectally PRN. *Peds.* < 2 y: 5 mg rectally PRN; *> 2 y:* 5 mg PO or 10 mg PR PRN
Notes: Do not use with an acute abdomen or bowel obstruction; do not chew tabs; do not give within 1 h of antacids or milk

Bismuth Subsalicylate (Pepto-Bismol, others)
Uses: Indigestion, nausea, and diarrhea
Dose: Adults. 2 tabs or 30 mL PO PRN. *Peds.* 3–6 y: 1/3 tab or 5 mL PO PRN; *6–9 y:* 2/3 tab or 10 mL PO PRN; *9–12 y:* 1 tab or 15 mL PO PRN

Bisoprolol (Zebeta)
Uses: HTN
Dose: 5–10 mg qd

Bitolterol (Tornalate)
Uses: Prophylaxis and treatment of asthma and reversible bronchospasm
Dose: Adults and children >12 y: 2 inhals q8h

Bleomycin (Blenoxane)
Uses: Treatment of cervical, ovarian, squamous cell, testicular cancer, and lymphoma; sclerotherapy of malignant pleural effusion
Dose: 0.25–0.5 U/kg/dose IV, IM, or SQ once or twice weekly
Notes: Pulmonary toxicity is increased with total doses of > 400 U

Brimonidine (Alphagan)
Uses: Glaucoma
Dose: 1 gt bid
Notes: Do not apply with soft contact lenses in place

■ Brinzolamide (Azopt)
Uses: Glaucoma
Dose: 1 gt in eye(s) tid

Bromocriptine (Parlodel)
Uses: Parkinsonian syndrome
Dose: Parkinson's: 1.25 mg PO bid initially, titrated to effect
Notes: Nausea and vertigo are common side effects

Buclizine (Bucladin-S Softabs)
Uses: Control of nausea, vomiting, and dizziness of motion sickness
Dose: 50 mg dissolved in mouth bid; 50 mg PO prophylactically 30 min before travel
Notes: Not safe in pregnancy; contains tartrazine, observe patient for allergic reactions

Budesonide (Rhinocort, Pulmicort)
Uses: Allergic and nonallergic rhinitis, asthma
Dose: Intranasal: 2 sprays/nostril bid or 4 sprays/nostril/d. *Aqueous:* 1 spray/nostril/d. *Oral inhaled:* 1–4 inhal bid. **Peds.** 1–2 inhal bid; rinse mouth after oral use Peds.

■ Bumetanide (Bumex)
Uses: Edema from CHF, hepatic cirrhosis, and renal disease
Dose: Adults. 0.5–2.0 mg PO daily; 0.5–1.0 mg IV q8–24h. **Peds.** 0.015–0.1 mg/kg/dose PO, IV, IM q6–24h
Notes: Monitor fluid and electrolyte status during treatment

■ Bupivacaine (Marcaine, Sensorcaine)
Uses: Local infiltration anesthesia, lumbar epidural.
Dose: Dependent on the procedure, vascularity of the tissues, depth of anesthesia, and degree of muscle relaxation required. Max infiltration dose in 70-kg adult is 70 mL of 0.25%

■ Buprenorphine (Buprenex) [C]
Uses: Relief of moderate-to-severe pain
Dose: 0.3 mg IM or slow IV push every 6 h PRN
Notes: May induce withdrawal syndrome in opioid-dependent subjects

■ Bupropion (Wellbutrin, Zyban)
Uses: Treatment of depression, adjunct to smoking cessation
Dose: *Depression:* 100–450 mg/d ÷ bid–tid. *Smoking:* 150 mg daily for 3 d, then 150 mg twice daily
Notes: Has been associated with seizures; avoid use of alcohol and other CNS depressants

■ Buspirone (BuSpar)
Uses: Short-term relief of anxiety
Dose: 5–10 mg PO tid
Notes: No abuse potential. No physical or psychologic dependence

■ Butalbital and Acetaminophen (Fioricet, Medigesic, Phrenilin, Phrenilin Forte, Sedapap-10, others)[C]
Uses: Tension headache, pain
Dose: 1–2 PO q4h PRN, max 6 tabs/d
Notes: Butalbital habit forming; *Medigesic caps:* butalbital 50 mg, caffeine 40 mg, and acetaminophen 325 mg; *Phrenilin Forte caps:* butalbital 50 mg and acetaminophen 650 mg; *Fioricet tabs:* butalbital 50 mg, caffeine 40 mg, and acetaminophen 325 mg; *Phrenilin tabs:* butalbital 50 mg and acetaminophen 325 mg; *Sedapap-10:* butalbital 50 mg and acetaminophen 650 mg.

■ Butalbital and Aspirin (Fiorinal, Lanorinal, Marnal, others) [C]
Uses: Tension headache, pain
Dose: 1–2 PO q4h PRN, max 6 tabs/d.

Notes: Butalbital habit-forming; *Fiorinal, Lanorinal, Marnal caps and tabs:* Butalbital 50 mg, caffeine 40 mg, and aspirin 325 mg

■ Butalbital, Aspirin, and Codeine (Fiorinal with codeine) [C]

Uses: Moderate pain
Dose: 1–2 PO q4h PRN, max 6/d
Notes: Butalbital may be habit-forming; may cause sedation; contains butalbital 50 mg, caffeine 40 mg, aspirin 325 mg, codeine 30 mg

■ Butorphanol (Stadol) [C]

Uses: Analgesic for moderate-to-severe pain; migraine headache
Dose: 1–4 mg IM or 0.5–2 mg IV every 3–4 h PRN; 1 spray in 1 nostril (1 mg) reevaluate in 60–90 min and repeat if needed; repeat 2-dose sequence PRN in 3–4 h
Notes: May induce withdrawal syndrome in opioid-dependent patients

■ Calcitriol (Rocaltrol)

Uses: Reduction of elevated PTH levels, hypocalcemia associated with dialysis
Dose: *Adults.* Renal failure 0.25 µg PO, qd ↑ 0.25 µg/d every 4–6 wk PRN; 0.5 µg 3 × a week IV, ↑ as needed. *Hyperparathyroidism:* 0.5–2.0 µg/d. *Peds.* Renal failure 15 ng/kg/d, ↑ PRN typical maintenance 30–60 ng/kg/d. *Hyperparathyroidism:* < 5 y, 0.25–0.75 µg/d; > 6 y, 0.5–2.0 µg/d
Notes: 1,25-dihydroxycholecalciferol, a vitamin D analogue; monitor dosing to keep calcium levels within normal range

■ Calcitonin (Cibacalcin, Miacalcin)

Uses: Paget's disease of bone; hypercalcemia; osteogenesis imperfecta, postmenopausal osteoporosis
Dose: Paget's salmon form: 100 U/d IM/SQ initially, 50 U/d or 50–100 U q1–3d maint. *Paget's human form:* 0.5 mg/d initially; Maint: 0.5 mg 2–3 times/wk or 0.25 mg/d, max: 0.5 mg bid. *Hypercalcemia salmon calcitonin:* 4 U/kg IM/SQ q12h; ↑ to 8 U/kg q12h, max: q6h. *Osteoporosis salmon calcitonin:* 100 U/d IM/SQ; Intranasal: 200 U = 1 nasal spray/d
Notes: Human (Cibacalcin) and salmon forms; human only approved for Paget's bone disease

■ Calcium Acetate

Uses: ESRD associated hyperphosphatemia
Dose: 2–4 tabs PO with meals
Notes: Can cause hypercalcemia, monitor levels

Calcium Carbonate (Alka-Mints, Caltrate, Tums, Os-Cal, others)

Uses: Hyperacidity associated with peptic ulcer disease, hiatal hernia, etc; calcium supplementation
Dose: From 500 mg–2.0 g PO PRN

Calcium Salts (chloride. gluconate) (See Cover)

Uses: Calcium replacement, ventricular fibrillation, electromechanical dissociation, management of hyperphosphatemia in ESRD. **ECC.** (1)Known/suspected hyperkalemia. (2) Hypocalcemia (eg, multiple transfusions). (3) Antidote for calcium channel blocker overdose.(4) Prophylactically before IV calcium channel blockers (prevent hypotension)
Dose: Adults. Replacement: 1–2 g PO qd. **ECC.** 8–16 mg/kg (usually 5–10 mL) IV slow push for hyperkalemia and calcium channel blocker overdose 2–4 mg/kg (usually 2 mL) IV before IV calcium blockers. **Peds.** Replacement: 200–500 mg/kg/24h PO or IV ÷ qid. **ECC.** Chloride: 20 mg/kg (0.2–0.25 mL/kg) slow push; repeat PRN. Gluconate: 60–100 mg/kg (0.6–1.0 mL/kg) IV slow push. Repeat for documented conditions
Notes: Calcium chloride contains 270 mg (13.6 mEq) elemental calcium per gram, and calcium gluconate contains 90 mg (4.5 mEq) elemental calcium per gram

■ Candesartan (Atacand)

Uses: Treatment of HTN
Dose: 2–32 mg/d, usual dose is 16 mg/d
Note: Monitor BP and titrate to effect; maximum BP response within 2 wk

Capsaicin (Zostrix, others)

Uses: Topical analgesic (postherpetic neuralgia, arthritis, postop pain)
Dose: OTC form, apply tid–qid

Captopril (Capoten)

Uses: Treatment of HTN, CHF, and diabetic nephropathy; **ECC.** To improve outcome after MI
Dose: Adults. HTN: Initially, 25 mg PO bid–tid; titrate to a maint dose every 1–2 wk by 25 mg increments per dose (max 450 mg/d) to desired effect. CHF: Initially, 6.25–12.5 mg PO tid; titrate to desired effect. **ECC.** 6.25 mg PO, ↑ to 25 mg tid and the 50 mg PO tid as tolerated. **Peds.** Infants < 2 mo: 0.05–0.1 mg/kg/dose PO tid–qid. Children: Initially, 0.15 mg/kg/dose PO; double q2h until BP is controlled, to max of 6 mg/kg/d; Maint: 0.5–0.6 mg/kg/d PO ÷ bid–qid
Notes: Caution in renal failure. Give 1 h before meals; can cause rash, proteinuria, and cough

■ Carbamazepine (Tegretol)
Uses: Epilepsy; trigeminal neuralgia
Dose: *Adults.* 200 mg PO bid initially; ↑ by 200 mg/d; usual 800–1200 mg/d.
Peds. 6–12 y: 100 mg/dose PO bid or 10 mg/kg/24h PO ÷ qd–bid initially; ↑ to a maint dose of 20–30 mg/kg/24h ÷ tid–qid
Notes: Can cause severe hematologic side effects; monitor CBC; monitor serum levels, (see Table A–22, page 675); generic products are not interchangeable

■ Carbidopa/Levodopa (Sinemet)
Uses: Parkinson's disease
Dose: Start at 10/100 PO bid–tid; titrate as needed
Notes: May cause psychiatric disturbances, orthostatic hypotension, dyskinesias, and cardiac arrhythmias

■ Carboplatin (Paraplatin)
Uses: Treatment of cervical, ovarian, and lung cancer
Dose: Varies with treatment protocol; 300–360 mg/m^2 on day 1 every 4 wk
Notes: May cause bone marrow suppression, vomiting, and anaphylaxis; follow platelet and neutrophil counts

■ Carisoprodol (Soma)
Uses: Adjunct to sleep and physical therapy for the relief of painful musculoskeletal conditions
Dose: 350 mg PO qid
Notes: Avoid alcohol and other CNS depressants; also available with 16-mg codeine/tab [C].

■ Carteolol (Cartrol, Ocupress Ophthalmic)
Uses: Treatment of HTN; opthalmic soln for increased intraocular pressure
Dose: 2.5–5 mg PO qd; ophthalmic 1 gt eye/eyes bid

■ Carvedilol (Coreg)
Uses: Treatment of HTN and CHF
Dose: *HTN:* 6.25–12.5 mg bid. *CHF:* 3.125–25 mg bid
Notes: Take with food to slow absorption and reduce incidence of orthostatic hypotension

■ Cefaclor (Ceclor)
Uses: Treatment of infections caused by susceptible bacteria involving the upper and lower respiratory tract, skin, bone, urinary tract, abdomen, and gynecologic system (*S aureus, S pneumoniae, H influenzae*).

Dose: Adults. 250–500 mg PO tid. *Peds.* 20–40 mg/kg/d PO ÷ tid
Notes: Second-generation cephalosporin; more gram-negative activity than first-generation cephalosporins

◼ Cefadroxil (Duricef, Ultracef)

Uses: Treatment of infections caused by susceptible strains of *Streptococcus, Staphylococcus, E coli, Proteus* and *Klebsiella* involving the skin, bone, upper and lower respiratory tract, and urinary tract
Dose: Adults. 500–1000 mg PO bid–qd. *Peds.* 30 mg/kg/d ÷ bid
Notes: First-generation cephalosporin.

◼ Cefazolin (Ancef, Kefzol)

Uses: Treatment of infections caused by susceptible strains of *Streptococcus, Staphylococcus, E coli, Proteus* and *Klebsiella* involving the skin, bone, upper and lower respiratory tract, and urinary tract
Dose: Adults. 1–2 g IV q8h. *Peds.* 50–100 mg/kg/d IV ÷ q8h
Notes: Widely used for surgical prophylaxis; first-generation cephalosporin

◼ Cefdinir (Omnicef)

Uses: Treatment of infections caused by susceptible bacteria involving the respiratory tract, skin, bone, urinary tract, meningitis, and septicemia
Dose: Adults. 300 mg PO bid or 600 mg PO qd. *Peds.* 7 mg/kg PO bid or 14 mg/kg PO qd
Notes: Third-generation cephalosporin

◼ Cefepime (Maxipime)

Uses: Treatment of UTIs and pneumonia caused by susceptible *S pneumoniae, S aureus, K pneumoniae, E coli, P aeruginosa,* and *Enterobacter* spp
Dose: 1–2 g IV q12h for 5–10 d; UTI 500 mg IV q12h
Notes: Fourth-generation cephalosporin; improved gram-positive coverage over third generation

◼ Cefixime (Suprax)

Uses: Treatment of infections caused by susceptible bacteria involving the respiratory tract, skin, bone, urinary tract, meningitis, and septicemia; single dose to treat gonorrhea
Dose: Adults. 200–400 mg PO bid–qd. *Peds.* 8 mg/kg/d PO ÷ bid–qd, 400 mg/max/d
Notes: Third-generation cephalosporin; use suspension to treat otitis media

◼ Cefmetazole (Zefazone)

Uses: Treatment of infections caused by susceptible bacteria involving the upper and lower respiratory tract, skin, bone, urinary tract, abdomen, and gynecologic system

Dose: Adults. treatment of infection, 1–2 g IV 8h; surgical prophylaxis, 2 g IV 30–90 min preop

Notes: Second-generation cephalosporin with more gram-negative activity than first-generation cephalosporins; has anaerobic activity

■ Cefonicid (Monocid)

Uses: Treatment of infections caused by susceptible bacteria: respiratory, skin, bone and joint, urinary, gynecologic, and septicemia

Dose: 1 g IM/IV q24h

Notes: Second-generation cephalosporin

■ Cefoperazone (Cefobid)

Uses: Treatment of infections caused by susceptible bacteria: respiratory, skin, urinary tract, sepsis; as a third generation cephalosporin, cefoperazone has activity against gram-negative bacilli (eg, *E coli, Klebsiella,* and *Haemophilus*) but variable activity against *Streptococcus* and *Staphylococcus* species; it has activity against *P aeruginosa,* but less than ceftazidime

Dose: Adults. 2–4 g/d, ÷ q12h IM/IV; 12 g/d max. *Peds.* 100–150 mg/kg/d ÷ q8–12h IM/IV

Notes: Third-generation cephalosporin; active against gram-negatives but variable activity against *Staphylococcus* and *Streptococcus;* some activity against *Pseudomonas*

■ Cefotaxime (Claforan)

Uses: Treatment of infections caused by susceptible bacteria involving the respiratory tract, skin, bone, urinary tract, meningitis, and septicemia

Dose: Adults. 1–2 g IV q4–12h. *Peds.* 100–200 mg/kg/d IV ÷ q6–8h

Notes: Third-generation cephalosporin

■ Cefotetan (Cefotan)

Uses: Treatment of infections caused by susceptible bacteria involving the upper and lower respiratory tract, skin, bone, urinary tract, abdomen, and gynecologic system

Dose: Adults. 1–2 g IV q12h. *Peds.* 40–80 mg/kg/d IV ÷ q12h

Notes: Second-generation cephalosporin; more gram-negative activity then first-generation cephalosporins; has anaerobic activity

■ Cefoxitin (Mefoxin)

Uses: Treatment of infections caused by susceptible bacteria involving the upper and lower respiratory tract, skin, bone, urinary tract, abdomen, and gynecologic system

Dose: Adults. 1–2 mg IV q6h. *Peds.* 80–160 mg/kg/d ÷ q4–6h

Notes: Second-generation cephalosporin; more gram-negative activity then first-generation cephalosporins; has anaerobic activity

■ Cefpodoxime (Vantin)
Uses: Treatment of infections caused by susceptible bacteria involving the respiratory tract (community-acquired pneumonia due to *S pneumonia* or non-β-lactamase *H influenzae,* otitis media, pharyngitis, tonsillitis, skin, bone, urinary tract, gonorrhea, meningitis, and septicemia)
Dose: Adults. 200–400 mg PO q12h. *Peds.* > 6 mo, 10 mg/kg/d PO ÷ bid
Notes: Second-generation cephalosporin; drug interactions with agents increasing gastric pH

■ Cefprozil (Cefzil)
Uses: Treatment of infections caused by susceptible bacteria involving the upper and lower respiratory tract, skin, bone, urinary tract, abdomen, and gynecologic system
Dose: Adults. 250–500 mg PO qd–bid. *Peds.* >6 mo, 7.5–15 mg/kg/d PO ÷ bid
Notes: Second-generation cephalosporin; more gram-negative activity then first-generation cephalosporins; use higher doses for otitis and pneumonia

■ Ceftazidime (Fortaz, Ceptaz, Tazidime, Tazicef)
Uses: Treatment of infections caused by susceptible bacteria involving the respiratory tract, skin, bone, urinary tract, meningitis, and septicemia
Dose: Adults. 1–2 g IV q8h. *Peds.* 30–50 mg/kg/d IV ÷ q8h
Notes: Third-generation cephalosporin; useful in patients with pseudomonal infections at risk for nephrotoxicity; empiric therapy in febrile granulocytopenic patients

■ Ceftibuten (Cedax)
Uses: Treatment of infections caused by susceptible bacteria involving the respiratory tract (bronchitis), skin, bone, urinary tract, meningitis, and septicemia
Dose: Adults. 400 mg/d PO. *Peds.* 9 mg/kg/d PO (400 mg max).
Notes: Third-generation cephalosporin; take before eating; little activity against *Streptococcus.*

■ Ceftizoxime (Cefizox)
Uses: Treatment of infections caused by susceptible bacteria involving the respiratory tract, skin, bone, urinary tract, meningitis, and septicemia
Dose: Adults. 1–2 g IV q12–8h. *Peds.* 150–200 mg/kg/d IV ÷ q6–8h
Notes: Third-generation cephalosporin

■ Ceftriaxone (Rocephin)
Uses: Treatment of infections caused by susceptible bacteria involving the respiratory tract, skin, bone, urinary tract, meningitis, chancroid, uncomplicated gonorrhea, and septicemia

Dose: Adults. 1–2 g IV q12–24h; GC and chancroid <45kg, 125 mg IM; > 45 kg, 250-mg IM single dose. *Peds.* 50–100 mg/kg/d IV ÷ q12–24h
Notes: Third-generation cephalosporin

■ Cefuroxime (Ceftin [oral], Zinacef [parenteral])
Uses: Treatment of infections caused by susceptible bacteria involving the upper and lower respiratory tract, skin, bone, urinary tract, abdomen, and gynecologic system
Dose: Adults. 750 mg–1.5 g IV q8h or 250–500 mg PO bid. *Peds.* 100–150 mg/kg/d IV ÷ q8h or 20–30 mg/kg/d PO ÷ bid
Notes: Second-generation cephalosporin; more gram-negative activity then first-generation cephalosporins; IV crosses the blood–brain barrier

■ Celecoxib (Celebrex)
Uses: Osteoarthritis and RA.
Dose: 100–200 mg qd or bid

■ Cephalexin (Keflex, Keftab)
Uses: Treatment of infections caused by susceptible strains of *Streptococcus, Staphylococcus, E coli, Proteus* and *Klebsiella* involving the skin, bone, upper and lower respiratory tract, and urinary tract
Dose: Adults. 250–500 mg PO qid. *Peds.* 25–100 mg/kg/d PO ÷ qid
Notes: First-generation cephalosporin

■ Cephapirin (Cefadyl)
Uses: Treatment of infections caused by susceptible strains of respiratory tract, skin, urinary tract, bone and joint, endocarditis, and sepsis (but not enterococcus); some gram-negatives
Dose: Adults. 1 g IM/IV q6h (12 g/d max). *Peds.* 10–20 mg/kg IM/IV q6h (4 g/24 d max)
Notes: First-generation cephalosporin

■ Cephradine (Velosef)
Uses: Treatment of susceptible bacterial infections, including group A β-hemolytic *Streptococcus*
Dose: Adults. 2–4 g/d in 4 ÷ doses (8 g/d max). *Peds.* > 9 mo: 25–100 mg/kg/d ÷ q6–12h (4 g/d max).
Notes: First-generation cephalosporin

■ Cetirizine (Zyrtec)
Uses: Allergic rhinitis and chronic urticaria
Dose: *Adults* and Children > 6 y: 5–10 mg/d

■ Charcoal, Activated (SuperChar, Actidose, Liqui-Char)
Uses: Emergency treatment for poisoning by most drugs and chemicals
Dose: *Adults. Acute intoxication:* 30–100 g/dose. *GI dialysis:* 25–50 g q4–6h.
Peds. Acute intoxication: 1–2 g/kg/dose. *GI dialysis:* 5–10 g/dose q4–8h
Notes: Administer with a cathartic; liquid dose forms are in sorbitol base; powder mixed with water; protect airway in lethargic or comatose patient

■ Chloral Hydrate (Noctec) [C]
Uses: Nocturnal and preoperative sedation
Dose: *Adults. Hypnotic:* Between 500 mg and 1 g PO or PR 30 min before sleep or procedure. *Sedative:* 250 mg PO or PR tid. *Peds. Hypnotic:* 50 mg/kg/24h PO or PR 30 min before sleep or procedure. *Sedative:* 25 mg/kg/24h PO or PR tid
Notes: Mix syrup in a glass of water or fruit juice

■ Chlorambucil (Leukeran)
Uses: Treatment of ovarian cancer, leukemia, and lymphoma
Dose: Initially, 0.1–0.2 mg/kg/d PO for 3–6 wk; then maint therapy with no more than 0.1 mg/kg/d

■ Chlordiazepoxide (Librium) [C]
Uses: Anxiety, tension, alcohol withdrawal
Dose: *Adults. Mild anxiety, tension:* 5–10 mg PO tid–qid or PRN. *Severe anxiety, tension:* 25–50 mg IM or IV tid–qid or PRN. *Alcohol withdrawal:* 50–100 mg IM or IV; repeat in 2–4 h if needed, up to 300 mg in 24 h; gradually taper daily. *Peds.* 0.5 mg/kg/24h PO or IM ÷ q6–8h
Notes: Reduce dose in elderly patients; absorption of IM doses can be erratic

■ Chlorothiazide (Diuril)
Uses: HTN, edema, CHF.
Dose: *Adults.* Between 500 mg and 1.0 g PO or IV qd–bid. *Peds.* 20–30 mg/kg/24h PO ÷ bid
Notes: Contra in anuria

■ Chlorpheniramine (Chlor-Trimeton, Others)
Uses: Seasonal rhinitis, allergic reactions
Dose: Adults. 4 mg PO or IV q4–6h or 8–12 mg PO bid of sustained release. *Peds.* 0.35 mg/kg/24h PO ÷ q4–6h or 0.2 mg/kg/24h SR
Notes: Anticholinergic side effects and sedation are common. Available in many OTC combinations (eg, acetaminophen, phenylephrine, pseudoephedrine)

■ Chlorpromazine (Thorazine)
Uses: Psychotic disorders, apprehension, intractable hiccups, control of nausea and vomiting
Dose: Adults. Acute anxiety, agitation: 10–25 mg PO or PR bid–tid. *Severe symptoms:* 25 mg IM, can repeat in 1 h, then 25–50 mg PO or PR tid. *Hiccups:* 25–50 mg PO bid–tid. *Peds.* 2.5–6.0 mg/kg/24h PO, PR or IM ÷ q4–8h
Notes: Beware of extrapyramidal side effects, sedation, has alpha-adrenergic blocking properties

■ Chlorpropamide (Diabinese)
Uses: Management of non-insulin-dependent DM
Dose: 100–500 mg qd
Notes: Use with caution in renal insufficiency

■ Chlorthalidone (Hygroton)
Uses: HTN, edema associated with CHF, steroid and estrogen therapy
Dose: Adults. 50–100 mg PO qd. *Peds.* 2 mg/kg/dose PO 3 × weekly or 1–2 mg/kg/d PO
Notes: Contra in anuric patients

■ Chlorzoxazone (Paraflex, Parafon Forte DSC)
Uses: Adjunct to rest and physical therapy for the relief of discomfort associated with acute, painful musculoskeletal conditions
Dose: Adults. 250–500 mg PO tid–qid. *Peds.* 20 mg/kg/d or 600 mg/m²/d ÷ in 3–4 doses

■ Cholecalciferol [Vitamin D3] (Delta D)
Uses: Dietary supplement for treatment of vitamin D deficiency
Dose: 400–1000 IU/d PO
Notes: 1 mg cholecalciferol = 40,000 IU of vitamin D activity

■ Cholera Vaccine
Uses: Cholera prophylaxis
Dose: Adults & Peds >10 y: 0.5 mL, 2 doses 1 wk to 1 mo or more apart.
Peds. 6 mo– 4 y: 0.2 mL ; 5–10 y: 0.3 mL schedule as adult
Notes: Inactivated Vibrio cholerae Inaba and Ogawa types

■ Cholestyramine (Questran)
Uses: Adjunctive therapy for the reduction of serum cholesterol in patients with primary hypercholesterolemia; relief of pruritus associated with partial biliary obstruction
Dose: Individualize dose to 4 g 1–6 × a day.
Notes: Mix 4 g cholestyramine in 2–6 oz of noncarbonated beverages

■ Ciclopirox (Loprox)
Uses: Topical fungal infections (tinea cruris, capitis, versicolor, and Candida)
Dose: Apply and massage into area bid.

■ Cilostazol (Pletal)
Uses: Peripheral vascular disease, with intermittent claudication
Dose: 100 mg PO bid (30 min before/2 h after meals; ↓ to 50 mg with inhibitors of CYP3A4 or CYP2C19

■ Cimetidine (Tagamet)
Uses: Duodenal ulcer; ulcer prophylaxis in hypersecretory states, such as trauma, burns, surgery, Zollinger–Ellison syndrome; and gastroesophageal reflux disease (GERD)
Dose: Adults. Active ulcer: 2400 mg/d IV cont inf or 300 mg IV q6–4h; 400 mg PO bid or 800 mg qhs. Maint therapy: 400 mg PO qhs. GERD: 800 mg PO bid; Maint 800 mg PO hs. **Peds.** Neonates: 10–20 mg/kg/24h PO or IV ÷ q4–6h. Children: 20–40 mg/kg/24h PO or IV ÷ q4–6h
Notes: Extend dosing interval with renal insufficiency; decrease dose in elderly patients

■ Ciprofloxacin (Cipro, Ciloxan Ophthalmic)
Uses: Broad-spectrum activity against a variety of gram-positive and gram-negative aerobic bacteria (UTI, prostatitis, sinusitis, skin, infectious diarrhea, osteomyelitis, ocular infections)
Dose: Adults. 250–750 mg PO q12h or 200–400 mg IV q12h. Ophthalmic **Dose:** 1–2 gtt in eye(s) q2h while awake for 2 d, then 1–2 gtt q4h while awake for 5d. **Peds.** Not recommended for use in children < 18 y, because of cartilage effects

Notes: Little activity against streptococci; drug interactions with theophylline, caffeine, sucralfate, and antacids. Nausea, vomiting, and abdominal discomfort are common side effects. Contra in pregnancy.

■ Ciprofloxacin and hydrocortisone (Cipro HC Otic)
Uses: Otitis externa (swimmers ear)
Dose: 3 gtt in ear bid–tid for 1 wk

■ Cisplatin (Platinol)
Uses: Treatment of cervical, ovarian, testicular, and other solid tumors
Dose: 20–70 mg/m^2 IV. Dose and duration of therapy is dependent on individual treatment protocols
Notes: Agent is nephrotoxic; hydrate patients with 1–2 L of fluid before infusion

■ Cisatracurium (Nimbex)
Uses: Muscle relaxant used in general anesthesia, endotracheal intubation
Dose: Adults. 0.15–0.2 mg/kg, IV then 0.03 mg/kg 40–60 min later to maintain block, followed by repeat doses of 0.03 mg/kg at 20-min intervals; *Inf:* After recovery from bolus, 3 µg/kg/min ICU: *Adults.* 0.1 mg/kg bolus; then 3 µg/kg/min IV, titrate; *Peds* 2–12 y: 0.1 mg/kg (block lasts about 28 min)

■ Citalopram (Celexa)
Uses: Treatment of depression
Dose: Initially, 20 mg per day, may be ↑ to 40 mg/d

■ Clarithromycin (Biaxin)
Uses: Treatment of upper and lower respiratory tract infections, skin, *H pylori* infections, and infections caused by nontuberculosis (atypical) *Mycobacterium;* prevention of Mac infections in HIV-infected individuals
Dose: Adults. 250–500 mg PO bid. *Mycobacterium:* 500–1000 mg PO bid. *Peds.* 7.5 mg/kg/dose PO bid
Notes: Increases theophylline and carbamazepine levels; avoid concurrent use with cisapride; causes metallic taste

■ Clemastine (Tavist [OTC])
Uses: Allergic rhinitis
Dose: 1.34– 2.68 mg (1–2 tabs) tid, max 8.04 mg/d

■ Clindamycin (Cleocin)

Uses: Susceptible strains of streptococci, pneumococci, staphylococci, and gram-positive and gram-negative anaerobes, no activity against gram-negative aerobes. Topical agent for severe acne, and vaginal infections

Dose: Adults. 150–450 mg PO qid; 300–600 mg IV q6h or 900 mg IV q8h. *Topical:* apply bid. *Vaginal:* 1 full applicator instilled hs for 1 wk. *Peds. Neonates:* 15–20 mg/kg/24h ÷ q6–8h. *Children > 1 mo:* 15–40 mg/kg/24h ÷ q6–8h,(4 g/d)

Notes: Beware of diarrhea that may represent pseudomembranous colitis caused by *C difficile*

■ Clonazepam (Klonopin) [C]

Uses: Lennox–Gastaut syndrome, akinetic and myoclonic seizures, absence seizures

Dose: Adults. 1.5 mg/d PO in 3 ÷ doses; increase by 0.5–1.0 mg/d every 3 d PRN ↑ to 20 mg/d. *Peds.* 0.01–0.05 mg/kg/24h PO ÷ tid; ↑ to 0.1–0.2 mg/kg/24h ÷ tid

Notes: CNS side effects including sedation

■ Clonidine (Catapres)

Uses: HTN, opioid and tobacco withdrawal

Dose: Adults. 0.10 mg PO bid adjusted daily by 0.1–0.2 mg increments (max 2.4 mg/d). *Peds.* 5–25 mg/kg/24h ÷ q6h

Notes: Dry mouth, drowsiness, sedation occur frequently; more effective for HTN when combined with diuretics, rebound HTN can occur with abrupt cessation of doses above 0.2 mg bid

■ Clonidine Transdermal (Catapres TTS)

Uses: HTN

Dose: Apply one patch every 7 d to a hairless area on the upper arm or torso; titrate according to individual therapeutic requirements.

Notes: TTS-1, TTS-2, TTS-3 (delivers 0.1, 0.2, 0.3 mg respectively of clonidine per day, for 1 wk). Doses above two TTS-3 are usually not associated with increased efficacy.

■ Clopidogrel (Plavix)

Uses: Reduction of atherosclerotic events

Dose: 75 mg/d

Notes: Prolongs bleeding time, use with caution in persons at risk of bleeding from trauma, etc

■ Clorazepate (Tranxene) [C]

Uses: Acute anxiety disorders, acute alcohol withdrawal symptoms, and adjunctive therapy in partial seizures.

Dose: Adults. 15–60 mg/d PO in single or ÷ doses. *Elderly and debilitated patients:* Initiate therapy at 7.5–15 mg/d in ÷ doses. *Alcohol withdrawal:* Day 1: Initially, 30 mg; followed by 30-60 mg in ÷ doses. Day 2: 45–90 mg in ÷ doses. Day 3: 22.5–45 mg in ÷ doses. Day 4: 15–30 mg in ÷ doses. **Peds.** 3.75–7.5 mg/dose bid, to a max of 60 mg/d ÷ bid–tid

Notes: Monitor patients with renal and hepatic impairment because drug may accumulate; CNS depressant effects

■ Clotrimazole (Lotrimin, Mycelex)
Uses: Treatment of candidiasis and tinea infections
Dose: *Orally:* One troche dissolved slowly in mouth 5 × a day for 14 d. *Vaginal:* Cream: One applicator qhs for 7–14 d; Tabs: 100 mg vaginally qhs for 7 d or 200 mg (2 tabs) vaginally qhs for 3 d or 500-mg tab vaginally hs for 3 d. *Topical:* Apply 3–4 times daily for 10–14 d
Notes: Oral prophylaxis commonly used in immunosuppressed patients

■ Cloxacillin (Cloxapen)
Uses: Treatment of respiratory, skin, bone, joint infections caused by susceptible strains of penicillinase-producing *Staphylococcus*
Dose: Adults. 250–500 mg PO qid. **Peds.** 50–100 mg/kg/d ÷ qid
Notes: Take on an empty stomach

■ Clozapine (Clozaril)
Uses: Severe schizophrenia that does not respond to standard therapy
Dose: Initially 25 mg qd–bid, increase dose to 300–450 mg/d over 2 wk. Maintain patient at lowest dose possible
Notes: Has limited distribution. Contact local pharmacy for drug availability. Monitor blood counts frequently because of the risk of agranulocytosis. May cause drowsiness and seizures.

■ Cocaine [C]
Uses: Topical anesthetic for mucous membranes
Dose: Apply topically lowest amount of topical soln that provides relief; 1 mg/kg max

■ Codeine [C]
Uses: Mild-to-moderate pain; symptomatic relief of cough
Dose: Adults. *Analgesic:* 15–60 mg PO, SQ/IM qid PRN. *Antitussive:* 5–15 mg PO or SQ q4h PRN. **Peds.** *Analgesic:* 0.5–1.0 mg/kg/dose PO or SQ q4–6h PRN. *Antitussive:* 1.0–1.5 mg/kg/24h ÷ q4h, max 30 mg/24h.
Notes: Most often used in combination with acetaminophen for pain or with agents such as terpin hydrate as an antitussive; 120 mg IM equivalent to 10 mg morphine IM

Colesevelam (Welchol)
Uses: Reduction of LDL cholesterol
Dose: 3 tabs PO bid with meals

Colchicine
Uses: Acute gout
Dose: Initially, 0.5–1.2 mg PO or IV, then 0.5–1.2 mg every 1–2 h until GI side effects develop (max of 8 mg/d)
Notes: Caution in elderly patients and patients with renal impairment. Colchicine 1–2 mg IV within 24–48 h of an acute attack can be diagnostic and therapeutic in a monoarticular arthritis

Colestipol (Colestid)
Uses: Adjunctive therapy for the reduction of serum cholesterol in patients with primary hypercholesterolemia
Dose: 15–30 g/d ÷ into 2–4 doses.
Notes: Do not use dry powder; mix with beverages, soups, cereals, etc

Cortisone
See Tables A–8 and A–33, pages 659 and 684.

Cromolyn Sodium (Intal, Nasalcrom, Opticrom)
Uses: Adjunct to the prophylaxis of asthma; prevention of exercise-induced asthma; allergic rhinitis; ophthalmic allergic manifestations
Dose: Adults & Peds. > 12 years. *Inhal:* 20 mg (as powder in cap) inhaled qid or metered-dose inhaler 2 puffs qid. *Oral:* 200 mg qid 15–20 min before meals, up to 400 mg qid. *Nasal instillation:* Spray once in each nostril 2–6 times daily. *Ophthalmic:* 1–2 gtt in each eye 4–6 × daily. *Peds.* Inhal: 2 puffs qid of metered-dose inhaler. *Oral:* Infants < 2 y: 20 mg/kg/d in 4 ÷ doses. 2–12 y: 100 mg qid before meals
Notes: Has no benefit in acute situations; may require 2–4 wk for maximal effect in perennial allergic disorders

Cyanocobalamin/Vitamin B$_{12}$
Uses: Pernicious anemia and other vitamin B$_{12}$ deficiency states
Dose: Adults. 100 mg, IM or SQ qd for 5–10 d, then 100 mg IM twice a week for 1 mo, then 100 mg IM monthly. *Peds.* 100 mg qd IM or SQ for 5–10 d, then 30–50 mg IM every 4 wk
Notes: Oral absorption highly erratic, altered by many drugs and not recommended; for use with hyperalimentation.

Cyclobenzaprine (Flexeril)
Uses: Muscle spasm associated with acute painful musculoskeletal conditions

Dose: 10 mg PO tid
Notes: Do not use for longer than 2–3 wk; has sedative and anticholinergic properties

■ Cyclopentolate (Cyclogyl)
Uses: Mydriasis and cycloplegia; useful before ocular exam; treatment of iritis
Dose: One gt 1% in eye(s), followed by a second application 5 min later; use 30–45 min before exam; iritis, apply tid

■ Cyclophosphamide (Cytoxan, Neosar)
Uses: Hodgkin's and non-Hodgkin's lymphomas, multiple myeloma, breast cancer, ovarian cancer, mycosis fungoides, neuroblastoma, retinoblastoma, acute leukemias, small-cell lung cancer, and allogeneic and autologous transplantation in high doses; severe rheumatologic disorders
Dose: 500–1500 mg/m^2 as a single dose at 2–4-wk intervals; 1.8 g/m^2 to 160 mg/kg (or approximately 12 g/m^2 in a 75-kg individual) in the bone marrow transplantation setting
Notes: Toxicity includes myelosuppression (leukopenia and thrombocytopenia), sterile hemorrhagic cystitis, SIADH, alopecia, and anorexia; nausea and vomiting are common. Hepatotoxicity and rarely interstitial pneumonitis may occur. Irreversible testicular atrophy may occur. Cardiotoxicity is rare. Second malignancies (bladder cancer and acute leukemias) have been reported; cumulative risk of 3.5% at 8 y, 10.7% at 12 y. Preventive measures to avoid hemorrhagic cystitis: continuous bladder irrigation and MESNA uroprotection.

■ Cyclosporine (Sandimmune, Neoral)
Uses: Prophylaxis of organ rejection in kidney, liver, heart, and bone marrow transplants in conjunction with adrenal corticosteroids; other autoimmune diseases
Dose: Adults & Peds. Oral: 15 mg/kg/d beginning 12 h prior to transplant; after 2 wk, taper the dose by 5 mg/wk to 5–10 mg/kg/d. IV: 5–6 mg/kg/d ÷ q12–24h. If the patient is unable to take the drug orally, give 1/2 of the oral dose IV, switch to PO as soon as possible
Notes: May elevate BUN and Cr, which may be confused with renal transplant rejection; should be administered in glass containers; has many drug interactions; **Neoral and Sandimmune are not interchangeable.**

■ Cyproheptadine (Periactin)
Uses: Allergic reactions; especially good for itching
Dose: Adults. 4 mg PO tid, max of 0.5 mg/kg/d. **Peds.** 2–6 y: 0.25/kg/24h ÷ tid–qid (max 12 mg/24h). 7–14 y: 0.25 mg/kg/24h ÷ tid–qid (max of 16 mg/24h)
Notes: Anticholinergic side effects and drowsiness common; may stimulate appetite in some patients

■ Cytomegalovirus Immune Globulin [CMV-IVIG] (Cytogam)

Uses: Attenuation of primary CMV disease associated with transplantation
Dose: Administered for 16 wk posttransplant, see product information for dosing schedule

■ Dacarbazine (DTIC-Dome)

Uses: Treatment of soft tissue and uterine sarcoma, melanoma, and Hodgkin's disease
Dose: Dependent on individual protocol
Notes: May cause myelosuppression

■ Daclizumab (Zenapax)

Uses: Prevention of acute organ rejection
Dose: *Adults & Peds.* 1 mg/kg IV per dose; first dose prior to transplant followed by 4 doses 14 d apart posttransplant

■ Dactinomycin (Cosmegen)

Uses: Treatment of Wilms' tumor, rhabdomyosarcoma, choriocarcinoma, testicular carcinoma, Ewing's sarcoma, and sarcoma botryoides
Dose: *Adults.* 0.5 mg/d IV for 5 d. *Peds.* 0.015 mg/kg/d IV for 5 d
Notes: Severe soft tissue damage may occur with extravasation

■ Dalteparin (Fragmin)

Uses: Prevent ischemic complications because of clot formation in patients on concurrent aspirin, prevention of DVT after surgery; *ECC.* ACS with non-Q wave or unstable angina
Dose: *DVT prophylaxis:* 2500–5000 IU SQ 1–2 h before surgery, then QD for 5–10 d. *Systemic anticoagulation:* 200 IU/kg/d SQ or 100 IU/kg SQ bid. *ECC.* 1 mg/kg bid SQ for 2–8 days with aspirin
Notes: Predictable antithrombotic effects eliminates need for laboratory monitoring

■ Dantrolene Sodium (Dantrium)

Uses: Treatment of spasticity due to upper motor neuron disorders (spinal cord injuries, strokes, cerebral palsy, or MS); treatment of malignant hyperthermia crisis
Dose: *Adults. Spasticity:* Initially, 25 mg PO qd, titrate to effect by 25 mg ↑ to max dose of 100 mg PO qid PRN. *Peds.* Initially, 0.5 mg/kg/dose bid, titrate by 0.5 mg/kg to effectiveness ↑ to max dose of 3 mg/kg/dose qid PRN. *Malignant hyperthermia: Adults & Peds.* Continuous rapid IV push beginning

at 1 mg/kg until symptoms subside or 10 mg/kg is reached. Postcrisis follow-up: 4–8 mg/kg/d in 3–4 ÷ doses for 1–3 d to prevent recurrence
Notes: Monitor ALT and AST closely

Daunorubicin (Cerubidine)
Uses: Leukemia
Dose: Varies with individual protocol
Notes: Severe tissue necrosis if extravasation occurs

Deferoxamine (Desferal)
Uses: Antidote for acute iron intoxication
Dose: Acute iron intoxication: 15 mg/kg/h IV 6 g/d max
Notes: IV preferred for symptomatic toxicity (coma, shock, acidosis, or severe GI bleeding) or serum iron level » 500 µg/dL. IM route can be used if symptoms absent

Delavirdine (Rescriptor)
Uses: HIV-1 infection in combination therapy
Dose: Adults. 400 mg PO tid

Demeclocycline (Declomycin)
Uses: Treatment of SIADH
Dose: 300–600 mg PO q12h
Notes: May cause DI

Desipramine (Norpramin)
Uses: Endogenous depression
Dose: 25–200 mg/d in single or ÷ doses; usually as a single dose hs
Notes: Many anticholinergic side effects, including blurred vision, urinary retention, and dry mouth

Desloratadine (Clarinex)
Uses: Symptoms of seasonal and perennial allergic rhinitis; chronic idio-pathic urticaria
Dose: Adults & Peds >12 y: 5 mg/d PO; in cases of hepatic/renal impair-ment, 5 mg PO qod

Desmopressin (DDAVP, Stimate)
Uses: DI; bleeding due to hemophilia A and type I von Willebrand's disease (parenteral); nocturnal enuresis

*Dose: DI: **Adults.*** intranasal, 0.1–0.4 mL (10–40 µg) daily in 2–3 ÷ doses. 0.5–1 mL (2–4 µg)/d IV/SQ in 2 ÷ doses. If converting from intranasal to parenteral dosing, use 1/10 of intranasal dose. ***Peds.*** *3 mo–12 y:* intranasal 0.05–0.3 mL daily in single or 2 doses. *Hemophilia A and von Willebrand's disease (type I):* ***Adults & Peds.*** > 10 kg: 0.3 mg/kg diluted to 50 mL with NSS infuse over 15–30 min. ***Peds.*** < 10 kg: Same as above with dilution to 10 mL with NS. *Nocturnal enuresis:* ***Peds.*** > 6 y: 20 µg (0.2 mL) qhs, adjust PRN 10–40 µg

Notes: In very young and old patients, adjust fluid intake to avoid water intoxication and hyponatremia

■ Dexamethasone, Systemic (Decadron, Dexasone, Others)
See Steroids, page 635.

■ Dexpanthenol (Ilopan-Choline, Ilopan)
Uses: Minimize paralytic ileus, treat postoperative distention
Dose: Adults. *Relief of gas:* 2–3 tabs PO tid. *Prevention of postoperative ileus:* 250–500 mg IM stat, repeat in 2 h, then q6h as needed. *Ileus:* IM: 500 mg stat, repeat in 2 h, followed by doses every 6 h, if needed
Notes: Do not use if obstruction is suspected

■ Dextran 40 (Macrodex, Rheomacrodex)
Uses: Plasma expander for adjunctive therapy in shock; prophylaxis of DVT and thromboembolism; adjunct in peripheral vascular surgery
Dose: Shock: 10 mL/kg infused rapidly with max dose of 20 mL/kg in the first 24 h; total daily dose beyond 24 h should not exceed 10 mL/kg and should be discontinued after 5 d. *Prophylaxis of DVT and thromboembolism:* 10 mL/kg IV on day of surgery followed by 500 mL IV daily for 2–3 d; then 500 mL IV every 2–3 d based on patient's risk factors for up to 2 wk
Notes: Observe for hypersensitivity reactions; monitor renal function and electrolytes

◤ Dextromethorphan (Vicks Formula 44,many others)
Uses: To control nonproductive cough
Dose: Adults. 10–20 mg PO q4h PRN. ***Peds.*** 1–2 mg/kg/24h ÷ tid–qid
Notes: May be found in many OTC combination products with guaifenesin, acetaminophen and pseudoephedrine

■ Dezocine (Dalgan)
Uses: Management of pain
Dose: 5–20 mg IM or 2.5–10 mg IV q2–4h PRN.

Notes: Narcotic agonist/antagonist; may cause withdrawal in patients dependent on narcotics

■ Diazepam (Valium) [C]
Uses: Anxiety, alcohol withdrawal, muscle spasm, status epilepticus, and preoperative sedation
Dose: Adults. Status epilepticus: 0.2–0.5 mg/kg/dose IV q15–30 min to 30 mg max. *Anxiety, muscle spasm:* 2–10 mg PO or IM q3–4h PRN. *Preoperative:* 5–10 mg PO or IM 20–30 min before procedure; can be given IV just before procedure. *Alcohol withdrawal:* Initially, 2–5 mg IV, may require up to 1000–2000 mg in 24-h period for severe withdrawal symptoms. *Peds. Status epilepticus:* < 5 y: 0.2–0.5 mg/kg/dose IV q15–30 min up to max of 5 mg; > 5 y: May administer up to max of 10 mg. *Sedation, muscle relaxation:* 0.04–0.2 mg/kg/dose q2–4h IM or IV up to max of 0.6 mg/kg in 8 h, or 0.12–0.8 mg/kg/24h PO ÷ tid–qid
Notes: Do not exceed 5 mg/min IV as respiratory arrest can occur; absorption of IM dose may be erratic

■ Diazoxide (Hyperstat, Proglycem)
Uses: Hypertensive emergencies; management of hypoglycemia owing to hyperinsulinism
Dose: Adults & Peds. Hypertensive crisis: 1–3 mg/kg/dose IV up to max of 150 mg IV; may repeat at 15-min intervals until desired effect is achieved. *Hypoglycemia:* 3–8 mg/kg/24h PO ÷ q8–12h. *Neonates. Hypoglycemia:* 10 mg/kg/24h ÷ in 3 equal doses; Maint: 3–8 mg/kg/24h PO in 2 or 3 equal doses
Notes: Sodium retention and hyperglycemia frequently occur; possible thiazide diuretic cross-hypersensitivity; cannot be titrated

■ Dibucaine (Nupercainal, [OTC])
Uses: Hemorrhoids and minor skin conditions
Dose: Insert into rectum with applicator bid and after each bowel movement

■ Diclofenac (Cataflam, Voltaren, Voltaren)
Uses: Treatment of arthritis (rheumatoid, osteoarthritis) and pain; ophthalmic as an adjunct to cataract surgery
Dose: 50–75 mg PO bid; ophthalmic 1 gt in eye qid 24 h postop for up to 2 wk

■ Dicloxacillin (Dynapen, Dycill)
Uses: Treatment of infections caused by susceptible strains of *S aureus* and *Streptococcus*
Dose: Adults. 250–500 mg qid. *Peds.* 12.5–25 mg/kg/d ÷ qid
Notes: Take on an empty stomach

■ Dicyclomine (Bentyl)
Uses: Treatment of functional irritable bowel syndromes
Dose: Adults. 20 mg PO qid titrated to max 160 mg/d or 20 mg IM q6h.
Peds. >6 mo: 5 mg/dose tid–qid; *Children:* 10 mg per dose tid–qid
Notes: Anticholinergic side effects may limit dose

■ Didanosine [ddI] (Videx)
Uses: Treatment of HIV infection in patients who are zidovudine intolerant
Dose: Adults. >60 kg: 400 mg PO qd or 200 mg PO bid. <60 kg: 250 mg PO qd or 125 mg PO bid. **Peds.** Dose by BSA (See package insert)
Notes: Reconstitute powder with water; side effects include pancreatitis, peripheral neuropathy, diarrhea, and headache; adults should take 2 tabs for each administration

■ Diflunisal (Dolobid)
Dose: Pain: 500 mg PO bid. *Osteoarthritis:* 500–1500 mg PO in 2–3 ÷ doses. Supplied tabs 250, 500 mg
Notes: May prolong prothrombin time

■ Digoxin (Lanoxin, Lanoxicaps)
Uses: CHF, atrial fibrillation and flutter, and paroxysmal atrial tachycardia.
ECC. Slow ventricular response in atrial fibrillation or flutter, second-line for PSVT
Dose: Adults. *PO digitalization:* 0.50–0.75 mg PO, then 0.25 mg PO q6–8h to a total dose between 1.0 and 1.5 mg. *IV/IM digitalization:* 0.25–0.50 mg IM/IV, then 0.25 mg q4–6h, total dose of about 1 mg. *Maint:* 0.125–0.500 mg PO/IM/IV qd (average daily dose 0.125–0.250 mg). **ECC.** Load 10–15 µg/kg IV. **Peds.** *Preterm infants:* Digitalization: 30 mg/kg PO or 25 mg/kg IV; give ½ of dose initially, then ¼ of dose at 8–to 12-h intervals for 2 doses. Maint: 10 mg/kg/24h PO or 6-8 mg/kg/24h IV ÷ q12h. *Term infants to 2 y:* Digitalization: 65–75 mg/kg PO or 50 mg/kg IV; give ½ of the dose initially, then ¼ of the dose at 8–12-h intervals for 2 doses. Maint: 15-20 mg/kg/24h PO or 12–15 mg/kg/24h IV ÷ q12h. *2–10 y:* Digitalization: 30–40 mg/kg PO or 25 mg/kg IV; give 1/2 dose initially, then ¼ of the dose at 8– to 12-h intervals for 2 doses. Maint: 8–10 mg/kg/24h PO or 6–8 mg/kg/24h IV ÷ q12h. *>10 y:* Same as for adults
Notes: Can cause heart block; low potassium can potentiate toxicity; reduce dose in renal failure; symptoms of toxicity include nausea and vomiting, headache, fatigue, visual disturbances (yellow-green halos around lights), and cardiac arrhythmias; IM inj can be painful and has erratic absorption

■ Digoxin Immune FAB (Digibind)
Uses: Treatment of life-threatening digoxin intoxication. **ECC.** Digoxin toxicity with uncontrolled life-threatening arrhythmias, shock, CHF. Hyperkalemia > 5 mEq/L with serum dig levels above 10–15 ng/mL.

Dose: Adults & Peds. Based on serum level and patient's weight. See dosing charts provided with the drug. Empiric where overdose is not known 20 vials (760 mg) IV in adults. *ECC.* Chronic intoxication: 3–5 vials may be effective. *Acute over dose:* Based on dose ingested (average dose is 10 vials (400 mg), but may require up to 20 vials (800 mg))

Notes: Each vial will bind approximately 0.6 mg of digoxin; in renal failure may require redosing in several days because of breakdown of the immune complex

■ Diltiazem (Cardizem, Dilacor)
Uses: Treatment of angina pectoris, prevention of reinfarction, HTN; atrial fibrillation or flutter, and paroxysmal SVT

Dose: Oral: 30 mg PO qid initially; titrate to 180–360 mg/d in ÷ doses as needed. *SR:* 60–120 mg PO bid, titrate to effect, max dose 360 mg/d. *Continuous dose:* 180–300 mg PO qd. *IV:* 0.25 mg/kg IV bolus over 2 min; may repeat dose in 15 min at 0.35 mg/kg. May begin cont inf of 5–15 mg/h. *ECC. Control ventricular rate in atrial fibrillation and flutter:* Use after adenosine to treat refractory PSVT in patients with narrow QRS complex and adequate BP. *Acute rate control:* 15–20 mg (0.25 mg/kg) IV over 2 min. Repeat in 15 min at 20–25 mg (0.35 mg/kg) over 2 min. *Maint:* 5–15 mg/h, titrated to heart rate.

Notes: Contra in sick-sinus syndrome, AV block, and hypotension. Cardizem CD and Dilacor XR are not interchangeable

■ Dimenhydrinate (Dramamine)
Uses: Prevention and treatment of nausea, vomiting, dizziness or vertigo of motion sickness

Dose: Adults. 50–100 mg PO q4–6h, max of 400 mg/d; 50 mg IM/IV PRN. *Peds.* 5 mg/kg/24h PO or IV ÷ qid

Notes: Anticholinergic side effects

■ Dimercaprol [BAL, British anti-Lewisite, dithioglycerol] BAL in Oil
Uses: Chelating agent antidote to arsenic, gold, mercury poisoning; adjunct to edetate calcium disodium in lead poisoning

Dose: Arsenic/gold poisoning: Mild: 2.5 mg/kg/dose q6h × 2 d, q12h on third day, daily × 10 d. Severe: 3 mg/kg/dose q4h × 2 d, q6h on third day, q12h × 10 d. *Mercury poisoning:* 5 mg/kg then 2.5 mg/kg/dose qd–bid × 10 d; Lead poisoning: 3–4 mg/kg/dose q4h × 5–7 d (with edetate calcium disodium)

■ Dimethyl Sulfoxide DMSO (Rimso 50)
Uses: Interstitial cystitis
Dose: Intravesical, 50 mL, retain for 15 min; repeat q2 wk until relief

■ Diphenhydramine (Benadryl, Others)
Uses: Allergic reactions, motion sickness, potentiate narcotics, sedation, cough suppression, treatment of extrapyramidal reactions

Dose: Adults. 25–50 mg PO, IV or IM bid–tid. *Peds.* 5 mg/kg/24h PO or IM ÷ q6h (max of 300 mg/d)

Notes: Anticholinergic side effects, including dry mouth, urinary retention; causes sedation; increase dosing interval in moderate-to-severe renal failure

■ Diphenoxylate with Atropine (Lomotil) [C]
Uses: Diarrhea
Dose: Adults. Initially 5 mg PO tid or qid until under control, then 2.5–5.0 mg PO bid. *Peds.* > 2 y: 0.3–0.4 mg/kg/24h ÷ bid–qid
Notes: Atropine-type side effects

■ Dipivefrin (Propine)
Uses: Open angle glaucoma
Dose: 1 gt into eye every 12 h

■ Dirithromycin (Dynabac)
Uses: Treatment of bronchitis, community-acquired pneumonia, and skin and skin structure infections
Dose: 500 mg PO qd for 7–14 d
Notes: Absorption is enhanced when taken with food

■ Disopyramide (Norpace)
Uses: Suppression and prevention of premature ventricular contractions
Dose: Adults. 400–800 mg/d ÷ q6h for regular release products and q12h for sustained release products. *Peds.* < 1 y: 10–30 mg/kg/24h PO. *1–4 y:* 10–20 mg/kg/24h PO. *4–12 y:* 10–15 mg/kg/24h PO. *12–18 y:* 6–15 mg/kg/24h PO
Notes: Anticholinergic side effects (urinary retention); negative inotropic properties may induce CHF; decrease dose in impaired hepatic function

■ Dobutamine (Dobutrex) (See Cover)
Uses: Short-term use in patients with cardiac decompensation secondary to depressed contractility.
Dose: Adults & Peds. Continuous IV infusion of 2.5–15 mg/kg/min; rarely 40 mg/kg/min may be required; titrate according to response; ECC. 2–20 µg/kg/min; titrate heart rate not > 10% of baseline *Peds. ECC.* Titrate to effect (initial dose 5–10 µg/kg/min). *Typical infusion dose:* 2 to 20 µg/kg/min
Notes: Monitor ECG for increase in heart rate, BP, and increased ectopic activity; monitor PWP and cardiac output

■ Docetaxol (Taxotere)
Uses: Breast and other cancers
Dose: 60–100 mg/m^2 IV every 3 wk based on protocol

Docusate Sodium (DOSS, Colace, Others)

Uses: Constipation-prone patient; adjunct to painful anorectal conditions (hemorrhoids)

Dose: Adults. 50–500 mg PO qd. **Peds.** *Infants to 3 y:* 10–40 mg/24h ÷ qd–qid. *3–6 y:* 20–60 mg/24h ÷ qd–qid. *6–12 y:* 40–120 mg/24h ÷ qd–qid

Notes: No significant side effects, no laxative action

Dolasetron (Anzemet)

Uses: Prevention of nausea and vomiting associated with chemotherapy

Dose: Adults & Peds. 1.8 mg/kg IV as a single dose. **Adults.** 100 mg PO as a single dose. **Peds.** 1.8 mg/kg PO up to 100 mg as a single dose

Notes: May cause prolongation of the QT interval

■ Dopamine (Intropin, Dopastat)

Uses: Short-term use in patients with cardiac decompensation secondary to decreased contractility; increases organ perfusion

Dose: Adults & Peds. 5 mg/kg/min by cont inf titrated by increments of 5 mg/kg/min to max of 50 mg/kg/min based on effect. **ECC. Adults.** Titrate to response

Low: 1–5 µg/kg/min ("renal doses"). *Moderate:* 5–10 µg/kg/min ("cardiac doses"). *High:* 10 to 20 µg/kg/min ("vasopressor doses"). *Pediatric:* Titrate to effect. Initial. 5–10 µg/kg/min; typical: 2–20 µg/kg/min. *Note:* If > 20 µg/kg/min is required, consider use of alternative adrenergic agent (eg, epinephrine)

Notes: Dose > 10 mg/kg/min may decrease renal perfusion; monitor urinary output; monitor ECG for increase in heart rate, BP, and increased ectopic activity; monitor PCWP and CO if possible

Dorzolamide (Trusopt)

Uses: Glaucoma

Dose: 1 gt in eye(s) tid

Dorzolamide and Timolol (Cosopt)

Uses: Glaucoma

Dose: 1 gt in eye(s) bid

■ Doxazosin (Cardura)

Uses: HTN and BPH

Dose: *HTN:* Initially 1 mg PO qd; may be increased to 16 mg PO qd. *BPH:* Initially 1 mg PO qd, may be increased to 8 mg PO qd

Notes: Doses > 4 mg increase the likelihood of excessive postural hypotension; use qhs dosing to limit

■ Doxepin (Sinequan, Adapin)
Uses: Depression or anxiety
Dose: 50–150 mg PO qd usually qhs but can be in ÷ doses
Notes: Anticholinergic, central nervous system, and cardiovascular side effects

■ Doxorubicin (Adriamycin)
Uses: Treatment of breast, endometrial, and ovarian cancer, and leukemia
Dose: 60–75 mg/m^2 IV as a single dose, at 21-d intervals
Notes: May cause myelosuppression and cardiotoxicity

■ Doxycycline (Vibramycin)
Uses: Broad-spectrum antibiotic including activity against *Rickettsia, Chlamydia,* and *M pneumoniae*
Dose: Adults. 100 mg PO q12h first day, then 100 mg PO qd or bid or 100 mg IV q12h. **Peds.** > 8 y: 5 mg/kg/24h PO up to a max of 200 mg/d, ÷ qd or bid
Notes: Useful for chronic bronchitis; tetracycline of choice for patients with renal impairment

■ Dronabinol (Marinol) [C]
Uses: Nausea and vomiting associated with cancer chemotherapy; appetite stimulation
Dose: Adults & Peds. Antiemetic: 5–15 mg/m^2/dose q4–6h PRN. **Adults.** Appetite: 2.5 mg PO before lunch and supper
Notes: Principal psychoactive substance present in marijuana; many CNS side effects

■ Droperidol (Inapsine)
Uses: Nausea and vomiting, premedication for anesthesia
Dose: Adults. *Nausea:* 1.25–2.5 mg IV PRN; *Premedication:* 2.5–10 mg IV. **Peds.** 0.1–0.15 mg/kg/dose
Notes: May cause drowsiness, moderate hypotension, and occasionally tachycardia.

■ Echothiophate iodine (Phospholine Ophthalmic)
Uses: Glaucoma
Dose: 1 gt eye(s) bid with one dose at hs

■ Econazole (Spectazole)
Uses: Treatment of most tinea, cutaneous *Candida,* and tinea versicolor infections

Dose: Apply to affected areas bid (qd for tinea versicolor) for 2–4 wk

Notes: Relief of symptoms and clinical improvement may be seen early in treatment, but course of therapy should be carried out to avoid recurrence

■ Edetate Calcium Disodium [Calcium EDTA] (Calcium Disodium Versenate)

Uses: Chelating agent for acute and chronic lead poisoning; aids diagnosis of lead poisoning

Dose: Adults. 2 g/day or 1.5 g/m^2/day ÷ dose q12–24h × 5 d; *Peds. Asymptomatic:* (lead levels > 55 µg/dL or lead levels 25–55 µg/dL with blood erythrocyte protoporphyrin level of 35 µg/dL and positive mobilization test) or symptomatic lead poisoning without encephalopathy and lead level < 100 µg/dL: 1 g/m^2/day IM/IV in ÷ doses q8–12h for 3–5 d (usually 5 d); max: 1 g/24 h or 50 mg/kg/d. *Symptomatic:* (encephalopathy and lead level > 100 µg/dL (treatment with calcium EDTA and dimercaprol is preferred): 250 mg/m^2 IM or intermittent IV infusion 4h after dimercaprol, then at 4-h intervals thereafter for 5 d (1.5 g/m^2/day); dose (1.5 g/m^2/d) can also be administered as a single IV cont inf over 12–24 h/day for 5 d; max: 1 g/24 h or 75 mg/kg/d.

Note: Course of therapy may be repeated in 2–3 wk until blood lead level is normal repeat course one time after at least 2 d (usually after 2 wk)

■ Edrophonium (Tensilon)

Uses: Diagnosis of myasthenia gravis; acute myasthenic crisis; curare antagonist; paroxysmal atrial tachycardia

Dose: Adults. Test for myasthenia gravis: 2 mg IV in 1 min; if tolerated, give 8 mg IV; a positive test is a brief increase in strength. *PAT:* 10 mg IV to a max of 40 mg. *Peds.* Test for myasthenia gravis: Total dose of 0.2 mg/kg. Give 0.04 mg/kg as a test dose. If no reaction occurs, give the remainder of the dose in 1-mg increments to a max of 10 mg

Notes: Can cause severe cholinergic effects; keep atropine available

■ Efavirenz (Sustiva)

Uses: HIV infections

Dose: Adults. 600 mg/d PO. *Peds.* Refer to product information; take hs, avoid high-fat meals

■ Enalapril (Vasotec)

Uses: HTN, CHF. *ECC.* To improve outcome in AMI

Dose: Adults. 2.5–5 mg/d PO titrated by effect to 10–40 mg/d as 1–2 ÷ doses, or 1.25 mg IV q6h. *ECC.* 2.5 mg PO single dose, increase to 20 mg PO bid. 1.25 mg IV over 5 min, then 1.25–5.0 MG IV every 6 h. *Peds.* 0.05–0.08 mg/kg/dose PO q12–24h

Notes: Initial dose can produce symptomatic hypotension, especially with concomitant diuretics; discontinue diuretic for 2–3 d before initiation if possible; monitor closely for increases in serum potassium; may cause a nonproductive cough

■ Enoxaparin (Lovenox)
Uses: Prevention of DVT. *ECC.* ACS with non-Q wave or unstable angina
Dose: 30 mg SQ bid. *ECC.* 1 mg/kg bid SQ for 2–8 days with aspirin
Notes: Does not significantly affect bleeding time, platelet function, PT or APTT

■ Entacapone (Comtan)
Uses: Treatment of Parkinson's disease
Dose: 200 mg administered concurrently with each levodopa/carbidopa dose to a max of 8 ×/d

■ Ephedrine
Uses: Acute bronchospasm, nasal congestion, hypotension, narcolepsy, enuresis, myasthenia gravis
Dose: Adults. 25–50 mg IM/SQ or 5–25 mg/dose slow IV every 10 min to max of 150 mg/d or 25–50 mg PO q3–4h PRN. *Peds.* 0.2–0.3 mg/kg/dose IM or IV q4–6h PRN

■ Epinephrine (Adrenalin, Sus-Phrine, others)
Uses: Cardiac arrest, anaphylactic reactions, acute asthma
Dose: Adults. Anaphylaxis: 0.3–0.5 mL of 1:1000 dilution SQ; may repeat q10–15 min to max of 1 mg/dose and 5 mg/d. *Asthma:* 0.3–0.5 mL of 1:1000 dilution SQ repeated at 20-min to 4-h intervals or 1 inhal (metered dose) repeated in 1–2 min or suspension 0.1–0.3 mL SQ for extended effect. *ECC. Cardiac arrest: IV dose:* 1.0 mg IV push, repeat every 3–5 min; doses up to (0.2 mg/kg) if 1 mg dose fails. *Infusion:* 30 mg epinephrine (30 mL of 1:1000 soln) to 250 mL NS or D_5W, run at 100 mL/h, titrate. *Endotracheal:* 2.0–2.5 mg in 20 mL NS. *Profound bradycardia/hypotension:* 2–10 µg/min (1 mg of 1:1000 in 500 mL NS, inf 1–5 mL/min). *Peds. ECC. Asystole, pulseless arrest:* First *dose:* 0.1 mg/kg IV (0.1 mL/kg of 1:10,000 "standard concentration"). Second and subsequent doses: 0.1 mg/kg IV (0.1 mL/kg of 1:1000 "high" concentration. Administer every 3–5 min during arrest; up to 0.2 mg/kg may be effective. *Endotracheal:* 0.1 mg/kg (0.1 mL/kg of 1:1000 ["high"] concentration) continue q3–5min of arrest until IV access achieved; then begin with first IV dose. *Symptomatic bradycardia:* 0.01 mg/kg IV (0.1 mL/kg of 1:10,000 ["standard"] concentration). *Continuous IV inf:* Begin with rapid inf, then titrate to response. Typical infusion: 0.1 to 1.0 µg/kg/min. (Higher doses may be effective)
Notes: Sus-Phrine offers sustained action; in acute cardiac settings can be given via endotracheal tube if a central line is not available

▪ Epoetin Alfa (Epogen, Procrit)

Uses: Treatment of anemia associated with chronic renal failure, zidovudine treatment in HIV-infected patients, and patients receiving cancer chemotherapy; reduction in transfusions associated with surgery
Dose: Adults & Peds. 50–150 U/kg 3 ×/wk; adjust the dose every 4–6 wk as needed. Surgery: 300 U/kg/d for 10 d before surgery
Notes: May cause HTN, headache, tachycardia, nausea, and vomiting; store in refrigerator

▪ Epoprostenol (Flolan)

Uses: Treatment of pulmonary HTN
Dose: 4 ng/kg/min IV cont inf; make adjustments based on clinical status and package insert guidelines
Notes: Availability through a pharmacy benefit manager

▪ Eprosartan (Teveten)

Uses: Treatment of HTN
Dose: 400–800 mg daily as single dose or bid.
Notes: Avoid use during pregnancy

▪ Eptifibatide (Integrilin)

Uses: Treatment of ACS, PCI
Dose: 180 µg/kg IV bolus, followed by 2 µg/kg/min cont inf. *ECC. ACS:* 180 µg/kg IV bolus then 2 µg/kg/min inf. *PCI:* 135 µg/kg IV bolus then 0.5 µg/kg/min inf; repeat bolus in 10 min

▪ Erythromycin (E-Mycin, Ilosone, Erythrocin, ERYC, Others)

Uses: Infections caused by Group A streptococci (*S pyogenes*), α-hemolytic streptococci and *N gonorrhoeae* infections in penicillin-allergic patients, *S pneumoniae*, *M pneumoniae*, and *Legionella*
Dose: Adults. 250–500 mg PO qid or between 500 mg and 1 g IV qid. *Peds.* 30–50 mg/kg/24h PO or IV ÷ q6h, to a max of 2 g/d
Notes: Frequent mild GI disturbances; estolate salt is associated with cholestatic jaundice; erythromycin base not well absorbed from the GI tract; some forms such as ERYC are better tolerated with respect to GI irritation; lactobionate salt contains benzyl alcohol, therefore use with caution in neonates; base formulation not absorbed and used as part of the "Nichols–Condon Bowel Prep"

▪ Erythromycin, Ophthalmic (Ilotycin)

Uses: Conjunctival infections
Dose: 0.5% oint, apply q6h

■ Esmolol (Brevibloc)

Uses: SVT and noncompensatory sinus tachycardia. *MOA:* β-Adrenergic blocking agent; class II antiarrhythmic

Dose: Adults & Peds. Initiate treatment with 500 µg/kg load over 1 min, then 50 µg/kg/min for 4 min; if inadequate response, repeat the loading dose and follow with Maint inf of 100 µg/kg/min for 4 min; titrate by repeating loading then incremental ↑ in the Maint dose of 50 µg/kg/min for 4 min until desired heart rate reached or BP decreases; average dose 100 µg/kg/min. *ECC.* All patients with suspected MI; may reduce chance of VF and reduce damage. Second line agents after adenosine, diltiazem, or digoxin to slow ventricular response in supraventricular tachyarrhythmias. Antihypertensive for hemorrhagic and ischemic stroke

Notes: Do NOT administer along with calcium channel blockers due to risk of hypotension

■ Estazolam (ProSom) [C]

Uses: Insomnia
Dose: 1–2 mg PO qhs PRN

■ Esterified Estrogens (Estratab, Menest)

Uses: Vasomotor symptoms, atrophic vaginitis, or kraurosis vulvae associated with menopause, female hypogonadism
Dose: Menopause: 0.3–1.25 mg daily; hypogonadism: 2.5 mg PO qd–tid

■ Esterified Estrogens with Methyltestosterone (Estratest)

Uses: Moderate-to-severe vasomotor symptoms associated with menopause, postpartum breast engorgement
Dose: 1 tab qd for 3 wk, then 1 wk off

■ Estradiol Topical (Estrace)

Uses: Atrophic vaginitis and kraurosis vulvae associated with menopause
Dose: 2–4 g daily 1–2 wk, then 1 g 1–3 ×/wk

■ Estradiol Transdermal (Estraderm)

Uses: Severe vasomotor symptoms associated with menopause; female hypogonadism
Dose: 0.05 system 2 ×/wk, adjust dose as necessary to control symptoms. Transdermal patches 0.05 mg, 0.1 mg (delivers 0.05 mg or 0.1 mg/24h)

■ Estramustine (Emcyt)
Uses: Advanced prostate cancer
Dose: 1 cap/22 lb body weight, ÷ tid–qid

■ Estrogen, Conjugated (Premarin)
Uses: Moderate-to-severe vasomotor symptoms associated with menopause; atrophic vaginitis; palliative therapy of advanced prostatic carcinoma; prevention of estrogen deficiency-induced osteoporosis
Dose: 0.3–1.25 mg/d PO cyclically; prostatic carcinoma requires 1.25–2.5 mg PO tid
Notes: Do not use in pregnancy; associated with an increased risk of endometrial carcinoma, gallbladder disease, thromboembolism, heart attach, stroke, and possibly breast cancer; generic products are not equivalent

■ Estrogen, Conjugated with Methylprogesterone (Premarin with Methylprogesterone)
Uses: Vasomotor symptoms associated with menopause
Dose: 1 tab qd

■ Estrogen, Conjugated with methyltestosterone (Premarin with methyltestosterone)
Uses: Moderate-to-severe vasomotor symptoms associated with menopause, postpartum breast engorgement
Dose: 1 tab qd for 3 wk, then 1 wk off

■ Ethacrynic Acid (Edecrin)
Uses: Edema, CHF, ascites, any time rapid diuresis is desired
Dose: **Adults.** 50–200 mg PO qd or 50 mg IV PRN. **Peds.** 1 mg/kg/dose IV. Repeated doses are not recommended
Notes: Contra in anuria; many severe side effects

■ Ethambutol (Myambutol)
Uses: Pulmonary tuberculosis and other mycobacterial infections
Dose: **Adults & Peds.** *> 12 y:* 15–25 mg/kg PO daily as single dose
Notes: May cause vision changes and GI upset

■ Ethanol [ethyl alcohol] Lavacol [OTC]
Uses: Antidote for ethylene glycol or methanol overdose
Dose: Load 0.6 g/kg IV, then 100–125 mg/kg/h IV to maintain blood levels of 100 mg/dL; 400 mL of a 5% sol in 1 h/max

Ethinyl Estradiol (Estinyl, Feminone)
Uses: Vasomotor symptoms associated with menopause, female hypogonadism
Dose: 0.02–1.5 mg/d ÷ qd–tid

Ethosuximide (Zarontin)
Uses: Absence seizures
Dose: *Adults.* 500 mg qd PO initially; increase by 250 mg/d every 4–7 d as needed. *Peds.* 20–40 mg/kg/24h PO qd to a max of 1500 mg/d
Notes: Blood dyscrasias, CNS and GI side effects may occur; use caution in patients with renal or hepatic impairment

Etidronate (Didronel)
Uses: Hypercalcemia of malignancy, hypertrophic ossification associated with spinal cord injury, Paget's disease, postmenopausal osteoporosis
Dose: *Hypercalcemia:* 7.5 mg/kg/d IV in NS over 2 h for 3 d, then 20 mg/kg/d PO for 1 mo. *Ossification:* 20 mg/kg/d for 2 wk, then 10 mg/kg/d for 10 wk

Etomidate (Amidate)
Uses: Induction during RSI and deep procedural sedation
Dose: 0.1 mg/kg slow IVP (procedural sedation); 0.3 mg/kg IVP for induction
Notes: May cause adrenal suppression, myoclonus, emesis; physician must be competent to provide deep procedural sedation and airway management

Etodolac (Lodine)
Uses: Treatment of arthritis and pain
Dose: 200–400 mg PO bid–qid

Etoposide (VePesid)
Uses: Treatment of gestational trophoblastic disease, ovarian, testicular, and lung cancer
Dose: 35–100 mg/m^2/d IV. Number of doses and duration of therapy is dependent on individual protocols
Notes: May cause bone marrow suppression; has low stability in concentrated solns

Famciclovir (Famvir)
Uses: Management of acute herpes zoster (shingles) and genital herpes infections
Dose: *Zoster:* 500 mg PO q8h. *Simplex:* 125–250 mg PO bid

Famotidine (Pepcid)
Uses: Short-term treatment of active duodenal ulcer and benign gastric ulcer; Maint therapy for duodenal ulcer, hypersecretory conditions, GERD, and heartburn
Dose: Adults. Ulcer: 20–40 mg PO hs or 20 mg IV q12h. *Hypersecretory:* 20–160 mg PO q6h. *GERD:* 20 mg PO bid; Maint 20 mg PO hs. *Heartburn:* 10 mg PO PRN heartburn. ***Peds.*** 1–2 mg/kg/d
Notes: Decrease dose in severe renal insufficiency

Felodipine (Plendil)
Uses: Treatment of HTN
Dose: 5–20 mg PO qd.
Notes: Closely monitor BP in elderly patients and patients with impaired hepatic function; doses of > 10 mg should not be used in these patients

Fenofibrate (Tricor)
Uses: Treatment of hypertriglyceridemia
Dose: Initial dose 67 mg/d. May be ↑ to 67 mg tid
Notes: Take with meals to increase bioavailability; May cause pancreatitis

Fenoldopam (Corlopam)
Uses: Treatment of hypertensive emergency
Dose: Initial dose 0.03–0.1 µg/kg/min IV cont inf, titrate to effect every 15 min with 0.05–0.1 µg/kg/min increments
Notes: Avoid concurrent use with β-blockers

Fenoprofen (Nalfon)
Uses: Treatment of arthritis and pain
Dose: 200–600 mg q4–8h, to a max of 3200 mg/d

Fentanyl (Sublimaze) [C]
Uses: Short-acting analgesic used in conjunction with anesthesia
Dose: Adults & Peds. 0.025–0.15 mg/kg IV/IM titrated to effect
Notes: Causes significant sedation

Fentanyl Transdermal System (Duragesic) [C]
Uses: Management of chronic pain
Dose: Apply patch to upper torso every 72 h. Dose is calculated from the narcotic requirements for the previous 24 h. Transdermal patches deliver 25 mg/h, 50 mg/h, 75 mg/h, 100 mg/h
Notes: 0.1 mg of fentanyl is equivalent to 10 mg of morphine IM

Fentanyl Transmucosal System (Actiq, Fentanyl Oralet) [C]
Uses: Induction of anesthesia and breakthrough cancer pain
Dose: Adults & Peds. *Anesthesia:* 5–15 µg/kg. *Pain:* 200 µg consumed over 15 min, titrate to appropriate effect

Ferrous Sulfate
Uses: Iron deficiency anemia; iron supplementation
Dose: Adults. 100–200 mg/d of elemental iron ÷ tid–qid. **Peds.** 1–2 mg/kg/24h ÷ qd–bid
Notes: May turn stools and urine dark; can cause GI upset, constipation; vitamin C taken with ferrous sulfate increases the absorption of iron especially in patients with atrophic gastritis

Fexofenadine (Allegra)
Uses: Relief of allergic rhinitis
Dose: Adults & Peds *> 12 y:* 60 mg bid

Filgrastim [G-CSF] (Neupogen)
Uses: To decrease the incidence of infection in febrile neutropenic patients and treatment of chronic neutropenia
Dose: Adults & Peds. 5 µg/kg/d SQ or IV as a single daily dose
Notes: May cause bone pain. Discontinue therapy when ANC > 10,000

Finasteride (Proscar, Propecia)
Uses: Treatment of benign prostatic hyperplasia and androgenetic alopecia
Dose: *BPH (Proscar):* 5 mg PO qd. *Alopecia (Propecia):* 1 mg PO qd
Notes: Will decrease prostate-specific antigen levels; may take 3–6 mo to see effect on urinary symptoms

Flavoxate (Urispas)
Uses: Symptomatic relief of dysuria, urgency, nocturia, suprapubic pain, urinary frequency, and incontinence
Dose: 100–200 mg PO tid–qid
Notes: May cause drowsiness, blurred vision, and dry mouth

Flecainide (Tambocor)
Uses: Life-threatening ventricular arrhythmias
Dose: 100 mg PO q12h; increase in increments of 50 mg q12h every 4 d to max of 400 mg/d

Notes: May cause new or worsened arrhythmias; therapy should be initiated in the hospital; may dose q8h if patient is intolerant or uncontrolled at q12h interval; drug interactions with propranolol, digoxin, verapamil, and disopyramide; may cause CHF

■ Fluconazole (Diflucan)
Uses: Oropharyngeal and esophageal candidiasis; cryptococcal meningitis; *Candida* infections of the lungs, peritoneum, and urinary tract; prevention of candidiasis in bone marrow transplant patients on chemotherapy or radiation; and candidal vaginitis
Dose: Adults. 100–400 mg PO or IV qd. *Vaginitis:* 150 mg PO as a single dose. *Peds.* 3–6 mg/kg PO or IV qd
Notes: Adjust dose in renal insufficiency; oral dosing produces the same blood levels as IV dosing, so the oral route should be used whenever possible

■ Fludarabine Phosphate (Fludara)
Uses: Treatment of leukemia
Dose: 25 mg/m^2 IV for 5 consecutive days. Give every 28 d
Notes: May cause severe bone marrow suppression and neurologic toxicity

■ Fludrocortisone Acetate (Florinef)
Uses: Partial treatment for adrenocortical insufficiency
Dose: Adults & Peds > 1 y: 0.05–0.1 mg PO qd. *Infants:* 0.1–0.2 mg PO qd
Notes: For adrenal insufficiency, must be used in conjunction with a glucocorticoid supplement; dosing changes based on plasma renin activity

■ Flumazenil (Romazicon)
Uses: Reverse benzodiazepine toxicity (do NOT use in tricyclic overdose or in unknown poisoning)
Dose: 0.2 mg IV over 15 s, dose may be repeated if the desired level of consciousness is not obtained to a max dose of 1 mg. *ECC.* 0.2 mg IV over 15 s, then 0.3 mg IV over 30 s; if no response, give third dose. *Third dose:* 0.5 mg IV given over 30 s, repeat once per min until response or total of 3 mg

■ Flunisolide (AeroBid)
Uses: Control of bronchial asthma in patients requiring chronic corticosteroid therapy
Dose: Adults. 2–4 inhals bid. *Peds.* 2 inhals bid
Notes: May cause oral candidiasis; not for acute asthma attack

Fluorouracil (Adrucil)
Uses: Management of carcinoma of the colon, rectum, breast, stomach, and pancreas
Dose: Varies with individual protocol

Fluoxetine (Prozac)
Uses: Treatment of depression, obsessive-compulsive disorders, and bulimia
Dose: Initially, 20 mg PO qd; titrate to a max of 80 mg/24h; doses of > 20 mg/d should be ÷. *Bulimia:* 60 mg/d in AM
Notes: May cause nausea, nervousness, and weight loss

Fluphenazine (Prolixin, Permitil)
Uses: Psychotic disorders
Dose: 0.5–10 mg/d in ÷ doses PO q6–8h; average Maint 5.0 mg/d or 1.25 mg IM initially then 2.5–10 mg/d in ÷ doses q6–8h PRN
Notes: Reduce dose in elderly patients; monitor LFTs ;may cause drowsiness; do not administer concentrate with caffeine, tannic acid, or pectin-containing products

Flurazepam (Dalmane) [C]
Uses: Insomnia
Dose: Adults & Peds. > 15 y: 15–30 mg PO qhs PRN
Notes: Reduce dose in elderly patients

Flurbiprofen (Ansaid)
Uses: Treatment of arthritis
Dose: 50–100 mg bid–qid, to a max of 300 mg/d

Flutamide (Eulexin)
Uses: Prostate cancer in combination with LHRH analogue
Dose: 3 (125 mg) caps PO q8h
Notes: Monitor LFTs

Fluticasone Nasal (Flonase)
Uses: Seasonal allergic rhinitis
Dose: 2 sprays per nostril qd; may reduce to 1 spray/d; max 4 sprays/d

Fluticasone Oral (Flovent, Flovent Rotadisk)
Uses: Chronic treatment of asthma

Dose: Adults and adolescents: 2–4 puffs bid. *Peds. 4–11 y:* 50 μg bid
Notes: Counsel patients carefully on use of device multidose inhaler 44, 110, or 220 μg/activation; Rotadisk dry powder 50, 100, and 250 μg/activation; risk of thrush

Fluvastatin (Lescol)
Uses: Adjunct to diet in the treatment of elevated total cholesterol
Dose: 20–40 mg PO qhs

Folic Acid
Uses: Macrocytic anemia
Dose: Adults. Supplement: 0.4 mg PO qd. *Pregnancy:* 0.8 mg PO qd. *Folate deficiency:* 1.0 mg PO qd–tid. **Peds.** *Supplement:* 0.04–0.4 mg/24h PO, IM, IV, or SQ *Folate deficiency:* 0.5–1.0 mg/24h PO, IM, IV or SQ

Fomepizole [4-methylpyrazole, 4-MP] Antizol
Uses: Ethylene glycol, methanol and propylene glycol toxicity
Dose: 15 mg/kg then 5 mg/kg in 12 h, then 10 mg/kg q12h until toxin cleared

Fomivirsen (Vitravene)
Uses: CMV retinitis in AIDS patients who do not respond to other therapies
Dose: 6.6 mg intraocular inj every other week for 2 wk followed by one inj once every 4 wk

Foscarnet (Foscavir)
Uses: Treatment of cytomegalovirus; acyclovir-resistant herpes infections
Dose: *Induction:* 60 mg/kg IV q8h for 14–21 d. *Maint:* 90–120 mg/kg IV qd (Monday–Friday)
Notes: Dose must be adjusted for renal function; nephrotoxic; monitor ionized calcium closely (causes electrolyte abnormalities); administer through a central venous catheter

Fosfomycin (Monurol)
Uses: Uncomplicated UTI in women
Dose: 3 g in water (one dose)

Fosinopril (Monopril)
Uses: HTN
Dose: Initially, 10 mg PO qd; may be increased to a max of 80 mg/d PO ÷ qd–bid

Notes: Decrease dose in elderly patients, unnecessary to adjust dose for renal insufficiency, may cause a nonproductive cough and dizziness

■ Fosphenytoin (Cerebyx)
Uses: Treatment of status epilepticus
Dose: Load: 15–20 mg PE/kg. *Maint:* 4–6 mg PE/kg/d
Notes: Dosed as phenytoin equivalents (PE); administer at < 150 mg PE/min to prevent hypotension

■ Furosemide (Lasix)
Uses: Edema, HTN, CHF. *ECC.* Acute pulmonary edema in BP > 90–100. Hypertensive emergencies or increased intracranial pressure
Dose: Adults. 20–80 mg PO or IV qd or bid. *ECC.* 0.5–1.0 mg/kg over 1–2 min. If no response, double the dose to 2.0 mg/kg over 1–2 min. *Peds.* 1 mg/kg/dose IV q6–12h; 2 mg/kg/dose PO q12h–24h
Notes: Monitor for hypokalemia; use with caution in hepatic disease; high doses of the IV form may cause ototoxicity

■ Gabapentin (Neurontin)
Uses: Adjunctive or supplementary therapy in the treatment of partial seizures
Dose: 900–1800 mg/d PO in 3 ÷ doses
Notes: It is not necessary to monitor serum gabapentin levels

■ Gallium Nitrate (Ganite)
Uses: Treatment of hypercalcemia of malignancy
Dose: 100–200 mg/m^2/d for 5 d
Notes: Can cause renal insufficiency; 1% acute optic neuritis

■ Ganciclovir (Cytovene, Vitrasert)
Uses: Treatment and prevention of cytomegalovirus (CMV) retinitis and prevention of CMV disease in transplant recipients.
Dose: Adults & Peds. IV: 5 mg/kg IV q12h for 14–21 d, then Maint of 5 mg/kg IV qd for 7 d/wk or 6 mg/kg IV qd for 5 d/wk. *Adults. PO:* Following induction, 1000 mg PO tid. Prevention: 1000 mg PO tid
Notes: Not a cure for CMV; granulocytopenia and thrombocytopenia are the major toxicities; inj should be handled with appropriate precautions; take caps with food

■ Gatifloxacin (Tequin)
Uses: Treatment of acute exacerbation of chronic bronchitis, sinusitis, community acquired pneumonia, UTIs

Dose: 400 mg/d PO or IV
Notes: Avoid use with antacids; do NOT use in children < 18 y, pregnant or lactating women; reliable activity against *S pneumoniae*

■ Gemfibrozil (Lopid)
Uses: Hypertriglyceridemia (types IV and V hyperlipoproteinemia)
Dose: 1200 mg/d PO in 2 ÷ doses 30 min before the AM and PM meals
Notes: Monitor liver function test and serum lipids during therapy; cholelithiasis may occur secondary to treatment; may enhance the effect of warfarin

■ Gentamicin (Garamycin)
Uses: Serious infections caused by susceptible *Pseudomonas, Proteus, E coli, Klebsiella, Enterobacter, Serratia,* and for initial treatment of gram-negative sepsis
Dose: Adults. 3–5 mg/kg/24h IV ÷ q8–24h. *Peds. Infants > 7 d:* 2.5 mg/kg/dose IV q12–24h. *Children:* 2.5 mg/kg/d IV q8h
Notes: Nephrotoxic and ototoxic; decrease dose with renal insufficiency; monitor creatinine clearance and serum concentration for dosing adjustments (see Tables A–24 and A–26, pages 676 and 678).

■ Gentamicin, Ophthalmic (Garamycin Ophthalmic)
Uses: Conjunctival infections
Dose: 0.3% oint apply bid or tid

■ Glimepiride (Amaryl)
Uses: Non-insulin-dependent DM
Dose: 1–4 mg/d

■ Glipizide (Glucotrol)
Uses: Non-insulin-dependent DM
Dose: 5–15 mg qd–bid

■ Glucagon (Generic)
Uses: Severe hypoglycemia in DM with sufficient liver glycogen stores.
ECC. Reverse effects of calcium channel blocker or β-blocker
Dose: Adults. 0.5–1.0 mg SQ, IM, or IV; repeat in 20 min PRN. *β-Blocker overdose:* 3–10 mg IV; repeat in 10 min PRN; may give as cont inf. *ECC.* 1–5 mg over 2–5 min. *Peds. Neonates:* 0.3 mg/kg/dose SQ, IM, or IV q4h PRN. *Peds.* 0.025–0.1 mg/kg/dose SQ, IM, or IV; repeat after 20 min PRN
Notes: Administration of glucose IV necessary; ineffective in states of starvation, adrenal insufficiency, or chronic hypoglycemia; hypotension

■ Glyburide (DiaBeta, Micronase)
Uses: Management of non-insulin-dependent DM
Dose: Nonmicronized: 1.25–10 mg qd–bid. *Micronized:* 1.5–6 mg qd–bid

■ Glycerin Suppository
Uses: Constipation
Dose: Adults. 1 adult suppository PR, PRN. *Peds.* 1 infant suppository PR, qd–bid PRN

■ Gonadorelin (Lutrepulse)
Uses: Primary hypothalamic amenorrhea
Dose: 5 µg IV q90min for 21 d using a Lutrepulse reservoir and pump
Notes: Risk of multiple pregnancies

■ Goserelin (Zoladex)
Uses: Treatment of advanced prostate cancer and endometriosis
Dose: 3.6 mg SQ every 28 d into the abdominal wall

■ Granisetron (Kytril)
Uses: Prevention of nausea and vomiting associated with emetogenic cancer therapy
Dose: Adults & Peds. 10 mg/kg IV 30 min before initiation of chemotherapy. *Adults.* 1 mg PO 1 h before chemotherapy, then q12 h

■ Guaifenesin (Robitussin, others)
Uses: Symptomatic relief of dry nonproductive cough; expectorant
Dose: Adults. 200–400 mg (10–20 mL) PO q4h. *Peds. 2–5 y:* 50–100 mg (2.5–5 mL) PO q4h. *6–11 y:* 100–200 mg (5–10 mL) PO q4h

■ Guaifenesin and Codeine (Robitussin ac, Brontex, Others) [C]
Uses: Antitussive with expectorant
Dose: Adults. 10 mL or 1 tab PO q6–8h. *Peds. 2–6 y:* 1–1.5 kg/kg codeine per day ÷ dose q4–6h. *6–12 y:* 5 mL q4h. *>12 y:* 10 mL q4h, max 60 mL/24h
Notes: Brontex tab contains 10 mg codeine; Brontex liquid 2.5 mg codeine/5 mL; others 10 mg codeine/5 mL

■ Guaifenesin and Dextromethorphan (many OTC brands)
Uses: Cough due to upper respiratory irritation
Dose: Adults & Peds > 12 y: 10 mL PO q6h. *Peds. 2–6 y:* 2.5 mL q6–8h, 10 mL/d max. *6–12 y:* 5 mL q6–8h, 20 mL max/d

Guanabenz (Wytensin)
Uses: HTN
Dose: Adults. Initially, 4 mg PO bid, increase by 4 mg/d increments at 1–2 wk intervals up to 32 mg bid. *Peds. > 12 y:* 0.5–4 mg/d initially, increase by 0.5–2 mg/d at 1-wk intervals up to 24 mg/d ÷ bid
Notes: Sedation, dry mouth, dizziness, and headache common

Guanadrel (Hylorel)
Uses: HTN
Dose: 5 mg PO bid initially, increase up to 10 mg/d weekly up to 75 mg PO bid
Notes: Interactions with tricyclic antidepressants; less orthostatic changes and impotence than guanethidine

Guanethidine (Ismelin)
Uses: HTN
Dose: Adults. Initially, 10–25 mg PO qd, ↑ dose based on response. *Peds.* 0.2 mg/kg/24h PO initially, ↑ by 0.2 mg/kg/24h increments q7–10d up to max dose of 3 mg/kg/24h
Notes: May produce orthostatic hypotension especially with diuretic use; may potentiate vasopressors; increased frequency of bowel movements and explosive diarrhea possible; interaction with tricyclic antidepressants reduces the effectiveness of guanethidine

Guanfacine (Tenex)
Uses: HTN
Dose: 1 mg qhs initially, increase by 1 mg/24h to max dose of 3 mg/24h; ÷ dose bid if BP increases at the end of the dosing interval
Notes: Use with thiazide diuretic is recommended; sedation, drowsiness common; rebound HTN may occur with abrupt cessation of therapy

Haemophilus B Conjugate Vaccine (ProHIBiT, Act-Hib, Pedvaxhib)
Uses: Routine immunization between the ages of 18 mo and 5 y against diseases caused by *Haemophilus influenzae* type B
Dose: Peds. 0.5 mL (25 mg) IM in deltoid or vastus lateralis
Notes: Booster not required; observe for anaphylaxis

Haloperidol (Haldol)
Uses: Management of psychotic disorders; schizophrenia; agitation; Tourette's disorders; hyperactivity in children
Dose: Adults. Moderate symptoms: 0.5–2.0 mg PO bid–tid. *Severe symptoms or agitation:* 3–5 mg PO bid–tid or 1–5 mg IM q4h PRN (max 100 mg/d).

Peds. 3–6 y: 0.01–0.03 mg/kg/24h PO qd. *6–12 y:* initially, 0.5–1.5 mg/24h PO, ↑ by 0.5 mg/24h to Maint of 2–4 mg/24h (0.05–0.1 mg/kg/24h) or 1–3 mg/dose IM q4–8h to a max of 0.1 mg/kg/24h. Tourette's up to 15 mg/24h PO
   Notes: Can cause extrapyramidal symptoms, hypotension; reduce dose in elderly patients

◼ Heparin Sodium
   Uses: Treatment and prevention of venous thrombosis and PE, AF with emboli formation, acute arterial occlusion. *ECC.* Adjuvant therapy in AMI. Begin heparin with fibrinolytics
   Dose: Adults. Prophylaxis: 3000–5000 units SQ q8–12h. *Treatment of thrombosis:* Loading dose of 50–75 units/kg IV, then 10–20 units/kg IV qh (adjust based on PTT). *ECC.* Bolus 60 IU/kg (max bolus: 4000 IU). Continue 12 IU/kg/h (max 1000 IU/h for patients > 70 kg) round to the nearest 50 IU. Adjust to maintain PTT 1.5 to 2.0 x control values for 48 h or until angiography.
   Peds. Infants: Load: 50 U/kg IV bolus, then 20 U/kg/h IV infusion. *Children:* Load: 50 U/kg IV then 15–25 U/kg/h cont inf or 100 U/kg/dose q4h IV intermittent bolus
   Notes: Follow PTT, thrombin time, or activated clotting time to assess effectiveness; heparin has little effect on the prothrombin time; with proper dose PTT is about 1½–2 × the control; can cause thrombocytopenia, follow platelet counts

◼ Hepatitis A Vaccine (Havrix)
   Uses: High-risk exposure to hepatitis A (travelers, health care workers, etc)
   Dose: Adults. 1 mL IM, booster 6–12 mo. *Peds.* 0.5 mL IM day 1 and 30, booster 6–12 mo

◼ Hepatitis B Immune Globulin (HyperHep, H-BIG)
   Uses: Exposure to HBsAg-positive materials: blood, plasma, or serum (accidental needlestick, mucous membrane contact, oral ingestion)
   Dose: Adults & Peds. 0.06 mL/kg IM, 5 mL max; within 24 h of needlestick or percutaneous exposure; within 14 d of sexual contact; repeat at 1 and 6 mo after exposure
   Notes: Administered in gluteal or deltoid muscle; if exposure continues should receive hepatitis B vaccine

◼ Hepatitis B Vaccine (Engerix-B, Recombivax HB)
   Uses: Prevention of type B hepatitis in high-risk individuals
   Dose: Adults. 3 IM doses of 1 mL each, the first 2 given 1 mo apart, the third 6 mo after the first. *Peds.* 0.5 mL IM dose given on the same schedule as adults
   Notes: IM injs for adults and older peds to be administered in the deltoid; other peds to be administered in anterolateral thigh; may cause fever, inj site soreness; derived from recombinant DNA technology

■ Hetastarch (Hespan)
Uses: Plasma volume expansion as an adjunct in treatment of shock due to hemorrhage, surgery, burns, and other trauma
Dose: 500–1000 mL (do not exceed 1500 mL/d) IV at a rate not to exceed 20 mL/kg/h
Notes: Not a substitute for blood or plasma; Contra in patients with severe bleeding disorders, severe CHF, or renal failure with oliguria or anuria

■ Hydralazine (Apresoline)
Uses: Moderate to severe HTN
Dose: Adults. 10 mg PO qid, increase to 25 mg qid to a max of 300 mg/d. *Peds.* 0.75–3 mg/kg/24h PO ÷ q12–6h
Notes: Caution with impaired hepatic function, CAD; compensatory sinus tachycardia can be eliminated with the addition of propranolol; chronically high doses can cause SLE-like syndrome; SVT can occur following IM administration

■ Hydrochlorothiazide (HydroDIURIL, Esidrix, Others)
Uses: Edema, HTN, CHF
Dose: Adults. 25–100 mg PO qd in single or ÷ doses. *Peds.* 2–3 mg/kg/24h PO ÷ bid
Notes: Hypokalemia is frequent; hyperglycemia, hyperuricemia, hyper-lipidemia, and hyponatremia are common side effects

■ Hydrochlorothiazide and Amiloride (Moduretic)
Uses: HTN, adjunctive therapy for CHF
Dose: 1–2 tabs PO qd
Notes: Should not be given to diabetics or patients with renal failure

■ Hydrochlorothiazide and Spironolactone (Aldactazide)
Uses: Edema (CHF, cirrhosis), HTN
Dose: 1–8 tabs (25–200 mg each component per day) 1–2 ÷ doses

■ Hydrochlorothiazide and Triamterene (Dyazide, Maxzide)
Uses: Edema, HTN
Dose: Dyazide: 1–2 caps PO qd–bid. *Maxzide:* 1 tab PO qd
Notes: Can cause hyperkalemia as well as hypokalemia; follow serum potassium levels

■ Hydrocortisone
See Steroids, page 636, and Tables A–8 and A–33, pages 659 and 684.

■ Hydrocodone and acetaminophen (Lorcet, Vicodin, others) [C]

Uses: Moderate to severe pain; hydrocodone has antitussive properties
Dose: 1–2 PO q4–6h PRN
Notes: Many different combinations; specify hydrocodone/acetaminophen
Dose: 2.5/500, 5/400, 5/500, 7.5/400, 10/400, 7.5/500, 7.5/650, 7.5/750, 10/325, 10/400, 10/500, 10/650. Elixir and soln 2.5 mg hydrocodone/167 mg acetaminophen per 5 mL

■ Hydrocodone and aspirin (Lortab ASA, others) [C]

Uses: Moderate-to-severe pain
Dose: 1–2 PO q4–6h PRN
Notes: 5 mg hydrocodone/500 mg aspirin per tab

■ Hydrocodone and guaifenesin (Hycotuss expectorant, others) [C]

Uses: Nonproductive cough associated with respiratory infection
Dose: Adults & Peds. > 12 y: 5 mL q4h, pc and hs. *Peds. <2 y:* 0.3 mg/kg/d ÷ qid. 2–12 y, 2.5 mL q4h pc and hs

■ Hydrocodone and homatropine (Hycodan, others) [C]

Uses: Relief of cough
Dose: Adults. 5–10 mg q4–6h. *Peds.* 0.6 mg/kg/d ÷ tid–qid
Notes: Dose based on hydrocodone; syrup 5-mg hydrocodone/5 mL; tab 5-mg hydrocodone

■ Hydrocodone and ibuprofen (Vicoprofen) [C]

Uses: Moderate to severe pain (less than 10 d).
Dose: 1–2 tabs q4–6h PRN
Notes: 7.5 mg hydrocodone/200 mg ibuprofen/tab

■ Hydrocodone and pseudoephedrine (Entuss-D, Histussin-D, others) [C]

Uses: Cough and nasal congestion
Dose: 5 mL qid, PRN
Notes: 5-mg hydrocodone/5 mL

■ Hydrocodone, chlorpheniramine, phenylephrine, acetaminophen, and caffeine (Hycomine)

Uses: Cough and symptoms of upper respiratory infections
Dose: 1 PO, q4h, PRN
Notes: 5-mg hydrocodone/tab

Hydromorphone (Dilaudid) [C]
Uses: Moderate-to-severe pain. Narcotic analgesic
Dose: 1–4 mg PO, IM, IV, or PR q4–6h PRN; 3 mg PR q6–8h PRN; ↓ with hepatic failure
Notes: 1.5 mg IM equivalent to 10-mg morphine IM

Hydroxyurea (Hydrea)
Uses: Treatment of cervical and ovarian cancer, melanoma, and leukemia adjunct in sickle cell anemia
Dose: Continuous therapy: 20–30 mg/kg PO qd; intermittent therapy: 80 mg/kg every 3 d

Hydroxyzine (Atarax, Vistaril)
Uses: Anxiety, tension, sedation, itching
Dose: Adults. Anxiety or sedation: 50–100 mg PO or IM qid or PRN (max of 600 mg/d). *Itching:* 25–50 mg PO or IM tid–qid. *Peds.* 0.6–1.0 mg/kg/24h PO or IM q6h
Notes: Useful in potentiating the effects of narcotics; not for IV use; drowsiness, anticholinergic effects are common

Hyoscyamine (Anaspaz, Cystospaz, Levsin, others)
Uses: Spasm associated with GI and bladder disorders
Dose: Adults. 0.125–0.25 mg (1–2 tabs) SL 3–4 times a day, pc and hs; 1 cap q12h (SR [Cystospaz-M, Levsinex])

Hyoscyamine, atropine, scopolamine, and Phenobarbital (Donnatal, others)
Uses: Irritable bowel, spastic colitis, peptic ulcer, spastic bladder
Dose: 0.125–0.25 mg (1–2 tabs) tid–qid, 1 cap q12h (SR), 5–10 mL elixir tid–qid or q8h

Ibuprofen (Motrin, Rufen, Advil, Others)
Uses: Treatment of inflammatory conditions (RA, others) arthritis and pain, fever, gout, dysmenorrhea
Dose: Adults. Pain, fever, dysmenorrhea: 200–400 mg PO q4–6h, max 1.2 g/d; inflammatory conditions 400–800 mg bid–qid, max 3.2 g/d. *Peds.* 4–10 mg/kg/dose in 3–4 ÷ doses. *RA:* 30–50 mg/kg/d ÷ qid, max 2.4 g/d

Ibutilide (Covert)
Uses: ECC. rapid conversion of AF or flutter
Dose: <60 kg: 0.01 mg/kg (max 1 mg). *>60 kg:* 1 mg IV over 10 min. May be repeated once if needed 10 min later

Notes: Do not administer Class I or III antiarrhythmics concurrently or within 4 h of ibutilide inf

■ Idarubicin (Idamycin)
Uses: Treatment of leukemia
Dose: 12 mg/m^2 daily for 3 d
Notes: Do not administer if bilirubin is > 5 mg/dL

■ Ifosfamide (Ifex)
Uses: Testicular, breast, sarcoma, and ovarian cancer
Dose: 1.2 g/m^2/d for 5 consecutive days. Repeat course every 3 wk
Notes: Causes hemorrhagic cystitis; hydrate patients well and administer with MESNA

■ Imipenem/Cilastatin (Primaxin)
Uses: Serious infections caused by a wide variety of susceptible bacteria; multiresistant infections, inactive against *S aureus,* group A and B streptococci, and others; empiric therapy of gram-negative sepsis in immunocompromised host
Dose: Adults. 250–500 mg (Imipenem) IV q6h. *Peds. < 3 y:* 100 mg/kg/24h IV ÷ q6h. *> 3 y:* 60 mg/kg/24h IV ÷ q6h
Notes: Seizures may occur if drug accumulates; adjust dose for renal insufficiency to avoid drug accumulation if CrCl < 70 mL/min

■ Imipramine (Tofranil)
Uses: Depression, enuresis
Dose: Adults. Hospitalized for severe depression: Start at 100 mg/24h PO or IV in ÷ doses, increase over several weeks to 250–300 mg/24h. *Outpatient:* 50–150 mg PO qhs not to exceed 200 mg/24h. *Peds. Antidepressant:* 1.5–5.0 mg/kg/24h ÷ tid. *Enuresis:* 10–25 mg PO qhs; ↑ by 10–25 mg at 1–2-wk intervals, treat for 2–3 mo, then taper
Notes: Do NOT use with MAO inhibitors; less sedation than amitriptyline

■ Immune Globulin IV (Gamimune N, Sandoglobulin, Gammar IV)
Uses: IgG antibody deficiency diseases (congenital agammaglobulinemia, common variable hypogammaglobulinemia; ITP
Dose: Adults & Peds. Immunodeficiency: 100–200 mg/kg IV monthly rate of 0.01–0.04 mL/kg/min to a max of 400 mg/kg/dose. *ITP:* 400 mg/kg/dose IV qd for 5 d. *BMT:* 500 mg/kg/wk
Notes: Adverse effects associated mostly with rate of infusion.

■ Indapamide (Lozol)
Uses: HTN, CHF.
Dose: 2.5–5.0 mg PO qd
Notes: Doses > than 5 mg do not have additional effects on lowering BP

■ Indinavir (Crixivan)
Uses: HIV infection as part of a two-drug (nucleosidase plus protease inhibitor) or three-drug (two nucleosidases plus protease inhibitor) treatment.
Dose: 800 mg PO q8h

■ Indomethacin (Indocin)
Uses: Arthritis and closure of the ductus arteriosus
Dose: Adults. 25–50 mg PO bid–tid, 200 mg/d max. *Infants:* 0.2–0.25 mg/kg/dose IV; may be repeated in 12–24 h for up to 3 doses
Notes: Monitor renal function

■ Infliximab (Remicade)
Uses: Treatment of moderate-to-severe Crohn's disease
Dose: 5 mg/kg IV inf, subsequent doses 2 and 6 wk after initial inf
Notes: May cause hypersensitivity reaction, made up of human constant and murine variable regions

■ Influenza Vaccine (Fluzone, FluShield, Fluvirin)
Uses: Prevent influenza in high-risk (chronic medical conditions, eg, heart disease, lung disease, or diabetes; with asthma; residents of chronic care facilities; any person > 50 y); health care workers or members of households who come into contact with these patients
Dose: Adults. 0.5 mL/dose IM. Optimal in the U.S. is Oct–Nov, protection begins 1–2 wk after and lasts up to 6 mo
Notes: Each year, specific vaccines manufactured based on predictions of the strains to be active in flu season (Dec–spring in U.S.). Whole or split virus usually given to adults; give peds < 13 y split virus or purified surface antigen form to ↓ febrile reactions

■ Insulins
Uses: DM that cannot be controlled by diet or oral hypoglycemic agents
Dose: Based on serum glucose levels; usually given SQ can also be given IV or IM (only regular insulin can be given IV) (See Table A–7, page 659). *General guidelines:* 0.5–1U/kg/d, ⅔ dose before breakfast, ⅓ before supper; adjust based on blood sugars over several days. Regular or rapid insulin should be dosed q4–6h, NPH or intermediate q8–12h. *Ketoacidosis:* Hydrate patient well with NS, 10 U regular insulin IV followed by inf 0.1 U/kg/h; optimum serum. *Glucose decline:* 50–100 mg/dL/h

Notes: The highly purified insulins provide an increase in free insulin; monitor these patients closely for several weeks when changing doses; most standard insulins 100 U/mL

■ Interferon Alpha (Roferon-A, Intron A)
Uses: Hairy cell leukemia, Kaposi's sarcoma, multiple myeloma, chronic myelogenous leukemia, renal cell carcinoma, bladder cancer, melanoma, and chronic hepatitis C
Dose: Alfa-2a (Roferon): 3 million IU daily for 16–24 wk SQ or IM. *Alfa-2b (Intron)*: 2 million IU/m^2 IM or SQ 3 ×/wk for 2–6 mo; intravesical 50–100 million IU in 50 mL NS weekly × 6
Notes: Systemic use may cause flu-like symptoms; fatigue is common; anorexia occurs in 20–30% of patients; neurotoxicity may occur at high doses; neutralizing antibodies can occur in up to 40% of patients receiving prolonged systemic therapy

■ Interferon Alpha and Ribavirin (Roferon-A, Intron A, Rebetron)
Uses: Chronic hepatitis C
Dose: Intron A: 3 million IU SQ 3 × with rebetol 1000–1200 mg ÷ PO bid for 24 wk
Notes: Supplied in combination with multidose pen injector for Intron A

■ Interferon Alfacon-1 (Infergen)
Uses: Management of chronic hepatitis C
Dose: 9 µg SQ 3 ×/wk
Notes: At least 48 h should elapse between injs

■ Ipecac Syrup
Uses: Treatment of drug overdose and certain cases of poisoning
Dose: Adults. 15–30 mL PO followed by 200–300 mL water; if no emesis occurs in 20 min, may repeat × 1. *Peds. 6–12 mo:* 5–10 mL PO followed by water. *1–12 y:* 15 mL PO followed by water
Notes: Do NOT use for ingestion of petroleum distillates, strong acid, base, or other corrosive or caustic agents; NOT for use in comatose or unconscious patients; caution in CNS depressant overdose

■ Ipratropium Bromide Inhalant (Atrovent)
Uses: Bronchospasm associated with COPD
Dose: Adults and children > 12 y: 2–4 puffs qid
Notes: Not for initial treatment of acute episodes of bronchospasm

■ Irbesartan (Avapro)
Uses: Treatment of HTN
Dose: 150 mg PO daily, may increased to 300 mg daily

■ Iron Dextran (Dexferrum)
Uses: Iron deficiency when oral supplementation is not possible
Dose: Based on estimate of iron deficiency (see package insert)
Notes: Must give a test dose because anaphylaxis is common (adult 0.5 mL, infants 0.25 mL; may be given deep IM using "Z-track" technique although IV route most preferred

■ Isoetharine (Bronkosol, Bronkometer)
Uses: Bronchial asthma and reversible bronchospasm
Dose: Adults & Peds. Nebulization: 0.25–1.0 mL diluted 1:3 with saline q4–6h. *Metered dose inhaler:* 1–2 inhals q4h

■ Isoniazid (INH)
Uses: Treatment of *Mycobacterium* sp infections
Dose: Adults. Active TB: 5 mg/kg/24h PO or IM qd (usually 300 mg/d). *Prophylaxis:* 300 mg PO qd for 6–12 mo. **Peds.** *Active TB:* 10–20 mg/kg/24h PO or IM qd to a max of 300 mg/d. *Prophylaxis:* 10 mg/kg/24h PO qd
Notes: Can cause severe hepatitis; given with other antituberculous drugs for active tuberculosis; IM route rarely used; to prevent peripheral neuropathy can give pyridoxine 50–100 mg/d

■ Isoproterenol (Isuprel, Medihaler-Iso)
Uses: Shock, cardiac arrest, AV nodal block, antiasthmatic. **ECC.** Refractory torsades de pointes unresponsive to magnesium sulfate. Temporary control of bradycardia in heart transplant patients. Class IIb at low doses for symptomatic bradycardias
Dose: Adults. Shock: 1–4 mg/min IV inf, titrated to effect. *AV nodal block:* 20–60 mg IV push; may repeat q3–5 min; 1–5 mg/min IV maint. *Inhal:* 1–2 inhals 4–6 ×/d.
ECC. 2–10 µg/min. Titrate to effect. **Peds. ECC.** 0.1–1.5 mg/kg/min IV inf, titrated to effect. *Inhal:* 1–2 inhals 4–6 ×/d
Notes: *Contraindications:* Tachycardia; pulse > 130 bpm may induce ventricular arrhythmias

■ Isosorbide Dinitrate (Isordil)
Uses: Angina pectoris.
Dose: *Acute angina:* 2.5–10.0 mg PO (chewable tab) or SL PRN q5–10 min; >3 doses should not be given in 15–30-min period. *Angina prophylaxis:* 5–60 mg PO tid

Notes: Nitrates should not be given on chronic q6h or qid basis because of development of tolerance; can cause headaches; usually need to give a higher oral dose to achieve same results as with sublingual forms

■ Isosorbide Monohydrate (ISMO)
Uses: Prevention of angina pectoris
Dose: 20 mg PO bid, with the 2 doses given 7 h apart or ER 30–120 mg PO qd

■ Isradipine (DynaCirc)
Uses: HTN
Dose: 2.5–5.0 mg PO bid

■ Itraconazole (Sporanox)
Uses: Treatment of systemic fungal infections caused by *Aspergillus, Blastomyces,* and *Histoplasma*
Dose: 200 mg PO or IV qd–bid
Notes: Administer with meals or cola; should not be used concurrently with H_2-antagonist, omeprazole, antacids

■ Japanese encephalitis vaccine (JE-VAX)
Uses: Active immunization against Japanese encephalitis
Dose: Peds > 3 y and *Adults.* 3 doses (1 mL) SQ days 0, 7, and 30; booster 2 y after primary series. *Peds* 1–3 y: 3 doses (0.5 mL) schedule as above
Notes: Recommended if > 1 mo in endemic areas

■ Kaolin-Pectin (Kaopectate)
Uses: Treatment of diarrhea
Dose: Adults. 60–120 mL PO after each loose stool or q3–4h PRN. *Peds. 3–6 y:* 15–30 mL/dose PO PRN. *6–12 y:* 30–60 mL/dose PO PRN

■ Ketamine (Ketalar) [C]
Uses: Short-acting anesthesia, short surgical procedures, dressing changes
Dose: Adults. 3–8 mg/kg IM or 1–4.5 mg/kg IV. *Induction dosage:* 1–2 mg/kg. *Peds.* 3–7 mg/kg IM or 0.5–2 mg/kg IV, use smaller doses (0.5–1 mg/kg) for sedation for minor procedures. *Maint: Adults & Peds.* ⅓–½ of initial dose

■ Ketoconazole (Nizoral)
Uses: Systemic fungal infections: candidiasis, chronic mucocutaneous candidiasis, blastomycosis, coccidioidomycosis, histoplasmosis, and paracoccid-

ioidomycosis; topical cream for localized fungal infections due to dermatophytes and yeast; rapid short-term treatment of prostate cancer where rapid reduction of testosterone is needed (ie, spinal cord compression)

Dose: Adults. *Oral:* 200 mg PO qd; increase to 400 mg PO qd for very serious infections; prostate cancer 400 mg PO tid (short term). *Topical:* Apply to affected area once daily. **Peds.** 3.3–6.6 mg/kg/24h PO qd

Notes: Associated with severe hepatotoxicity; monitor LFTs closely throughout course of therapy; drug interaction with any agent increasing gastric pH preventing absorption of ketoconazole; may enhance oral anticoagulants; may react with alcohol to produce disulfiram-like reaction

■ Ketoprofen (Orudis)
Uses: Treatment of arthritis and pain
Dose: 25–75 mg PO tid–qid, to a max of 300 mg/d

■ Ketorolac (Toradol)
Uses: Treatment of arthritis and pain
Dose: 15–30 mg IV/IM q6h or 10 mg PO qid
Notes: Do NOT use for longer than 5 d

■ Ketorolac (Acular Ophthalmic)
Uses: Itching associated with seasonal allergic conjunctivitis
Dose: 1 gt in eye(s) qid

■ Ketotifen (Zaditor)
Uses: Ophthalmic antihistamine, H1 blocker
Dose: Allergic conjunctivitis. **Adults.** 1 ggt in eye/s q8–12h

■ Labetalol (Trandate, Normodyne) (see Cover)
Uses: HTN, hypertensive emergencies **ECC.** see Esmolol, page 568
Dose: Adults. *HTN:* Initially, 100 mg PO bid; then 200–400 mg PO bid. *Hypertensive emergency:* 20–80 mg IV bolus, then 2 mg/min IV inf, titrated to effect. **ECC.** 10 mg IV push over 1–2 min; Repeat or double dose every 10 min (150 mg max); or initial bolus, then 2–8 µg/min. **Peds.** *Oral:* 3–20 mg/kg/d in ÷ doses. *Hypertensive emergency:* 0.4–3 mg/kg/h IV cont inf

■ Lactobacillus (Lactinex Granules)
Uses: Control of diarrhea, especially after antibiotic therapy
Dose: Adults & Peds > 3 y: 1 packet, 2 caps, or 4 tabs with meals or liquids tid

■ Lactulose (Chronulac, Cephulac)
Uses: Hepatic encephalopathy; laxative; constipation
Dose: Adults. Acute hepatic encephalopathy: 30–45 mL PO q1h until soft stools are observed, then tid–qid. *Chronic laxative therapy:* 30–45 mL PO tid–qid; adjust the dose every 1–2 d to produce 2–3 soft stools qd. *Rectally:* 200 g diluted with 700 mL of water instilled into the rectum. *Peds. Infants:* 2.5–10 mL/24h ÷ tid–qid. *Children:* 40–90 mL/24h ÷ tid–qid
Notes: Can cause severe diarrhea

■ Lamivudine (Epivir, Epivir-HBV)
Uses: Treatment of HIV infection when therapy is warranted based on clinical and/or immunologic evidence of disease progression, and chronic hepatitis B
Dose: HIV: Adults & Peds >12 y: 150 mg PO bid. *Peds* <12 y: 4 mg/kg twice daily. *HBV:* 100 mg/d
Notes: Used in combination with zidovudine; use with caution in pediatric patients because of an increased incidence of pancreatitis

■ Lamotrigine (Lamictal)
Uses: Treatment of partial seizures
Dose: Adults. Initially 50 mg PO qd, then 50 mg PO bid for 2 wk, then maint 300–500 mg/d ÷ bid. *Peds.* 0.15 mg/kg in 1–2 ÷ doses for week 1 and 2, then 0.3 mg/kg for weeks 3 and 4, then maint dose of 1 mg/kg/d in 1–2 ÷ doses
Notes: May cause rash and photosensitivity; the value of therapeutic monitoring has not been established

■ Lansoprazole (Prevacid)
Uses: Treatment of duodenal ulcers, *H pylori* infection, erosive esophagitis, and hypersecretory conditions
Dose: 15–30 mg/d PO

■ Latanoprost (Xalatan)
Uses: Glaucoma that does not respond to standard therapies
Dose: 1 gt eye(s) qhs
Notes: May darken light irides

■ Leflunomide (Arava)
Uses: Treatment of active RA
Dose: 100 mg PO once daily for 3 d, followed by 10–20 mg/d
Notes: Pregnancy category X-DO NOT USE; monitor ALT

■ Lepirudin (Refludan)
Uses: Management of heparin-induced thrombocytopenia
Dose: Bolus of 0.4 mg/kg IV, followed by 0.15 mg/kg cont inf
Notes: Monitor aPTT 4 h into initial inf and at least daily; adjust dose based on aPTT ratio; maintain aPTT ratio of 1.5–2.0

■ Leucovorin Calcium (Wellcovorin)
Uses: Overdoses of folic acid antagonist
Dose: **Adults & Peds.** *Methotrexate rescue:* 10–100 mg/m^2/dose IV or PO q3–6h. *Adjunct to antimicrobials:* 5–10 mg PO qd
Notes: Many dosing schedules exist for Leucovorin rescue following methotrexate therapy

■ Leuprolide (Lupron Depot)
Uses: Treatment of prostate cancer, endometriosis, and central precocious puberty (CPP)
Dose: **Adults.** *Prostate:* 7.5 mg IM monthly of depot, 22.5 mg 3-mo depot or 30 mg 4-mo depot. *Endometriosis (depot only):* 3.75 mg IM as a single monthly dose. **Peds.** CPP: 50 mg/kg/d SQ inj; titrate ↑ by 10 mg/kg/d until total down regulation is achieved. *Depot:* <25 kg: 7.5 mg IM every 4 wk. 25–37.5 kg: 11.25 mg IM every 4 wk. >37.5 kg: 15 mg IM every 4 wk

■ Levalbuterol (Xopenex)
Uses: Treatment and prevention of bronchospasm
Dose: 0.63 mg nebulized every 6–8 h
Notes: Therapeutically active R-isomer of albuterol

■ Levamisole (Ergamisol)
Uses: Adjuvant therapy of node-positive colon cancer (in combination with 5-FU)
Dose: 50 mg PO q8h for 3 d every 14 d during 5-FU therapy
Notes: Toxicity includes nausea and vomiting, diarrhea, abdominal pain, taste disturbance, anorexia, hyperbilirubinemia, disulfiram-like reaction on alcohol ingestion, minimal bone marrow depression, fatigue, fever, and conjunctivitis

■ Levetiracetam (Kappra)
Uses: Treatment of partial onset seizures
Dose: 500 mg PO bid, may be increased to a max of 3000 mg/d
Notes: May cause dizziness and somnolence; may impair coordination

Levobunol (Betagan Liquifilm Ophthalmic, others)
Uses: Glaucoma
Dose: 1–2 gtt in eye(s) bid.

Levocabastine (Livostin)
Uses: Allergic seasonal conjunctivitis
Dose: 1 gt in eye(s) qid up to 4 wk

Levofloxacin (Levaquin)
Uses: Treatment of lower respiratory tract infections, sinusitises, and UTIs
Dose: 250–500 mg/d PO or IV
Notes: Reliable activity against *S pneumoniae,* drug interactions with cation-containing products

Levonorgestrel Implants (Norplant)
Uses: Prevention of pregnancy
Dose: Implant 6 caps in the midforearm
Notes: Prevents pregnancy for up to 5 y; caps may be removed if pregnancy is desired

Levorphanol (Levo-Dromoran) [C]
Uses: Moderate-to-severe pain
Dose: 2 mg PO or SQ PRN

Levothyroxine (Synthroid)
Uses: Hypothyroidism
Dose: Adults. 25–50 mg/d PO or IV initially; increase by 25–50 mg/d every mo. *Usual dose:* 100–200 mg/d. **Peds.** 0–1 y: 8–10 mg/kg/24h PO or IV qd. *1–5 y:* 4–6 mg/kg/24h PO or IV qd. *>5 y:* 3–4 mg/kg/24h PO or IV qd
Notes: Titrate dose based on clinical response and thyroid function tests; dose can be increased more rapidly in young to middle-aged patients

Lidocaine (Xylocaine)
Uses: Local anesthesia; treatment of cardiac arrhythmias, ***ECC.*** Cardiac arrest from VF/VT. Stable VT, wide-complex tachycardias of uncertain type, wide-complex PSVT
Dose: Adults. Arrhythmias: 1 mg/kg (50–100 mg) IV bolus, then 2–4 mg/min IV infusion, should repeat bolus after 5 min. Local anesthesia: Infiltrate a few mL of a 0.5–1.0% soln max 3 mg/kg/dose (See Table A–22, page 675). ***ECC.*** *Cardiac arrest from VF/VT:* Initial *dose:* 1.0–1.5 mg/kg IV. *Refractory VF:* May give additional 0.5–0.75 mg/kg IV push, repeat in 5–10 min, max total dose is 3 mg/kg. A single dose of 1.5 mg/kg IV in cardiac arrest is acceptable.

Endotracheal administration: 2–4 mg/kg. *Perfusing arrhythmia:* Stable VT, wide complex tachycardia or uncertain type, significant ectopy: 1.0–1.5 mg/kg IV push. Repeat 0.5–0.75 mg/kg q5–10 min; max total dose, 3 mg/kg. *Main inf:* 1–4 mg/min (30–50 μg/min). **Peds.** *Arrhythmias:* 1 mg/kg dose IV bolus, then 20–50 mg/kg/min IV infusion. *Local anesthetic:* Infiltrate a few mL of a 0.5–1.0% soln, with a max of 3 mg/kg/dose

Notes: Epinephrine may be added for local anesthesia to prolong effect and help decrease bleeding; for IV forms, dose reduction is required with liver disease, CHF; dizziness, paresthesias, and convulsions are associated with toxicity

■ Lidocaine 5%/(ELA-Max)
Uses: Topical anesthetic: Adjunct to phlebotomy or invasive dermal procedures

Dose: Apply a ¼ in. thick layer to intact skin at least 30 min before procedure; do not apply over area larger than 100 cm² in children

■ Lidocaine/Prilocaine (EMLA)
Uses: Topical anesthetic; adjunct to phlebotomy or invasive dermal procedures

Dose: Adults. *EMLA cream and anesthetic disc (1 g/10 cm²):* Thick layer of cream 2–2.5 g applied to intact skin, cover with an occlusive dressing (Tegaderm) for at least 1 h. *Anesthetic disc:* 1 g per 10 cm² for at least 1 h. **Peds.** *Max dose ≤ to 3 mo or < 5 kg:* 1 g/10 cm² for 1 h. *3–12 mo and > 5 kg:* 2 g/20 cm² for 4 h. *1–6 y and > 10 kg:* 10 g per 100 cm² for 4 h. *7–12 y and > 20 kg:* 20 g/200 cm² for 4 h

Notes: Longer contact time gives greater effect

■ Lindane (Kwell)
Uses: Head lice, crab lice, scabies

Dose: Adults & Peds. *Cream or lotion:* Apply thin layer after bathing and leave in place for 24h; pour on laundry. *Shampoo:* Apply 30 mL and develop lather with warm water for 4 min; comb out nits

Notes: Caution with overuse, may be absorbed into blood; wash clothing and bedding as well

■ Linezolid (Zyvox)
Uses: Infections caused by gram-positive bacteria, including vancomycin-resistant and methicillin-resistant strains

Dose: 400–600 mg IV or PO q12h

Notes: A reversible, inhibitor of MAO; therefore avoid foods that contain tyramine; avoid cough and cold products containing pseudoephedrine or phenylpropanolamine

Lepirudin (Refludan)
Uses: Heparin-induced thrombocytopenia
Dose: Bolus 0.4 mg/kg IV, then 0.15 mg/kg inf; ↓ dose and rate if CrCl < 60 mL/min
Notes: Adjust dose based on aPTT; maintain aPTT ratio of 1.5–2.0

Loxapine (Loxitane)
Uses: Psychotic disorders
Dose: 10 mg PO bid, ↑ until symptoms controlled; range 60–100 mg/d ÷ doses bid–qid; 250 mg/d. *Max:* 12.5–50 mg IM q4–6h, change to PO ASAP

Liothyronine (Cytomel)
Uses: Hypothyroidism
Dose: Adults. Initially 25 mg/24h, then titration q1–2 wk according to clinical response and thyroid function tests to maint of 25–75 mg PO qd. *Peds.* Initially 5 mg/24h, then titration by 5 mg/24h increments at 1–2-wk intervals. *Maint:* 25–75 mg/24h PO qd
Notes: Reduce dose in elderly patients; monitor thyroid function test

Lisinopril (Prinivil, Zestril)
Uses: Treatment of HTN, heart failure, and AMI. *ECC.* Improve outcome after MI
Dose: 5–40 mg/24h PO qd–bid. *ECC.* AMI 5 mg within 24 h of MI, then 5 mg after 24 h, 10 mg after 48 h, then 10 mg qd.
Notes: Dizziness, headache, and cough are common side effects; DO NOT use in pregnancy

Lithium Carbonate (Eskalith, others)
Uses: Manic episodes of manic–depressive illness; maint therapy in recurrent disease
Dose: Acute mania: 600 mg PO tid or 900 mg slow release bid. *Maint:* 300 mg PO tid–qid
Notes: Dose must be titrated; follow serum levels (Table A–22, page 675); common side effects are polyuria, tremor. Contra in patients with severe renal impairment; sodium retention or diuretic use may potentate toxicity.

Lodoxamide (Alomide Ophthalmic)
Uses: Seasonal allergic conjunctivitis
Dose: Adults & Peds > 2 y: 1–2 gtt in eye(s) qid up to 3 mo

Lomefloxacin (Maxaquin)
Uses: Treatment of UTI and lower respiratory tract infections caused by gram-negative bacteria; prophylaxis in transurethral procedures

Dose: 400 mg PO qd
Notes: May cause severe photosensitivity

■ Loperamide (Imodium)
Uses: Diarrhea
Dose: Adults. 4 mg PO initially, then 2 mg after each loose stool, up to 16 mg/d. *Peds.* 0.4–0.8 mg/kg/24h PO ÷ q6–12h until diarrhea resolves or for 7 d max
Notes: Do NOT use in acute diarrhea caused by *Salmonella, Shigella,* or *Clostridium difficile*

■ Loracarbef (Lorabid)
Uses: Treatment of infections caused by susceptible bacteria involving the upper and lower respiratory tract, skin, bone, urinary tract, abdomen and gynecologic system
Dose: Adults. 200–400 mg PO bid. *Peds.* 7.5–15 mg/kg/d PO ÷ bid
Notes: Has more gram-negative activity then first-generation cephalosporins

■ Loratadine (Claritin)
Uses: Treatment of allergic rhinitis
Dose: 10 mg/d PO
Notes: Take on empty stomach

■ Lorazepam (Ativan, Alzapam) [C]
Uses: Anxiety and anxiety mixed with depression; preop sedation; control of status epilepticus
Dose: Adults. Anxiety: 0.5–1.0 mg PO bid–tid. *Preop:* 0.05 mg/kg up to max of 4 mg IM 2 h before surgery. *Insomnia:* 2–4 mg PO qhs. *Status epilepticus:* 2.5–10 mg/dose IV repeated at 15–20-min interval PRN. *Peds. Status epilepticus:* 0.05 mg/kg/dose IV repeated at 15–20-min interval PRN
Notes: Decrease dose in elderly patients; may take up to 10 min to see effect when given IV

■ Losartan (Cozaar)
Uses: Treatment of HTN
Dose: 25–50 mg PO qd–bid
Notes: Do NOT use in pregnancy; symptomatic hypotension may occur in patients on diuretics

■ Lovastatin (Mevacor)
Uses: Adjunct to diet for the reduction of elevated total and LDL cholesterol levels in patients with primary hypercholesterolemia (types IIa and IIb)

Dose: 20 mg/d PO with evening meal; increase at 4-wk intervals to max 80 mg/d

Notes: Patient should be maintained on standard cholesterol-lowering diet throughout treatment; monitor LFTs every 6 wk during first year of therapy; headache and GI intolerance common

■ Magaldrate (Riopan, Lowsium)

Uses: Hyperacidity associated with peptic ulcer; gastritis, and hiatal hernia
Dose: 1–2 tabs PO or 5–10 mL PO between meals and hs
Notes: Less than 0.3 mg sodium/tab or teaspoon; do NOT use in renal insufficiency

■ Magnesium Citrate

Uses: Vigorous bowel prep; constipation
Dose: Adults. 120–240 mL PO PRN. *Peds.* 0.5 mL/kg/dose, up to max 200 mL PO
Notes: Do NOT use in renal insufficiency, intestinal obstruction

■ Magnesium Hydroxide (Milk of Magnesia)

Uses: Constipation
Dose: Adults. 15–30 mL PO PRN. *Peds.* 0.5 mL/kg/dose PO PRN
Notes: Do NOT use in renal insufficiency or intestinal obstruction

■ Magnesium Oxide (Uro-Mag, Mag-Ox 400, Maox)

Uses: Replacement for low plasma levels
Dose: 400–800 mg/d ÷ qd–qid
Notes: May cause diarrhea

■ Magnesium Sulfate

Uses: Replacement for low plasma levels; refractory hypokalemia and hypocalcemia; preeclampsia and premature labor. *ECC.* Cardiac arrest associated with torsades de pointes or suspected hypomagnesemic state. Refractory VF. Life-threatening ventricular arrhythmias due to digitalis toxicity, tricyclic overdose. Consider prophylactic administration in hospitalized patients with AMI

Dose: Adults. Supplement: 1–2 g IM or IV; repeat dosing based on response and continued hypomagnesemia. *Preeclampsia, premature labor:* 1–4 g/h IV infusion. *ECC. Cardiac arrest:* 1–2 g IV push (2–4 mL of a 50% soln) diluted in 10 mL of D_5W. *AMI:* Load: 1–2 g, mixed in 50–100 mL of D_5W, over 5–60 min IV. Follow with 0.5–1.0 g/h IV for up to 24 h. *Torsades de pointes:* Load: 1–2 g mixed in 50–100 mL of D_5W, over 5–60 min IV. Follow with 1–4 g/h IV (titrate dose to control the torsades). *Peds.* 25–50 mg/kg/dose IM or IV q4–6h for 3–4 doses; may repeat if hypomagnesemia persists
Notes: Reduce dose with low urine output or renal insufficiency

◼ Mannitol

Uses: Osmotic diuresis (cerebral edema, oliguria, anuria, myoglobinuria, etc), bowel prep. **ECC.** Increased intracranial pressure in management of neurologic emergencies

Dose: Adults. *Diuresis:* 0.2 g/kg/dose IV over 3–5 min; if no diuresis within 2 h, discontinue. **ECC.** 0.5–1.0 g/kg over 5–10 min. Additional doses of 0.25–2g/kg can be given q4–6h as needed. Use in conjugation with oxygenation and ventilation. **Peds.** *Diuresis:* 0.75 g/kg/dose IV over 3–5 min; if no diuresis within 2 h, discontinue. **Adults & Peds.** *Cerebral edema:* 0.25 g/kg/dose IV push repeated at 5-min intervals PRN; ↑ incrementally to 1 g/kg per dose PRN intracranial HTN

Notes: Caution with CHF or volume overload

◼ Maprotiline (Ludiomil)

Uses: Depressive neurosis; manic–depressive illness; major depressive disorder; anxiety associated with depression

Dose: 75–150 mg/d qhs, max of 300 mg/d

Notes: Contra with MAO inhibitors or seizure history; for patients > 60 y, give only 50–75 mg/d; anticholinergic side effects

◼ Measles, Mumps and Rubella Vaccine [MMR] M-M-R II

Uses: Measles, mumps, and rubella prophylaxis

Dose: Peds 15 mo: SQ in outer aspect of the upper arm

◼ Meclizine (Antivert)

Uses: Motion sickness, vertigo associated with diseases of the vestibular system

Dose: Adults & Peds > 12 y: 25 mg PO tid–qid PRN

Notes: Drowsiness, dry mouth, blurred vision commonly occur

◼ Medroxyprogesterone (Provera, Depot Provera, Others)

Uses: Secondary amenorrhea and abnormal uterine bleeding owing to hormonal imbalance, endometrial cancer, contraceptive

Dose: *Secondary amenorrhea:* 5–10 mg PO qd for 5–10 d. Abnormal uterine bleeding: 5–10 mg PO qd for 5–10 d beginning on the 16th or 21st d of menstrual cycle. *Endometrial cancer:* 400–1000 mg IM/wk

Notes: Contra with past thromboembolic disorders or with hepatic disease

◼ Megestrol Acetate (Megace)

Uses: Treatment of breast and endometrial cancer; appetite stimulation in cancer and HIV-related cachexia

Dose: Cancer: 40–320 mg/d PO in ÷ doses. *Appetite stimulant:* 80 mg PO qid

Meloxicam (Mobic)
Uses: Treatment of osteoarthritis
Dose: 7.5–15 mg/d PO

Melphalan (Alkeran)
Uses: Treatment of breast and ovarian cancer, and multiple myeloma
Dose: 6 mg/d PO as single dose or 16 mg/m^2 IV every 2 wk for 4 doses
Notes: Monitor blood counts closely

Meperidine (Demerol) [C]
Uses: Relief of moderate-to-severe pain
Dose: Adults. 50–100 mg PO or IM q3–4h PRN. *Peds.* 1–1.5 mg/kg/dose PO or IM q3–4h PRN
Notes: 75 mg IM equivalent to 10-mg morphine IM; beware of respiratory depression. A useful preprocedure sedative, particularly in children, is a so-called cardiac cocktail, consisting of 30 mg Demerol, 6.25 mg Thorazine, and 6.25 mg Phenergan (per 30-lb body weight) given IM

Mepivacaine (Carbocaine, Isocaine, Polocaine)
Uses: Local anesthesia by nerve block; infiltration in dental procedures
Dose: See Table A–32, page 683

Meprobamate (Equanil, Miltown) [C]
Uses: Short-term relief of anxiety
Dose: 200–400 mg PO tid–qid; sustained release 400–800 mg PO bid
Notes: May cause drowsiness

Mercaptopurine (Purinethol)
Uses: Treatment of leukemia
Dose: Adults & Peds. 2.5 mg/kg/d PO

Meropenem (Merrem)
Uses: Serious infections caused by a wide variety of bacteria including intraabdominal and polymicrobial; bacterial meningitis
Dose: Adults. 1 g IV q8h. *Peds.* 20–40 mg/kg IV q8h
Notes: Adjust dose for renal function; less seizure potential than imipenem

Mesalamine (Rowasa, Asacol, Pentasa)
Uses: Treatment of mild-to-moderate distal ulcerative colitis, proctosigmoiditis, or proctitis

Dose: Retention enema hs daily or insert 1 suppository bid. *Oral:* 800–1000 mg PO tid–qid

■ Mesna (Mesnex)

Uses: Reduce the incidence of ifosfamide-induced hemorrhagic cystitis
Dose: 20% of the ifosfamide dose (+/-) IV at the time of ifosfamide inf and 4 and 8 h after, for a total dose equal to 60% of the ifosfamide dose

■ Mesoridazine (Serentil)

Uses: Schizophrenia; acute and chronic alcoholism; chronic brain syndrome
Dose: 25–50 mg PO or IV tid initially; titrate to max of 300–400 mg/d
Notes: Low incidence of extrapyramidal side effects

■ Metaproterenol (Alupent, Metaprel)

Uses: Bronchodilator for asthma and reversible bronchospasm
Dose: **Adults.** *Inhal:* 1–3 inhals q3–4h to max of inhals 12/24 h; allow at least 2 min between inhals. *Oral:* 20 mg q6–8h. **Peds.** *Inhal:* 0.5 mg/kg/dose up to max of 15 mg/dose inhaled q4–6h by nebulizer or 1–2 puffs q4–6h. **Peds.** *Oral:* 0.3–0.5 mg/kg/dose q6–8h
Notes: Fewer β-1 effects than isoproterenol and longer acting

■ Metaraminol (Aramine)

Uses: Prevention and treatment of hypotension due to spinal anesthesia
Dose: **Adults.** *Prevention:* 2–10 mg IM q10–15min PRN. *Treatment:* 0.5–5 mg IV bolus followed by IV inf of 1–4 mg/kg/min titrated to effect. **Peds.** *Prevention:* 0.1 mg/kg/dose IM PRN. *Treatment:* 0.01 mg/kg IV bolus followed by IV inf of 5 mg/kg/min titrated to effect
Notes: Allow 10 min for max effect; employ other shock management techniques such as fluid resuscitation as needed; may cause cardiac arrhythmias

■ Metaxalone (Skelaxin)

Uses: Relief of painful musculoskeletal conditions
Dose: 800 mg PO tid–qid

■ Metformin (Glucophage)

Uses: Treatment of non-insulin-dependent DM
Dose: Initial dose of 500 mg PO bid; may be increased to a max daily dose of 2500 mg
Notes: Administer with the morning and evening meals; may cause lactic acidosis; do not use if the creatinine is > 1.3 in females or > 1.4 in males

■ Methadone (Dolophine) [C]
Uses: Severe pain; detoxification and maint of narcotic addiction
Dose: Adults. 2.5–10 mg IM q8h or 5–15 mg PO q8h (titrate as needed). ***Peds.*** 0.7 mg/kg/24h PO or IM ÷ q8h
Notes: Equianalgesic with parenteral morphine; long half-life; increase dose slowly to avoid respiratory depression

■ Methenamine (Hiprex, Urex, others)
Uses: Suppression or elimination of bacteriuria associated with chronic and recurrent infections of the urinary tract
Dose: *Initial:* bid–qid. *Maint:* 2–4 tabs/d in ÷ doses
Notes: Contra in patients with renal insufficiency, severe hepatic disease, and severe dehydration

■ Methimazole (Tapazole)
Uses: Hyperthyroidism; preparation for thyroid surgery or radiation
Dose: Adults. Initial: 15–60 mg/d PO ÷ tid. Maint: 5–15 mg PO qd. ***Peds.*** Initial: 0.4–0.7 mg/kg/24h PO ÷ tid. Maint: 0.2 mg/kg/d ÷ tid
Notes: Follow patient clinically and with thyroid function tests

■ Methocarbamol (Robaxin)
Uses: Relief of discomfort associated with painful musculoskeletal conditions.
Dose: Adults. 1.5 g PO qid for 2–3 d, then 1 g PO qid maint therapy; IV form rarely indicated. ***Peds.*** 60 mg/kg/24h PO ÷ qid
Notes: Can discolor urine; may cause drowsiness or GI upset; Contra with myasthenia gravis

■ Methohexital (Brevital)
Common Uses: Deep procedural sedation
Dose: 0.75 mg/kg IVP in adults; 20 mg/kg PR for pediatric radiologic sedation (Closely monitor throughout!)
Notes: May cause sudden apnea and hypotension; laryngospasm; hiccups; seizures. Physicians must be competent in deep procedural sedation and airway management (see Section VIII, 13. p 464)

■ Methotrexate (Folex)
Uses: ALL, AML, leukemic meningitis, trophoblastic tumors (chorioepithelioma, choriocarcinoma, chorioadenoma destruens, hydatidiform mole), breast cancer, Burkitt's lymphoma, mycosis fungoides, osteosarcoma, head and neck cancer, Hodgkin's and non-Hodgkin's lymphoma, lung cancer, psoriasis, and rheumatoid arthritis

Dose: *Cancer:* "conventional dose": 15–30 mg PO or IV 1–2/wk every 1–3 wk; "intermediate dose": 50–240 mg or 0.5–1 g/m² IV once every 4 d to 3 wk, "high dose": 1–12 g/m² IV once every 1–3 wk; 12 mg/m² (max 15 mg) intrathecally, weekly until the CSF cell count returns to normal. *RA:* 7.5 mg/wk PO as a single dose or 2.5 mg q12h PO for 3 doses/wk

Notes: Toxicity includes myelosuppression, nausea and vomiting, anorexia, mucositis, diarrhea, hepatotoxicity (transient and reversible; may progress to atrophy, necrosis, fibrosis, cirrhosis), rashes, dizziness, malaise, blurred vision, renal failure, pneumonitis, and, rarely, pulmonary fibrosis. Chemical arachnoiditis and headache may occur with intrathecal delivery. "High-dose" therapy requires leucovorin rescue to prevent severe hematologic and mucosal toxicity (see page 591); monitor blood counts and methotrexate levels carefully

■ Methoxamine (Vasoxyl)

Uses: Support, restoration, or maint of BP during anesthesia; for termination of some episodes of paroxysmal SVT

Dose: *Adults. Anesthesia:* 10–15 mg IM; if emergency exists, 3–5 mg slow IV push. *Paroxysmal SVT:* 10 mg by slow IV push. **Peds.** 0.25 mg/kg/dose IM or 0.08 mg/kg/dose slow IV push

Notes: IM dose requires 15 min to act; use 5–10 mg phentolamine locally in case of extravasation; interaction with MAO inhibitors and TCAs to potentiate methoxamine effect

■ Methyldopa (Aldomet)

Uses: Essential HTN

Dose: *Adults.* 250–500 mg PO bid–tid (max 2–3 g/d) or 250 mg to 1 g IV q4–8h. **Peds.** 10 mg/kg/24h PO in 2–3 ÷ doses (max 40 mg/kg/24h ÷ q6–12h) or 5–10 mg/kg/dose IV q6–8h to a total dose of 20–40 mg/kg/24h

Notes: Do NOT use in presence of patients with liver disease; can discolor urine; initial transient sedation or drowsiness occurs frequently

■ Methylene Blue (Urolene Blue)

Uses: Cyanide poisoning and drug-induced methemoglobinemia, indicator dye

Dose: *Adults & Peds.* 1–2 mg/kg IV over several min; repeat in 1 h PRN

■ Methylergonovine (Methergine)

Uses: Prevention and treatment of postpartum hemorrhage caused by uterine atony

Dose: 0.2 mg IM after delivery of placenta, may repeat at 2–4-h intervals or 0.2–0.4 mg PO q6–12h for 2–7 d

Notes: IV doses should be given over a period of not less than 1 min with frequent BP monitoring

■ **Methylprednisolone (Solu-Medrol)**
See Steroids, page 635, and Table A–8, page 659

■ **Metoclopramide (Reglan, Clopra, Octamide)**
Uses: Relief of diabetic gastroparesis; symptomatic GERD; relief of cancer chemotherapy-induced nausea and vomiting
Dose: Adults. Diabetic gastroparesis: 10 mg PO 30 min ac and hs for 2–8 wk PRN; or same dose given IV for 10 d, then switch to PO. *GERD:* 10–15 mg PO 30 min ac and hs. *Antiemetic:* 1–3 mg/kg/dose IV 30 min before antineoplastic agent, then q2h for 2 doses, then q3h for 3 doses. *Peds. GERD:* 0.1 mg/kg/dose PO qid. *Antiemetic:* 2 mg/kg/dose IV on same schedule as adults
Notes: Dystonic reactions common with high doses that can be treated with IV diphenhydramine (Benadryl); can also be used to facilitate small bowel intubation and radiologic evaluation of the upper GI tract

■ **Metolazone (Diulo, Zaroxolyn)**
Uses: Mild-to-moderate essential HTN; edema of renal disease or cardiac failure
Dose: Adults. HTN: 2.5–5 mg PO daily. *Edema:* 5–20 mg PO daily. *Peds.* 0.2–0.4 mg/kg/d PO ÷ q12h–qd
Notes: Monitor fluid and electrolyte status of patient during treatment

■ **Metoprolol (Lopressor, Toprol XL) (See Cover)**
Uses: Treatment of HTN, angina, and AMI. *ECC.* see Esmolol, page 568
Dose: Angina: 50–100 mg PO bid. *HTN:* 100–450 mg PO qd. *AMI:* 5 mg IV × 3 doses, then 50 mg PO q6h × 48 h, then 100 mg PO bid. *ECC. Adults.* 5 mg slow IV Q 5 min, total 15 mg

■ **Metronidazole (Flagyl)**
Uses: Amebiasis, trichomoniasis, *C difficile,* and anaerobic infections
Dose: Adults. Anaerobic infections: 500 mg IV q6–8h. *Amebic dysentery:* 750 mg PO qd for 5–10 d. *Trichomoniasis:* 250 mg PO tid for 7 d or 2 g PO in 1 dose. *C difficile:* 500 mg PO or IV q8h for 7–10 d. *Peds. Anaerobic infections:* 30 mg/kg/24h PO or IV ÷ q6h. *Amebic dysentery:* 35–50 mg/kg/24h PO in 3 ÷ doses for 5–10 d
Notes: For *Trichomonas* infections, also treat partner; ↓ dose in hepatic failure; no activity against aerobic bacteria; use in combination in serious mixed infections; may cause disulfiram-like reaction.

■ **Mexiletine (Mexitil)**
Uses: Suppression of symptomatic ventricular arrhythmias
Dose: Administer with food or antacids; 200–300 mg PO q8h, max 1200 mg/d

Notes: Not to be used in cardiogenic shock, second- or third-degree AV block if no pacemaker; may worsen severe arrhythmias; monitor liver function during therapy; drug interactions with hepatic enzyme inducers and suppressors requiring dosing changes

Mezlocillin (Mezlin)
Uses: Infections caused by susceptible strains of gram-negative bacteria including *Klebsiella, Proteus, E coli, Enterobacter, P aeruginosa,* and *Serratia* involving the skin, bone, respiratory tract, urinary tract, abdomen, and septicemia
Dose: Adults. 3 mg IV q4–6h. **Peds.** 200–300 mg/kg/d ÷ q4–6h
Notes: Often used in combination with aminoglycosides

Miconazole (Monistat)
Uses: Severe systemic fungal infections including coccidioidomycosis, candidiasis, cryptococcosis, and others; various tinea forms; cutaneous candidiasis; vulvovaginal candidiasis; tinea versicolor
Dose: Adults. Systemic: from 200–3600 mg/24h IV based on diagnosis ÷ into 3 doses. *Topical:* Apply to affected area twice daily for 2–4 wk. *Intravaginally:* Insert 1 full applicator or suppository hs for 7 d. **Peds.** 20–40 mg/kg/24h IV ÷ q8h
Notes: Antagonistic to amphotericin-B in vivo; rapid IV inf may cause tachycardia or arrhythmias; may potentiate warfarin drug activity

■ Midazolam (Versed) [C]
Uses: Preoperative sedation; conscious sedation for short procedures; induction of general anesthesia
Dose: Adults. 1–5 mg IV or IM, titrate dose to effect. **Peds.** *Conscious sedation:* 0.08 mg/kg IM. *General anesthesia:* 0.15 mg/kg IV followed by 0.05 mg/kg/dose q2min for 1–3 doses as needed to induce anesthesia
Notes: Monitor patient for respiratory depression; may produce hypotension in conscious sedation

Miglitol (Glyset)
Uses: Treatment of Type 2 DM
Dose: Initial 25 mg PO tid taken at the first bite of each meal; Maint 50–100 mg tid with meals
Notes: May be used alone or in combination with sulfonylureas; can cause GI disturbances

Milrinone (Primacor)
Uses: CHF
Dose: Loading dose of 50 mg/kg, followed by a cont inf of 0.375–0.75 mg/kg/min
Notes: Carefully monitor fluid and electrolyte status

Mineral Oil
Uses: Constipation
Dose: *Adults.* 15–45 mL PO PRN. *Peds* > 6 y: 10–20 mL PO bid

Minoxidil (Loniten, Rogaine)
Uses: Severe HTN; treatment of male and female pattern baldness
Dose: *Adults.* Oral: 2.5–10 mg PO bid–qid. *Topical Rogaine:* Apply bid to affected area. *Peds.* 0.2–1 mg/kg/24h ÷ PO q12–24h
Notes: Pericardial effusion and volume overload may occur; hypertrichosis after chronic use

Mirtazapine (Remeron)
Uses: Treatment of depression
Dose: 15 mg PO qhs, up to 45 mg qhs
Notes: Do NOT ↑ dose at intervals of less than 1–2 wk

Misoprostol (Cytotec)
Uses: Prevention of NSAID-induced gastric ulcers
Dose: 200 µg PO qid with meals; in females, start on 2nd or 3rd day of next normal menstrual period

Mitomycin (Mutamycin)
Uses: Treatment of breast, cervical, ovarian cancer, and GI adenocarcinomas; intravesical for bladder cancer
Dose: 20 mg/m^2 IV as a single dose every 6–8 wk; bladder cancer 20–40 mg in 40 mL of NSS via a urethral catheter once a week for 8 wk, followed by monthly treatments for 1 y
Notes: May cause cumulative myelosuppression

Mitoxantrone (Novantrone)
Uses: Treatment of leukemia, lymphoma, prostate and breast cancer
Dose: 12 mg/m^2/d IV infusion for 2–3 d of each chemotherapy cycle
Notes: Causes severe myelosuppression

Mivacurium (Mivacron)
Uses: Adjunct to general anesthesia or mechanical ventilation
Dose: *Adults.* 0.15 mg/kg/dose IV, may need to repeat at 15-min intervals. *Peds.* 0.2 mg/kg/dose IV, may need to repeat at 10-min intervals

Moexipril (Univasc)
Uses: Treatment of HTN
Dose: 7.5–30 mg in 1–2 ÷ doses administered 1 h before meals

■ Molindone (Moban)
Uses: Management of psychotic disorders
Dose: 5–100 mg PO tid–qid

■ Montelukast (Singulair)
Uses: Prophylaxis and treatment of chronic asthma
Dose: Adults > 15 y: 10 mg PO daily taken in the evening *Peds.* 6–14 y:
5 mg PO daily taken in the evening. *2–5 y:* 4 mg/d PO taken in the evening
Notes: NOT for acute asthma attacks

■ Moricizine (Ethmozine)
Uses: Treatment of ventricular arrhythmias
Dose: 200–300 mg PO tid

■ Morphine Sulfate [C] (See Cover)
Uses: Relief of severe pain. *ECC.* Chest pain and anxiety associated with AMI
or cardiac ischemia. Acute cardiogenic pulmonary edema (if BP is adequate)
Dose: Adults. Oral: 10–30 mg q4h PRN; SR tabs 30–60 mg q8–12h.
IV/IM: 2.5–15 mg q4h PRN. *ECC.* 2–4 mg IV (over 1–5 min) every 5–30 min.
Peds. 0.1–0.2 mg/kg/dose IM/IV q2–4h PRN up to max 15 mg/dose
Notes: Large number of narcotic side effects; may require scheduled dos-
ing to relieve severe chronic pain

■ Moxifloxacin (Avelox)
Uses: Treatment of acute sinusitis, acute bronchitis, and community-
acquired pneumonia
Dose: 400 mg/d
Notes: Active against gram-negative bacteria and *S pneumoniae;* interactions with Mg-, Ca-, Al-, and Fe-containing products and Class IA and III
antiarrhythmic agents

■ Mupirocin (Bactroban)
Uses: Treatment of impetigo; eradication of MRSA nasal carrier state
Dose: Topical: apply small amount to affected area. *Nasal:* apply twice
daily in the nostrils
Notes: Do NOT use concurrently with other nasal products

■ Muromonab-CD3 (Orthoclone OKT3)
Uses: Treatment of acute rejection following organ transplantation
Dose: 5 mg IV qd for 10–14 d
Notes: This is a murine antibody; may cause significant fever and chills
after the first dose

Mycophenolate Mofetil (CellCept)
Uses: Prevention of organ rejection following transplantation
Dose: 1 g PO bid
Notes: Used in conjunction with corticosteroids and cyclosporine

Nabumetone (Relafen)
Uses: Arthritis and pain
Dose: 1000–2000 mg/d ÷ qd–bid

Nadolol (Corgard)
Uses: HTN and angina, prevention of migraines
Dose: 40–80 mg qd; 160 mg/d max

Nafcillin (Nallpen)
Uses: Treatment of infections caused by susceptible strains of *S aureus* and *Streptococcus*
Dose: *Adults.* 250–500 mg (1 g max) PO q4–6h; 1–2 g IV q4–6h; 500 mg IM q4–6h. *Peds.* 50–200 mg/kg/d ÷ q4–6h (max 12 g/d); 50–100 mg/kg/d ÷ q6h
Notes: No adjustments for renal function

Nalbuphine (Nubain)
Uses: Moderate-to-severe pain
Dose: 10–20 mg IM, IV, SQ q4–6h PRN
Notes: Causes CNS depression and drowsiness; Caution in patients receiving opiate drugs

Nalidixic Acid (NegGram)
Uses: UTIs caused by susceptible strains of *Proteus, Klebsiella, Enterobacter,* and *E coli* but not *Pseudomonas*
Dose: *Adults.* 1 g PO qid for 7–14 d. *Peds.* 55 mg/kg/24h in 4 ÷ doses
Notes: Resistance emerges within 48 h in significant percentage of trials; may enhance effect of oral anticoagulants; may cause CNS adverse effects which reverse on discontinuation of the drug

Naloxone (Narcan)
Uses: Reversal of narcotic effect. *ECC.* Reverse effects of narcotic toxicity, including respiratory depression, hypotension, and hypoperfusion
Dose: *Adults.* 0.4–2.0 mg IV, IM or SQ q5min, max dose of 10 mg. *ECC.* 0.4–2.0 mg IV q2min; up to 10 mg over < 30 min. *Peds.* 0.01 mg/kg/dose IV, IM, or SQ; may repeat IV q3min for 3 doses PRN. *ECC. Bolus IV:* For total re-

versal of narcotic effects (smaller doses may be used if total reversal not required), as follows: Birth–5 y (≤ 10 kg): 0.1 mg/kg; ≥ 5 (or > 20 kg): 2.0 mg. May be necessary to repeat doses frequently. *Cont inf:* 0.04–0.16 mg/kg/h

Notes: May precipitate acute withdrawal in addicts; if no response after 10 mg, suspect a nonnarcotic cause

Naltrexone (ReVia)
Uses: Treatment of alcoholism and narcotic addiction
Dose: 50 mg PO qd
Notes: May cause hepatotoxicity; do NOT give until opioid-free for 7–10 d

Naphazoline and Pheniramine (Naphcon-A Ophthalmic, Others)
Uses: Ocular congestion and itching
Dose: 1–2 gtt in eye(s) q3–4h

Naproxen (Naprosyn, Anaprox)
Uses: Treatment of arthritis and pain
Dose: **Adults & Peds** > 12 y: 200–500 mg bid–tid, to a max of 1500 mg/d

Naratriptan (Amerge) See Table A–35, page 687

■ Nedocromil (ophthalmic) Alocril
Uses: Mast cell stabilizer used in allergic conjunctivitis
Dose: Adults. *Ophthalmic:* 1–2 gtt in eye(s) bid

Nedocromil (Tilade)
Uses: Management of mild-to-moderate asthma
Dose: 2 inhals 4 ×/d

Nefazodone (Serzone)
Uses: Treatment of depression
Dose: Initially, 100 mg PO bid; usual effective range is 300–600 mg/d in 2 ÷ doses
Notes: May cause postural hypotension and allergic reactions

Nelfinavir (Viracept)
Uses: HIV infection
Dose: Adults. 750 mg PO tid or 1250 mg PO bid. **Peds.** 20–30 mg/kg PO tid; with food

■ Neomycin
   Uses: Hepatic coma; preop bowel prep; minor skin infections
   Dose: **Adults.** 3–12 g/24h PO in 3–4 ÷ doses. **Peds.** 50–100 mg/kg/24h PO in 3–4 ÷ doses
   Notes: Part of Nichols-Condon bowel prep

■ Neomycin, Polymyxin-B Bladder Irrigant Soln
   Uses: Continuous irrigant for prophylaxis against bacteriuria and gram-negative bacteremia associated with indwelling catheter use
   Dose: 1-mL irrigant added to 1-L 0.9% NaCl; continuous irrigation of the bladder with 1–2 L of soln/24 h.
   Notes: Potential for bacterial or fungal superinfection; possibility for neomycin-induced ototoxicity or nephrotoxicity

■ Neomycin, Polymyxin-B and Dexamethasone, (Maxitrol)
   Uses: Steroid-responsive ocular conditions with bacterial infection
   Dose: 1–2 gtt in eye(s) q4–6h; apply oint in eye 3–4 ×/d
   Notes: Should be used under supervision of ophthalmologist

■ Neomycin, Polymyxin-B, and Hydrocortisone (Cortisporin Ophthalmic and Otic, Others)
   Uses: Superficial bacterial infections of the eye or external auditory canal by organisms sensitive to neomycin or polymyxin and associated with inflammation; suspension used in the treatment of infections in mastoidectomy and fenestration cavities
   Dose: **Adults & Peds.** Ophthalmic: oint, apply every 3–4 h; suspension 1 gt q3–4h. Otic: 3–4 gtt into external auditory canal tid–qid
   Notes: Use suspension in cases of ruptured ear drum. Limit use to < 10 d; ocular use should be used under supervision of ophthalmologist

■ Neomycin, Polymyxin-B and Prednisolone (Poly-Pred)
   Uses: Steroid-responsive ocular conditions with bacterial infection
   Dose: 1–2 gtt in eye(s) q4–6h; apply oint in eye 3–4 ×/d
   Notes: Should be used under supervision of ophthalmologist.

■ Nevirapine (Viramune)
   Uses: HIV infection
   Dose: **Adults.** 200 mg/d for 14 d; then 200 mg bid. **Peds.** < 8 y: 4 mg/kg/d for 14 d; then 7 mg/kg bid. > 8 y: 4 mg/kg/d for 14 d; then 4 mg/kg bid; give without regard to food
   Notes: WARNING: Reports of fatal hepatotoxicity even after short-term use; severe life-threatening skin reactions (Stevens–Johnson, toxic epidermal necrolysis and hypersensitivity reactions; monitor closely during first 8 wk of treatment

■ Niacin (Nicolar)

Uses: Adjunctive therapy in patients with significant hyperlipidemia who do not respond adequately to diet and weight loss

Dose: 1–2 g PO tid with meals; up to 8 g/d

Notes: Upper body and facial flushing and warmth following dose; may cause GI upset and pruritus

■ Nicardipine (Cardene)

Uses: Chronic stable angina, HTN

Dose: Oral: 20–40 mg PO tid. *SR:* 30–60 mg PO bid. *IV:* 0.5–15 mg/h continuous IV inf. Titrate to desired BP

Notes: Oral to IV conversion: 20 mg tid = 0.5 mg/h; 30 mg tid = 1.2 mg/h; 40 mg tid = 2.2 mg/h

■ Nicotine Gum (Nicorette, Nicorette DS)

Uses: See Nicotine, Transdermal

Dose: 9–12 pieces/d PRN. Max 30 pieces/d

Notes: Patients must stop smoking and perform behavior modification for max effect

■ Nicotine Nasal Spray (Nicotrol NS)

Uses: Aid to smoking cessation for the relief of nicotine withdrawal

Dose: 0.5 mg/actuation

Notes: Patients must stop smoking and perform behavior modification for max effect

■ Nicotine, Transdermal (Habitrol, Nicoderm, Nicotrol, ProStep)

Uses: Aid to smoking cessation for the relief of nicotine withdrawal

Dose: Individualized to the patient's needs; apply 1 patch (14–22 mg qd), and taper over 6 wk

Notes: Nicotrol to be worn for 16 h to mimic smoking patterns; others worn for 24 h; patients must stop smoking and perform behavior modification for max effect

■ Nifedipine (Procardia, Procardia XL, Adalat, Adalat CC)

Uses: Vasospastic or chronic stable angina; HTN

Dose: Adults. 10–30 mg PO q8h, max 180 mg/d, or SR tabs 30–90 mg/d. *Peds.* 0.6–0.9 mg/kg/24h ÷ tid–qid

Notes: Headaches common on initial treatment; reflex tachycardia may occur; Adalat CC and Procardia XL are NOT interchangeable dosing forms

■ Nilutamide (Nilandron)
Uses: Combination with surgical castration for the treatment of metastatic prostate cancer
Dose: 300 mg/d in ÷ doses for the first 30 d, then 150 mg/d
Notes: Toxicity can include hot flashes, loss of libido, impotence, diarrhea, nausea, vomiting, gynecomastia, hepatic dysfunction (Follow LFTs), and interstitial pneumonitis

■ Nimodipine (Nimotop)
Uses: Prevention of vasospasms following subarachnoid hemorrhage
Dose: 60 mg PO q4h for 21 d
Notes: Contents of cap may be extracted and administered through an NG tube if the cap cannot be swallowed whole

■ Nisoldipine (Sular)
Uses: Treatment of HTN
Dose: 10–60 mg/d PO
Notes: Do NOT take with grapefruit juice or high-fat meal

■ Nitrofurantoin (Macrodantin, Furadantin)
Uses: UTIs
Dose: Adults. Suppression: 50–100 mg PO qd. *Treatment:* 50–100 mg PO qid. *Peds.* 5–7 mg/kg/24h in 4 ÷ doses
Notes: GI side effects common; should be taken with food, milk, or antacid; macrocrystals (Macrodantin) cause less nausea than other forms of drug, may cause pulmonary fibrosis

■ Nitroglycerin (Nitrostat, Nitrolingual, Nitro-Bid Oint, Nitro-bid IV, Nitrodisc, Transderm-Nitro) (See Cover)
Uses: Angina pectoris; acute and prophylactic therapy; CHF, BP control, pulmonary HTN in children. *ECC.* Chest pain of suspected cardiac origin. Unstable angina. Complications of AMI, including CHF, left ventricular failure. Hypertensive crisis or urgency with chest pain
Dose: Adults. SL: 1 tab (0.3, 0.4, 0.6 mg) SL. q5min PRN × 3 doses. *Translingual:* 1–2 doses sprayed under tongue q5min PRN × 3 doses. *Oral:* 2.5-, 6.5-, or 9-mg SR cap or tab PO tid. *IV:* 5–20 μg/min titrated to effect 200 μg/min max. *Topical:* 1–2 in. oint to chest wall q6h, then wipe off at night. *Transdermal:* 0.2–0.4 mg/h, titrated to 0.4–0.8 mg/h; patches deliver in 24 h: 2.5, 5, 7.5, 10 or 15 mg; keep patch off 10–12 h each day. *ECC.* IV bolus: 12.5–25 μg. Inf at 10–20 μg/min. Route of choice for emergencies. Use IV sets provided by manufacturer. *Subinguinal route:* 0.3–0.4 mg, repeat q5min. *Aerosol spray:* Spray for 0.5–1.0 s at 5-min intervals. *Peds.* 1 μg/kg/min IV titrated to effect, max 5 μg/kg/min

Notes: Tolerance to nitrates develops with chronic use after 1–2 wk; this can be avoided by providing a nitrate-free period each day; shorter acting nitrates should be used on a tid basis, and long-acting patches and oint should be removed before bedtime to prevent the development of tolerance

■ Nitroprusside (Nipride, Nitropress)

Uses: Hypertensive crisis, aortic dissection, pulmonary edema. Reduce afterload in CHF and acute pulmonary edema.

Dose: Adults & Peds. 0.5–10 µg/kg/min IV inf titrated to desired effect. **ECC.** 0.10 µg/kg/min, titrate up to 5.0 µg/kg/min. Use inf pump; hemodynamic monitoring for optimal safety

Notes: Thiocyanate, the metabolite, is excreted by the kidney; thiocyanate toxicity occurs at plasma levels of 5–10 mg/dL; if used to treat aortic dissection, a β-blocker must be used concomitantly

■ Nizatidine (Axid)

Uses: Treatment of duodenal ulcers

Dose: Active ulcer: 150 mg PO bid or 300 mg PO qhs. *Maint:* 150 mg PO qhs

■ Norepinephrine (Levophed)

Uses: Acute hypotensive states. **ECC.** Severe cardiogenic shock and significant hypotension. Last resort for ischemic heart disease and shock

Dose: Adults. 8–12 µg/kg/min IV titrated to desired effect. **ECC.** 0.5–1.0 µg/min titrated to 30 µg/min. *Peds.* 0.1 µg/kg/min IV titrated to effect. **ECC.** Initial 0.1–2 (g/kg/min to effect

Notes: Do NOT administer with alkaline solns. Correct blood volume depletion as much as possible before initiation of vasopressor therapy; drug interaction with TCA, leading to severe profound HTN. Infuse into large vein to avoid extravasation; phentolamine 5–10 mg/10 mL NS injected locally is antidote to extravasation

■ Norfloxacin (Noroxin, Chibroxin Ophthalmic)

Uses: Complicated and uncomplicated UTIs resulting from a wide variety of gram-negative bacteria, and prostatitis; topical for ocular infections

Dose: Adults. 400 mg PO bid; ophthalmic 1–2 gtt qid; if severe use up to q2h. *Peds.* NOT recommended for use in patients < 18 y

Notes: NOT for use in pregnancy; drug interactions with antacids, theophylline, and caffeine

■ Nortriptyline (Aventyl, Pamelor)

Uses: Endogenous depression

Dose: 25 mg PO tid–qid; doses > 100 mg/d are NOT recommended
Notes: Many anticholinergic side effects including blurred vision, urinary retention, dry mouth

■ Nystatin (Mycostatin, Nilstat)
Uses: Treatment of mucocutaneous *Candida* infections (thrush, vaginitis)
Dose: **Adults.** *Oral:* 400,000–600,000 U PO "swish and swallow" qid or troche 200,000 U 1–2 dissolved in mouth. *Vaginal:* 1 tab inserted into vagina qhs. *Topical:* Apply bid–tid to affected area (cream, oint or powder). **Peds.** *Infants:* 200,000 U PO q6h. *Children:* See adult.
Notes: Not absorbed orally, therefore NOT effective for systemic infections

■ Octreotide Acetate (Sandostatin)
Uses: Suppresses or inhibits severe diarrhea associated with carcinoid and vasoactive intestinal tumors
Dose: **Adults.** 100–600 mg/d SQ in 2–4 ÷ doses. **Peds.** 1–10 mg/kg/24h SQ in 2–4 ÷ doses
Notes: May cause nausea, vomiting, and abdominal discomfort

■ Ofloxacin (Floxin, Ocuflox Ophthalmic)
Uses: Infections of the lower respiratory tract, skin and skin structure, and urinary tract, prostatitis, uncomplicated gonorrhea, and *Chlamydia* infections; topical for bacterial conjunctivitis and otitis externa
Dose: **Adults.** 200–400 mg PO bid or IV q12h. **Adults & Peds** > 1 y ophthalmic: 1–2 gtt in eye(s) q2–4h for 2 d, then qid for 5 additional days. **Peds.** Systemic administration should not be used in children < 18 y. *1–12 y otic:* 5 gtt in ear bid for 10 d. *> 12 y and* **Adults** *otic:* 10 gtt in ear bid for 10 d
Notes: May cause nausea, vomiting, diarrhea, insomnia and headache; drug interactions with antacids, sucralfate, and iron- and zinc-containing products that decrease the absorption of ofloxacin; may increase theophylline levels

■ Olanzapine (Zyprexa)
Uses: Treatment of psychotic disorders
Dose: Titrate up to max of 20 mg/d
Notes: May take many weeks to titrate to therapeutic dose; cigarette smoking will ↓ levels

■ Olopatadine (Patanol)
Uses: Allergic conjunctivitis, H_1 receptor antagonist
Dose: 1–2 gtts in eye/s bid, q6–8h

■ Olsalazine (Dipentum)
Uses: Maint of remission of ulcerative colitis
Dose: 500 mg PO bid
Notes: Take with food; may cause diarrhea

■ Omeprazole (Prilosec)
Uses: Treatment of duodenal and gastric ulcers, Zollinger–Ellison syndrome, GERD, and *H pylori* infections
Dose: 20-40 mg PO qd–bid
Notes: Combination therapy necessary for *H pylori*

■ Ondansetron (Zofran)
Uses: Prevention of nausea and vomiting associated with cancer chemotherapy and postoperative nausea and vomiting
Dose: Adults & Peds. *Chemotherapy:* 0.15 mg/kg/dose IV before chemotherapy, then repeated 4 and 8 h after the first dose or 4–8 mg PO tid, administer first dose 30 min before chemotherapy. **Adults.** *Postop:* 4 mg IV immediately before induction or postop
Notes: May cause diarrhea and headache

■ Orphenadrine (Norflex)
Uses: Treatment of muscle spasms
Dose: 60–100 mg bid
Notes: Dose dependent on route of administration

■ Oseltamivir (Tamiflu)
Uses: Treatment of influenza A and B
Dose: 75 mg bid for 5 d

■ Oprelvekin (Neumega)
Uses: Prevent severe thrombocytopenia due to chemotherapy
Dose: Adults. 50 µg/kg/d SQ for 10–21 d. **Peds.** 75–100 µg/kg/d SQ for 10–21d. *< 12:* Use only in clinical trials

■ Oxacillin (Bactocill, Prostaphlin)
Uses: Treatment of infections caused by susceptible strains of *S aureus* and *Streptococcus*
Dose: Adults. 1–2 mg IV q4–6h. **Peds.** 150–200 mg/kg/d IV q4–6h

■ Oxaprozin (Daypro)
Uses: Treatment of arthritis and pain
Dose: 600–1200 mg qd

■ Oxazepam (Serax) [C]
Uses: Anxiety; acute alcohol withdrawal; anxiety with depressive symptoms
Dose: 10–15 mg PO tid–qid; severe anxiety and alcohol withdrawal may require up to 30 mg qid
Notes: Oxazepam is one of the metabolites of diazepam (Valium)

■ Oxcarbazepine (Trileptal)
Uses: Treatment of partial seizures
Dose: Adults. 300 mg, increase dose weekly to a usual dose of 1200–2400 mg/d. ***Peds.*** 8–10 mg/kg PO bid, 600 mg/d max; increase dose weekly to target maint dose
Notes: May cause hyponatremia

■ Oxybutynin (Ditropan, Ditropan XL)
Uses: Symptomatic relief of urgency, nocturia, and incontinence associated with neurogenic or reflex neurogenic bladder
Dose: Adults & Peds > 5 y: 5 mg PO tid–qid. ***Adults.*** ER 5 mg PO qd; can ↑ to 30 mg PO, qd (5 and 10 mg/tab) ***Peds*** 1–5 y: 0.02 mg/kg/dose bid–qid (syrup 5 mg/5 mL)
Notes: Anticholinergic side effects (dry mouth, constipation, dry eyes, somnolence, others)

■ Oxycodone (OxyContin, Roxicodone, Others) [C]
Uses: Moderate-to-severe pain usually in combination with other analgesics
Dose: Adults. 5 mg PO q4–6h PRN; 10–40 mg PO q12h SR. ***Peds. 6–12 y:*** 1.25 mg PO q6h PRN. *>12 y:* 2.5 mg PO q6h PRN
Notes: SR (OxyContin) 10, 20, 40, 80 mg; liq 5 mg/5mL, soln 20 mg/mL

■ Oxycodone and Acetaminophen (Percocet, Tylox) [C]
Uses: Moderate-to-severe pain
Dose: Adults. 1–2 tabs/caps PO q4–6h PRN (Specify oxycodone/acetaminophen dose). ***Peds.*** 0.05–0.15 mg/kg/dose q4–6h, max 5 mg/dose (based on oxycodone)
Notes: Supplied as (Percocet: oxycodone/acetaminophen, 2.5 mg/325 mg, 5 mg/325 mg, 7.5mg/500 mg, 10 mg/500 mg; Tylox: 5-mg oxycodone, 500-mg acetaminophen) soln 5-mg oxycodone/325-mg acetaminophen/5 mL

■ Oxycodone and Aspirin (Percodan, Percodan-Demi) [C]
Uses: Moderate-to-moderately severe pain
Dose: Adults. 1–2 tabs/caps PO q4–6h PRN. ***Peds.*** 0.05–0.15 mg/kg/dose q4–6h, max 5 mg/dose (based on oxycodone)
Notes: *Percodan:* 4.5-mg oxycodone hydrochloride 0.38-mg oxycodone terephthalate, 325-mg aspirin. *Percodan-Demi:* 2.25-mg oxycodone hydrochloride, 0.19-mg oxycodone terephthalate, 325-mg aspirin

■ Oxymorphone (Numorphan) [C]
Uses: Treatment of moderate-to-severe pain, sedative
Dose: 0.5 mg IM, SQ, IV initially, 1–1.5 mg q4–6h PRN. *PR:* 5 mg q4–6h PRN
Notes: Chemically related to hydromorphone

■ Oxytocin (Pitocin, Syntocinon)
Uses: Induction of labor; control of postpartum hemorrhage
Dose: 0.001–0.002 U/min IV titrate to effect, max 0.02 U/min
Notes: Can cause uterine rupture and fetal death; monitor vital signs closely

■ Paclitaxel (Taxol)
Uses: Treatment of ovarian cancer
Dose: 135 mg/m^2 IV q3wk
Notes: May cause severe neutropenia

■ Pancreatin/Pancrelipase (Pancrease, Cotazym)
Uses: For deficiencies in exocrine pancreatic secretions (CF, chronic pancreatitis, other pancreatic insufficiency), and for steatorrhea of malabsorption syndrome
Dose: Adults & Peds. 1–3 caps (tabs) with meals and snacks may be increased up to 8 caps (tabs)
Notes: Avoid antacids; may cause nausea, abdominal cramps, or diarrhea; do not crush or chew EC products

■ Pancuronium (Pavulon)
Uses: Aids in the treatment of patients on mechanical ventilator, intraoperative muscle relaxation
Dose: Adults. 2–4 mg IV q2–4h PRN. ***Peds.*** 0.02–0.10 mg/kg/dose q2–4h PRN
Notes: Patient must be intubated and on controlled ventilation; use adequate amount of sedation or analgesia

■ Paregoric [C]
Uses: Diarrhea, pain and neonatal withdrawal syndrome
Dose: Adults. 5–10 mL qd–qid PRN
Notes: Contains opium

■ Paroxetine (Paxil)
Uses: Depression
Dose: 20–50 mg PO as a single daily dose

■ Pantoprazole (Protonix)
Uses: GERD
Dose: 40 mg/d PO
Notes: Delayed-release tab, therefore do not crush or chew tab

■ Pemirolast (Alamast)
Uses: Allergic conjunctivitis
Dose: 1–2 qtt in each affected eye qid response in days, occasionally 1 mo

■ Penbutolol (Levatol)
Uses: HTN
Dose: 20–40 mg qd

■ Penicillamine [d-3-Mercaptovaline] (Cuprimine, Depen)
Uses: Chelating agent used in Wilson's disease, cystinuria, lead and arsenic poisoning, primary biliary cirrhosis
Dose: *Lead poisoning:* **Adults.** 250 mg/dose q8–12h. **Peds.** 25–40 mg/kg/d 3 ÷ doses. *Arsenic poisoning:* **Peds.** 100 mg/kg/day in ÷ doses q6h for 5 d; max: 1 g/day
Notes: Continue until blood lead level is < 60 µg/dL

■ Penicillin G Aqueous (Potassium or Sodium) (Pfizerpen, Pentids)
Uses: Most gram-positive infections (except penicillin-resistant staphylococci), including those caused by streptococci, *N meningitidis,* syphilis, clostridia, corynebacteria, and some coliforms
Dose: **Adults.** 400,000–800,000 units PO qid; IV doses vary greatly depending on indications. *Range:* 1.2–24 million U/d. **Peds.** *Newborns < 1 wk:* 25,000–50,000 U/kg/dose IV q12h. *Infants 1 wk–1 mo:* 25,000–50,000 U/kg/dose IV q8h. *Children:* 100,000–300,000 U/kg/24h IV ÷ q4h
Notes: Watch for hypersensitivity reactions; drug of choice for group A streptococcal infections and syphilis

■ Penicillin G Benzathine (Bicillin)
Uses: Useful as a single-dose treatment regimen for streptococcal pharyngitis, rheumatic fever and glomerulonephritis prophylaxis, and syphilis.
Dose: **Adults.** 1.2–2.4 million U deep IM inj q2–4 wk. **Peds.** 50,000 U/kg/dose to a max of 2.4 million U/dose deep IM inj q2–4wk
Notes: Sustained action with detectable levels up to 4 wk; considered drug of choice for treatment of noncongenital syphilis; Bicillin L-A contains the benzathine salt only; Bicillin C-R contains a combination of the benzathine and procaine salts and is used for most acute strep infections (300,000 U procaine with 300,000 U benzathine/mL or 900,000 U benzathine with 300,000 U procaine/2 mL)

■ Penicillin G Procaine (Wycillin, Others)

Uses: Moderately severe infections caused by penicillin G-sensitive organisms that respond to low persistent serum levels (syphilis, uncomplicated pneumococcal pneumonia)

Dose: Adults. 300,000–1.2 million U/d IM ÷ qd–bid. *Peds.* 25,000–50,000 U/kg/d IM ÷ qd–bid

Notes: A long-acting parenteral penicillin; blood levels ≤ 15 h; give probenecid at least 30 min before administration of penicillin to prolong action

■ Penicillin V (Pen-Vee K, Veetids, Others)

Uses: Most gram-positive infections (except penicillin-resistant staphylococci), including those caused by streptococci, *N meningitidis,* syphilis, clostridia, corynebacteria, and some coliforms

Dose: Adults. 250–500 mg PO q6h. *Peds.* 25–50 mg/kg/24h PO in 4 ÷ doses

Notes: A well-tolerated oral penicillin; 250 mg = 400,000 U

■ Pentamidine Isethionate (Pentam 300, NebuPent)

Uses: Treatment and prevention of *P carinii* pneumonia

Dose: Adults & Peds. 4 mg/kg/24h IV daily for 14–21 d. *Adults. Prevention:* 300 mg once every 4 wk, administered via nebulizer

Notes: Monitor patient for severe hypotension following IV administration; associated with pancreatic islet-cell necrosis leading to hypoglycemia and hyperglycemia; monitor hematology labs for leukopenia and thrombocytopenia

■ Pentazocine (Talwin) [C]

Uses: Moderate-to-severe pain

Dose: 30 mg IM or IV; 50–100 mg PO q3–4h PRN

Notes: 30–60 mg IM equianalgesic to 10-mg morphine IM; associated with considerable dysphoria

■ Pentobarbital (Nembutal, others) [C]

Uses: Insomnia, convulsions, induced coma following severe head injury

Dose: Adults. Sedative: 20–40 mg PO or PR q6–12h. *Hypnotic:* 100–200 mg PO or PR qhs PRN. *Induced coma:* load 3–5 mg/kg IV 3 1, then maint 2–3.5 mg/kg/dose IV q1h PRN to keep level between 25–40 mg/mL. *Peds. Hypnotic:* 2–6 mg/kg/dose PO qhs PRN. *Induced coma:* See adult.

Notes: Can cause respiratory depression; may produce hypotension when used IV for cerebral edema; tolerance to sedative-hypnotic effect acquired within 1–2 wk

■ Pentosan Polysulfate Sodium (Elmiron)

Uses: Bladder pain and discomfort associated with interstitial cystitis

Dose: 100 mg PO tid

Notes: Alopecia, diarrhea, nausea, and headaches have been reported

Pentoxifylline (Trental)
Uses: Intermittent claudication
Dose: 400 mg PO tid with meals
Notes: Treat for at least 8 wk to see full effect

Pergolide (Permax)
Uses: Parkinson's disease
Dose: Initially 0.05 mg PO tid, titrated every 2–3 d to desired effect
Notes: May cause hypotension during initiation of therapy

Perindopril (Aceon)
Uses: Treatment of HTN and CHF
Dose: 4–8 mg daily
Notes: Avoid taking with food

Permethrin (Elimite, Nix)
Uses: Eradication of lice
Dose: Adults & Peds. Lice: Saturate hair and scalp with cream rinse; allow to remain in hair for 10 min before rinsing out. *Scabies:* Apply cream over entire body; rinse after 8–14 h

Perphenazine (Trilafon)
Uses: Psychotic disorders, intractable hiccups, severe nausea
Dose: Antipsychotic: 4–8 mg PO tid, max 64 mg/d. *Hiccups:* 5 mg IM q6h PRN or 1 mg IV at not less than 1–2 mg/min intervals up to 5 mg

Phenazopyridine (Pyridium)
Uses: Symptomatic relief of discomfort from lower urinary tract irritation
Dose: Adults. 200 mg PO tid. *Peds* 6–12 y: 12 mg/kg/24h PO in 3 ÷ doses
Notes: GI disturbances; causes red-orange urine color, which can stain clothing

Phenobarbital [C]
Uses: Seizure disorders, insomnia, anxiety
Dose: Adults. Sedative-hypnotic: 30–120 mg PO or IM qd PRN. *Anticonvulsant:* Load 10–12 mg/kg in 3 ÷ doses, then 1–3 mg/kg/24h PO, IM, or IV. *Peds. Sedative-hypnotic:* 2–3 mg/kg/24h PO or IM qhs PRN. *Anticonvulsant:* Load 15–20 mg/kg ÷ into 2 equal doses 4 h apart, then 3–5 mg/kg/24h PO ÷ in 2–3 doses
Notes: Tolerance develops to sedation; paradoxical hyperactivity seen in pediatric patients; long half-life allows single daily dosing

Phenylephrine (Neo-Synephrine)
Uses: Treatment of vascular failure in shock, hypersensitivity, or drug-induced hypotension; nasal congestion; mydriatic

Dose: **Adults.** *Mild-to-moderate hypotension:* 2–5 mg IM or SQ elevates BP for 2 h; 0.1–0.5 mg IV elevates BP for 15 min. *Severe hypotension/shock:* Infusion at 100–180 mg/min; after BP stabilized, maint rate of 40–60 mg/min. *Nasal congestion:* 1–2 sprays into each nostril PRN. **Adults & Peds** > 1: *Mydriasis:* 1 gt 2.5–10% soln in eye(s) 30 min before procedure; may repeat in 10–60 min if needed. **Peds.** *Hypotension:* 5–20 mg/kg/dose IV q10–15 min or 0.1–0.5 mg/kg/min IV infusion titrated to desired effect. *Nasal congestion:* 1 spray into each nostril q3–4h PRN. **Peds** < 1: *Mydriasis:* 1 gt 2.5% soln in eye(s) 30 min before procedure

Notes: Promptly restore blood volume if loss has occurred; use caution in patients with hyperthyroidism, bradycardia, partial heart block, myocardial disease, or severe arteriosclerosis; use large veins for infusion to avoid extravasation; phentolamine 10 mg in 10–15 mL saline for local inj as antidote for extravasation; activity potentiated by oxytocin, MAOIs, and TCA

■ Phenytoin (Dilantin)

Uses: Tonic–clonic and partial seizures

Dose: **Adults & Peds.** *Load:* 15–20 mg/kg, IV at a max inf rate of 25 mg/min or orally in 400-mg doses at 4-h intervals. **Adults.** *Maint:* 200 mg PO or IV bid or 300 mg qhs initially then follow serum level. **Peds.** *Maint:* 4–7 mg/kg/24h PO or IV ÷ qd–bid

Notes: Caution with cardiac depressant side effects, especially with IV administration; follow levels as needed (see Table A–22, page 675); nystagmus and ataxia are early signs of toxicity; gum hyperplasia occurs with long-term use; avoid use of oral suspension if possible because of erratic absorption; avoid use in pregnancy

■ Physostigmine (Antilirium)

Uses: Antidote for TCA, atropine, and scopolamine overdose

Dose: **Adults.** 2 mg IV/IM q15min. **Peds.** 0.01–0.03 mg/kg/dose IV q15–30 min

Notes: Rapid IV administration associated with convulsions; cholinergic side effects; may cause asystole

■ Phytonadione [Vitamin K] (AquaMEPHYTON, Others)

Uses: Coagulation disorders caused by faulty formation of factors II, VII, IX, and X, hyperalimentation

Dose: Adults & Peds. *Anticoagulant-induced prothrombin deficiency:* 2.5–10.0 mg PO or IV slowly. *Hyperalimentation:* 10 mg IM or IV every week. *Infants:* 0.5–1.0 mg/dose IM, SQ, or PO

Notes: With parenteral treatment, usually see first change in prothrombin in 12–24 h; anaphylaxis can result from IV dosing; should be administered slowly IV

■ Pilocarpine (Salagen Oral, Ocusert Pilo-20, Ocusert Pilo-40, Others)

Uses: Glaucoma and to reverse cycloplegia; radiation-induced xerostomia
Dose: Reversal mydriasis: 1 gt 1% soln to eye. *Glaucoma:* 1–2 gtt hydrochloride soln up to 6 ×/d; titrate based on pressures; 0.5-in. ribbon into eye qhs. Ocusert: 1 in eye weekly
Notes: Ocusert implant system releases 20 or 40 µg/h over 1 wk.

■ Pindolol (Visken)

Uses: Treatment of HTN
Dose: 5–10 mg bid

■ Pioglitazone (Actos)

Uses: Management of Type 2 DM
Dose: 15–45 mg/d

■ Pipecuronium (Arduan)

Uses: Adjunct to general anesthesia
Dose: Adults. 50–100 mg/kg IV. *Peds.* 40–57 mg/kg IV

■ Piperacillin (Pipracil)

Uses: Infections caused by susceptible strains of gram-negative bacteria, including *Klebsiella, Proteus, E coli, Enterobacter, P aeruginosa,* and *Serratia* involving the skin, bone, respiratory tract, urinary tract, abdomen, and septicemia
Dose: Adults. 3 g IV q4–6h. *Peds.* 200–300 mg/kg/d IV ÷ q4–6h
Notes: Often used in combination with aminoglycosides

■ Piperacillin/Tazobactam (Zosyn)

Uses: Treatment of infections caused by susceptible strains of gram-negative bacteria including *Klebsiella, Proteus, E coli, Enterobacter, P aeruginosa,* and *Serratia* involving the skin, bone, respiratory tract, urinary tract, abdomen, and septicemia
Dose: Adults. 3.375–4.5 g IV q6h
Notes: Often used in combination with aminoglycosides

■ Pirbuterol (Maxair)

Uses: Prevention and reversal of bronchospasm
Dose: Adults & Peds > 12 y: 2 inhals q4–6h, max of 12 inhals/d

■ Piroxicam (Feldene)
Uses: Treatment of arthritis and pain
Dose: 10–20 mg qd

■ Plasma Protein Fraction (Plasmanate, others)
Uses: Shock and hypotension
Dose: Adults. 250–500 mL IV initially (not 0.10 mL/min); subsequent inf should depend on clinical response. *Peds.* 10–15 mL/kg/dose IV; subsequent inf should depend on clinical response
Notes: Hypotension associated with rapid infusion; 130–160 mEq sodium/L; not a substitute for red cells

■ Plicamycin (Mithracin)
Uses: Hypercalcemia of malignancy
Dose: 25 mg/kg/d IV for 3–4 d

■ Pneumococcal Vaccine, Polyvalent (Pneumovax-23)
Uses: Immunization against pneumococcal infections in patients predisposed to or at high risk of acquiring these infections (ie, before elective splenectomy)
Dose: Adults & Peds > 2 y: 0.5 mL IM
Notes: Do not vaccinate during immunosuppressive therapy

■ Pneumococcal 7-Valent Conjugate Vaccine (Prevnar)
Uses: Immunization against pneumococcal infections in infants and children
Dose: 0.5 mL IM per dose; series consists of 3 doses; first dose at 2 mo with subsequent doses every 2 mo

■ Polio Vaccine [Poliovirus Vaccine (inactivated), IPV, Poliomyelitis Vaccine, Salk Vaccine] (IPOL)
Uses: Active immunization for polio
Dose: Initial: 3 doses 0.5 mL SQ; first 2 doses at 8-wk intervals; third dose 6–12 (preferred) mo after the second dose. *Booster dose:* Children who received 3-dose primary series in early childhood should receive booster of 0.5 mL before entering school. If third dose of primary series administered after 4th birthday, a booster not required at school entry

■ Polyethylene Glycol-Electrolyte Soln (Go-LYTLEY, CoLyte)
Uses: Bowel cleansing before examination or surgery
Dose: Adults. Following 3–4 h fast, the patient must drink 240 mL of soln q10min until 4 L is consumed. *Peds.* 25–40 mL/kg/h over 4–10 h

Notes: First bowel movement should occur in approximately 1 h; may cause some cramping or nausea

■ Potassium Citrate (Urocit-K)
Uses: Alkalinize urine, prevention of urinary stones (uric acid), calcium stones if hypocitraturic; urinary alkalinizer
Dose: 10–20 mEq PO tid with meals, max 100 mEq/d
Notes: *Tabs:* 540 mg = 5 mEq, 1080 mg = 10 mEq

■ Potassium Citrate and Citric Acid (Polycitra-K)
Uses: Alkalinize urine, prevention of urinary stones (uric acid), calcium stones if hypocitraturic; urinary alkalinizer
Dose: 10–20 mEq PO tid with meals, max 100 mEq/d
Notes: *Soln:* 10 mEq/5 mL. *Powder:* 30 mEq/packet

■ Potassium Iodide [Lugol's soln] (SSKI, Thyro-Block)
Uses: Radiation exposure, thyroid crisis, reduction of vascularity before thyroid surgery, thin bronchial secretions
Dose: *Radiation emergency:* 100 mg PO. *Preop thyroidectomy:* **Adults & Peds.** 50–250 mg PO tid (2–6 gtt strong iodine soln); administer for 10 d before surgery. *Thyroid crisis:* **Adults & Peds** > 1 y: 300 mg (6 gtt SSKI q8h). *Infants < 1 y:* 1/2 dose
Notes: SSKI = 1 g/mL, Lugol's = 100 mg/mL.
Notes: Usually indicated for radiation exposure > 100 rad adults, > 50 rad children

■ Potassium Supplements
Uses: Prevention or treatment of hypokalemia
Dose: **Adults.** 20–100 mEq/d PO ÷ qd–bid; IV 10–20 mEq/h, max 40 mEq/h and 150 mEq/d (monitor frequent potassium levels when using high-dose IV infusions). **Peds.** Calculate potassium deficit; 1–3 mEq/kg/d PO ÷ qd–qid; IV max dose 0.5–1 mEq/kg/h
Notes: Dosing ranges based on clinical conditions. See Table A–36, page 688 for oral agents. Can cause GI irritation; powder and liquids must be mixed with beverage (unsalted tomato juice, etc); use cautiously in renal insufficiency, and along with NSAIDs and ACE inhibitors; chloride salt recommended in co-existing alkalosis; for coexisting acidosis, use acetate, bicarbonate, citrate or gluconate salt

■ Pramipexole (Mirapex)
Uses: Treatment of Parkinson's disease
Dose: 1.5–4.5 mg/d; titrated slowly

Pramoxine with Hydrocortisone (Proctofoam-HC, Anusol-HC, Others)

Uses: Relief of pain and itching from external and internal hemorrhoids and anorectal surgery

Dose: 1 suppository every AM and hs and following each bowel movement; apply cream, oint, gel or spray, freely to anal area q6–12h

Notes: Anusol-HC/Proctofoam HA contains 1% hydrocortisone

Pravastatin (Pravachol)

Uses: Reduction of elevated cholesterol levels

Dose: 10–40 mg PO qhs

Prazepam (Centrax) [C]

Uses: Anxiety disorders

Dose: 5–10 mg PO tid–qid, or 20–50 mg PO as single hs dose to minimize daytime drowsiness

Prazosin (Minipress)

Uses: HTN and CHF

Dose: **Adults.** 1 mg PO tid; to total daily dose of 20 mg/d PRN. **Peds.** 5-25 mg/kg/dose q6h

Notes: Can cause orthostatic hypotension, so the patient should take the first dose hs; tolerance develops to this effect; tachyphylaxis may result

Prednisone

See Steroids, page 635, and Table A–8, page 659.

Prednisolone

See Steroids, page 635, and Table A–8, page 659.

Prednisolone, Ophthalmic (AK-Pred Ophthalmic, Pred-Forte Ophthalmic, Others)

Uses: Iritis, postop inflammation, palpebral and bulbar conjunctivitis, chemical, radiation or thermal injury, corneal abrasion

Dose: 1–2 gtt in eye(s) qh during day and q2h at night until inflammation subsides; then 1 gt q4h

Notes: Can increase intraocular pressure, cause cataracts, and worsen herpes keratitis

■ Probenecid (Benemid)

Uses: Gout, maint of serum levels of penicillins or cephalosporins
Dose: Adults. Gout: 0.25 g bid for 1 wk; then 0.5 g PO bid. *Antibiotic effect:* 1–2 g PO 30 min before dose of antibiotic. *Peds.* 25 mg/kg, then 40 mg/kg/d PO ÷ qid.

■ Procainamide (Pronestyl, Procan) (See Cover)

Uses: Treatment of supraventricular and ventricular arrhythmias. *ECC.* Recurrent VT not controlled by Lidocaine. Refractory PSVT. Refractory VF/ pulseless VT. Stable wide-complex tachycardia of unknown origin. AF with rapid rate in WPW
Dose: Adults. Chronic dosing: 50 mg/kg/d PO in ÷ doses q4–6h. *ECC. Recurrent VF/VT:* 20 mg/min IV (max total 17 mg/kg). In urgent situations up to 50 mg/min to a total dose of 17 mg/kg. *Other indications:* 20 mg/min IV until one of the following occurs: (1) Arrhythmia suppression, (hypotension), (2) QRS widens by more than 50%, (3) Total dose of 17 mg/kg is given. *Maint:* 1–4 mg/min. *Peds. ECC.* 3–6 mg/kg/dose IV over 5 min, then 20–80 mg/kg/min IV inf. *Maint:* 15–50 mg/kg/24h PO ÷ q3–6h
Notes: Can cause hypotension and a lupus-like syndrome; dose adjustment renal impairment; see Table A–22, page 675

■ Prochlorperazine (Compazine)

Uses: Nausea, vomiting, agitation, psychotic disorders
Dose: Adults. Antiemetic: 5–10 mg PO tid–qid or 25 mg PR bid or 5–10 mg IM q4–6h. *Antipsychotic:* 10–20 mg IM acutely or 5–10 mg PO tid–qid for maint. *Peds.* 0.1–0.15 mg/kg/dose IM q4–6h or 0.4 mg/kg/24h PO ÷ tid–qid
Notes: Much larger dose may be required for antipsychotic effect; extrapyramidal side effects common; treat acute extrapyramidal reactions with diphenhydramine

■ Procyclidine (Kemadrin)

Uses: Treatment of Parkinson's syndrome
Dose: 2.5 mg PO tid
Notes: Contra for glaucoma patients

■ Promethazine (Phenergan)

Uses: Nausea, vomiting, motion sickness
Dose: Adults. 12.5–50 mg PO, PR, or IM bid–qid PRN. *Peds.* 0.1–0.5 mg/kg/dose PO or IM q4–6h PRN
Notes: High incidence of drowsiness

■ Propafenone (Rythmol)

Uses: Treatment of life-threatening ventricular arrhythmias
Dose: 150–300 mg PO q8h
Notes: May cause dizziness, unusual taste, and first-degree heart block

■ Propantheline (Pro-Banthine)

Uses: Symptomatic treatment of small intestine hypermotility, spastic colon, ureteral spasm, bladder spasm, and pylorospasm

Dose: Adults. 15 mg PO ac and 30 mg PO hs. *Peds.* 1.5–3.0 mg/kg/24h PO ÷ tid–qid

Notes: Anticholinergic side effects such as dry mouth, blurred vision are common

■ Proparacaine (Alcaine, Ocu-Caine, Ophthetic, RO-Parcaine)

Uses: Topical anesthetic for ophthalmology procedures (cornea and conjunctiva)

Dose: Adults & Peds. Surgery: 1 gtt 0.5% sol in eye q5–10min × 5–7 doses. *Tonometry, etc:* 1–2 gtt 0.5% soln before procedure

■ Propofol (Diprivan)

Uses: Induction or maint of anesthesia; continuous sedation in intubated patients, deep procedural sedation

Dose: Anesthesia: 20–40 mg q10min until induction onset, then 50 200 mg/kg/min cont inf. *ICU sedation:* 5-50 mg/kg/min cont inf. *Deep procedural sedation:* 0.5 mg/kg IVP wait 60 90 s for response (*Note:* Physician must be competent in deep procedural sedation and airway management; sudden apnea and hypotension common! Formulated in soybean oil and egg emulsion—Do NOT give to anyone with allergies to eggs or soybeans. (See Section VIII, 13, page 464)

Notes: 1 mL of propofol contains 0.1 g of fat; may increase serum triglycerides when administered for extended periods

■ Propoxyphene and Aspirin (Darvon Compound-65, Darvon-N with Aspirin) [C]

Uses: Mild-to-moderate pain

Dose: 1–2 PO q4h PRN

Notes: Darvon: Propoxyphene HCl cap 65 mg. *Darvon-N:* Propoxyphene napsylate 100-mg tab. *Darvocet-N:* Propoxyphene napsylate 50 mg/acetaminophen 325 mg. *Darvocet-N 100:* Propoxyphene napsylate 100 mg/acetaminophen 650 mg. Darvon Compound-65: Propoxyphene HCl 65-mg/aspirin 389-mg/caffeine 32-mg caps. *Darvon-N with aspirin:* Propoxyphene napsylate 100 mg/aspirin 325 mg

■ Propranolol (Inderal)

Uses: HTN, angina, MI prophylaxis, arrhythmias (atrial fibrillation and flutter, others) essential tremor, pheochromocytoma, thyrotoxicosis, migraine prevention, *ECC.* See esmolol.

Dose: ***Adults.*** *Angina:* 80–320 mg PO qd ÷ bid–qid or 80–160 mg SR qd.
Arrhythmia: 10–80 mg PO tid–qid or 1 mg IV slowly, repeat q5min up to 5 mg.
HTN: 40 mg PO bid or 60–80 mg SR qd, increase weekly to max 640 mg/d.
Hypertrophic subaortic stenosis: 20–40 mg PO tid–qid. MI: 180–240 mg PO ÷
tid–qid. *Migraine prophylaxis:* 80 mg/d ÷ qid–tid, increase weekly to max
160–240 mg/d ÷ tid–qid; wean off if no response in 6 wk. *Pheochromocytoma:*
30–60 mg/d ÷ tid–qid. *Thyrotoxicosis:* 1–3 mg IV single dose; 10–40 mg PO
q6h. *Tremor:* 40 mg PO bid, increase as needed to max 320 mg/d. ***ECC.*** 0.1
mg/kg slow IV push, ÷ 3 equal doses 2–3 min intervals, max 1 mg/min. Repeat
after 2 min, PRN. ***Peds.*** *Arrhythmia:* 0.5–1.0 mg/kg/d ÷ tid–qid, ↑ as needed
q3–7d to max 60 mg/d; 0.01–0.1 mg/kg IV over 10 min, max dose 1 mg. *HTN:*
0.5–1.0 mg/kg ÷ bid–qid, ↑ as needed q3–7d to 2 mg/kg/d max

■ Propylthiouracil [PTU]
Uses: Hyperthyroidism
Dose: ***Adults.*** 100 mg PO q8h ↑ to 1200 mg/d); after euthyroid (6–8 wk),
taper dose by ⅓ q4–6wk to a maint dose of 50–150 mg/24h; treatment is often
discontinued in 2–3 y. ***Peds.*** *Initial:* 5–7 mg/kg/24h PO ÷ q8h. *Maint:* of ⅓–⅔
of initial dose
Notes: Follow patient clinically; monitor thyroid function tests

■ Protamine Sulfate
Uses: Reversal of heparin effect
Dose: ***Adults & Peds.*** Based on amount of heparin reversal desired; given
slow IV, 1 mg will reverse approximately 100 U of heparin given in the preceding 3–4h to max dose of 50 mg
Notes: Follow coagulation studies; may have anticoagulant effect if given
without heparin

■ Pseudoephedrine (Sudafed, Novafed, Afrinol)
Uses: Decongestant
Dose: ***Adults.*** 30–60 mg PO q6–8h; SR caps 120 mg PO q12h. ***Peds.***
4 mg/kg/24h PO ÷ qid
Notes: Contra in patients with HTN or CAD and in patients taking MAO
inhibitors; an ingredient in many cough and cold preparations

■ Psyllium (Metamucil, Serutan, Effer-Syllium)
Uses: Constipation, diverticular disease of the colon
Dose: 1 tsp (7 g) in a glass of water qd–tid
Notes: Do NOT use if bowel obstruction is suspect; one of the safest laxa-
tives; psyllium in effervescent (Effer-syllium) form usually contains potassium
and should be used with caution in patients with renal failure

Pyrazinamide
Uses: Treatment of active tuberculosis
Dose: Adults. 20–35 mg/kg/24h PO ÷ tid–qid, max dose is 3 g/d. *Peds.* 15–30 mg/kg/d PO ÷ bid or qd
Notes: May cause hepatotoxicity; use in combination with other antituberculosis drugs

Pyridoxine (Vitamin B$_6$)
Uses: Treatment and prevention of vitamin B$_6$ deficiency
Dose: Deficiency: 2.5–10.0 mg PO qd. *Drug-induced neuritis:* 50 mg PO qd

Quazepam (Doral) [C]
Uses: Insomnia
Dose: 7.5–15 mg PO qhs PRN
Notes: ↓ dose in elderly patients

Quinapril (Accupril)
Uses: HTN
Dose: 10–80 mg PO qd in single dose

Quinidine (Quinidex, Quinaglute)
Uses: Prevention of tachydysrhythmias
Dose: Adults. PACs, PVCs: 200–300 mg PO tid–qid. *Conversion of atrial fibrillation or flutter:* Use after digitalization, 200 mg q2–3h for 8 doses; then ↑ daily dose to max of 3–4 g or until normal rhythm. *Peds.* 30 mg/kg/24h PO in 4–5 ÷ doses
Notes: Contra in digitalis toxicity, AV block; follow serum levels if available (see Table A–22, page 675); extreme hypotension seen with IV administration. Sulfate salt contains 83% quinidine, gluconate salt is 62% quinidine

Quinine Sulfate (Generic)
Uses: Suppression/treatment of chloroquine-resistant *P falciparum* malaria
Dose: Adults. 650 mg q8h × 7 d PO with another agent. *Peds.* 25 mg/kg/day ÷ doses q8h × 7 d; 650 mg/dose max

Quinupristin/Dalfopristin (Synercid)
Uses: Infections caused by vancomycin-resistant *Enterococcus faecium,* and other gram-positive organisms
Dose: Adults & Peds. 7.5 mg/kg IV q8–12h
Notes: Administer through central line if possible; NOT compatible with saline or heparin, therefore flush IV lines with dextrose

■ Rabeprazole (Aciphex)
Uses: Peptic ulcers, GERD, and hypersecretory conditions
Dose: 20 mg/d; may be ↑ to 60 mg/d
Notes: Do NOT crush tabs

■ Rabies Immune Globulin (Bayrab, Imogam Rabies-HT) (See Appendix)
Uses: Postexposure prophylaxis of individuals exposed to the virus
Dose: See Table A–2, page 652.

■ Rabies Vaccine [HFCV,RVA, PCEC] Imovax Rabies I.D. Vaccine, Imovax Rabies Vaccine, Rabies Vaccine Adsorbed (RVA), RabAvert (See Table A–2, page 652)
Uses: Rabies immunization; postexposure immunization (with local treatment and immune globulin)
Dose: Preexposure: See Table A–2, page 652. *Postexposure:* See Table A–2, page 652.
Notes: HFCV (Imovax) given IM, (Imovax ID) given ID, RVA given IM. Purified chick embryo cell (PCEC. RabAvert given IM)

■ Raloxifene (Evista)
Uses: Prevention of osteoporosis
Dose: 60 mg/d

■ Ramipril (Altace)
Uses: HTN and heart failure. *ECC.* Improve outcome after MI
Dose: 2.5–20 mg/d PO ÷ qd–bid. *ECC.* 2.5 mg PO single dose, increase to 5 mg PO bid
Notes: May use in combination with diuretics; may cause a nonproductive cough

■ Ranitidine (Zantac)
Uses: Duodenal ulcer, active benign ulcers, hypersecretory conditions, GERD
Dose: Adults. Ulcer: 150 mg PO bid, 300 mg PO qhs, or 50 mg IV q6–8h; or 400 mg IV/d cont inf. *Maint:* 150 mg PO qhs. *Hypersecretion:* 150 mg PO bid. *Peds.* 0.1–0.8 mg/kg/dose IV q6–8h or 1.25–2.0 mg/kg/dose PO q12h
Notes: ↓ dose with renal failure; note oral and parenteral doses are different

■ Rapacuronium (Raplon)
Uses: Muscle relaxer, adjunct to general anesthesia, endotracheal intubation

*Dose: **Adults.*** Intubation, short surgical procedures: 1.5–2.5 mg/kg. Repeat up to 3 maint. of 0.5 mg/kg IV (not IM): ***Peds.*** *1 mo– 12 y:* 2 mg/kg, repeat dosing not recommended. *13–17 y:* Use adult guidelines if child physically mature

■ Rimexolone (Vexol Ophthalmic)
Uses: Postop inflammation and uveitis
Dose: Adults & Peds > 2 y: *Uveitis:* 1–2 gtt q1h daytime and q2h at night, can taper to 1 gt q4h; postop 1–2 gtt qid for up to 2 wk
Notes: Should taper dose to zero

■ Repaglinide (Prandin)
Uses: Management of Type 2 DM
Dose: 0.5–4 mg ac

■ Respiratory Syncytial Virus Immune Globulin [RSV-IGIV] RespiGam
Uses: Prevent serious RSV respiratory infection (< 24 mo with BPD or prematurity (< 35 wk gestation)
Dose: 750 mg/kg/mo as follows: 1.5 ml /kg/h × 15 min, then 3 mL/kg/h × 15 min then at 6 mL/kg/h until complete dose

■ Reteplase (Retavase) (See Cover)
Uses: Thrombolytic after AMI
Dose: ECC. 10 U IV over 2 min, 2nd dose 30 min later of 10 U IV over 2 min. NS flush before and after each bolus

■ Rh$_o$(D) Immune Globulin [RhoGAM] WinRho SD, WinRho SDF
Uses: Prevention of Rh isoimmunization in nonsensitized Rho(D) antigen-negative women within 7 H of after a variety of conditions and treatment of ITP in nonsplenectomized Rho(D) antigen-positive patients
Dose: See package insert, based on Rh status and conditions of patient and fetus. *Treatment of ITP:* IV: Initial: 25–50 μg/kg based on Hg concentration. Maint: 25–60 μg/kg based on response

■ Ribavirin (Virazole, Rebetron)
Uses: Treatment of infants and children with respiratory syncytial virus infection; treatment of hepatitis C
Dose: RSV: 6 g in 300 mL of sterile water inhaled over 12-18 h. *Hepatitis C:* 600 mg PO bid in combination with interferon alfa-2b

Notes: Aerosolized by a SPAG generator; may accumulate on soft contact lenses; monitor Hgb and Hct frequently; pregnancy test every month

Rifampin (Rifadin)
Uses: Tuberculosis, treatment, and prophylaxis of *N meningitidis, H influenzae,* or *S aureus* carriers
Dose: **Adults.** *N meningitidis and H influenzae carrier:* 600 mg PO qd 3–4 d. *Tuberculosis:* 600 mg PO or IV qd or twice weekly with combination therapy regimen. **Peds.** 10–20 mg/kg/dose PO or IV qd–bid
Notes: Multiple side effects; causes orange-red discoloration of bodily secretions including tears; never used as a single agent to treat active tuberculosis infections

Rifampin, Isoniazid, and Pyrazinamide (Rifater)
Uses: Active TB
Dose: Based on weight:44 kg = 4 tabs, 45–54 kg = 5 tabs, 55 kg = 6 tabs, in a single daily dose

Rifapentine (Priftin)
Uses: Treatment of tuberculosis
Dose: *Intensive phase:* 600 mg PO twice weekly for 2 mo; separate doses by ≥ 3 d. *Continuation phase:* 600 mg/wk
Notes: Has similar adverse effects and drug interactions as rifampin

Rimantadine (Flumadine)
Uses: Prophylaxis and treatment of influenza A virus infections
Dose: **Adults.** 100 mg PO bid. **Peds.** 5 mg/kg PO qd, not to exceed 150 mg/d

Risedronate (Actonel)
Uses: Prevention and treatment of postmenopausal osteoporosis
Dose: 5 mg/d PO with 6–8 oz of water
Notes: Take 30 min before first food or drink of the day; interaction with calcium supplements; may cause GI distress and arthralgia

Risperidone (Risperdal)
Uses: Management of psychotic disorders
Dose: 1–8 mg PO bid

Ritonavir (Norvir)
Uses: HIV in combination with two or three other agents
Dose: 600 mg PO bid with food

Rizatriptan (Maxalt) See Table A–35, page 687

Rocuronium (Zemuron)
Uses: Skeletal muscle relaxation as an adjunct to general anesthesia, endotracheal intubation
Dose: Adults. Intubation: Initial: 0.45–0.6 mg/kg (provides 22–31 min relaxation); 0.9–1.2 mg/kg max. Maint. 0.1–0.2 mg/kg; *Rapid sequence intubation:* 0.6–1.2 mg/kg. *Inf:* 0.01–0.012 mg/kg/min IV: *Peds. Initial:* 0.6 mg/kg. *Maint:* 0.075–0.125 mg/kg

Rofecoxib (Vioxx)
Uses: Osteoarthritis, acute pain, and primary dysmenorrhea
Dose: 12.5–50 mg/d
Notes: Alert patients to be aware of GI ulceration or bleeding

Rosiglitazone (Avandia)
Uses: Treatment of type 2 DM
Dose: 4–8 mg/d PO or in 2 ÷ doses
Notes: May be taken with or without meals

Salmeterol (Serevent)
Uses: Treatment of asthma and exercise-induced bronchospasm
Dose: 2 inhals bid

Saquinavir (Fortovase, Invirase)
Uses: HIV in combination with two or three other agents
Dose: Fortovase: 1200 mg tid after meals. *Invirase:* 600 mg PO tid after meals

Sargramostim [GM-CSF] (Prokine, Leukine)
Uses: Treatment of myeloid recovery following bone marrow transplantation
Dose: Adults & Peds. 250 mg/m^2/d IV for 21 d
Notes: May cause bone pain

Scopolamine, Transdermal (Transderm-Scop)
Uses: Prevention of nausea and vomiting associated with motion sickness; preop control of secretions
Dose: Transderm-Scop: Apply 1 patch behind the ear every 3 d; 0.3–0.65 IM/IV/SQ repeat PRN q4–6h
Notes: May cause dry mouth, drowsiness, and blurred vision

Secobarbital (Seconal) [C]
Uses: Insomnia
Dose: Adults. 100 mg PO, or IM qhs PRN. *Peds.* 3–5 mg/kg/dose PO or IM qhs PRN
Notes: Beware of respiratory depression; tolerance acquired within 1–2 wk

Selegiline (Eldepryl)
Uses: Parkinson's disease
Dose: 5 mg PO bid
Notes: May cause nausea and dizziness

Sertraline (Zoloft)
Uses: Treatment of depression
Dose: 50–200 mg/d PO
Notes: Can activate manic/hypomanic state; has caused weight loss in clinical trials

Sibutramine (Meridia)
Uses: Management of obesity
Dose: 10–15 mg/d
Notes: Use with low-calorie diet, monitor BP

Sildenafil (Viagra)
Uses: Erectile dysfunction
Dose: 25–100 mg 1 h prior to sexual activity, max dosing is once daily
Notes: Do not take with nitrates in any form; no fatty food; adjust dose in persons > 65 y

Silver Nitrate
Uses: Prevention of ophthalmia neonatorium due to GC; removal of granulation tissue cauterization of wounds
Dose: Adults & Peds. Apply to moist surface 2–3 × a week for several weeks or until desired effect. *Peds.* Newborns apply 2 gtt into conjunctival sac immediately after birth

Silver Sulfadiazine (Silvadene)
Uses: Prevention of sepsis in second-degree and third-degree burns
Dose: Adults & Peds. Aseptically cover affected area with thin coating bid
Notes: Can have systemic absorption with extensive application; must be aggressively debrided daily

■ Simethicone (Mylicon)
Uses: Symptomatic treatment of flatulence
Dose: *Adults & Peds.* 40–125 mg PO pc and hs PRN

■ Simvastatin (Zocor)
Uses: Reduction of elevated cholesterol levels
Dose: 5–40 mg PO qhs

■ Sirolimus (Rapamune)
Uses: Prophylaxis of organ rejection
Dose: 2 mg/d PO
Notes: Dilute in water or orange juice; do NOT drink grapefruit juice while on sirolimus; take 4 h after cyclosporin

■ Sodium Bicarbonate
Uses: Alkalinization of urine, renal tubular acidosis (RTA), treatment of metabolic acidosis. **ECC.** Specific adult indications: Class I (usually indicated) if known preexisting hyperkalemia. Class IIa (accepted, possibly controversial) if known preexisting bicarbonate-responsive acidosis (eg, diabetic ketoacidosis); tricyclic antidepressant overdose; alkalinize urine in aspirin overdose. Class IIb (accepted, but may not help, probably not harmful) if prolonged resuscitation with effective ventilation; upon return of spontaneous circulation after long arrest interval. Class III (harmful) in hypoxic lactic acidosis (eg, cardiac arrest and CPR without intubation).
Peds indications: Treatment of severe metabolic acidosis (documented or following prolonged arrest) unresponsive to oxygenation and hyperventilation. Treatment of hyperkalemia, tricyclic antidepressant toxicity
Dose: *Adults. Metabolic acidosis:* 2–5 mEq/kg IV over 8 h and PRN based on acid/base status. *Alkalinize urine:* 4 g (48 mEq) PO, then 1–2 g q4h; adjust based on urine pH. *Chronic renal failure:* 1–3 mEq/kg/d. *Distal RTA:* 1 mEq/kg/d PO. **ECC.** IV inf. 1 mEq/kg IV bolus. Repeat half this dose q10min thereafter. If rapidly available, use ABG analysis to guide therapy. **Peds.** *Chronic renal failure:* see Adult. *Distal RTA:* 2–3 mEq/kg/d PO. *Proximal RTA:* 5–10 mEq/kg/d titrate based on serum bicarbonate levels. *Urine alkalinization:* 84–840 mg/kg/d (1–10 mEq/kg/d) ÷ doses; adjust based on urine pH. **ECC.** 1 mEq/kg. Dose may be calculated to correct 1/4–1/2 of base deficit
Notes: 1 g neutralizes 12 mEq of acid; in infants, do not exceed 10 mEq/min inf. Supplied as IV inf, powder, and tabs: 300 mg = 3.6 mEq; 325 mg = 3.8 mEq; 520 mg = 6.3 mEq; 600 mg = 7.3 mEq; 650 mg = 7.6 mEq

■ Sodium Citrate (Bicitra)
Uses: Alkalinization of urine; dissolve uric acid and cysteine stones
Dose: *Adults.* 2–6 tsp (10–30 mL) diluted in 1–3 oz of water pc and hs.
Peds. 1–3 tsp (5–15 mL) diluted in 1–3 oz of water pc and hs

Notes: Do NOT give to patients on aluminum-based antacids. Contra in patients with severe renal impairment of sodium-restricted diets

■ Sodium Polystyrene Sulfonate (Kayexalate)
Uses: Treatment of hyperkalemia
Dose: Adults. 15–60 g PO or 30–60 g PR q6h based on serum K. *Peds.* 1 g/kg/dose PO or PR q6h based on serum K
Notes: Can cause hypernatremia; given with agent such as sorbitol (mixed in 20–100 mL of 70% soln) to promote movement through bowel

■ Sorbitol (Generic)
Uses: Constipation. Cathartic used in conjunction with sodium polystyrene sulfonate or charcoal
Dose: Constipation: Adults & Peds > 12 y: 30–150 mL of a 20–70% soln PRN. *With sodium polystyrene sulfonate:* 15 mL 70% sol PO until diarrhea occurs (10–20 mL/2 h) or 20–100 mL PO. *With sodium polystyrene sulfonate resin with charcoal: Adults.* 4.3 mL/kg 70% sorbitol with 1 g/kg activated charcoal PO. *Peds.* 4.3 mL/kg 35% sorbitol with 1 g/kg activated charcoal

■ Sotalol (Betapace)
Uses: Treatment of ventricular arrhythmias
Dose: 80 mg PO bid; may be ↑ to 240–320 mg/d
Notes: Dose should be adjusted for renal insufficiency

■ Sparfloxacin (Zagam)
Uses: Community-acquired pneumonia, acute exacerbations of chronic bronchitis
Dose: 400 mg PO on day 1, then 200 mg q24h for a total of 10 days; ↓ dose in renal dysfunction
Notes: MUST protect from sunlight up to 5 days after last dose. Do NOT administer with drugs that prolong QT internal

■ Spironolactone (Aldactone)
Uses: Treatment of hyperaldosteronism, essential HTN, edematous states (CHF, cirrhosis), polycystic ovary
Dose: Adults. 25–100 mg PO qid. *Peds.* 1–3.3 mg/kg/24h PO ÷ bid–qid
Notes: Can cause hyperkalemia and gynecomastia; avoid prolonged use; diuretic of choice for cirrhotic edema and ascites

■ Stavudine (Zerit)
Uses: Advanced HIV disease MOA: Reverse-transcriptase inhibitor

Dose: Adults. 60 kg: 40 mg bid. *< 60 kg:* 30 mg bid; ↓ dose in renal failure C/CI: [C, +]. **Supplied:** Caps 15, 20, 30, 40 mg; soln 1 mg/mL
   Notes: Lactic acidosis and severe hepatomegaly with steatosis and pancreatitis reported

■ Steroids, Systemic

The following relates only to the commonly used systemic glucocorticoids.
   Uses: Endocrine disorders (adrenal insufficiency), rheumatoid disorders, collagen-vascular diseases, dermatologic diseases, allergic states, edematous states (cerebral, nephrotic syndrome), immunosuppression for transplantation, hypercalcemia, malignancies (breast, lymphomas), preop (in any patient who has been on steroids in the previous year, known hypoadrenalism, preop for adrenalectomy); inj into joints/tissue
   Dose: Varies with use and institutional protocols. Some commonly used doses are: *Adrenal insufficiency, acute (Addisonian crisis).* **Adults.** Hydrocortisone 100 mg IV q8h; then 300 mg/d ÷ q8h; convert to 50 mg PO q8h × 6 doses, taper to 30–50 mg/d ÷ bid. **Peds.** *Hydrocortisone:* 1–2 mg/kg IV; then 150–250 mg/d ÷ tid. *Adrenal insufficiency, chronic (physiologic replacement):* May also need mineralocorticoid supplementation such as DOCA. **Adults.** Hydrocortisone 20 mg PO qAM, 10 mg PO qPM; cortisone 0.5–0.75 mg/kg/d ÷ bid; cortisone 0.25–0.35 mg/kg IM qd. Dexamethasone· 0.03–0.15 mg/kg/d or 0.6–0.75 mg/m²/d in ÷ q6–12h PO, IM, IV. **Peds.** Hydrocortisone 0.5–0.75 mg/kg/d PO tid; hydrocortisone succinate 0.25–0.35 mg/kg/d IM. *Asthma, Acute:* **Peds.** Prednisolone 1–2 mg/kg/d or prednisone 1–2 mg/kg/d ÷ qd–bid for up to 5 d; prednisolone 2–4 mg/kg/d IV ÷ tid. *Congenital adrenal hyperplasia:* **Peds.** Initially hydrocortisone 30–36 mg/m²/d PO ÷ ⅓ dose qAM, ⅔ dose qPM; Maint: 20–25 mg/m²/d ÷ bid. *Extubation/airway edema:* Dexamethasone 0.5–1 mg/kg/d IM/IV ÷ 6h, start beginning 24 h before extubation; continue 4 additional doses. *Immunosuppressive/antiinflammatory:* **Adults** and older **Peds.** Hydrocortisone: 15–240 mg PO, IM, IV q12h; methylprednisolone: 4–48 mg/d PO; taper to lowest effective dose; methylprednisolone sodium succinate 10–80 mg IM qd. **Adults.** Prednisone or prednisolone 5–60 mg/d PO, ÷ qd–qid. Infants and younger children: 2.5–10 mg/kg/d hydrocortisone PO ÷ q6–8h; 1–5 mg/kg/d IM/IV ÷ bid/qd. *Nephrotic syndrome:* Children: prednisolone or prednisone 2 mg/kg/d PO ÷ tid–qid until urine is protein-free for 5 d, use up to 28 d; for persistent proteinuria, 4 mg/kg/dose PO qod max 120 mg/d for an additional 28 d; Maint: 2 mg/kg/dose qod for 28 d; taper over 4–6 wk (max 80 mg/d). *Septic shock:* **Adults.** Hydrocortisone 500 mg–1 g IM/IV q2–6h. **Peds.** Hydrocortisone 50 mg/kg IM/IV, repeat q4–24h PRN. *Status asthmaticus:* **Adults & Peds.** Hydrocortisone 1–2 mg/kg/dose IV q6h; then by 0.5–1 mg/kg q6h. *Rheumatic disease* (adults): Intraarticular: Hydrocortisone acetate 25–37.5 mg large joint; 10–25 mg small joint; methylprednisolone acetate 20–80 mg large joint, 4–10 mg small joint. *Intrabursal:* Hydrocortisone acetate 25–37.5 mg. *Intraganglia:* Hydrocortisone acetate 25–37.5 mg. *Tendon sheath:* Hydrocortisone acetate 5–12.5 mg. *Perioperative steroid coverage:* Hydrocortisone 100 mg IV night before surgery, 1 h preop, intraoperatively, and 4, 8,

and 12 h postop; POD No. 1: 100 mg IV q6h; POD No. 2: 100 mg IV q8h; POD No. 3: 100 mg IV q12h; POD No. 4: 50 mg IV q12h; POD No. 5: 25 mg IV q12h; then, resume prior oral dosing if chronic use or discontinue if only perioperative coverage is required. *Cerebral edema:* Dexamethasone 10 mg IV; then 4 mg IV q4–6h

Notes: See Table A–8, page 659. All can cause hyperglycemia, "steroid psychosis," adrenal suppression; never acutely stop steroids, especially if chronic treatment; taper dose. Hydrocortisone succinate administered systemically, acetate form intraarticular

■ Steroids, Topical
Uses: Topical therapy of a variety of inflammatory and pruritic dermatologic conditions that respond to corticosteroid therapy
Dose: Application based on individual agent (See Table A–33, page 684).

■ Streptokinase (Streptase, Kabikinase) (See Cover)
Uses: Coronary artery thrombosis; acute massive PE; DVT; some occluded vascular grafts; **ECC.** See Alteplase, page 526
Dose: *PE:* Loading dose of 250,000 IU IV through a peripheral vein over 30 min, then 100,000 IU/h IV for 24–72 h. *DVT or arterial embolism:* Load as with PE, then 100,000 IU/h IV for 72 h. **ECC.** 1.5 million IU in a 1 h inf
Notes: If maint inf is not adequate to maintain thrombin clotting time 2–5 × control, refer to package insert for adjustments

■ Succimer (Chemet)
Uses: Chelating agent for lead poisoning in **Peds** with blood levels > 45 µg/dL
Dose: **Adults & Peds.** 30 mg/kg/d ÷ doses q8h × 5 d, then 20 mg/kg/d × 14

■ Succinylcholine (Anectine, Quelicin, Sucostrin)
Uses: Adjunct to general anesthesia to facilitate endotracheal intubation and to induce skeletal muscle relaxation during surgery or mechanically supported ventilation
Dose: **Adults.** 0.6 mg/kg IV over 10–30 s followed by 0.04–0.07 mg/kg as needed to maintain muscle relaxation. **Peds.** 1–2 mg/kg/dose IV followed by 0.03–0.06 mg/kg/dose at intervals of 10–20 min
Notes: May precipitate malignant hyperthermia; respiratory depression or prolonged apnea may occur; many drug interactions potentiating activity of succinylcholine; observe for cardiovascular effects; use only freshly prepared solns

■ Sucralfate (Carafate)
Uses: Treatment of duodenal ulcers, gastric ulcers

Dose: Adults. 1 g PO qid, 1 h before meals and hs. *Peds.* 40–80 mg/kg/d ÷ q6h

Notes: Treatment should be continued for 4–8 wk unless healing is demonstrated by radiograph or endoscopy; constipation is the most frequent side effect

■ Sufentanil (Sufenta) [C]

Uses: Analgesic adjunct to maintain balanced general anesthesia

Dose: Adjunctive: 1–8 mg/kg with nitrous oxide/oxygen. Maint of 10–50 mg PRN. *General anesthesia:* 8–30 mg/kg with oxygen and a skeletal muscle relaxant. Maint of 25–50 mg PRN

Notes: Respiratory depressant effects persisting longer than the analgesic effects; 80 × more potent than morphine

■ Sulfacetamide

Uses: Conjunctival infections

Dose: 10% oint apply qid and qhs; 10-, 15-, 30% soln for keratitis apply q2–3h depending on severity

■ Sulfasalazine (Azulfidine)

Uses: Ulcerative colitis

Dose: Adults. 1–2 g PO initially, increase to max of 8 g/d in 3–4 ÷ doses; Maint 500 mg PO qid. *Peds.* 40–60 mg/kg/24h PO ÷ q4–6h initially. Maint 20–30 mg/kg/24h PO ÷ q6h.

Notes: Can cause severe GI upset; discolors urine

■ Sulfinpyrazone (Anturane)

Uses: Acute and chronic gout

Dose: 100–200 mg PO bid for 1 wk, then increase as needed to Maint of 200–400 mg bid

■ Sulindac (Clinoril)

Uses: Treatment of arthritis and pain

Dose: 150–200 mg bid

■ Sulfisoxazole (Gantrisin, others)

Uses: Acute uncomplicated UTIs

Dose: Adults. Between 500 mg and 1 g PO qid. *Peds* > 2 mo: 120–150 mg/kg/24h PO ÷ q4–6h

Notes: Avoid use in last half of pregnancy (causes fetal hyperbilirubinemia)

Sumatriptan (Imitrex) See Table A–35, page 687

Tacrine (Cognex)
Uses: Treatment of mild-to-moderate dementia
Dose: 10–40 mg PO qid
Notes: May cause elevations in transaminases; LFTs should be monitored regularly

Tacrolimus [FK 506] (Prograf)
Uses: Prophylaxis of organ rejection
Dose: IV: 0.05–0.1 mg/kg/d as cont inf. *PO:* 0.15–0.3 mg/kg/d ÷ into 2 doses
Notes: May cause neurotoxicity and nephrotoxicity

Tamoxifen (Nolvadex)
Uses: Adjuvant treatment of breast cancer
Dose: 10–20 mg PO bid
Notes: May increase the risk of secondary uterine cancer

Tamsulosin (Flomax)
Uses: Treatment of benign prostatic hyperplasia
Dose: 0.4– 0.8 mg qd

Telmisartan (Micardis)
Uses: Treatment of HTN
Dose: 40–80 mg/d
Notes: Avoid use during pregnancy

Temazepam (Restoril) [C]
Uses: Insomnia
Dose: 15–30 mg PO qhs PRN
Notes: Reduce dose in elderly patients

Tenecteplase (TNKase)
Uses: Reduction of mortality associated with AMI
Dose: 30– 50 mg IV; see product information for weight-based dosing

Teniposide (Vumon)
Uses: Treatment of leukemia
Dose: 165 mg/m^2 IV twice weekly for 8–9 doses

■ Terazosin (Hytrin)
Uses: Treatment of HTN and benign prostatic hyperplasia
Dose: Initially 1 mg PO hs; titrate ↑ to max of 20 mg PO qhs
Notes: Hypotension and syncope following first dose; dizziness, weakness, nasal congestion, peripheral edema common; often used with thiazide diuretic

■ Terbutaline (Brethine, Bricanyl)
Uses: Reversible bronchospasm (asthma, COPD); inhibition of labor
Dose: *Adults. Bronchodilator:* 2.5–5 mg PO qid or 0.25 mg SQ, may repeat in 15 min (max 0.5 mg in 4 h). *Metered dose inhaler:* 2 inhals q4–6h. *Premature labor:* 10–80 mg/min IV infusion for 4h, then 2.5 mg PO q4–6h until term. *Peds. Oral:* 0.05–0.15 mg/kg/dose PO tid; max 5 mg/24h
Notes: Caution with diabetes, HTN, hyperthyroidism; high doses may precipitate β_1-adrenergic effects

■ Terconazole (Terazol 7)
Uses: Vaginal fungal infections
Dose: 1 applicator intravaginally qhs for 7 d

■ Tetanus immune globulin [TIG] BayTet
Uses: Tetanus immunization
Dose: Prophylaxis: Adults. 250 units IM. *Peds.* 4 units/kg. *Treatment: Adults.* 3000–6000 units IM. *Peds.* 500–3000 units
Notes: Consider local infiltration around wound. TIG preferred over tetanus antitoxin for treatment of active tetanus; used in unclean, nonminor wound where history of tetanus toxoid is unknown or inadequate (ie < 3 doses of tetanus toxoid)

■ Tetanus Toxoid
Uses: Protection against tetanus
Dose: See Table A–34, page 686 for tetanus prophylaxis

■ Tetracaine (Pontocaine)
Uses: Topical ocular anesthesia; spinal anesthesia; topical anesthesia for skin and mucous membranes
Dose: Ophthalmic: ½–1 in. oint in lower conjunctival fornix or 1–2 ggt. *Topical mucous membranes:* Apply 2% PRN, 20 mg max. *Topical for skin:* Apply PRN

■ Tetracycline (Achromycin V, Sumycin)
Uses: Broad-spectrum antibiotic treatment against *Staphylococcus, Streptococcus, Chlamydia, Rickettsia,* and *Mycoplasma*

Dose: Adults. 250–500 mg PO bid–qid. *Peds* > 8 y: 25–50 mg/kg/24h PO q6–12h. Do NOT use in children < 8 y

Notes: Can stain enamel and depress bone formation in children; caution with use in pregnancy. Do NOT use in presence of impaired renal function (see Doxycycline, page 564)

■ Theophylline (Theolair, Theo-Dur, Somophyllin, Others)
Uses: Asthma, bronchospasm.
Dose: Adults. 24 mg/kg/24h PO ÷ q6h; SR products may be ÷ q8–12h.
Peds. 16 mg/kg/24h PO ÷ q6h; SR products may be ÷ q8–12h
Notes: See drug levels in Table A–22, page 675; many drug interactions; side effects include nausea, vomiting, tachycardia, and seizures

■ Thiamine (Vitamin B$_1$)
Uses: Thiamine deficiency (beriberi); alcoholic neuritis; Wernicke's encephalopathy
Dose: Adults. Deficiency: 100 mg IM qd for 2 wk, then 5–10 mg PO qd for 1 mo. *Wernicke's encephalopathy:* 100 mg IV 3 1 dose, then 100 mg IM qd for 2 wk. *Peds.*10–25 mg IM qd for 2 wk, then 5–10 mg/24h PO qd for 1 mo
Notes: IV thiamine administration associated with anaphylactic reaction; must be given slowly IV

■ Thiethylperazine (Torecan)
Uses: Nausea and vomiting
Dose: 10 mg PO, PR or IM qd–tid
Notes: Extrapyramidal reactions may occur

■ Thioridazine (Mellaril)
Uses: Psychotic disorders; short-term treatment of depression, agitation, organic brain syndrome
Dose: Adults. Initial: 50–100 mg PO tid. Maint: 200–800 mg/24h PO in 2–4 ÷ doses. *Peds* > 2 y: 1–2.5 mg/kg/24h PO ÷ bid–tid
Notes: Low incidence of extrapyramidal effects.

■ Thiothixene (Navane)
Uses: Psychotic disorders
Dose: Adults & Peds > 12 y: *Mild-to-moderate psychosis:* 2 mg PO tid. *Severe psychosis:* 5 mg PO bid; ↑ to max dose of 60 mg/24h PRN. *IM use:* 16–20 mg/24h ÷ bid–qid; max 30 mg/d. *Peds* < 12 y: 0.25 mg/kg/24h PO ÷ q6–12h
Notes: Drowsiness and extrapyramidal side effects most common

■ Thyroid [Thyroid Extract]
Uses: Replacement in hypothyroidism
Dose: 30 mg/d PO, titrate 30 mg/d over several weeks. maint 60–120 mg/d

■ Tiagabine (Gabitril)
Uses: Adjunctive therapy in treatment of partial seizures
Dose: Initially 4 mg/d, ↑ by 4 mg during 2nd week; ↑ by 4–8 mg/d until clinical response is achieved; max dose 32 mg/d
Notes: Withdraw gradually; used in combination with other anticonvulsants

■ Ticarcillin (Ticar)
Uses: Infections caused by susceptible strains of gram-negative bacteria including *Klebsiella, Proteus, E coli, Enterobacter, P aeruginosa,* and *Serratia* involving the skin, bone, respiratory tract, urinary tract, abdomen, and septicemia
Dose: *Adults.* 3 g IV q4–6h; *Peds.* 200–300 mg/kg/d IV ÷ q4–6h
Notes: Often used in combination with aminoglycosides

■ Ticarcillin/Potassium Clavulanate (Timentin)
Uses: Infections caused by susceptible strains of gram-negative bacteria (*Klebsiella, Proteus, E coli, Enterobacter, P aeruginosa,* and *Serratia*) involving the skin, bone, respiratory tract, urinary tract, abdomen, and septicemia
Dose: *Adults.* 3.1 g IV q4–6h. *Peds.* 200–300 mg/kg/d IV ÷ q4–6h
Notes: Often used in combination with aminoglycosides

■ Ticlopidine (Ticlid)
Uses: Reduce the risk of thrombotic stroke
Dose: 250 mg PO bid
Notes: Should be administered with food

■ Timolol (Blocadren, Timoptic)
Uses: Treatment of HTN and MI; glaucoma
Dose: *HTN:* 10–20 mg bid. *MI:* 10 mg bid. *Ophthalmic:* 0.25% 1 gt bid; ↓ to qd when controlled; use 0.5% if needed; 1 gt gel qd
Notes: Timoptic XE (0.25, 0.5%) is a gel-forming soln

■ Tioconazole (Vagistat)
Uses: Vaginal fungal infections
Dose: 1 applicator intravaginally hs (single dose)

■ Tirofiban (Aggrastat) (see Cover)
Uses: Management of ACS, PCI
Dose: *ECC.* Initial 0.4 µg/kg/min for 30 min, followed by 0.1 µg/kg/min
Notes: Adjust dose in renal insufficiency; use in combination with heparin

■ Tizanidine (Zanaflex)
Uses: Antispasmodic (eg, MS, spinal cord injury)
Dose: 4 mg PO initially q6–8h, 3 doses or 36 mg/d max, ↑ PRN 2–4 mg increments, no single dose > 12 mg

■ Tobramycin (Nebcin)
Uses: Serious gram-negative infections, especially *Pseudomonas*
Dose: Based on renal function 2 mg/kg IV load followed 1.5 mg/kg IV q8h; refer to Aminoglycoside Dosing, Tables A–24 and A–26, pages 676 and 678
Notes: Nephrotoxic and ototoxic; decrease dose with renal insufficiency; monitor creatinine clearance and serum concentrations for dosing adjustments; see Table A–24, page 676

■ Tobramycin Ophthalmic (Tobrex)
Uses: Ocular bacterial infections
Dose: 0.3% oint apply q3–8h or 0.3% soln apply 1–2 gtt q1–4h based on severity of infection

■ Tobramycin and Dexamethasone Ophthalmic (Tobradex)
Uses: Ocular bacterial infections associated with significant inflammation
Dose: 0.3% oint apply q3–8h or soln 0.3% apply 1–2 gtt q1–4h

■ Tocainide (Tonocard)
Uses: Suppression of ventricular arrhythmias including PVCs, and VT
Dose: 400–600 mg PO q8h
Notes: Properties similar to lidocaine; ↓ dose in renal failure; CNS and GI side effects are common

■ Tolazamide (Tolinase)
Uses: Management of non-insulin-dependent DM
Dose: 100–500 mg qd

■ Tolazoline (Priscoline)
Uses: Persistent pulmonary vasoconstriction and HTN of the newborn, peripheral vasospastic disorders

Dose: Adults. 10–50 mg IM/IV/SQ qid. *Neonates.* 1–2 mg/kg IV over 10–15 min, followed by 1–2 mg/kg/h

Tolbutamide (Orinase)
Uses: Management of non-insulin-dependent DM
Dose: 500–1000 mg bid

Tolmetin (Tolectin)
Uses: Treatment of arthritis and pain
Dose: 200–600 mg tid, to a max of 2000 mg/d

Topiramate (Topamax)
Uses: Treatment of partial onset seizures
Dose: Total dose 400 mg/d. See product information of 8-wk titration schedule
Notes: May precipitate kidney stones

Torsemide (Demadex)
Uses: Edema, HTN, CHF, and hepatic cirrhosis
Dose: 5–20 mg/d PO or IV

Tramadol (Ultram)
Uses: Management of moderate-to-severe pain
Dose: 50-100 mg PO q4–6h PRN, not to exceed 400 mg/d

Trandolapril (Mavik)
Uses: Treatment of HTN, CHF, left-ventricular systolic dysfunction, post AMI
Dose: HTN: 2–4 mg/d. *CHF/LV dysfunction:* 4 mg/d

Trazodone (Desyrel)
Uses: Major depression
Dose: 50–150 mg PO qd–qid; max 600 mg/d
Notes: May take 1–2 wk for symptomatic improvement; anticholinergic side effects

Triamcinolone (inhal, nasal) (Nasacort, Nasacort AQ)
Uses: Seasonal and perennial allergic rhinitis
Dose: Peds >12 y & *Adults. Intranasal:* 2 sprays in each nostril qd. may ↑ in 4–7 d to 4 sprays/d or 1 spray qid in each nostril

■ Triamcinolone (inhal, oral) Azmacort
Uses: Asthma
Dose: Peds >12 y & *Adults.* 2 inhals tid–qid, 16 inhals/day max. *Peds.*
6–12 y: 1–2 inhals tid–qid, 12 inhals/d max

■ Triamterene (Dyrenium)
Uses: Edema associated with CHF, cirrhosis
Dose: 100–300 mg/24h PO ÷ qd–bid
Notes: Can cause hyperkalemia; blood dyscrasias, liver damage, and
other reactions

■ Triazolam (Halcion) [C]
Uses: Insomnia
Dose: 0.125–0.5 mg PO qhs PRN
Notes: Additive CNS depression with alcohol and other CNS depressants

■ Triethanolamine Polypeptide Oleate (Cerumenex Otic)
Uses: Removal of symptomatic ear wax, ceruminolytic
Dose: Adults & Peds. Fill ear canal and insert cotton plug; allow to remain
15–30 min, then flush ear with water

■ Trifluoperazine (Stelazine)
Uses: Psychotic disorders
Dose: Adults. 2–10 mg PO bid. *Peds* 6–12 y: 1 mg PO qd–bid, gradually
↑ to 15 mg/d
Notes: Decrease dose in elderly and debilitated patients; oral concentrate
must be diluted to 60 mL or more before administration

■ Trifluridine (Viroptic)
Uses: Herpes simplex keratitis and conjunctivitis
Dose: 1 gt q2h (max 9 gtt/d); decrease to 1 gt q4h after healing begins; treat
up to 14 d

■ Trihexyphenidyl (Artane)
Uses: Parkinson's disease
Dose: 2–5 mg PO qd–qid
Notes: Contra in narrow angle glaucoma

■ Trimethaphan (Arfonad)
Uses: Controlled hypotension during surgery; treatment of hypertensive
crisis; treatment of pulmonary edema with pulmonary HTN and systemic HTN;
dissecting aortic aneurysm

Dose: Adults. 0.3–6 mg/min IV inf titrated to effect; *Peds.* 50–150 mg/kg/min IV inf

Notes: Additive effect with other antihypertensive agents; vasopressors may be used to reverse hypotension if required; phenylephrine is vasopressor of choice for reversal of effects

■ Trimethobenzamide (Tigan)
Uses: Nausea and vomiting
Dose: Adults. 250 mg PO or 200 mg PR or IM tid–qid PRN. *Peds.* 20 mg/kg/24h PO or 15 mg/kg/24h PR or IM in 3–4 ÷ doses (NOT recommended for infants)
Notes: In the presence of viral infections, may contribute to Reye's syndrome; may cause Parkinsonian-like syndrome

■ Trimethoprim (Trimpex, Proloprim)
Uses: UTIs caused by susceptible gram-positive and gram-negative organisms
Dose: 100 mg PO bid or 200 mg PO qd
Notes: Reduce dose in renal failure

■ Trimethoprim-Sulfamethoxazole (Co-trimoxazole Bactrim, Septra)
Uses: UTIs, otitis media, sinusitis, bronchitis, *Shigella, P carinii, Nocardia*
Dose: Adults. 1 double strength (DS) tab PO bid or 5–10 mg/kg/24h (based on trimethoprim component) IV in 3–4 ÷ doses. *P carinii:* 15–20 mg/kg/d IV or PO (trimethoprim component) in 4 ÷ doses. *Peds.* 8–10 mg/kg/24h (trimethoprim) PO ÷ into 2 doses or 3–4 doses IV; do NOT use in newborn
Notes: Synergistic combination; ↓ dosage in renal failure

■ Trimipramine (Surmontil)
Uses: Treatment of depression
Dose: 75–300 mg PO qhs

■ Tropicamide (Mydriacyl)
Uses: Ocular exam; mydriatic and cycloplegic
Dose: 1–2 gtt of 0.5–1% soln 30 min before exam; repeat q30min PRN
Notes: Effects last 4–6 h

■ Urokinase (Abbokinase)
Uses: PE, DVT, restore patency to IV catheters, coronary artery thrombosis
Dose: Adults & Peds. Systemic effect: 4400 IU/kg IV over 10 min, followed by 4400 IU/kg/h for 12 h. *Restore catheter patency:* Inject 5000 IU into catheter and gently aspirate.

Notes: Do NOT use systemically within 10 d of surgery, delivery, or organ biopsy

■ Valacyclovir (Valtrex)
Uses: Treatment of herpes zoster
Dose: 1 g PO tid

■ Valproic Acid and Divalproex (Depakene and Depakote)
Uses: Epilepsy, mania, and prophylaxis of migraines
Dose: Adults & Peds. Seizures: 30–60 mg/kg/24h PO ÷ tid. *Mania:* 750 mg in 3 ÷ doses, ↑ to a max of 60 mg/kg/d. *Migraines:* 250 mg bid, increased to 1000 mg/d
Notes: Monitor LFTs and follow serum levels; concurrent use of phenobarbital and phenytoin may alter serum levels of these agents

■ Valsartan (Diovan)
Uses: HTN
Dose: 80 mg/d
Notes: Use with caution with potassium-sparing diuretics or potassium supplements

■ Vancomycin (Vancocin, Vancoled)
Uses: Serious infections resulting from methicillin-resistant staphylococci and in enterococcal endocarditis in combination with aminoglycosides in penicillin-allergic patients; oral treatment of *C difficile* pseudomembranous colitis
Dose: Adults. 1 g IV q12h; for colitis 250–500 mg PO q6h. *Peds* (NOT neonates): 40 mg/kg/24h IV in ÷ doses q12–6h
Notes: Ototoxic and nephrotoxic; not absorbed orally, provides local effect in gut only; IV dose must be given slowly over 1 h to prevent "red-man syndrome"; adjust dose in renal failure; see Table A–23 and page 676.

■ Varicella Virus Vaccine [Chicken Pox Vaccine, Varicella-Zoster Vaccine] (Varivax)
Uses: AAP recommends vaccination for all healthy children 12 mo–18 y; if 12 mo–13 y who have not been immunized or have not had chickenpox should receive 1 vaccination. Children 3–18 y require 2 vaccinations 4–8 wk apart
Dose: Give SQ: *Peds* 12 mo–12 y: 0.5 mL. *Adults & Peds* > 12 y: 2 doses of 0.5 mL 4–8 wk apart
Notes: The vaccine has been added to childhood immunization schedule for infants 12–28 mo and peds 11–12 y who have not been vaccinated or who have not had the disease; recommended to be given with MMR vaccine

■ Varicella-Zoster Immune Globulin [VZIG]
Uses: Immunization of immunodeficient patients after varicella exposure
Dose: Deep IM: 125U/10 kg (22 lb), 625 units (5 vials) max; mini dose 125 U
Note: Most effective if begun within 96 h of exposure; alternative: treat varicella, if it occurs, with IV acyclovir

■ Vasopressin (Antidiuretic Hormone) (Pitressin)
Uses: Treatment of DI; gaseous GI tract distention; severe GI bleeding
Dose: Adults & Peds. DI: 2.5–10 U SQ or IM tid–qid or 1.5–5.0 U IM q1–3d of the tannate. *GI bleed:* 20 U in 50–100-mL D_5W or NS given IV over 15–30 min
Notes: Should be used with caution with any vascular disease

■ Vecuronium (Norcuron)
Uses: Skeletal muscle relaxation during surgery or mechanical ventilation
Dose: Adults & Peds. 0.08–0.1 mg/kg IV bolus. Maint of 0.010–0.015 mg/kg after 25–40 min followed with additional doses every 12–15 min
Notes: Drug interactions leading to increased effect of vecuronium include aminoglycosides, tetracycline, and succinylcholine; less cardiac effects then pancuronium

■ Venlafaxine (Effexor)
Uses: Treatment of depression
Dose: 75–225 mg/d ÷ into 2–3 equal doses

■ Verapamil (Calan, Isoptin) (See Cover)
Uses: Supraventricular tachyarrhythmias (PAT, Wolff–Parkinson–White syndrome, atrial flutter or fibrillation); vasospastic (Prinzmetal's) and unstable (crescendo, preinfarction) angina; chronic stable angina (classical effort-associated); HTN; *ECC.* Second line for PSVT with narrow QRS complex and adequate BP
Dose: Adults. Tachyarrhythmias: 5–10 mg IV over 2 min (may repeat in 30 min). *Angina:* 240–480 mg/24h ÷ in 3–4 doses. *HTN:* 80–180 mg PO tid or SR tab 240 mg PO qd. *ECC.* 2.5–5.0 mg IV over 1–2 min. Repeat 5–10 mg, if needed, in 15–30 min (30 mg max). *Alternative:* 5 mg bolus q15min to total dose of 30 mg. *Peds.* <1 y: 0.1–0.2 mg/kg IV over 2 min (may repeat in 30 min). *1–15 y:* 0.1–0.3 mg/kg IV over 2 min (may repeat in 30 min). Do NOT exceed 5 mg
Notes: Use caution with elderly patients; reduce dose in renal failure; constipation is a common side effect

■ Vidarabine (Vira-A)
Uses: Herpes simplex keratitis and conjunctivitis

Dose: Apply oint 5 ×/d ÷q3–4h; after healing begins, decrease to bid for up to 7 d

■ Vinblastine (Velban)
Uses: Hodgkin's disease, lymphoma, and testicular and ovarian cancer
Dose: On the basis of protocol; typical dosing 4–12 mg/m^2 q7–10d or 5-d cont inf 1.4–1.8 mg/m^2/d
Notes: May cause neutropenia; reduce dose after radiation exposure

■ Vincristine (Oncovin)
Uses: Cervical and ovarian cancer, sarcoma, leukemia, and Hodgkin's disease
Dose: Varies with protocol 1.4–2 mg/m^2 IV once a week
Notes: May cause severe extravasation

■ Vitamin B$_{12}$
See Cyanocobalamin, page 554.

■ Vitamin K
See Phytonadione, page 619.

■ Warfarin Sodium (Coumadin)
Uses: Prophylaxis and treatment of PE and venous thrombosis, AF with embolization, other postop uses
Dose: Adults. Need to individualize dose to keep INR level at 2–3; some mechanical heart valves require INR to be 2.5–3.5; initially, 10–15 mg PO, IM, or IV qd for 1–3 d; then maint, 2–10 mg PO, IV, or IM qd; follow INR levels during initial phase to guide dosing. ***Peds.*** 0.05–0.34 mg/kg/24h PO, IM, or IV qd. Follow PT closely to adjust dose
Notes: Follow INR while on maint dose; beware of bleeding caused by over anticoagulation (PT > 3 × control); caution patient on effects of taking Coumadin with other medications, especially aspirin; to rapidly correct over-anticoagulation, use vitamin K or fresh frozen plasma or both; highly teratogenic, do not use in pregnancy

■ Witch Hazel (Tucks Pads)
Uses: After bowel movement cleansing to decrease local irritation or relieve hemorrhoids; after anorectal surgery and episiotomy
Dose: Apply as needed

■ Yellow Fever Vaccine (YF-VAX)
Uses: Immunization against yellow fever
Dose: 0.5 mL SC × 1 dose

■ Zafirlukast (Accolate)
Uses: Prophylaxis and chronic treatment of asthma
Dose: 20 mg bid
Notes: Not for acute exacerbations of asthma, Contra in nursing women

■ Zalcitabine (Hivid)
Uses: HIV infection in patients intolerant to zidovudine and didanosine
Dose: 0.75 mg PO tid
Notes: May be used in combination with zidovudine; may cause peripheral neuropathy

■ Zaleplon (Sonata)
Uses: Insomnia
Dose: 5–20 mg qhs PRN

■ Zanamivir (Relenza)
Uses: Treatment of influenza
Dose: 2 inhals (10 mg) bid
Notes: Uses a diskhaler for administration

■ Zidovudine (Retrovir)
Uses: Management of HIV infections
Dose: Adults. 200 mg PO tid or 300 mg PO bid or 1–2 mg/kg/dose IV q4h.; Pregnancy: 100 mg PO 5 ×/d until labor; during labor 2 mg/kg over 1 h followed by 1 mg/kg/h until clamping of the umbilical cord. ***Peds.*** 720 mg/m^2/24h PO ÷ 5 ×/d

■ Zidovudine and Lamivudine (Combivir)
Uses: HIV infections
Dose: Adults & ***Peds*** > 12 y. 1 tab bid; ↓ dose in renal failure
Notes: An alternative to ↓ number of caps for combination therapy with the two agents. WARNING—Neutropenia, anemia, lactic acidosis, and hepatomegaly with steatosis

■ Zileuton (Zyflo)
Uses: Prophylaxis and chronic treatment of asthma
Dose: 600 mg qid
Notes: MUST take on a regular basis; does NOT treat acute exacerbation

■ **Zolmitriptan (Zomig) See Table A–35, page 687**

■ **Zolpidem (Ambien) [C]**
Uses: Short-term treatment of insomnia
Dose: 5–10 mg PO qhs PRN

■ **Zonisamide (Zonegran)**
Uses: Partial seizures
Dose: Initial 100 mg/d; may be ↑ to 400 mg/d
Notes: Contra in persons with hypersensitivity to sulfonamides

Appendix

TABLE A–1. THROMBOLYTIC INDICATIONS/DOSING/CONTRAINDICATIONS

■ **Thrombolytic indications for MI (all must be present)**
1. Within 12 h of symptom onset
2. ≥ 1 mm ST-segment elevation[a] in two or more continuous leads **or** new LBBB
3. Absence of cardiogenic shock
4. Absence of contraindications (see below)

■ **Thrombolytic dosing for acute MI**[b]
TPA: If ≥ 65 kg; 100 mg/3 h. (60 mg/h 1; 20 mg/h 2; 20 mg/h 3)
   If < 65 kg: 1.25 mg/kg over 3 h.
Streptokinase: 1.5 million U IV as a continuous infusion up to 60 min.
TNKase: All given as a bolus over 5 s:
   < 60 kg: 30 mg
   ≥ 60 kg < 70 kg: 35 mg
   ≥ 70 kg < 80 kg: 40 mg
   ≥ 80 kg < 90 kg: 45 mg
   ≥ 90 kg: 50 mg

■ **Contraindications for thrombolytic therapy**
1. Major surgery within 10 days[c] (eg, CABG, obstetric delivery, organ biopsy, previous puncture of noncompressible vessels)
2. Trauma within 10 days[c]
3. GI or GU bleeding within 10 days[c]
4. h/o hemorrhagic stroke[d]
5. Sys BP ≥ 180 mm Hg or dias BP ≥ 110 mm Hg
6. High likelihood of left heart thrombus (eg, mitral stenosis with atrial fibrillation)
7. Acute pericarditis
8. Subacute bacterial endocarditis
9. Hemostatic defects (eg, severe hepatic or renal disease)
10. Diabetic hemorrhagic retinopathy or other hemorrhagic ophthalmic condition
11. Septic thrombophlebitis including occluded AV fistula at seriously infected site
12. Warfarin anticoagulation
13. Any other potential source of significant bleeding

■ **Treatment of reperfusion arrhythmias:**
Symptomatic bradycardia (increased pain, cardiogenic shock):
1. Atropinee 1 mg IV, may repeat × 1
2. Aminophylline[e] 100 mg/min IV, max 250 mg until convert to NSR (*Ann Intern Med* 1995;7:509)
3. Repeat ECG
4. Synchronized transcutaneous or transjugular pacing PRN as bridge to cath lab for refractory symptomatic bradycardia
Ventricular tachycardia:
1. R/O a-fib with RVR
2. Lidocaine 1.5 mg/kg IV bolus, then 2–4 mg/min gtt. May repeat bolus × 1.[f]

(continued)

TABLE A–1. *(Continued)*

■ **Emergency treatment of bleeding complications of antithrombotic therapy**

Minor external bleeding	Manual pressure
All others	Immediate cessation of fibrinolytic agent, aspirin, heparin
	Protamine (1 mg/100 U heparin) IV slowly over 1–3 min; max 50 mg
	T&C 4U PRBC, 4U FFP, platelets
	Check PTT, CBC, and fibrinogen
	Volume replacement with crystalloid and blood as necessary
	Call cardiologist and consult hematologist.
	FFP for serious bleeding.
	For ICH, secure airway, CT head and consult neurosurgeon

ª**Beware:** Cardiac aneurysm after previous MI may give permanent ST elevation outside the context of acute ischemia.
ᵇDosing schedule taken from The University of Pittsburgh Medical Center Pharmacy.
ᶜSome studies use 6 weeks.
ᵈh/o nonhemorrhagic stroke is only a relative contraindication.
Age > 75 is no longer considered a contraindication, although the risk of intracranial bleeding is increased.
ᵉCaution when treating bradycardia associated with MIs in the LAD distribution, which supplies His bundle; increasing AV conduction may increase degree of block in His bundle and actually exacerbate bradycardia.
ᶠAmiodarone 150 mg IV over 10–15 min. is an alternative if time available, then start gtt; 300 mg IV push for unstable V-tach.
Note: Direct coronary angioplasty has compared favorably with thrombolytic therapy for the treatment of AMI, especially in centers with significant experience.
LBBB = left bundle branch block; CABG = coronary artery bypass graft; GI = gastrointestinal; GU = genitourinary; AV = arterovenous; ECG = electrocardiogram; R/O = rule out; RVR = rapid ventricular response; T&C = type and cross-match; PRBC = packed red blood cells; PTT = partial thromboplastin time; FFP = fresh-frozen plasma; ICH = intracranial hemorrhage; CT = computed tomography.

TABLE A–2. RABIES TREATMENT RECOMMENDATIONS—UNITED STATES

Status of Vaccination	Modality of Treatment	Treatment Regimen
No previous vaccination	Cleaning of wound	Clean all wounds with soap and water. If available use a virucidal agent to irrigate wounds (eg, povidine–iodine solution)
	Rabies immune globulin (RIG)	20 IU/kg body weight should be infiltrated around the wound(s) if feasible anatomically. The remainder should be given IM at a site distant from the vaccine.
	Rabies vaccine	Given IM (deltoid) on days 0, 3, 7, 14, 28.
Received previous vaccination	Wound care	Same as above.
	Rabies immune globulin	Do not administer.
	Rabies vaccine	Given IM (deltoid) on days 0 & 3.

TABLE A–2. *(Continued)*

Type of Animal	Assessment and Disposition of Animal	Recommendations for Postexposure Prophylaxis
Dogs, cats and ferrets	Healthy and available for 10 days observation	Individual should not start prophylaxis unless animal develops clinical signs of rabies (If during the 10 days animal develops signs of rabies begin prophylaxis. In addition, euthanize and test animal.)
	Rabid or suspected rabid Unknown secondary to animal not available	Immediate vaccination recommended. Contact local health department.
Skunks, raccoons, foxes, other carnivores, and bats	Suspect as rabid unless animal is already proven to be negative for rabies by laboratory tests	Immediate vaccination recommended.
Livestock, small rodents, lagomorphs (rabbits and hares), large rodents (woodchucks and beavers), and other animals	Consider on an individual basis	**Consult local health department** Bites of squirrels, hamsters, guinea pigs, gerbils, chipmunks, rats, mice, other small rodents, rabbits, and hares rarely require rabies postexposure prophylaxis.

Reproduced, with permission, from Updated rabies postexposure prophylaxis guidelines. *MMWR* 1999; 48 (no. RR-1): 1–21.

TABLE A–3. HELPFUL INTERNET LINKS

■ **Problem: How do I get started?**
Where can I find applications?

General	**Palmgear** http://www.palmgear.com	
	First and most complete.	
	Handango http://www.handango.com/	
	Includes PalmOS, PocketPC, PSion and RIM applications.	
Medical	**PDAMD** http://www.pdamd.com/	
	Best forums, good reviews and articles	
	Handheldmed http://www.handheldmed.com	
	Useful collection of resources	
Emergency	**Emerg Doc Palm** http://www.jimthompson.net/palmpda	

How can I keep up to date?

Applications	**Peripheral Brain List** http://pbrain.hypermart.net/medapps.html	
	Current and annotated list of the best applications	
	PDAMD Forum http://www.pdamd.com/vertical/forums/list.php?f=2	
	Lively and helpful discussions.	

(continued)

TABLE A–3. *(Continued)*

News	**Epocrates DocAlerts** http://www.epocrates.com
	Self-updating. Has drug, bug, and news applications.
	Avantgo http://www.avantgo.com
	Self-updating. Has hundreds of channels, most not medical.
	BMC Research
Journals	**Mobile Channels** http://www.handheldmed.com/mobilecontent.php
	Self-updating. Table of contents service for *Annals of Emergency Medicine* and 25 other journals
	JournalToGo http://www.journaltogo.com/
	Self-updating. Article summaries; Emergency Medicine covers 11 journals
	Wiley InterScience MobileEdition http://www.avantgo.com
	Select journals to receive after installing.
	PDAs in the Health Literature http://educ.ahsl.arizona.edu/pda/art.htm
	Bibliography from MEDLINE and eight other databases on use of PDAs in medicine and consumer health

■ **Problem: How can I make my palmtop more useful?**
Medical Calculators

Ob-Gyn	**PregCalc Pro** http://www.medicaltoolbox.com/products/PregCalcPro/
	PregTrak http://www.stacworks.com
	\$\$ Calculate due date; track patients
EBM	**MedCalc**
	MedMath
	MedRules
	Free. Calculate 40–70 common formulae
Drips	**InfusiCalc** http://www.users.bigpond.com/aetherpalm
	\$\$ Highly recommended.
	Wizard Drip Calculator http://www.medicalwizards.com/i2_drips.htm
	\$\$ Easy to use
Other	**ABG Pro**
	Free. Analyze Arterial Blood Gases
	ToxWizard http://www.medicalwizards.com/i2_tozwizard.htm
	\$\$. Calculate antidotes; poison management guide
	STAT GrowthCharts
	Free. Child growth norms
	STAT Cardiac Clearance
	Free. Is patient cleared for surgery cardiac-wise?
	STAT Cardiac Risk
	Free. Heart disease risk.

Reference Guides

Drugs	**Epocrates qRX** http://www.epocrates.com
	Johns Hopkins Antibiotic Guide http://hopkins-abxguide.org/main.cfm
	Free, although both track statistical data
	DrDrugs http://www.Skyscape.com
	Physicians Drug Handbook http://www.Skyscape.com
	\$\$. More thorough, links to medical texts.
Bugs	**Epocrates qID** http://www.epocrates.com
	Free. Infections/antibiotics guide
	Infectious Diseases Notes http://www.pdamedsolutions.com/
	\$\$. Exhaustive Rx guide to infections and normal flora

TABLE A–3. *(Continued)*

Dictionaries	**Taber's Medical Dictionary** http://www.Skyscape.com
	    $$ 55,000 words.
	Dorland's Pocket Medical Dictionary http://www.Skyscape.com
	    $$ Can cross-link to drug and medical references

Emergency Med	**Pepid** http://www.pepid.com
	    $$ Versions for students, nurses, interns, etc
	5MEC http://www.Skyscape.com or http://www.Handheldmed.com
	    $$ Text of Five Minute Emergency Consult

Med Ref	**5MCC** http://www.Skyscape.com or http://www.Handheldmed.com

Patient Management

Tests	**TestTrakker** http://www.cedarcovetech.com/ $$. Status of tests, searchable
Charting	**DigitalAssist** http://www.digitalassist.net/ $$. For ER physicians. Haven't seen any reviews.

Billing And Coding

ICD	**ICD-Notes** http://www.med-notes.com **Stat-Coder** http://www.statcoder.com/ **MD-Coder** http://www.mobiledesigntech.com/product/mdcoder30.htm $$. 15,000+ ICD9/CM diagnosis codes lookup/tracking
Other	**STAT E&M Coder** http://www.statcoder.com/eandm.htm Evaluation and Management

■ **Problem: How can palmtops help my patients?**

PatientWare

Images	**Netter** http://www.graphicwitness.com/netter/gallery/
	Grey's Anatomy http://www.bartleby.com/107/
	Vesalius http://www.vesalius.com/
	    Use Fireviewer or AlbumToGo to move explanatory pictures to your
	    palmtop

Pill reminders	On-Time-Rx 1.3
	MiniRX 1.0 http://www.handango.com
	    Encourage patients with palmtops and complex medication schedules
	    to have reminders

Personal med
record
	My Medical Records
	Health Empowerment Tools 1.4
	4T Medical http://www.handango.com
	    Encourage patients with palmtops to have medical information in an
	    accessible location.

$$—Commercial or shareware applications
Free—freeware; may collect information about use patterns

TABLE A–4. MINI-MENTAL STATUS EXAMINATION

	Maximum Possible Score	Score
Orientation		
What is the: (year) (season) (date) (day) (month)?	5	( )
Where are we: (state) (county) (town) (hospital) (floor)?	5	( )
Registration		( )
Name 3 objects; ask patient to repeat.	3	
Attention and calculation		( )
The serial 7 test; 1 point for each correct. Stop after 5 answers.	5	
Option: spell "world" backwards.		
Recall	3	( )
Ask for the 3 objects repeated above.		
1 point scored for each correct object recalled.		
Language	9	( )
Name a pencil and watch	(2 points)	
Repeat the following, "No if's, ands, or buts."	(1 point)	
Follow 3 stage command: "Take a paper in your right hand, fold it in half, and put it on the floor."	(3 points)	
Read and follow the following printed command: "Close your eyes"	(1 point)	
Write a sentence	(1 point)	
Copy design	(1 point)	
Scoring: A score of less than 24 may suggest the presence of delirium, dementia, or another problem affecting mental status and may indicate the need for further evaluation.	30 possible	

Orientation: Ask for the date. Specifically ask for any omitted information. One point for each correct.

Registration:

Ask permission to test memory. Name 3 unrelated objects clearly and slowly about 1 second apart. After you have said all three, ask the patient to repeat. The first repetition determines the score. Keep repeating the items up to six times until the patient can repeat all three. (Patient must learn this to test recall)

Attention and calculation: Ask the patient to begin with 100 and count backwards by 7. Stop after 5 subtractions and score correct answers. If the patient cannot calculate, ask him to spell "world" backwards. The score is the number of letters in correct order.

Recall: Ask the patient if he can recall the 3 words previously asked to remember. Score 0–3.

Language: Naming: Show the patient a wrist watch and pencil and ask name. Score 0–2.

Repetition: Ask the patient to repeat a sentence. Allow one trial. Score 0 or 1.

3-Stage command: Give the patient a piece of paper and repeat the command. Score 1 point for each portion of the command correctly performed.

Reading: Print clearly a piece of paper in large letters the command, "Close your eyes." Ask the patient to read and perform the command. Score one point if the eyes are closed.

Writing: Five the patient a blank piece of paper and ask him to write a sentence of his own choosing. It must contain a subject and a verb to be scored 1 point. Punctuation does not matter for scoring purposes.

Copying: On a clean piece of paper, draw intersecting pentagons, each side out inch, and ask the patient to copy exactly. All 10 angles must by present and the two figures must intersect to score one point. Any rotation of the figures or tremor is ignored.

Modified with permission, from Folstein ME: Mini-mental state: A practical method for grading the cognitive state of patients for the clinician. *J Psychiatr Res* 1975;12:189.

TABLE A–5. GENERALIZATION SUMMARY OF FEATURES OF DELIRIUM, DEMENTIA, AND PSYCHIATRIC DISORDERS

Features of Delirium, Dementia, and Psychiatric Disorders	Delirium	Dementia	Psychiatric Disorders
Onset	Sudden	Insidious	Sudden
Course over 24 h	Fluctuating	Stable	Stable
Consciousness	Reduced or clouded	Alert	Alert
Attention	Disordered	Normal early in clinical course	May be disordered
Cognition	Disordered	Impaired	May be impaired
Orientation	Impaired	Often impaired	May be impaired
Hallucinations	Visual or auditory	Often absent	Usually auditory
Delusions	Transient, poorly organized	Usually absent	Sustained
Movement	Asterixis, tremor may be may be present	Usually absent; if present usually from another condition	Absent

Modified, with permission, from Lipowski Z. Delirium in the elderly patient. *N Engl J Med* 1989;20:578

TABLE A–6. QUICK CONFUSION SCALE (QCS) FOR SCREENING FOR COGNITIVE IMPAIRMENT[a]

Item	Score Number correct (Highest number in category indicates correct response; decreased scoring number indicates increased number or errors)	Weight Multiply item score by weight	Total
What year is it now?	0 or 1 (score 1 if correct, 0 if incorrect)	×2	
What month is it?	0 or 1 (score 1 if correct, 0 if incorrect)	×2	
Repeat this phrase after me and remember it: John Brown, 42 Market Street, New York			
About what time is it? (Answer correct within the hour)	0 or 1 (score 1 if correct, 0 if incorrect)	×2	
Count backward from 20 to 1.	0, 1, or 2 (score 2 if correct; 1 if one error, score 0 if more than 2 errors)	×1	
Say the months in reverse	0, 1, or 2 (score 2 if correct; 1 if one error, score 0 if more than 2 errors)	×1	
Repeat memory phrase (Each underlined portion is worth 1 point)	0, 1, 2, 3, 4, or 5 (score 5 if correctly performed; each error drops score by one)	×1	
Final score is sum of the totals			

[a]The Quick Confusion Scale scores over a 1–15 range, with 15 being the top score. Like the MMSE, it is a screening examination for cognitive impairment to detect deficits in orientation, memory, and attention that might not be detected in routine examination. Correlation with the MMSE is good and it is quicker to administer at the bedside. A score of 11 or less correlates with a score of less than 24 on the MMSE and may indicate the need for further patient testing and evaluation. Like the MMSE, there is a correlation on scoring with educational level.
Reprinted, with permission, from Huff JS, Farace E, Brady WJ, Kheir J, Shawver G. The quick confusion scale in the ED: Comparison with the mini-mental state examination. Am J Emerg Med 2001;19(6):461–464.

TABLE A–7. INSULINS.

Type of Insulin	Onset (h)	Peak (h)	Duration (h)	Compatible to Mix with
■ Rapid-acting				
Aspart (Novolog)	0.25	0.5–1.5	3–5	All
Lispro (Humalog)	0.25	0.5–1.5	3–4	All
Regular Iletin II	0.5–1	5–10	6–8	All
Humulin R	0.5–1	5–10	6–8	All
Novolin R	0.5–1	5–10	6–8	All
■ Intermediate-acting				
NPH Iletin II	1–1.5	4–6	24	Regular
Humulin N	1–1.5	4–6	24	Regular
Novolin N	1–1.5	4–6	24	Regular
Lente Iletin II	1–2.5	7.5	24	Regular, Semilente
■ Long-acting				
Humulin U	4–8	10–30	36	Regular
Ultralente	4–8	10–30	36	Regular
Insulin Glargine (Lantus)	1–1.5	Peakless	24	Do not mix with other insulins
■ Combinations				
Humulin 70/30	0.5	4–8	24	
Novolin 70/30	0.5	4–8	24	

Reproduced, with permission, from Haist SA, Robbins JB, Gomella LG, eds. *Internal Medicine On Call*, 3rd ed. McGraw-Hill, 2002.

TABLE A–8. COMPARISON OF GLUCOCORTICOIDS.

Drug (Trade)	Equivalent Dose (mg)	Anti-inflammatory Potency	Mineralocorticoid Potency
■ Short-acting			
Cortisone (Cortone)	25	0.8	2
Hydrocortisone (Cortef)	20	1	2
■ Intermediate-acting			
Methylprednisolone (Medrol)	4	5	0
Prednisone (Deltasone)	5	4	1
Prednisolone (Delta-Cortef)	5	4	1
Triamcinolone	4	5	0
■ Long-acting			
Betamethasone (Celestone)	0.6–0.75	20–30	0
Dexamethasone (Decadron)	0.75	20–30	0

Reproduced, with permission, from Haist SA, Robbins JB, Gomella LG, eds. *Internal Medicine On Call*, 3rd ed. McGraw-Hill, 2002.

TABLE A–9. ANGIOTENSIN-CONVERTING ENZYME INHIBITORS.[a,b,c,d]

Drug (Trade)	Hypertension	Heart Failure	Left Ventricular Dysfunction
Benazepril (Lotensin)	10–40 mg/day divided qd-bid		
Captopril (Capoten)	25–50 mg bid–tid	6.25–25 mg tid	Titrate to 50 mg tid
Enalapril (Vasotec)	5–40 mg/d divided q day–bid	2.5–10 mg bid	Titrate to 10 mg bid
Fosinopril (Monopril)	10–40 mg q day	10–40 mg q day	
Lisinopril (Prinivil, Zestril)	10–40 mg q day	5–20 mg q day	
Moexipril (Univasc)	7.5–30 mg/d divided q day–bid		
Perindopril (Aceon)	4–16 mg/d	4 mg/d	
Quinapril (Accupril)	10–80 mg q day	5–20 mg bid	
Ramipril (Altace)	2.5–20 mg/d divided q day–bid	1.25–5 mg bid	
Trandolapril (Mavik)	2–8 mg/d	1 mg/d	

Notes:
[a] Pro-drugs (metabolized to active agent): Benazepril, Enalapril, Fosinopril, Moexipril, Perindopril, Quinapril, Ramipril, Trandolapril.
[b] Persistent, nonproductive cough has occurred with the use of *all* ACE inhibitors. Cough typically resolves within 1–4 days after therapy is discontinued. Angiotensin-II receptor antagonists are less frequently associated with cough.
[c] Coadministration of ACE inhibitors with potassium preparations may result in elevated serum potassium concentrations.
[d] Strictly contraindicated in pregnancy. Women of child-bearing age should be warned regarding risk of teratogenicity and use of ACE inhibitors.
Reproduced with permission from Haist SA, Robbins JB, Gomella LG, eds. *Internal Medicine On Call*, 3rd ed. McGraw-Hill, 2002.

TABLE A–10. ANGIOTENSIN RECEPTOR ANTAGONISTS.

Drug (Trade)	Daily Dosage Range	Renal Dysfunction	Product Availability (mg)
Candesartan (Atacand)	8–32 mg/d	No adjustment necessary	Tablets 4, 8, 16, 32
Eprosartan (Teveten)	400–800 mg/d	No adjustment necessary	Tablets 400, 600
Irbesartan (Avapro)	140–300 mg/d	No adjustment necessary	Tablets 75, 150, 300
Irbesartan/ Hydrochlorothiazide (Avalide)	1–2 tablets/d	HCTZ not recommended in severe impairment	Tablets Irbesartan 150/HCTZ 12.5 Irbesartan 300/HCTZ 12.5
Losartan (Cozaar)	25–100 mg/d or bid	No adjustment necessary	Tablets 25, 50
Losartan/ Hydrochlorothiazide (Hyzaar)	50/12.5 mg 1–2/d 100 mg/25 mg/d	HCTZ not recommended in severe impairment	Tablets Losartan 50/HCTZ 12.5 Losartan 100/HCTZ 25
Telmisartan (Micardis)	20–80 mg/d	No adjustment necessary	Tablets 40, 80
Valsartan (Diovan)	80–320 mg/d	Decrease dose if ClCr < 10 mL/min	Capsules 80, 160
Valsartan/ Hydrochlorothiazide (Diovan HCT)	1–2 capsules/d	HCTZ not recommended in severe impairment	Tablets Valsartan 80/HCTZ 12.5 Valsartan 160/HCTZ 12.5

ClCr – creatinine clearance.
Reproduced with permission from Haist SA, Robbins JB, Gomella LG, eds. *Internal Medicine On Call*, 3rd ed. McGraw-Hill, 2002.

TABLE A–11. ANTISTAPHYLOCCOCCAL PENICILLINS.[a,b]

Drug (Brand)	Dosage	Dosing Interval	Supplied	Notes
Oxacillin (Bactocill)	1–2 g	4–6 h	Injection	
Nafcillin (Nafcil, Unipen)	1–2 g	4–6 h	Injection	No dosage adjustments for renal function
Cloxacillin (Cloxapen, Tegopen)	250–500 mg	6 h	Oral	Administer on an empty stomach
Dicloxacillin (Dynapen, Dycill)	250–500 mg	6 h	Oral	Administer on an empty stomach

[a] **Indications:** Treatment of infections caused by susceptible strains of *Staphylococcus* and *Streptococcus*.
[b] **Actions:** Bactericidal: Inhibits cell wall synthesis.
Reproduced with permission from Haist SA, Robbins JB, Gomella LG, eds. *Internal Medicine On Call*, 3rd ed. McGraw-Hill, 2002.

TABLE A–12. EXTENDED-SPECTRUM PENICILLINS.[a,b,c]

Drug (Brand)	Dose	Dosing Interval	mEq Na⁺ Per Gram	Notes
Ticarcillin (Ticar)	3 g	4–6 h	5.2	May cause hypokalemia/sodium overload, acquired platelet dysfunction with the potential for bleeding to occur
Ticarcillin-clavulanate (Timentin)	3.1 g	4–6 h	4.75	Clavulanate is a β-lactamase inhibitor
Mezlocillin (Mezlin)	3 g	4–6 h	1.85	Activity against Enterobacteriaceae
Piperacillin (Pipracil)	3 g	4–6 h	1.85	Best activity against *Pseudomonas*
Piperacillin-tazobactam (Zosyn)	3.375 g	6 h		Tazobactam is a β-lactamase inhibitor (Does not improve activity against *Pseudomonas* when compared to piperacillin without tazobactam)

[a] **Indications:** Treatment of infections caused by susceptible gram-negative bacteria (including *Klebscherichia Proteus, E. coli, Enterobacter, P aeruginosa, Serratia*) involving the skin, bone and joints, respiratory tract, urinary tract, abdomen, and vascular system.

[b] **Actions:** Bactericidal, inhibits cell wall synthesis.

[c] **Notes:** These agents are often used in combination with an aminoglycoside to treat *P aeruginosa* and in neuropenic patients with a fever. Dosage adjustment necessary in renal impairment.

Reproduced with permission from Haist SA, Robbins JB, Gomella LG, eds. *Internal Medicine On Call*, 3rd ed. McGraw-Hill, 2002.

TABLE A–13. BETA-ADRENERGIC BLOCKING AGENTS. [a,b,c,d]

Drug (Trade)	Receptor	Angina	Hypertension	Myocardial Infarction	Congestive Heart Failure
Acebutolol (Sectral)	B_1, ISA		200–400 mg bid		
Atenolol (Tenormin)	B_1	50–100 mg q day	50–100 mg q day	5 mg IV × 2 doses, then 50 mg PO bid	
Betaxolol (Kerlone)	B_1		10–20 mg q day		
Bisoprolol (Zebeta)	B_1		5–10 mg q day		
Carteolol (Cartrol)	B_1, B_2, ISA		2.5–5 mg q day		
Carvedilol (Coreg)	B_1, B_2, α (See p 568)		6.25–25 mg bid		3.125–25 bid
Esmolol (Brevibloc)					
Labetalol (Trandate, Normodyne)	B_1, B_2, α_1		100–400 mg bid		
Metoprolol (Lopressor, Toprol XL)	B_1	50–100 mg bid	100–450 mg q day	5 mg IV × 3 doses, then 50 mg PO qbh × 48 h, then 100 mg PO bid	6.25–50 mg bid or 12.5–200 mg XL q day
Nadolol (Corgard)	B_1, B_2	40–80 mg q day	40–80 mg q day		

(continued)

TABLE A-13. *(Continued)*

Drug (Trade)	Receptor	Angina	Hypertension	Myocardial Infarction	Congestive Heart Failure
Penbutolol (Levatol)	B₁, B₂, ISA		20–40 mg q day		
Pindolol (Visken)	B₁, B₂, ISA		5–10 mg bid		
Propranolol (Inderal)	B₁, B₂	160 mg SR qd	120–160 mg SR qd	60 mg tid–qid	
Sotalol (Betapace)	(See p 634)				
Timolol (Blocadren)	B₁, B₂		10–20 mg bid	10 mg bid	

ISA = intrinsic sympathomimetic activity.

Other Uses: Cardiac Arrhythmias: Various agents and doses

Migraine Prophylaxis: Atenolol 50–100 mg/d **or**
   Nadolol 40–80 mg/d **or**
   [c]Propranolol 80–240 mg/d

Essential Tremor: Propranolol 40 mg bid; maximal dose 320 mg/d

Adjunctive Therapy: Pheochromocytoma (after α-adrenergic drugs are added)
   Hyperthyroidism (propranolol)
   Rebleeding of esophageal varices in cirrhotic patients and alcohol withdrawal (atenolol)

Precautions:

[a] Use with caution in diabetic patients. May blunt symptoms/signs of acute hypoglycemia; nonselective agents may potentiate insulin-induced hypoglycemia. Beta-blockade also reduces the release of insulin in response to hyperglycemia.

[b] May increase serum lipid concentrations. May not be as pronounced with agents having intrinsic sympathomimetic activity.

[c] Use with caution in patients with CHF (decreased myocardial contractility) and chronic obstructive pulmonary diseases (potential blockade of B₂ receptors).

[d] When discontinuing chronically administered β-blockers, particularly in patients with ischemic heart disease, reduce dose gradually, especially with agents with a short half-life (propranolol, metoprolol).

[e] FDA-approved indication.

Reproduced, with permission, from Haist SA, Robbins JB, Gomella LG, eds. *Internal Medicine On Call*, 3rd ed. McGraw-Hill, 2002.

TABLE A–14. FIRST-GENERATION CEPHALOSPORINS.[a,b,c]

Drug (Brand)	Dose	Dosing Interval	Supplied	Notes
Cefadroxil (Duricef, Ultracef)	500 mg–1 g	12–24 h	Capsules, tablets	
Cefazolin (Ancef, Ketzol)	1–2 g	8 h	Injection	For surgical prophylaxis most widely used antibiotic
Cephalexin (Keflex)	250–500 mg	qid	Capsules, tablets	
Cephalothin (Keflin)	1–2 g	6 h	Injection	
Cephapirin (Cefadyl)	1–2 g	6 h	Injection	
Cephradine (Velosef)	250–500 mg 1 g	qid 6 h	Capsules Injection	

[a] **Indications:** Treatment of infections caused by susceptible strains of *Streptococcus, Staphylococcus, Escherichia coli, Proteus,* and *Klebsiella* involving the skin, bone and joints, upper and lower respiratory tract, and urinary tract.
[b] **Actions:** Bactericidal: inhibits cell wall synthesis.
[c] **Dosage adjustments:** Necessary in renal impairment.
Reproduced, with permission, from Haist SA, Robbins JB, Gomella LG, eds. *Internal Medicine On Call,* 3rd ed. McGraw-Hill, 2002.

TABLE A–15. SECOND-GENERATION CEPHALOSPORINS.[a,b,c,d]

Drug (Brand)	Dose	Dosing Interval	Supplied	Notes
Cefaclor (Ceclor)	250–500 mg	8 h	Capsules Tablets	
Cefamandole (Mandol)	1–2 g	4–6 h	Injection	
Cefmetazole (Zefazone)	1–2 g	8 h	Injection	Activity against anaerobes
Cefonicid (Monocid)	1–2 g	24 h	Injection	
Cefoletan (Cefotan)	1–2 g	12 h	Injection	Activity against anaerobes
Cefoxitin (Metoxin)	1–2 g	6 h	Injection	Best activity against anaerobes
Cefprozil (Cefzil)	250–500 mg	qd–bid	Tablets	Use higher doses for otitis and pneumonia
Cefuroxime (Zinacef, Ceftin)	750 mg–1.5 g 250–500 mg	8 h bid	Injection Tablets	Ceftin should be taken with food
Loracarbef (Lorabid)	200–400 mg	bid	Capsules	Similar to cefaclor

[a] **Indications:** Treatment of infections caused by susceptible bacteria involving the upper and lower respiratory tract, skin, bone, urinary tract, abdomen, and female reproductive system.
[b] **Actions:** Bactericidal; inhibits cell wall synthesis.
[c] **Notes:** More active than 1st-generation agents against *Haemophilis, Escherichia coli, Klebsiella* spp., and *Proteus mirabilis.* Risk of hypoprothrombinemia or bleeding has been associated with cephalosporins containing a N-methylthiotetrazole (NMTT) side chain. These agents include cefotetan, cefmetazole, and cefoperazone (3rd-generation). Administration of vitamin K will prevent clinical bleeding associated with these drugs for patients with vitamin K deficiency.
[d] Dosage adjustment necessary in renal impairment.
Reproduced, with permission, from Haist SA, Robbins JB, Gomella LG, eds. *Internal Medicine On Call,* 3rd ed. McGraw-Hill, 2002.

TABLE A–16. THIRD- AND FOURTH-GENERATION CEPHALOSPORINS.[a,b,c]

Drug (Brand)	Dose	Interval	Supplied	Notes
Cefdinir (Omnicef)	300–600 mg	12–24 h	Capsules	
Cefepime[d] (Maxipime)	1–2 g	12 h	Injection	
Cefixime (Suprax)	200–400 mg	12–24 h	Tablets, suspension	Use suspension for otitis media
Cefoperazone (Cefobid)	1–2 g	12 h	Injection	See Footnote[c], Table A–15
Cefotaxime (Claforan)	1–2 g	4–8 h	Injection	Crosses the blood–brain barrier
Cefpodoxime (Vantin)	200–400 mg	12 h	Tablets	Drug interations with agents increasing the gastric pH
Ceftazidime (Fortaz, Ceptaz) (Tazidime, Tazicef)	1–2 g	8 h	Injection	Best activity against *Pseudomonas.* Crosses the blood–brain barrier.
Ceftibuten (Cedax)	400 mg	12 h	Capsule	Take on an empty stomach
Ceftizoxime (Cefizox)	1–2 g	8–12 h	Injection	
Ceftriaxone (Rocephin)	1–2 g	12–24 h	Injection	Treatment of choice for gonorrhea. Crosses the blood–brain barrier.

[a] *Indications:* Treatment of infections caused by susceptible bacteria involving the respiratory tract, skin, bone and joints, and urinary tract; treatment of meningitis, febrile neutropenia, and septicemia.

[b] *Actions:* Bactericidal; inhibits cell wall synthesis.

[c] *Notes:* Less active against gram-positive cocci than 1st- and 2nd-generation agents. Increased activity against gram-negative aerobes *(Enterobacteriaceae including Enterobacter and Serratia)* due to increased stability to β-lactamases. May be used in combination with an aminoglycoside. Dosage adjustment necessary in renal impairment.

[d] *Notes:* 4th-generation cephalosporin.

Reproduced with permission from Haist SA, Robbins JB, Gomella LG, eds. *Internal Medicine On Call,* 3rd ed. McGraw-Hill, 2002.

TABLE A-17. NONSTEROIDAL ANTIINFLAMMATORY DRUGS.[a]

Drug (Trade)	Arthritis	Analgesia	Dysmenorrhea	Maximum Daily Dose (mg)
■ **Salicylates**[b]				
Diflunisal[c] (Dolobid)	500 mg bid–tid	500 mg bid–tid		1500
■ **Acetic acids**[b]				
Diclofenac (Cataflam, Voltaren)	50–75 mg bid–tid	50 mg tid	50 mg tid	200
Etodolac (Lodine)	200–400 mg bid–tid	200–400 mg q6–8h		1200
Indomethacin (Indocin)	25–50 mg bid–tid			200 or SR 150
Ketorolac (Toradol)		IV/IM 15–30 mg q 6h; PO 10 mg q hr		IV: 120; PO: 40; do not use for more than 5 days
Nabumetone (Relafen)	1000–2000 mg/d divided qd–bid			2000
Sulindac (Clinoril)	150–200 mg bid			400
Tolmetin (Tolectin)	200–600 mg tid			2000
■ **Oxicams**[b]				
Piroxicam (Feldene)	10–20 mg qd			20
■ **Propionic acids**[b]				
Fenoprofen (Nalfon)	300–600 mg tid–qid	200 mg q4–6h		3200
Flurbiprofen (Ansaid)	50–100 mg bid–qid			300

(continued)

667

TABLE A-17. *(Continued)*

Drug (Trade)	Arthritis	Analgesia	Dysmenorrhea	Maximum Daily Dose (mg)
Ibuprofen (Advil, Motrin)	400–800 mg tid–qid	400 mg q4–6h	400 mg q4h	3200
Ketoprofen (Orudis)	50–75 mg tid–qid	25–50 mg q6–8h		300
Meloxicam[d,e] (Mobic)	7.5–15 mg q day			
Naproxen (Naprosyn)	250–500 mg bid	250 mg q6–8h	250 mg q6–8h	1500
Naproxen sodium (Aleve, Anaprox)	275–550 mg bid	275 mg q6–8h	275 mg q6–8h	1375
Oxaprozin (Daypro)	600–1200 mg q day			1200
■ Selective COX-2 Inhibitors				
Celecoxib[e,f] (Celebrex)	100 mg bid or 200 mg qd (osteoarthritis) 100–200 mg bid (rheumatoid arthritis)			400
Rofecoxib[f] (Vioxx)	12.5–25 mg qd	50 mg q day × 5 days	50 mg qd × 5 days	50

[a] Can cause renal insufficiency/failure, especially in the elderly. **Do not** take in the third trimester of pregnancy.
[b] Chronic use can cause gastrointestinal bleeding from gastroduodenal ulceration. Inhibits platelet aggregation except for meloxicam.
[c] First dose 1000 mg, then 500 mg bid–tid.
[d] Inhibits COX-2 more than COX-1.
[e] Dosage for familial adenomatous polyposis is 400 mg bid.
[f] Does not inhibit platelet aggregation.
Reproduced with permission from Haist SA, Robbins JB, Gomella LG, eds. *Internal Medicine On Call*, 3rd ed. McGraw-Hill, 2002.

668

TABLE A–18. OPHTHALMIC AGENTS.

Drug (Trade)	Strength (%)	Dosing Schedule
Agents for Glaucoma		
Alpha₂ Adrenergic Agonists		
Brimonidine (Alphagan)	0.2	1 gtt tid
Apraclonidine (Iopidine)	0.5, 1.0	1–2 gtts tid (0.5%), 1 gtt 1 h prior to surgery (1.0%)
Dipivefrin (Propine)	0.1	1 gtt q12h
Beta-Blockers		
Betaxolol (Betoptic-S. Betoptic)	0.25, 05	1 gtt bid
Levobunol (Betagan Liquifilm)	0.25, 0.5	1 gtt qd–bid
Metipranolol (OptiPranolol)	0.3	1 gtt bid
Timolol–(Timoptic)	0.25, 0.5	1 gtt qd–bid
Carteolol (Ocupress)	1.0	1 gtt bid
Levobetaxolol (Betaxon)	0.5	1 gtt bid
Carbonic Anhydrase Inhibitors		
Brinzolamide (Azopt)	1.0	1 gtt tid
Dorzolamide (Trusopt)	2.0	1 gtt tid
Miotics, Cholinesterase Inhibitors		
Carbachol (Isopto Carbachol)	0.75–3	1–2 gtts tid
Physostigmine (Isopto Eserine)	0.25, 0.5	2 gtts up to qid
Demecarium (Humorsol)	0.125, 0.25	1–2 gtts twice weekly, up to 1–2 gtts bid
Echothiophate iodine (Phospholine iodide)	0.03, 0.06, 0.125, 0.25	1 gtt bid
Pilocarpine (Isopto Carpine, Pilocar)	0.25–10	1–2 gtts up to 6 × per day
(Pilopine HS gel)	4.0	0.5 in. q hs

(continued)

TABLE A–18. *(Continued)*

Drug (Trade)	Strength (%)	Dosing Schedule
Prostaglandin Agonists		
Latanoprost[b] (Xalatan)	0.005	1 gtt q hs
Combination Agents		
Dorzolamide and Timolol (Cosopt)	2/0.5	1 gtt bid
Antibiotics		
Bacitracin (See p 535)		
Chloramphenicol (AK-Chlor)	oint/sol	1–2 gtts or 0.5 in. q3–4h
Ciprofloxacin (Ciloxan)	solution	1–2 gtts 4–6 × per day
Erythromycin (AK-Mycin, Ilotycin)	ointment	0.5 in. 2–8 × per day
Gentamicin (Garamycin)	oint/sol	1–2 gtts or 0.5 in. 2–3 × per day, up to q3–4h
Neomycin, Polymyxin B, Hydrocortisone 1% (Cortisporin)	sus	1–2 gtts q3–4h
Sulfacetamide Sodium (Sodium Sulamyd, Bleph 10)	10–30% oint/sol	1–2 gtts q1–3h or 0.5 in. qd–qid
Tobramycin (Tobrex)	oint/sol	1–2 gtts or 0.5 in. 2–3 × per day, up to q3–4h
Antiinflammatory		
NSAIDs		
Diclofenac (Voltaren)	0.1	1 gtt qid (postop inflammation following cataract surgery)
Flurbiprofen (Ocufen)	0.03	1 gtt q4h × 3 days (ocular inflammation)
Ketorolac (Acular)	0.5	1 gtt qid (relieves itching due to seasonal allergic conjunctivitis)
Corticosteroids		
Dexamethasone (AK-Dex, others)	0.05 (oint), 0.1 (sol)	1–2 gtts or 0.5 in. tid–qid
Fluorometholone (FML, Flarex)	0.1	1–2 gtts bid–qid

Prednisolone (AK-Pred, Pred Forte)	0.12, 0 125, 1.0	1–2 gtts q1h day, q 2 night until response, then 1 gtt Q 4 hr
Rimexolone (Vexol)	1	1–2 gtts q1h to qid
Decongestant/Anti-allergy		
Ketotifen[c] (Zaditor)	0.025	1 gtt bid–tid
Levocabastine (Livostin)	0.05	1 gtt qid
Lodoxamide (Alomide)	0.1	1–2 gtts qid
Naphazoline and Antazoline (Albalon-A)	0.05/0.5	1–2 gtts tid–qid
Naphazoline and Pheniramine Acetate (Naphcon A)	0.025/0.3	1–2 gtts tid–qid
Mast Cell Stabilizers		
Nedocromil sodium (Alocril)	2%	1–2 gtts bid
Pemirolast potassium (Alamast)	0.1%	1–2 gtts qid
Combination Agents (also see Glaucoma)		
Gentamicin and Prednisolone (Pred-G)	Oint/sol	0.5 in. bid–tid (oint), 1–2 gtts q2–4h up to q2h (sol)
Neomycin & Dexamethasone (Dex-Neo-Dex)	Oint/sol	0.5 in. tid–qid (oint), 1–2 gtts q3–4h (sol)
Neomycin, Polymyxin, Hydrocortisone (Cortisporin)	Oint/sol	0.5 in q day–qid (oint), 1–2 gtts bid–qid
Neomycin, Polymyxin, & Dexamethasone (Maxitrol)	Oint/sol	0.5 in. tid–qid (oint), 1–2 gtts q4–6h (sol)
Neomycin, Polymyxin, & Prednisolone (Poly-Pred)	Oint/sol	0.5 in. tid–qid (oint), 1–2 gtts q4–6h (sol)
Sulfacetamide & Prednisolone (Blephamide)	Oint/sol	0.5 in. qd–qid (oint), 1–3 gtts q2–3h

[a] Systemic absorption may cause bradycardia.
[b] May darken light irides.
[c] Wait at least 10 min before putting in contact lens.
Reproduced with permission from Haist SA, Robbins JB, Gomella LG, eds. *Internal Medicine On Call*, 3rd ed. McGraw-Hill, 2002.

TABLE A–19. SULFONYLUREA AGENTS.[a,b]

Drug (Trade)	Duration of Activity (hr)	Equivalent Dose (mg)	Dosing Schedule
■ **First-generation**			
Acetohexamide (Dymelor)	24	500	250–1500 mg qd
Chlorpropamide (Diabinese)	≥ 60	250	100–500 mg qd
Tolazamide (Tolinase)	12–24	250	100–500 mg qd
Tolbutamide (Orinase)	6–12	1000	500–1000 mg bid
■ **Second-generation**			
Glipizide[c] (Glucotrol, Glucotrol-XL)	10–16	10	5–15 mg qd–bid
Glyburide non-micronized[d] (DiaBeta, Micronase)	24	5	1.25–10 mg qd–bid
Glyburide micronized[d] (Glynase)	24	3	1.5–6 mg qd–bid
Glimepiride (Amaryl)	24	2	1–4 mg qd 8 mg qd[e]

[a] **Indications:** Management of non-insulin-dependent diabetes mellitus (NIDDM).
[b] **Actions:** Stimulates the release of insulin from the pancreas; increase insulin sensitivity at peripheral sites; reduces glucose output from the liver.
[c] **Glipizide:** Give approximately 30 min before a meal. Divide total daily doses when doses exceed 15 mg. Maximum daily recommended daily dose is 40 mg.
[d] **Glyburide:** Administer with first main meal. Maximum recommended daily dose nonmicronized, 20 mg; micronized, 12 mg.
[e] Given with the first main meal in patients receiving low-dose insulin.
Reproduced with permission from Haist SA, Robbins JB, Gomella LG, eds. *Internal Medicine On Call*, 3rd ed. McGraw-Hill, 2002.

TABLE A–20. PROTON PUMP INHIBITORS.[a,b,c]

	Duodenal Ulcer	Gastric Ulcer	Hypersecretory Conditions	GERD Healing	GERD Maintenance	Helicobacter pylori Eradication
Esomeprazole (Nexium)[b] —Delayed-release capsules: 20, 40 mg				20–40 mg qd × 4–8 wks	20 mg qd	40 mg qd; Amoxicillin 1 g bid, & Clarithromycin 500 mg bid × 10 days
Lansoprazole (Prevacid) —Delayed-release capsules: 15, 30 mg	15 mg qd × 4 wks	30 mg qd × 8 wks	60 mg qd up to 90 mg bid (divide doses >120 mg/d)	15–30 mg qd × 8 wks	15 mg qd	30 mg bid; Amoxicillin 1 g bid; & Clarithromycin 500 mg bid × 14 days
Omeprazole (Prilosec) —Delayed-release capsules: 10, 20, 40 mg	20 mg qd × 4–8 wks	40 mg qd × 4–8 wks	60 mg qd up to 120 mg tid (divide doses 80 mg/d)	20–40 mg qd × 4–8 wks	20 mg qd	20 mg bid; Amoxicillin 1 g bid & Clarithromycin 500 mg bid × 10 days OR 40 mg q day & Clarithromycin 500 mg tid × 14 days
Pantoprazole (Protonix)[c] —Delayed-release tablet: 40 mg				40 mg × 8 wks		
Rabeprazole (Aciphex) —Delayed-release tablet: 20 mg	20 mg qd × 4 wks	60 mg qd	20 mg × 4–8 wks	20 mg qd		

[a] All products are delayed-release formulations. Swallow whole—do not crush or chew.
[b] If patient has difficulty swallowing the capsule, open delayed-release capsule and mix the pellets inside the capsule in 1 tablespoon of applesauce. Swallow immediately—do not chew or crush pellets.
[c] Pantoprazole is now available in an IV formulation.

Reproduced with permission from Haist SA, Robbins JB, Gomella LG, eds. *Internal Medicine On Call*, 3rd ed. McGraw-Hill, 2002.

TABLE A–21. HMG-COA REDUCTASE INHIBITORS.[a,b,c]

	Dose	Comparative Dosages	Hydrophilic/ Lipophilic	Metabolism	LFT Monitoring
Atorvastatin (Lipitor) Tablet: 10, 20, 40, 80 mg	10–80 mg/d	5 mg	Lipophilic	P450 3A4	Baseline or elevation of dose, 12 wks, semiannually
Flurvastatin (Lescol) Capsule: 20, 40 mg	20–80 mg/d	20 mg	Lipophilic	P450 2C9	Baseline or elevation of dose, 12 wks, semiannually
Lovastatin (Mevacor) Tablet: 10, 20 40 mg	10–80 mg/d	20 mg	Lipophilic	P450 3A4	Baseline or elevation of Dose, 6 wks, 12 wks, semiannually
Pravastatin (Pravachol) Tablet: 10, 20, 40 mg	10–40 mg/d	20 mg	Hydrophilic	Not extensively metabolized	Baseline or elevation of dose, 12 wks
Simvastatin (Zocor) Tablet: 10, 20, 40, 80 mg	10–80 mg/d	10 mg	⁻Lipophilic	P450 3A4	Baseline or elevation of dose, semiannually

[a] Pregnancy category X.
[b] Maximum response occurs in 4–6 weeks.
[c] Counsel patients to report unexplained muscle pain, tenderness or weakness due to risk of myopathy, or jaundice and abdominal pain due to the risk of hepatic injury.
LFT = liver function test.
Reproduced with permission from Haist SA, Robbins JB, Gomella LG, eds. *Internal Medicine On Call*, 3rd ed. McGraw-Hill, 2002.

TABLE A–22. NONANTIBIOTIC DRUG LEVELS.[a]

Drug	Therapeutic Level	Toxic Level
Carbamazepine	8.0–12.0 µg/mL	> 15.0 µg/mL
Digoxin	0.8–2.0 ng/mL	> 2.0 ng/mL
Ethanol		>80–100 mg/100 mL (legally intoxicated)
		100–200 mg/100 mL (labile)
		150–300 mg/100 mL (confusion)
		250–400 mg/100 mL (stupor)
		350–500 mg/100 mL (coma)
		> 450 mg/100 mL (death)
Ethosuximide	40–100 µg/mL	> 150 µg/mL
Lidocaine	1.5–6.5 µg/mL	> 6.5 µg/mL
Lithium	0.6–1.2 mmol/L	> 2.0 mmol/L
Phenobarbital	15.0–40.0 µg/mL	> 45.0 µg/mL
Phenytoin (total)	10.0–20.0 µg/mL	> 20.0 µg/mL
Phenytoin (free)	1–2 µg/mL	> 2.0 µg/mL
Procainamide	4.0–10.0 µg/mL	> 16.0 µg/mL
N-acetylprocainamide (NAPA-active metabolite of procainamide)	5.0–30.0 µg/mL	> 40.0 µg/mL
Quinidine	3.0–5.0 µg/mL	> 7 µg/mL
Salicylate	20–30 µg/mL	40–50 µg/mL
Tacrolimus	5–15 ng/mL	
Theophylline	5–15 µg/mL	> 20.0 µg/mL
Valproic acid	50–100 µg/mL	> 150 µg/mL

[a] Each lab may have its own set of values that vary slightly from those given.
Modified and reproduced with permission from Gomella LG, ed. *Clinician's Pocket Reference*, 9th ed. McGraw-Hill, 2002.

TABLE A–23. THERAPEUTIC DRUG LEVELS: ANTIBIOTICS.

Antibiotic	Trough (µg/mL) Maintain Below Upper Limit	Peak (µg/mL)
Amikacin	5.0–7.5	25–35
Gentamicin	1.0–2.0	5–8
Gentamicin (24-h dosing with normal renal function)	1.0–2.0	>10
Tobramycin	1.0–2.0	5–8
Tobramycin (24-h dosing with normal renal function)	1.0–2.0	>10
Vancomycin	5.0–10.0	20–40

Modified and reproduced, with permission, from Gomella LG, ed. *Clinician's Pocket Reference,* 9th ed. McGraw-Hill, 2002.

TABLE A–24. AMINOGLYCOSIDE DOSING IN ADULTS: EVERY 8- OR 12-H DOSING (FOR DAILY DOSING OF GENTAMICIN AND TOBRAMYCIN SEE PAGES 577 AND 642, RESPECTIVELY).

1. Select the loading dose:
Gentamicin 1.5–2.0 mg/kg
Tobramycin 1.5–2.0 mg/kg
Amikacin 5.0–7.5 mg/kg

2. Calculate the estimated creatinine clearance (CrCl) based on serum creatinine (SCr), age, and weight (kg); **or** order a formal creatinine clearance, if time permits.

$$\text{CrCl for male} = \frac{(140 - \text{age}) \times (\text{weight in kg})}{(\text{SCr}) \times (72)} \times 100.$$

CrCl for female = 0.85 × (CrCl male)

3. By using Table A–25, p 677, you can now select the maintenance dose (as a percentage of the chosen loading dose) most appropriate for the patient's renal function based on CrCl and dosing interval. Shaded areas are the percentages and intervals suggested for any given creatinine clearance. For patients over 60 years old, it is recommended to give the dose no more frequently than every 12 h.

4. Empiric dosing, as above, is used to begin therapy. Serum levels (see Table A–23, p 676) should be monitored and adjustments made in the dosing based on the drug levels for optimal therapy.

See Table A–23, p 676, for the trough and peak levels of the aminoglycosides gentamicin, tobramycin, and amikacin. Peak levels should be drawn 30 min after the dose is completely infused; trough levels should be drawn 30 min prior to dose. As a general rule, draw the peak and trough around the fourth maintenance dose. Therapy can be initiated with the recommended guidelines. These **calculations are not valid for netilmicin.** Modified and reproduced, with permission, from Gomella LG, ed. *Clinician's Pocket Reference,* 9th ed. McGraw-Hill, 2002.

TABLE A–25. AMINOGLYCOSIDE DOSING: PERCENTAGE OF LOADING DOSE REQUIRED FOR DOSAGE INTERVAL SELECTED.

Creatinine Clearance (mL/min)	Dosing Interval (h)		
	8	12	24
90	90%[a]	—	—
80	88	—	—
70	84	—	—
60	79	91%	—
50	74	87	—
40	66	80	—
30	57	72	92%
25	51	66	88
20	45	59	83
15	37	50	75
10	29	40	64
7	24	33	55
5	20	28	48
2	14	20	35
0	9	13	25

[a] Shaded areas indicate suggested dosage intervals.
Reproduced, with permission, from Hull JH, Sarubbi FA: Gentamicin serum concentrations: Pharmacokinetic predictions. *Ann Intern Med* 1976;85:183–189.

TABLE A–26. AMINOGLYCOSIDE DOSING: ONCE-DAILY DOSING OF GENTAMICIN AND TOBRAMYCIN (*NOT* AMIKACIN).

Several studies suggest that larger doses of aminoglycosides given once daily are just as effective, and less toxic, than conventional dosing given three times a day. Once-daily dosing of gentamicin and tobramycin regimens takes advantage of concentration-dependent killing through the optimization of peak concentration/MIC rations. In addition, there are potential cost savings for nursing, pharmacy, and laboratory personnel.

Inclusion Criteria: All patients ordered aminoglycosides for prophylaxis, empiric therapy, or documented infection. (Aminoglycosides are usually indicated as synergistic or adjunctive therapy with other antibiotics as double coverage for gram-negative infections.)

Exclusion Criteria: 1. Patients with ascites

2. Patients with burns on > 20% of body surface

3. Pregnant patients

4. Patients receiving dialysis

5. Patients with gram-positive bacterial endocarditis

6. Pediatric patients

Initial Dose: Doses will be based on **dosing body weight** (DBW), ideal body weight plus 40% of estimated adipose tissue mass (*see Dosing Guidelines*). Patients with estimated CrCl ≥ 40 mL/min/1.73 m^2 will receive initial gentamicin dose of 7 mg/kg-DBW, infused over 30 min. Patients with estimated creatinine clearances < 40 mL/min/1.73 m^2 will receive an initial gentamicin dose of 3 mg/kg, infused over 30 min.

Monitoring: Two random concentrations will be obtained to monitor. Once-daily dosing of gentamicin and tobramycin:

The *1st random* concentration will be drawn *4 h*[a] after completion of the *1st* dose. The average 4-h random sample, with a 7 mg/kg dose will be 13–15 mg/L 4 h after a 30-minute infusion.

Note: The therapeutic drug monitoring lab should be notified that the expected gentamicin/ tobramycin level will be greater than 10 mg/L.[b]

The *2nd random* concentration will be drawn *12 h* after completion of the *1st* dose.

Subsequent Doses: SCr/BUN should be measured at baseline and 2 times per week thereafter. Subsequent doses will be the same as the initial dose, but the dosing intervals will be adjusted to achieve troughs ≤*1 mg/L*. Appropriate dosing intervals include every 24, 36, or 48 h.

Initial Dosing Guidelines for Adults:

1. Estimate CrCl using *actual body weight* (ABW) for nonobese patients; in obese patients (> *125% IBW*) use DBW (see below for equation).

$$\text{Males CrCl} = \frac{(140 - \text{Age}) \times \text{ABW}}{}\qquad \text{Females CrCl} = \text{CrCl} \times 0.85$$

2. Estimate body surface area (BSA) using the Mosteller equation:

$$\text{BSA (m}^2) = \frac{\sqrt{\text{Ht(cm)} \times \text{Wt (kg)}}}{60} \quad \text{(Mosteller; } N \text{ Engl J Med 1987;317:109}$$

3. Calculate standardized creatinine clearance:

$$\text{CrCl}_{(\text{Std})} = \text{CrCl} \times \frac{1.73 \text{ m}^2}{\text{BSA}}$$

4. Determine IBW:

IBW (kg) = 50 (kg) + (2.3 (kg) × each in. over 5 ft) male
= 45 (kg) + (2.3 (kg) × each in. over 5 ft) female

TABLE A–26. *(Continued)*

5. Calculate DBW:

   DBW = IBW + 0.4 (ABW – IBW)

   (*if ABW < IBW, then DBW = ABW*)

6. Calculate the patient's dose based on DBW:

   (a) If $CrCl_{(std)} \geq 40$ mL/min/1.73 m^2, then give 7 mg/kg—DBW.

   (b) If $CrCl_{(std)} < 40$ mL/min/1.73 m^2, then give 3 mg/kg—DBW.

Dilute dose in 100 mL of either 5% Dextrose or Normal Saline and infuse over 30 minutes.

Order two random concentrations at **4 and 12 h** after the end of 1st dose. *Notify lab of the patient's name to allow for proper dilution of sample.*

[a] The rationale for the 4-hour sample versus a "peak" is to determine the serum concentration after the distribution phase. A study (Jennings HJ, Davis GA, June 2000) was conducted at the University of Kentucky Medical Center that demonstrated a prolonged distribution phase following a 7 mg/kg dose in trauma surgery patients.

[b] If the serum concentration following a 7 mg/kg dose requires > 48 h to decline to 1 mg/L, then 3 mg/kg or conventional dosing may be warranted. Some patients may have a prolonged "drug-free" period that may warrant conventional dosing to maintain concentrations. Patients should not receive a single dose of 7 mg/kg more frequently than every 24 hours until more studies are available.

MIC = minimal inhibitory concentration; CrCl = creatinine clearance; SCr = serum creatinine; BUN = blood urea nitrogen; IBW = ideal body weight

Modified and reproduced, with permission, from Davis GA: *Clinical Pharmacokinetics Service Policy and Procedural Manual,* 23rd ed. University of Kentucky Medical Center, 2000.

TABLE A–27. FAHRENHEIT/CELSIUS TEMPERATURE CONVERSION.

°F	°C	°C	°F
95.0	35.0	35.0	95.0
96.0	35.5	35.5	95.9
97.0	36.1	36.0	95.8
98.0	36.6	36.5	97.7
98.6	37.0	37.0	98.6
99.0	37.2	37.5	99.5
100.0	37.7	38.0	100.4
101.0	38.3	38.5	101.3
102.0	38.8	39.0	102.2
103.0	39.4	39.5	103.1
104.0	40.0	40.0	104.0
105.0	40.5	40.5	104.9
106.0	41.1	41.0	105.8
$°C = (°F - 32) \times 5/9$			$°F = (°C \times 95) + 32$

Modified and Reproduced, with permission, from Gomella LG, ed. *Clinician's Pocket Reference,* 9th ed. McGraw-Hill; 2002.

TABLE A–28. POUNDS/KILOGRAMS WEIGHT CONVERSION.

lb	kg	kg	lb
1	0.5	1	2.2
2	0.9	2	4.4
4	1.8	3	6.6
6	2.7	4	8.8
8	3.6	5	11.0
10	4.5	6	13.2
20	9.1	8	17.6
30	13.6	10	22.0
40	18.2	20	44.0
50	22.7	30	66.0
60	27.3	40	88.0
70	31.8	50	110.0
80	36.4	60	132.0
90	40.9	70	154.0
100	45.4	80	176.0
150	68.2	90	198.0
200	90.8	100	220.0
	$kg = lb \times 0.454$		$lb = kg \times 2.2$

Reproduced, with permission, from Gomella LG, ed. *Clinician's Pocket Reference*, 9th ed. McGraw-Hill, 2002.

TABLE A–29. GLASGOW COMA SCALE.[a]

Parameter	Response		Score
Eyes	Open	Spontaneously	4
		To verbal command	3
		To pain	2
		No response	1
Best motor response	To verbal command	Obeys	6
	To painful stimulus	Localizes pain	5
		Flexion-withdrawal	4
		Decorticate (flex)	3
		Decerebrate (extend)	2
		No response	1
Best verbal response		Oriented, converses	5
		Disoriented, converses	4
		Inappropriate responses	3
		Incomprehensible sounds	2
		No response	1

[a]The Glasgow Coma Scale (EMV Scale) is a fairly reliable and objective way to monitor changes in levels of consciousness. It is based on eye opening, motor responses, and verbal responses (EMV). A person's EMV score is based on the total of the three different responses. The score ranges from 3 (lowest) to 15 (highest). Modified and reproduced, with permission, from Gomella LG, ed. *Clinician's Pocket Reference*, 9th ed. McGraw-Hill, 2002.

TABLE A–30. ENDOCARDITIS PROPHYLAXIS.[a,b]

■ **Dental and upper respiratory procedures**

Oral

Amoxicillin[c]	2 g PO 1 h before procedure
Penicillin allergy:	
Clindamycin	600 mg PO 1 h before procedure **or**
Cephalexin[d] OR Cefadroxil[d] **or**	2 g PO 1 h before procedure
Azithromycin or Clarithromycin	500 mg PO 1 h before procedure

Parenteral

Ampicillin	2 g IV or IM 30 min before procedure
Penicillin allergy:	
Clindamycin **or**	600 mg IV within 30 min before procedure
Cefazolin[d]	1 g IV or IM within 30 min before procedure

■ **Gastrointestinal and genitourinary procedures[a]**

Oral

Amoxicillin[c]	2 g PO 1 h before procedure

Parenteral[c]

Ampicillin *plus/minus*	2 g IV or 1 IM within 30 min before procedure
Gentamicin	1.5 mg/kg (120 mg maximum dose) IV or IM 30 min before procedure

Penicillin allergy:[e]

Vancomycin *plus/minus*	1 g IV infused *slowly over 1 h* beginning 1 h before procedure
Gentamicin	1.5 mg/kg (120 maximum dose) IV or IM 30 min before procedure

[a]For patients with previous endocarditis, valvular heart disease, prosthetic heart valves, or complex cyanotic congenital heart disease (eg, tetralogy of Fallot), the risk is considered high. The risk is also considered high enough to treat in patients with other forms of congenital heart disease (but not uncomplicated secundum atrial septal defect), acquired valvular disease (eg, rheumatic heart disease), hypertrophic cardiomyopathy, and mitral valve prolapse with regurgitation or thickened valve leaflets. Viridans streptococci are the most likely cause of bacterial endocarditis after dental or upper respiratory procedures; enterococci are the most common cause of endocarditis after gastrointestinal or genitourinary procedures.

[b]For a review of the risk of bacteremia and endocarditis with various procedures, see Dajani AS, Taubert KA, Wilson W et al: Prevention of bacterial endocarditis: Recommendations by the American Heart Association. *JAMA* 1997;277:1794; and Durack DT: Prophylaxis of infective endocarditis. In: Mandell GL, Bennet JE, Dolin R, eds. *Principles and Practice of Infectious Diseases*, 5th ed. Churchill Livingstone; 2000:917. Among dental procedures, tooth extraction and gingival surgery (including implant placement) are thought to have the highest risk for bacterial endocarditis (Durack DT: Antibiotics for prevention of endocarditis during dentistry: Time to scale back? *Ann Intern Med* 1998;129:829.

[c]Amoxicillin is recommended because of its excellent bioavailability and good activity against streptococci and enterococci.

[d]Not recommended for patients with a history of immediate-type allergic reaction to penicillin (eg, urticaria, angioedema, anaphylaxis).

[e]Gentamicin should be added for patients with a high risk for bacterial endocarditis (see footnote a). High-risk patients given parenteral ampicillin before the procedure should receive a dose of ampicillin 1 g IV or IM or a dose of amoxicillin 1 g PO 6 h after the first dose.

Modified and reproduced, with permission, from *Med Lett* 1999;41:80.

TABLE A–31. SPECIMEN TUBES FOR VENIPUNCTURE.[a]

Tube Color	Additives	General Use
Red	None	Clot tube to collect serum for chemistry, cross-matching, serology
Red and black (hot pink)	Silicone gel for rapid clot	As above, but not for osmolality or blood bank work
Blue	Sodium citrate (binds calcium)	Coagulation studies (best kept on ice, not for fibrin split products)
Blue/yellow label		Fibrin split products
Royal blue		Heavy metals, arsenic
Purple	Disodium EDTA (binds calcium)	Hematology, not for lipid profiles
Green	Sodium heparin	Ammonia, cortisol, ionized calcium (best kept on ice)
Green/glass beads		LE prep
Gray	Sodium fluoride	Lactic acid
Yellow	Transport medium	Blood cultures

[a] Individual labs may vary slightly from these listings.
Reproduced, with permission, from Gomella LG, Lefor AT: *Surgery On Call,* 3rd ed. McGraw-Hill, 2001.

TABLE A–32. LOCAL ANESTHETIC COMPARISON CHART FOR COMMONLY USED INJECTABLE AGENTS.

Agent	Proprietary Names	Onset	Duration	Maximum Dose mg/kg	Volume in 70-kg Adult[a]
Bupivacaine	Marcaine, Sensoricaine	7–30 min	5–7 h	3	70 mL of 0.25% solution
Lidocaine	Xylocaine, Anestacon	5–30 min	2 h	4	28 mL of 1% solution
Lidocaine with epinephrine (1:200:000)		5–30 min	2–3 h	7	50 mL of 1% solution
Mepivacaine	Carbocaine	5–30 min	2–3 h	7	50 mL of 1% solution
Procaine	Novocaine	Rapid	30 min–1 h	10–15	70–105 mL of 1% solution

[a]To calculate the maximum dose if the patient is not a 70 kg adult, use the fact that a 1% solution has 10 mg of drug per milliliter.
Reproduced, with permission, from Gomella LG, Haist S, eds. *Clinician's Pocket Reference*, 9th ed. McGraw-Hill, 2002.

TABLE A–33. TOPICAL STEROID PREPARATIONS (SEE PAGE 636 FOR ADDITIONAL INFORMATION)

Agent	Common Trade Names	Potency	Apply
Aclometasone dipropionate	Aclovate, cream, oint 0.05%	Low	bid/tid
Amcinonide	Cyclocort, cream, lotion, oint 0.1%	High	bid/tid
Betamethasone			
Betamethasone valerate	Valisone cream, lotion 0.01%	Low	qd/bid
Betamethasone valerate	Valisone cream, 0.01, 0.1%, oint, lotion 0.1%	Intermediate	qd/bid
Betamethasone dipropionate	Diprosone cream (0.05%)	High	qd/bid
	Diprosone aerosol (0.1%)		
Betamethasone dipropionate, augmented	Diprolene oint, gel 0.05%	Ultra high	qd/bid
Clobetasol propionate	Temovate cream, gel, oint, scalp, soln 0.05%	Ultra high	bid (2 wk max)
Clocortolone pivalate	Cloderm cream 0.1%	Intermediate	qd–qid
Desonide	DesOwen, cream, oint, lotion 0.05%	Low	bid–qid
Desoximetasone			
Desoximetasone 0.05%	Topicort LP cream, gel 0.05%	Intermediate	
Desoximetasone 0.25%	Topicort cream, oint	High	
Dexamethasone base	Aeroseb-Dex aerosol 0.01%	Low	bid–qid
	Decadron cream 0.1%		
Diflorasone diacetate	Psorcon cream, oint 0.05%	Ultrahigh	bid/qid
Fluocinolone			
Fluocinolone acetonide 0.01%	Synalar cream, soln 0.01%	Low	bid/tid
Fluocinolone acefonide 0.025%	Synolar oint, cream 0.025%	Intermediate	bid/tid

Fluocinolone acetonide 0.2%	Synalar-HP cream 0.2%	High	bid/tid
Fluocinonide 0.05%	Lidex, anhydrous cream, gel, soln 0.05%	High	bid/tid oint
	Lidex-E aqueous cream 0.05%		
Flurandrenolide	Cordran cream, oint 0.025% cream, lotion, oint 0.05% tape, 4 μg/cm²	Intermediate	bid/tid
		Intermediate	bid/tid
		Intermediate	qd
Fluticasone propionate	Activate cream 0.05%, oint 0.005%	Intermediate	bid
Halobetasol	Cutivate cream, oint 0.05%	Very High	bid
Halcinonide	Halog cream 0.025%, emollient base 0.1% cream, oint, solution 0.1%	High	qd/tid
Hydrocortisone			
Hydrocortisone	Cortisone, Caldecort, Hycort, Hytone, etc. aerosol 1%, cream: 0.5, 1, 2.5%, gel 0.5% oint 0.5, 1, 2.5%, lotion 0.5, 1, 2.5% paste 0.5% soln 1%	Low	tid/qid
Hydrocortisone acetate	Corticaine cream, oint 0.5, 1%	Low	tid/qid
Hydrocortisone butyrate	Locoid oint, soln 0.1%	Intermediate	bid/tid
Hydrocortisone valerate	Westcort cream, oint 0.2% oint, lotion 0.025%	Intermediate	bid/tid
Mometasone furoate	Elacon 0.1% cream, oint, lotion	Intermediate	qd
Prednicarbate	Dermalop 0.1% cream	Intermediate	bid
Triamcinolone			
Triamcinolone acetonide 0.025%	Aristocort, Kenalog cream	Low	tid/qid
Triamcinolone acetonide 0.1%	Aristocort, Kenalog cream, oint, lotion 0.1% Aerosol 0.2 mg/2-sec spray	Intermediate	tid/qid
Triamcinolone acetonide 0.5%	Aristocort, Kenalog cream, oint 0.5%	High	tid/qid

Reproduced, with permission, from Gomella LG, Haist S. eds. *Clinician's Pocket Reference*, 9th ed. McGraw-Hill, 2002.

TABLE A–34. TETANUS PROPHYLAXIS.

History of Absorbed Tetanus Toxoid Immunization	Clean, Minor Wounds		All Other Wounds[a]	
	Td[b]	TIG[c]	Td[b]	TIG[c]
Unknown or <3 doses	Yes	No	Yes	Yes
<3 doses[d]	No[e]	No	No[f]	No

[a] Such as, but not limited to, wounds contaminated with dirt, feces, soil, saliva, etc; puncture wounds; avulsions; and wounds resulting from missiles, crushing, burns, and frostbite.

[b] Td = tetanus-diphtheria toxoid (adult type), 0.5 mL IM.
- For children <7 y of age, DPT (DT, if pertussis vaccine is contraindicated) is preferred to tetanus toxoid alone.
- For persons >7 years of age. Td is preferred to tetanus toxoid alone.
- DT = diphtheria-tetanus toxoid (pediatric) used for those who cannot receive pertussis.

[c] TIG = tetanus immune globulin, 250 U IM.

[d] If only three doses of fluid toxoid have been received, then a fourth dose of toxoid, preferably an absorbed toxoid, should be given.

[e] Yes, if >10 y since last dose.

[f] Yes, if >5 y since last dose.

Source: Based on guidelines from the Centers for Disease Control and reported in *MMWR*.

TABLE A-35. SEROTONIN 5-HT$_1$ RECEPTOR AGONISTS[a,b]

Drug	Initial Dose	Repeat Dose	Max Dose/24hrs	Supplied
Almotriptan (Axert)	6.25 or 12.5 mg PO	×1 in 2 h	25 mg	Tabs 6.25, 12.5 mg
Frovatriptan (Frova)	2.5 mg PO	in 2 h	7.5 mg	Tabs 2.5 mg
Naratriptan (Amerge)	1 or 2.5 mg PO[c]	in 4 h	5 mg	Tabs 1, 2.5 mg
Rizatriptan (Maxalt)	5 or 10 mg PO[d]	in 2 h	30 mg	Tabs 5, 10 mg Disintegrating Tabs 5, 10 mg
Sumatriptan (Imitrex)	25, 50, or 100 mg PO	in 2 h	200 mg	Tabs 25, 50 mg
	5–20 mg intranasally	in 2 h	40 mg	Nasal spray 5, 20 mg
	6 mg SC	in 1 h	12 mg	Inj 12 mg/mL
Zolmitriptan (Zomig)	2.5 or 5 mg PO	in 2 h	10 mg	Tabs 2.5, 5 mg

[a]**Precautions/Contraindication:** [C,M]: Ischemic heart disease, coronary artery vasospasm, Prinzmetal's angina, uncontrolled HTN, hemiplegic or basilar migraine, ergots, use of another serotonin agonist within 24 hrs, use with MAOI

[b]**Side Effects:** dizziness, somnolence, paresthesias, nausea, flushing, dry mouth, coronary vasospasm, chest tightness, HTN, GI upset

[c]Reduce dose in mild renal and hepatic insufficiency (2.5 mg/d MAX); Contraindicated with severe renal (CrCl <15 mL/min) or hepatic impairment

[d]Initiate therapy at 5 mg PO (15 mg/d MAX) in patients receiving propranolol

Reproduced, with permission, from Gomella LG, Haist, SA. eds. *Clinicians Pocket Drug Reference 2003.* McGraw Hill, 2003.

TABLE A–36. SOME COMMON ORAL POTASSIUM SUPPLEMENTS (SEE PAGE 622)

Brand Name	Salt	Form	mEq potassium/ Dosing Unit
Glu-K	Gluconate	Tablet	2 mEq/tablet
Kaochlor 10%	KCl	Liquid	20 mEq/15 mL
Kaochlor S-F 10% (sugar-free)	KCl	Liquid	20 mEq/15 mL
Kaochlor Eff	Bicarbonate/ KCl/citrate	Effervescent tablet	20 mEq/tablet
Kaon elixir	Gluconate	Liquid	20 mEq/mL
Kaon	Gluconate	Tablets	5 mEq/tablet
Kaon-Cl	KCl	Tablet, SR	6.67 mEq/tablet
Kaon-Cl 20%	KCl	Liquid	40 mEq/15 mL
KayCiel	KCl	Liquid	20 mEq/15 mL
K-Lor	KCl	Powder	15 or 20 mEq/pocket
Klorvess	Bicarbonate/KCl	Liquid	20 mEq/15 mL
Klotrix	KCl	Tablet, SR	10 mEq/tablet
K-lyte	Bicarbonate/ citrate	Effervescent tablet	25 mEq/tablet
K-Tab	KCl	Tablet, SR	10 mEq/tablet
Micro-K	KCl	Capsules, SR	8 mEq/capsule
Slow-K	KCl	Tablet, SR	8 mEq/tablet
Tri-K	Acetate/bicar- bonate and citrate	Liquid	45 mEq/15 mL
Twin-K	Citrate/gluconate	Liquid	20 mEq/5 mL

SR = sustained release.
Reproduced, with permission, from Gomella LG, Haist S, eds. *Clinician's Pocket Reference,* 9th ed. McGraw-Hill, 2002.

Subject Index

Note: Page numbers followed by the letter "*t*" indicates tables; those followed by the letter "*f*" indicate figures.

A

Abacavir, 522
Abbokinase, 645–646
Abciximab, 523
Abdominal pain, 1–6
  in children, 3, 221–223
  differential diagnosis of, 2–3
  indications for urgent surgery in, 5*t*
  laboratory studies and imaging in, 4
  physical findings in, 3*t*, 3–4
  in pregnancy, 169
  treatment plan in, 4–6
Abdominal trauma
  blunt, 253–256
    differential diagnosis of, 253–254
    laboratory studies and imaging in, 254–255
    physical findings in, 254
    treatment plan in, 255–256
  in electrical injury, 268, 269
Abelcet, 531
Abortion
  spontaneous, 168, 171
  threatened, 169, 171, 212
Abscess
  cutaneous, differential diagnosis of, 190
  drainage of, 417–418
    complications of, 418
    indications and contraindications for, 417
    procedure in, 417–418
  facial, localized, 71, 72
  oropharyngeal, respiratory distress in, 175
  perinephric, 208
  peritonsillar, 193, 194
  retropharyngeal, 193, 194
  scrotal, 177, 178, 179
Abuse
  of children. *See* Child abuse
  of older people. *See* Elder abuse
Acarbose, 523
Accolate, 649

Accupril, 627
Acebutolol, 523, 663*t*
Aceon, 618, 660*t*
Acetaminophen, 523
  with butalbital, 540
  with butalbital and caffeine, 523
  with codeine, 523
  overdose of, 316–318
    differential diagnosis of, 316
    laboratory studies and imaging in, 317
    physical findings in, 316–317
    treatment plan in, 317–318
Acetazolamide, 524
  in altitude illness, 17
Acetic acid, 667*t*
  and aluminum acetate, 524
Acetohexamide, 524, 672*t*
Acetone toxicity, 320
Acetylcysteine, 524
  in acetaminophen overdose, 317–318
N-Acetylprocainamide, therapeutic and toxic levels of, 675*t*
Achromycin V, 639–640
Acid-base disorders, 7–10, 381, 382*t*
  differential diagnosis of, 7–9
  laboratory studies and imaging in, 10
  physical findings in, 9–10
  treatment plan in, 10
Acid-fast stain, 377
Acid ingestion. *See* Caustic and corrosive ingestion
Acidosis, 7*t*, 381, 382*t*
  cardiac arrest in, 45
  diabetic ketoacidosis, 77
  differential diagnosis of, 76
Aciphex, 628, 673*t*
Aclometasone dipropionate, 684*t*
Aclovate, 684*t*
Acrodermatitis, differential diagnosis of, 73
Act-Hib, 579

ACTH
  serum levels, 377
  stimulation test, 377
Actidose, 548
Actiq, 572
Activase, 526
Activate, 685*t*
Actonel, 630
Actos, 620
Acular, 670*t*
  ophthalmic, 589
Acyclovir, 524
  in herpes zoster oticus, 92
Adalat, 609
Adalat CC, 609
Adapin, 564
Adenocard, 524–525
Adenosine, 524–525
Adhesive "skin glue" for wound closure, 458
Adrenalin, 566
Adrenergic receptors
  α_1 blockers, 512
  α_2 agonists as ophthalmic agents, 669*t*
  β blockade. *See* Beta-blockers
Adrenocorticotropic hormone. *See* ACTH
Adriamycin, 564
Adrucil, 574
Advil, 583, 668*t*
AeroBid, 573
Aeroseb-Dex, 684*t*
Afrinol, 626
Agenerase, 531
Aggrastat, 642
Aging. *See* Geriatric problems
Agitation
  drug-induced, 324
  in ventilator patients, 496–498
    differential diagnosis of, 497
    laboratory studies and imaging in, 498
    physical findings in, 497
    treatment plan in, 498
Airway management in anaphylaxis, 19